DRUGS, SOCIETY, AND HUMAN BEHAVIOR

DRUGS, SOCIETY, & HUMAN BEHAVIOR

OAKLEY RAY, Ph.D.

Professor, Department of Psychology, Vanderbilt University;
Associate Professor, Department of Pharmacology,
Vanderbilt University School of Medicine;
Chief, Mental Health and Behavioral Sciences Unit,
Veterans Administration Hospital,
Nashville, Tennessee

THIRD EDITION

with 54 illustrations

The C. V. Mosby Company

ST. LOUIS • TORONTO • LONDON   1983

MOSBY

A TRADITION OF PUBLISHING EXCELLENCE

Editor: Nancy K. Roberson
Assistant editor: Michelle Turenne
Editing supervisor: Peggy Fagen
Manuscript editor: Patricia Gayle May
Book design: Nancy Steinmeyer
Cover design: Diane Beasley
Production: Jeanne A. Gulledge
Cover illustrations by Robert Maust and Richard Wachter

THIRD EDITION

The C.V. Mosby Company
11830 Westline Industrial Drive, St. Louis, Missouri 63141

Library of Congress Cataloging in Publication Data

Ray, Oakley Stern.
　　Drugs, society, and human behavior.

　　Bibliography: p.
　　Includes index.
　　　1. Drugs. 2. Drug abuse. 3. Drugs—Physiological effect. I. Title. [DNLM: 1. Behavior—
Drug effects. 2. Substance abuse. 3. Drugs.
4. Pharmacology. 5. Psychopharmacology. QV
77 R264d]
HV5801.R35 1983　　　615'.1　　　82-8203
ISBN 0-8016-4092-X

GW/VH/VH 9 8 7 6 5 4 3 2　　　05/A/642

my high . . .
MY STUDENTS

. . . substances which act on the brain
mock at all obstacles which oppose their extension.
Their attraction grows slowly,
silently, but surely.

Phantastica
L. Lewin, 1931

Men are qualified for civil liberty in exact proportion to their
disposition to put moral chains upon their own appe-
tites. . . . Society cannot exist unless a controlling power upon
will and appetite be placed somewhere, and the less of it
there is within, the more there must be without. It is ordained
in the eternal constitution of things, that men of intemperate
minds cannot be free. Their passions forge their fetters.

Edmund Burke, 1791

PREFACE

I **am really pleased** to be writing a third edition of a book dealing with drugs, drug use, and drug users. Pleased because it may mean that I'm on the right track. Since the first edition was published in 1972 many books concerned with these issues have come and gone. Most of them proposed solutions to either the social or personal problems that accompanied increasing drug use. As the first edition suggested, there are no final solutions to these problems; there are only approaches to be taken, perspectives to be viewed, actions to be accomplished. The separation of fact from fantasy, the effervescent from the evermore, and rhetoric from reason is especially difficult in this emotion-filled area that impacts on each of our lives. The primary emphasis here is to do just that—to separate and discuss facts and themes that will enable the reader to reach a rational point of view on drug-taking behavior.

In addition to continuing the historical perspective on the psychosocial issues raised by advances in pharmacology and changes in society, this edition incorporates the many scientific and technical advances that have occurred since publication of the second edition. New topics have been included, such as the effect of drugs on sexual behavior, pregnancy, and sports. The consumer—of both legal and illegal drugs—is an important, recurring topic. To accomplish all these things, I hope to partially fill the void at the center of the triangle formed by the fields of pharmacology, psychology, and history. This book will not make you an expert in these areas, but the material should be of considerable value to the pharmacologist, the psy-chologist and the social historian. The material presented here is an amalgamation of the facts, attitudes, opinions and perspectives necessary to understand what psychoactive drugs do, how they do it, who uses them and why.

Also new to this edition is the inclusion of the "Checklist for Knowledge of and Interest in Drugs and Drug Use." Found in the final section and easily removable, the checklist may be used as a tool to secure student appraisal of knowledge and interest in various topics and issues. When used at the beginning of a semester or quarter, it can assist in appraising student interest and understanding to facilitate the planning of course organization and emphasis. The checklist also provides the student with an orientation to the breadth of the area of drugs and drug use.

A drug has no effect in isolation—the effect is always on an individual, a unique person in a particular environment. To comprehend the kinds of effects a drug can have on behavior, you must not only learn about the drug but also know much about the drug user and his society, now and in historical perspective. Drug use is very much a part of our cultural history, and some of our scientific technological progress has come as a result of the push for more and newer psychoactive drugs. An understanding of the history of our present drugs and our present drug use is essential to appreciate the changes now rapidly occurring.

Many people believe that the current pattern of drug use (drug misuse?) is an unusual phenomenon, a new experience for our civilization. Some have suggested that this increased drug use is a cancer that can be removed from our life—through laws or education—without affecting the fabric of our society. Contrary to this belief, one of my conclusions is that the pattern of drug use now seen in our country is an integral part of our developing culture, and to eliminate it would require major changes in some of our beliefs and attitudes, changes that many may not support.

Usually in a preface some mention is made of the groups that might be particularly interested in the book. Originally the book was aimed at a college population for use in a course I teach entitled "Drugs and Behavior." In introducing that course and now the third edition of this book, I say that no prior information is needed. We're going to start from scratch and do two things. First, the material will cover all that most people need and want to know about drugs and drug use—legal and illegal. Second, enough background and basic material will be presented so that the reader will be better able to understand the whys and wherefores of new drugs, new uses, and new patterns of use as they come on the scene.

Referencing a book such as this is difficult. I have referenced quotes and also facts and opinions that do not appear either in the already cited material or in one of the standard books in this area. It should be clear that neither the form of presentation, the opinions, nor the conclusions represent the views of the Veterans Administration.

To write a book is to realize that no man is an island and that there is no way to acknowledge all the support and help given by others—some by doing, some by being. Many thanks to Dave Shepard. Most of all—hugs and kisses and kudos to Lori Wingett. Through it all and in spite of it all, as she typed and retyped, referenced and rereferenced—she kept talking to me! Amazing. For my research and clinical colleagues and for all the others who helped—much love and many many thanks.

Oakley Ray

CONTENTS

ix

DRUGS, SOCIETY, AND HUMAN BEHAVIOR

UNIT 1

INTRODUCTION

CHAPTER 1

DRUG USE:
AN OVERVIEW

CUT IT ANY WAY YOU WANT TO—drug use is here. It's not "in," "out," "cool," or anything else—drug use *is*. Drug use has lost the frenzy it had in the psychedelic sixties and the anxiety it aroused in the seventies. Drug use is housebroken—it's tolerated by many, condemned by some, profitable to a few, but illicit drug use has found a niche in our culture.

That fact must astound and amaze anyone over 40, baffle and infuriate those over 50, and confirm the fact for those over 60 that the world is, indeed, on the fast track to the nether world. If you talk to the very young—the early teens—drugs are an everyday part of their life, in and out of health classes: No big deal! High school and college students may have some appreciation of the transition period they have lived through, but for many, drugs are like sex: something that agitates their parents, upsets their teachers, but is to be enjoyed mostly in a low-keyed way. The young adults saw the changes exploding around them as they grew up. They were part of it—maybe on one side, maybe on the other, maybe on both sides. They were the ones who knew there was a war on—the battle was over their minds and bodies. They saw some fall, they saw some falter, but most of all, they saw nearly all of their friends and fellows make it through.

The question is, of course: Is the war over, or is there just a lull in the fighting? What are the peace terms? Who won? Maybe some answers will stand out for you by the time you reach Chapter 20. It should be clear that the drug use of the sixties and seventies changed our society and that the bubbling social milieu in those years influenced our patterns of drug use.

This chapter sets the stage for what is to follow. It provides a perspective through which the panorama of drugs and drug users needs to be viewed. This chapter also provides a form, a structure, so that our peripatetic view does not become just a rapidly moving kaleidoscope.

The increase in drug use and misuse can be viewed as part of two rapidly developing revolutions: a cultural revolution and a biological revolution. It is not possible here to examine all the ramifications of the many rapid advances in the field of biology, but special note should be made of two of the broad issues. First, it is no longer clear that all biomedical advances are seen as good for society. Until recently every step forward was clearly in the direction of solving a problem for which most people agreed a solution was needed. Now, certain advances have given us the capability of accomplishing things that do not clearly solve one of society's problems.[1]

This realization leads us directly to the second point. It is now obvious that the advances in biology and the biomedical fields have had very broad impact on our society—on our mores, on the way we view man. Rather than just improving the quality of living that exists at the time of the breakthrough, these advances sometimes greatly change the character of our culture.

Many cultural changes have resulted from some of the advances in the field of pharmacology. By reviewing these changes it is possible to set the scene for a consideration of our present use of drugs. The influence of some of these advances has been so great that they must be called revolutionary.

PHARMACOLOGICAL REVOLUTIONS

The first revolution is the one that brought the major communicable diseases well under control. The use of vaccines, which began with Pasteur, Jenner, and Koch in the nineteenth century and is still continuing with the development of the rubella (measles) vaccine, has certainly had a major impact on our society. There are now 24 established and effective vaccines. In 1954 there were over 18,000 cases of paralytic polio; in 1971 only 19 cases occurred. The measles vaccine, first mass-produced in the United States in 1969, is 93% to 95% effective in preventing the disease in children. So it seems clear that another hurdle in the path of growing up is almost demolished. Students today don't know what a quarantine sign is—they've never seen one! Diphtheria and whooping cough are words that the pediatrician mumbles as he inoculates the baby. Protracted absence from school, long-term after-effects from childhood disease, death of a young child—all these are not now part of our culture, gone because of the development of techniques that can prevent most of the serious childhood diseases. Unfortunately, all these things may come back again. As if to prove the point that biological and cultural factors continually interact, a 1975 survey found that two thirds of the preschool children had not been immunized against polio, measles, rubella, mumps, or tetanus.[2]

The second pharmacological revolution resulted from the introduction of sulfa drugs, penicillin, and broad-spectrum antibiotic agents. Proved first in war, they continue to save and prolong lives in peacetime. This change in mortality and in the role of hospitals is ongoing. The increase in longevity (and thus the number of "senior citizens") and the use of hospitals as places in which to be treated and recover from illness are clearly shaping our economy and our politics (a la Medicare and Medicaid).

These two revolutions may be too pervasive and too close to home to impress anyone. This is not the case with the third pharmacological revolution: the advent of tranquilizers for the treatment of the mentally ill (Chapter 13). The rapid development of tranquilizers in the early 1950s and the beginning of their widespread use in 1954 have resulted in many cultural effects. One of the most interesting, but little studied, cultural results was the realization that the tranquilizers are used for their effect on the mind, not on the body. The first two revolutions were aimed at restoring the physiological homeostasis that we call physical health. The tranquilizers introduced to the public the concept that drugs which act on the mind could be used to return one's mental health to normal. Not much was said about this different effect because mental illness was viewed as a disease, and tranquilizers were acting the *same way* as an antibiotic—to remove the disease!

The impact on our mental hospital population was more obvious. Between 1955 and 1975 there was a 65% decrease in the number of individuals in mental hospitals in spite of an increasing population. The return of these individuals to the community and the prevention of hospitalization for others have had a major effect on the methods and models developed in the 1960s and 1970s for the delivery of mental health services. The singular effectiveness of tranquilizers, followed by considerable success with antidepressant agents in the late 1950s, clearly made chemotherapy the only effective procedure available for the treatment of severely disturbed individuals.

The fourth pharmacological revolution is still in process. Although its ultimate effect cannot be known now, some of its possible impact can be predicted with moderate confidence. This revolution is the development of the oral contraceptive. Still in preliminary stages are the "day-after" pill, pills for men, and sustained-release agents that would be effective for months or years. What additional impact these drugs will have cannot be predicted, but for the millions of American women who have used oral contraceptives, there has been a change in many attitudes and behaviors. How greatly the concept of "sex without worry" will accelerate certain trends in our society that were already obvious in the 1950s cannot be determined. It seems reasonable, though, that the decline of the family as the basic unit of our social structure and the development of equal rights for women are both considerably advanced when sex without pregnancy becomes easier.

Of more interest here, however, is the fact that *for the first time* potent chemicals clearly labeled as drugs were being widely used by healthy people because of their social convenience. No longer were we eliminating infection to have a healthy body, neither were we reducing anxiety to have a better functioning mind. Now we added a drug to alter a healthy body and mind because of the convenience it offered in interpersonal contacts. This was a major shift in our thinking about drugs and was a result of, and a part of, the evolving credit card culture—instant pleasure!

There are three pharmacological revolutions that have been repeatedly predicted. One is the development of euphoriants. We have moved from drugs to cure the body, through drugs to cure the mind, to drugs that alter the body for our convenience and pleasure. The next step would be compounds that deliver the pleasure themselves. Why wake up in the morning and just feel good? Why not feel *really great?* Ecstatic! In 1949 one writer phrased it:

> And a time may come when people take Benzedrine in a suitably flavored drink for breakfast instead of coffee or tea, and before luncheon conferences instead of a cocktail. One day, maybe we'll have to test students for Benzedrine before exams, the way we test race horses. It is doubtful that Benzedrine will ever be considered good form on the race track or in athletic events, but a time may come when, like liquor, it will be quite all right socially if you carry it like a gentleman.[3]

It may come. With the development of drugs that are specific in their neural and behavioral effects, it may soon be possible to select the effect we want. As that happens, we'll all turn on . . . easily, and regularly. Aldous Huxley foretold it in *Brave New World*,[4] and one article said that it was here:

> The age of euphorigens is upon us. . . . Over the next few years a wide variety of drugs that produce euphoria will be available for use. The questions about who will be in charge of them, when they will be used, and how they will be used reach beyond the purview of laboratory investigators and psychiatrists. Whether they can ever be used effectively except on a periodic basis awaits further research.[5]

Another drug revolution frequently mentioned is the development of chemicals that will increase our learning ability—smart pills![6,7] If learning is, as it seems to be, dependent on the availability of certain neural connections in the central nervous system *and* on the effectiveness of those connections, then certain drugs should be potentially capable of increasing the efficiency of the neural connections that exist. Work with animals indicates that this is a real possibility.[8] Drug facilitation of learning in animals suggests that some (much, most?) of the variability in learning ability in humans may be eliminated. Interestingly, though, it may be the less bright who will be affected most by the drugs.

The social changes such a development suggests are immense. The one remaining legal basis for discrimination in this country is intelligence. The brighter people have the opportunity for education, better jobs, better salaries, and so on. If drugs could possibly make 80% to 90% of the population bright enough to benefit from a college education and to hold down high-level positions, how would we pick who gets the chance? Or would we see that everyone gets paid the same no matter what he does?

A final pharmacological revolution is control of the aging process. Aging must be the result of biochemical changes. If so, it doesn't seem too remote to use chemicals to slow, stop, reverse(?) those biochemical changes that we call aging. Talk about changes in society! Maybe we would add it to our drinking water as we do chlorine and fluoride and "stop" everyone at the age they are now, or maybe at 18 or 21 everyone gets a 20-year supply, or maybe. . . . Students reading this book will certainly be in this revolution and in making the decisions about how to use, when to use, and with whom to use the antiaging drugs.

There are many revolutions in pharmacology that could be (and have been) predicted. No one knows, of course, what will happen, but the changes in social values and attitudes discussed here make it likely that there will be a very great increase in the use of psychoactive drugs by normal people in the next 20 years.[9]

CULTURAL CHANGE

> There is a revolution under way. It is not like revolutions of the past. It has originated with the individual and with culture. . . . It is now spreading with amazing rapidity, and already our laws, institutions, and social structure are changing in consequence.[10]

The present comes so quickly now that it's difficult to remember the past. When the rate of change in a society is slow, certain truths are self-evident and affect everyone's behavior. With moderate cultural movement the future is predictable. It is easy to feel secure extrapolating from where we are to where we will be in 10 to 20 or 50 years. With a predictable future you can make plans, follow through with them, and expect them to work out. As a guide to what you should plan for and educate for, you look to the past and see where society has been. With a slow rate of social change, your personal and society's history are important in planning for the future.

It's hard to keep track of all the social "revolutions" that have occurred since World War II. There were so many, and they came so fast, they seem to meld together. America bounded out of the war with a belief in the future that was untarnished by minor setbacks such as an Iron Curtain, the Korean War, and an economic recession here and there. Everything seemed to be moving up after the depression of the thirties and the war of the forties. This was the time to make it big, to make up for not having, for sacrificing.

The bright-eyed boys and girls who applauded the American flag when it appeared in the movies during the world war grew up, got married, and moved to the suburbs. These were the men in the gray flannel suits, and they *knew* progress was the most important product—their own progress. They knew where they were headed. They were after goodies. The formula was simple: hard work leads to advancement, which leads to more goodies, which. . . . Hard work and time, take aim and GO! Two cars, one acre, and zero crab grass! This *was* the good life—and their kids would have it even better! When the harvest is good and the barns are full, even the tight people loosen up. It was Fat City! The children of the late fifties grew up with everything. Honesty in history so all would know that the heroes of old had clay feet. Television so you could learn that there were better lives and that people would work hard to make you happy. Sit tight, do nothing, let me entertain you. A *real* hero—assassinated. *Fight in Vietnam? Why? We've no business there. Because your country says to. My country? Ha!* And the chickens come home to roost.

The rate of social change was fueled to a high level by modern educational techniques and new technological capability. With a high rate of cultural change, the past is less relevant to the present than ever before. The future is less easily predicted from the past or the present. The technological civilization that bloomed in the fifties and sixties had a major impact on human relationships.[11] Even though "the roots of the technocracy reach deep into our cultural past and are ultimately entangled in the scientific world-view of the Western tradition,"[12,p.7] there is always the danger that technocracy will destroy the factors that brought it into being.

The main feature of technological society is . . . creative destruction. It not only destroys habits, beliefs, and institutions inherited from the past, but those which were created only yesterday. In a society where memory is an irritant because it impedes progress, concepts like "tradition" or categories like "the past" are mostly meaningless.[13]

The guys in the button-down collars did it. They got what they wanted, and some that they didn't ask for. The world was no longer predictable; there were no more heroes. But the organization men of the 1950s and 1960s had made an affluent society. This is an important determiner of the Aquarian and the hang-loose ethics. Because it was possible to live adequately with very little work (and if you've always had everything, it seems easier to give it up than if you never had it), and because there was little training for achievement, the Protestant Ethic fast disappeared. This belief in self-restraint, drive, and hard work as the way to get ahead and be happy was gone for many people. Why work hard to have leisure time to enjoy life when you can work less, have more leisure time, and still survive?

I'll tell you what I think of hard work and conformity and your system. You tell me and teach me to think for myself. You stress the rights of the individual. So what if I mess around, my television tells me "nice people do get VD." Look at you, dad. What did all that hard work get you? A crummy house in suburbia—big deal. I want to do my own thing—be myself. I'm not sure who I am—but I know I'm not what you think I am. Don't tie me down. I'm not German or English or Italian or black. Don't tell me about my heritage, my roots. I'm a person, a unique individual, and I'm going to find me.

Becoming an adult is a tricky business in the most stable of settings. Becoming independent and establishing a unique identity is especially difficult in changing times. Social adolescence is one big double bind, a period in which almost everything told to the youth is contradictory, double-edged. *Be yourself—but don't let your hair grow down to your shoulders. Do what you want to do with your life, pick your profession—but don't pick your courses in school; they know best. Learn some responsibility—here's your allowance. Dress sexy, look sexy—but don't go all the way.*

The period of social adolescence has reached an uncontrollable duration. In this period between puberty and the termination of schooling the individual is treated as an adult in some respects, since physically he is an adult, but not in others, since he is still not emotionally or financially independent. The social adolescent is given many of the advantages of being an adult, but he doesn't have to work for them, and he keeps the advantages of being young.[14]

The young do learn some things. They did listen to the messages we sent them every day. They didn't rebel against the establishment; they outdid the establishment. What the over-30 and over-40 groups were doing, the under-30 and under-20 groups did better! People wonder where the young get their ideas. People forget that the young are still learning rules to live by and forming basic beliefs about the way the world is and how it ought to be. The young get their ideas from the older generation, its ads, its behavior, whether the older generation knows it or not.

The magic word in the sixties and early seventies was alienation. Alienation may be inevitable in a technologically oriented bureaucracy. Regardless, clearly more and more people at all ages felt that they could no longer exert any influence on the social institutions that determine the options which are open to them in life. When an individual feels that his life is not predictable, partly because of groups and ideas beyond his influence and control, he has three options. He can drop out, as the hippies and many drug users did. They were just saying, "If I can't help make the rules I'm to live by, I won't play your game. You've been telling me for years that I should think for myself. Why get uptight when I do?" Another option is taken by those who think they know what changes they want. They don't just want a say in making the rules, they want certain rules—now! These were the social activists of the right and the left. Their aim was to establish certain premises as basic to the game, and they were willing to ruin the game if they couldn't have their way. The final group consisted of the activists of the middle, those who tried to initiate change within the system. The Peace Corps volunteers, the McCarthyites, the Robert Kennedy student workers all fit into this slice of the pie. There is, always, a large silent majority at all ages, and the most that can be said of them is that they are at least satisfied enough with the status quo not to actively try to change it.

With no meaningful history and no foreseeable future, what's there to grab hold of? The only thing to hold onto is the here and now, the immediate experience. And that's what it was all about—the NOW generation. What's in the NOW? Experiences. What are experiences made of? Actions, sensations.

Maybe religion, maybe Christ is the way, maybe I'll know the real me. Maybe Buddhism, meditation, ummm—don't worry, I'll find me. Who am I anyway? What meaning is there to anything? It's not out there—everyone is a double-dealer, a money-grabber. Maybe drugs are the answer. What are you talking about? There's no answer—there's not even a question. I don't know where I've been or where I'm going, but I'm going to grab what I can. You only go around once—reach out with gusto—experience it—try anything once, or twice—enjoy, man, enjoy. The only thing that counts is the NOW.

You're doing what, Dad? Leaving Mom? Right on! That makes us alike—we're all doing our own thing. Somehow, though, it's not as much fun when you're doing it too. You smoke dope, too?! You're making it hard for me to tell you what a lousy materialistic world you've made when you're on my side of the fence. Yeah, maybe you're right—we're doing it more but enjoying it less. Doing what? Everything. Hard to get too excited about the boy or girl next door when the door is always open, and, besides, I've been watching it and doing it since I was—I dunno how old.

If I can do dope and almost anything I want with almost anyone I want, and still be "straight," I might as well admit the mainstream has shifted. If I wade just a little—maybe a 9-to-5 job—I'll be in the swift current. It is kind of fun to be doing something different—but why are we nine-to-fivers supporting all those bums who don't work?

When you reject the hardworking fifties, you appear in the live-and-let-live sixties. Being, not having, was a basic component of the youth philosophy. You can *be* only if you've experienced—yourself, your environment, the world around you. Individualism in clothes, in actions, in thoughts are all components of the Aquarian philosophy. Give to others as Aquarius the water-bearer gives; but first know yourself, be yourself, experience yourself, through drugs if necessary.

Was this attitude, this philosophy, this emphasis on the NOW a cancer growing in society, a foreign body that didn't represent the mainstream of our culture? Hardly. The grab-what-you-can-when-you-can approach to life is but one aspect of the credit card culture—instant pleasure! No need now to work and worry to earn your pleasure; if you like it, charge it! Why wait? Have it now with a small down payment and 36 easy monthly installments.

The poets and the physicists know about the real world. And they both said it well. William Butler Yeats said it in 1894 in a poem, "The Land of Heart's Desire": "When we are young we long to tread a way none trod before."[15, p.876] Newton's third law said the same thing, and it is true with people, too: for every action there is a reaction. How do you reject the "loosey-goosey" sixties and early seventies? How do you find a new way?

To reject the NOW you have to tighten your belt and aim for something, and that's what we started to do in the late 1970s; we reacted to the changes of the sixties. The reaction began slowly—the shift to conservatism was small, and economic growth slowed. The expansion of individual liberties and civil rights, which was nothing more than the political expression of the "do-your-own-thing" philosophy, faltered and bogged down. The slowing was, in part, to digest the big changes that society had swallowed since the late 1950s.

At the turn of the decade society burped! The growing malaise and discontent and the need for a reduction in tension exploded in an orgasm of political and social changes that brought relief to many. Even as the slowdown developed in the early 1980s, the mood of the country changed. A mid-1981 poll found that 46% of Americans were optimistic about the future and believed that life would be even better in 5 years. In 1979, only 24% were optimistic about the future.[16] A study of above-average high school students in late 1981 found a 20% to 30% increase in conservatism compared to 1 or 2 years earlier.[17] *Yeah, drugs came in with a bang in the sixties—so did easy sex. Like you said—it's easier to give something up when you've always had it than if you had to work for it. It is kind of nice every once in a while to dress up and go some place different for a meal—hamburgers do get boring after a while. Really.*

What has changed since the 1950s? We had our revolution, our counterculture—now we're in a counterrevolution. What was radical is now de rigeur.

Transitions are always fun and exciting—as well as anxiety-arousing and sometimes flammable. Sometimes things are confusing if you haven't kept your eye on the pendulum: February 1981—Leveling Off of Drug Use Among Students[18]; July 1981—Teen-Agers Call Illicit Drugs One of Life's Commonplaces[19]; July 1981—Youths Regard Illicit Drugs as Harmful[20]; August 1981—Teen-Age Drug Use Declining, Congress Told[21]. Don't you just love it? Drugs are no big deal—they're like the boy or girl next door, always there, and the door is open.

How do you react to: *"I'm a unique individual—I'm going to find the real me"*? You look for commonalities, for roots, " . . . for cultural identity, sense of one's place in history, and pride in one's race and heritage. . . ."[22,p.3] It's not just blacks, all of us are wondering who we are, where we came from—and why. The action-reaction and the idea of a transition period are nowhere more clear than in the area of love and marriage. Who would have believed that in 1981 there was *both* "a steady increase in the number of persons living in unmarried cohabitation [formerly called "living in sin"] . . . and the marriage rate continued a climb that began in 1976."[23,p.63]

Once changed, nothing can ever be as it was before. Not people, not institutions, not societies. We are more conservative today than yesterday and will probably be more so tomorrow. But a conservative today is almost a flaming liberal of 1950. With each phase we move three steps in one direction, and in the next move two steps back. Sometimes things go too far, so there is no back stepping. It may be true with the family, which seems to be following the dodo bird.

Everywhere you look the action-reaction has occurred. The traditional religions and God of our forefathers shifted to social psychology and ecumenicalism, where they were saying that the differences they used to teach really weren't all that important. As the rock on which the churches stood was rapidly eroded, a new fundamentalistic, charismatic, pentecostal, full-gospel revival exploded on the scene. From God to god-is-dead to *God!* in 20 years.[24]

Universities used to be hallowed halls covered with slow-growing ivy and filled with pipe-smoking, deep-thinking scholars. College students in the 1950s were studied and described as "politically disinterested, apathetic, and conservative."[25] The students changed, the universities changed; federal money and a young faculty made many colleges active and activist. Marijuana replaced the ivy, joints replaced the pipes, and twelve credits "just for the experience of being" pushed deep thoughts to the background. The faculty aged, money grew tight, the students changed again—and so did the colleges. More required courses, more concern about education than with degrees.[26]

Some cycles seem out of phase—but that must be just because we don't understand them. The pragmatic attitude toward science and technology in the mid-1950s turned into a passionate embrace with Sputnik, rockets, satellites, and the race to put man on the moon. Science flourished in the sixties, and the counterreaction began to build. The facts of science were rejected. The honesty of scientists was denied. There was an increase in the mid-seventies in interest, involvement, and belief in the supernatural. A mid-1977 survey showed that less than half of American adults had confidence in those in the medical profession and what they say about disease—down 30% from 1966.[2] As noted earlier they put their behavior where their beliefs were—they ignored vaccinations, changed state laws so cancer "cures" labeled as worthless by experts could be legal.

No one can be sure where we are headed. None of the dynamics, the rules, the principles that influence society has changed—everything is just speeded up. Speeded up because of the revolution in communications—satellites let us *see* the other side of the world as it's happening—no more slow boats to China. The information explosion feeds in. Everybody knows more about everything, it seems. In science, the amount of information now doubles every 5 to 10 years. In the early part of the century it took 50 years.[27] Hang on tight—we're moving fast. No one knows where we'll be in 5 or 10 years—but we do know it won't be here.

DRUG-TAKING BEHAVIOR

In recent years there has been a tremendous increase in illegal drug use by individuals with healthy minds and bodies. These drugs are not used to improve physical health or to reduce symptoms of mental illness. How should we view this current upsurge in drug-taking behavior? What purpose does it serve? Why does it persist?

A neutral view suggests that this nonclinical drug-taking behavior can be seen as problem-solving behavior. Our society is searching for, and finding, new solutions to both old and new problems. Some of our difficulties develop because we have yet to reach an acceptable social standard on these new ways of solving problems. Finding a cultural norm in the area of drug use is particularly important, since, as new drugs are produced, both the amount and pervasiveness of drug use will increase.

Why do people take drugs? Is drug taking a unique phenomenon? Are there no counterparts to it in our society? One fact that must be understood is that *drug taking is behavior!* As such it follows the same rules and principles as any other behavior. The most basic principle is that behavior persists when it either increases the individual's pleasure or reduces his discomfort. That is, people don't use just any old drug; they take only those which pro-

vide *for them* either a positive, satisfying, pleasurable effect or a decrease in their discomfort. And of those drugs which do increase pleasure or decrease discomfort, the particular ones selected must be acceptable within the individual's cultural group.

Many people refer to *psychological dependence* on a drug. The term is a poor one, since it suggests, incorrectly, that there is something unique about drug use. If the term is used, it should refer to one of two aspects of behavior. Psychological dependence may indicate the importance of a drug, or the use of a drug, as a life-organizing factor. The heroin addict organizes his world around ensuring the availability of an adequate supply of heroin. Some suburbanites refer to their daily life events as before or after cocktail parties. Many students keep track of their lives as so many days before or after an activity such as a big date, a concert series, or a sports event. When the term is used this way, most of us are probably psychologically dependent on some activity as one of the primary organizing factors in our life.

Sometimes psychological dependence on drugs refers to the prominent role of drug use in the individual's repertoire of coping mechanisms. How does the person handle a stressful situation? Use drugs. Occupy free time? Use drugs. Search out pleasure? Use drugs. For many young people it is possible to substitute music, sex, sports, or other activities for drugs. The basic message here is that there is nothing unusual or unique about drug use; drug-taking behavior is like all other behaviors.

As with other behaviors, there are multiple causes underlying a person's drug-taking behavior. To look for a single reason for drug taking is to whistle in the wind. Studies with animals show that susceptibility to narcotic addiction is, in part, genetically determined, and strains of animals have been bred that are either very easy or very difficult to addict.[28] Similarly, strains of animals have been developed that prefer alcohol over water for drinking, although most animals will select water if given a choice.[29] There are suggestions that alcoholism in humans is partly based on the individual's heredity.[30] Drug taking (regardless of whether there is a genetic predisposition) is like other behaviors in that it is the result of a complex interaction of past experiences and present environment. Many scientists believe that a single common mechanism might underlie several types of habitual behavior such as cigarette smoking, use of narcotics, over-eating, and jogging.[31]

The primary point, again, is that drug-taking behavior is not unique; it is like any other behavior. An appreciation of this goes a long way toward taking a rational look at current drug use. For example, a more common set of behaviors that approximates drug-taking behavior in motivation and effect is the "neuroses." Drug-taking behavior can be viewed as cut from the same cloth as neurotic behavior. The two have many similar characteristics, and possibly over the next several years some of the more traditional neurotic symptoms will gradually be replaced by drug taking. It may be that drug taking will just be superimposed on neurotic behavior, or vice versa. It follows that the same kinds of concern should be shown toward drug taking as toward neurotic patterns of behavior.

As is true of neurotic behavior, illegal drug taking offers the individual both benefits and disadvantages. The benefit is usually some short-term gain such as a more positive feeling or a decrease in discomfort. The disadvantages are multiple but more remote in time. For one, there is a decrease in a chance of reaching long-term, permanent solutions to the underlying problems. There is also, in our society, a probable decrease in the rewards an individual can obtain if he persists in repeated drug taking.

If this is a reasonable way of viewing drug taking, then the concern many people have about drug use should perhaps be shifted to include the fact that drug taking *may* have negative effects on the individual *only* when it becomes the dominant mode of problem solving. Taking drugs does solve some immediate problems! It offers the individual short-term solutions. However, it may have adverse long-term effects either by preventing a better solution or by causing new problems to arise. In the case of some drugs, used in certain ways, it seems that adverse long-term effects are not only possible but almost inevitable for most people.

PSYCHOACTIVE DRUG EFFECTS

Thus far, the term "drug" has been used to indicate the generality of what has been said; the foregoing statements are true of all psychoactive drugs. There are so many kinds and classes of psychoactive drugs that to attempt to specify a few of them would be of little value. Are there any other general statements that can be made about psychoactive drugs—those compounds which alter consciousness and affect mood? In fact, there are four basic principles that seem to apply to all these drugs.

First, *drugs*, per se, *are not "good" or "bad."* There are no "bad drugs." When drug abuse is talked about, it is the behavior, the way the drug is being used, that is being referred to. The labeling of a particular use of a drug as an "abuse" requires the adoption of a particular set of values. All drugs, like most other things, can be used in ways that our society labels *bad* or *good*. These labels, though, have a way of shifting—sometimes gradually, sometimes rapidly.

This is not just a semantic matter. Some things can probably be labeled bad by everyone's standards: cancer, a tidal wave, and so forth. In most self-selected human behaviors there are both positive and negative factors to be considered before choosing to participate. Usually the more information available, the more the decision will be in line with what the individual really wants. You may agree to go for an automobile trip, taking a chance on becoming a statistic, but then change your mind when you see the car is in poor mechanical condition. You didn't want to take *that big* a chance!

Different factors will be given different weight by different people. Usually there are two phases in reaching a decision: is the behavior something that can even be conceived? If conceivable, do the advantages outweigh the disadvantages? Most 50-year-olds cannot conceive of ever skydiving; it's an unthinkable thing. For many 20-year-olds, however, it is something to be thought about, the pros and cons considered, and a real decision reached. To do this rationally, much information is needed.

The same is true with drugs. Using amphetamines under any conditions may be unthinkable and, since it's also illegal, labeled bad by some people. To many young people "using amphetamines" is a real possibility when the dose, the way the drug is taken, and the reason it's to be taken are brought into the picture. To label a drug "bad" categorically solves nothing and convinces no one.

A second basic, and often forgotten, fact about psychoactive drugs is that *every drug has multiple effects*. Although a user may focus on a single aspect of a drug's effect, clearly we do not yet have compounds that alter only one aspect of consciousness. That a drug usually has many *different* effects on the individual using it might be expected from the fact that most drugs act at many different places in the brain.

This brings us to a third principle about psychoactive drug effects. *The effects of a drug depend on the amount the individual has taken*. This relationship between dose and effect works in two ways. By increasing the dose, there is usually an accentuation of effects noticed at lower drug levels. Also, and frequently this is a more important relationship, at different dose levels there is often a change in the kind of effect, an alteration in the quality of the experience. Varying doses, then, can change not only the magnitude but also the character of the drug effect. Do certain dose levels constitute an abuse of a drug while other dose levels do not?

The fourth item of general relevance about psychoactive compounds is that *their effect, in part, depends on the individual's history and expectations*. Since these drugs act to alter consciousness and thought processes, the effect they have on an individual depends on what was there initially. The attitude an individual has can have a major effect on his perception of the drug experience. The fact that some people can experience a *real* high when smoking oregano and dry oak tree leaves—thinking it's good marijuana—should come as no surprise to anyone who has arrived late at a swinging cocktail party and found himself turned on after one martini rather than the usual two or three. It is not possible, then, to talk about many of the effects of these drugs independent of the user's attitude and the setting.

If there is one point about which every student of the drugs agrees, it is that there is no such thing as the drug experience per se—no experience which the drugs, as it were, merely secrete. Every experience is a mix of three ingredients: drug, set (the psychological makeup of the individual) and setting (the social and physical environment in which it is taken).[32,p.158]

Reviewing some of the basic points before moving on to talk about society and the extent of psychoactive drug use, it seems well supported that the current increase in drug-taking behavior reflects (mainly) a general cultural change in the direction of beginning to see drugs as acceptable ways of solving problems. The answers drugs provide are usually only short-term solutions and may prevent the individual from finding a permanent, non-drug resolution to the problem.

Drugs have multiple effects that vary with the amount of the drug used and the personality of the user, as well as his expectancies about the effects of the drug. The reason people initially take drugs recreationally varies considerably, but, at a very fundamental level, it is either to obtain a pleasurable experience or to reduce unhappiness. Whether a person decides to use drugs to solve problems depends on his background, his present environment, and the availability of drugs.

Drug availability is a secondary point here. If drugs were the problem, the issue could be handled by shutting off the supply—a big job, perhaps one with undesirable social effects, but actually possible. The problem, though, is people, not drugs. Individuals are looking for rapid solutions to problems, and drugs are one of the options our society makes available.

DRUGS AND DRUG USE TODAY

If the pharmacological and cultural revolution encourage drug use, if drug use supports and extends the revolutions, and if many deny the Protestant Ethic as a philosophy of life while substituting the Aquarian and hang-loose ethics, there should be widespread use of psychoactive drugs today. And there is.

Four classes comprise the commercially available and legal psychoactive drugs. The group of compounds most people think of as "drugs" are the prescription drugs. These are chemicals that require a physician's prescription to purchase legally. About 30% of all prescriptions are for drugs that act on the brain, making this class of compounds the most commonly prescribed group.

Another group of psychoactive agents are those called over-the-counter (OTC) drugs. These drugs are intended for temporary medication of minor illnesses and are considered safe for use without a physician's supervision if the instructions on the label are followed carefully. Unfortunately this is frequently not done, and the potential dangers of these drugs are not appreciated.

The third class of mood- and consciousness-altering chemicals legally available in this country includes the social drugs: alcohol, caffeine, and nicotine. Some governmental control is exerted over the purchase of products containing alcohol and nicotine, but in spite of these restrictions, the legal social drug business is extremely large.

The last group of psychoactive compounds is quite different from other agents that are manufactured and merchandised for their psychoactive effect. This final group includes many compounds and items sold for nondrug purposes that, under some conditions, do have effects on mood and awareness. Substances such as airplane glue, certain herbs like nutmeg, and the seeds from some morning glory plants all have been used for their psychoactive properties.

There are also illegal psychoactive drugs, such as marijuana, heroin, and LSD, and legal psychoactive drugs used illegally, as happens with the street use of narcotics, stimulants, and depressants. It is the use of these drugs that causes the most hubbub, anxiety, and activity in our society. It is not at all clear that the illegal use of psychoactive drugs causes the most problems—social, personal, or medical. Prevention of misuse and abuse of any drug—legal or illegal, approved or disapproved— is where our time and effort should be spent.

With drugs and other psychoactive agents readily available and a large amount of money spent each year on these compounds, it would be expected that a very high percentage of the population uses one type of drug or another. Excluding the social drugs and agents that are marketed for nondrug purposes, a good place to start looking at drug use in the United States today is your drug cabinet.

TABLE 1-1 Past year pattern of use of medically prescribed psychotherapeutic drugs by drug class*

	Percentage distributions for drug class				
	Antianxiety agents	Hypnotics	Daytime sedatives	Anti-depressants	Anti-psychotics
Did not use	88.9	97.4	98.7	97.9	98.7
Used	11.1	2.6	1.3	2.1	1.3
Used less than 30 days total	5.5	1.6	0.5	0.4	0.6
Daily use for more than 4 months	2.2	0.5	0.6	1.0	0.4

From Mellinger, G., and Balter, M.: Prevalence and patterns of use of psychotherapeutic drugs: results from a 1979 national survey of American adults. In Tognoni, G., Ballantuono, C., and Lader, M., editors: Epidemiological impact of psychotropic drugs: proceedings of international seminar on epidemiological impact of psychotropic drugs, Amsterdam, 1981, Elsevier/North-Holland Biomedical Press.

*Nonhospital use only.

TABLE 1-2 Prevalence of past year use of medically prescribed psychotherapeutic drugs by drug class, age, and sex*

Drug class and sex	% using during past 12 months in age/sex group				
	18-34	35-49	50-64	65-79	All
Antianxiety agents					
Men	4.1	8.1	12.4	9.1	7.5
Women	7.9	16.6	19.5	18.7	14.1
Hypnotics					
Men	0.8	0.7	4.1	5.3	2.1
Women	1.7	2.4	3.5	6.5	3.0
Daytime sedatives					
Men	0.5	0.4	1.3	0.8	0.7
Women	1.5	1.4	2.4	2.6	1.9
Antidepressants					
Men	0.3	1.8	1.9	2.8	1.3
Women	2.1	1.1	4.7	4.1	2.8
Antipsychotics					
Men	0.8	0.4	2.0	1.1	1.0
Women	1.8	2.1	0.6	1.2	1.5
Any of the five classes					
Men	6.1	9.7	18.3	16.2	11.0
Women	13.3	21.4	26.5	27.5	20.2

From Mellinger, G., and Balter, M.: Prevalence and patterns of use of psychotherapeutic drugs: results from a 1979 national survey of American adults. In Tognoni, G., Bellantuono, C., and Lader, M., editors: Epidemiological impact of psychotropic drugs: proceedings of international seminar on epidemiological impact of psychotropic drugs, Amsterdam, 1981, Elsevier/North-Holland Biomedical Press.
*Nonhospital use only.

Count the number of different drugs you have stashed away. It will probably surprise you—the leftover drugs from last winter's colds and other illnesses, plus the basic "necessary" drugs, plus. . . . One study[33] found an average of 12 drugs per household—and the average age of the drugs was almost 20 months. Forty-one percent of the households said that someone was using the drug other than the person for whom it was prescribed. Of these drugs about 1 in 4 were those acting on the central nervous system.

There is much discussion over whether Americans are overmedicated. Do physicians prescribe, and do we take, too many psychoactive drugs? There is no way to determine what "the correct level of psychotherapeutic drug use" should be, but there are some data[34] that you should know. Table 1-1 shows the percentage of adults in the United States who were users of five classes of psychotherapeutic drugs and an indication of their pattern of drug use in the year preceding the 1979 survey. It is clear that *most* people don't use any of these drugs. Of those who do, *most* use them for short periods of time. The group around which most of the media and medical debate has revolved are the 2.2% who used antianxiety agents daily for more than 4 months (see Chapter 13).

It is perhaps of more than passing interest to review the pattern of drug use in Table 1-2, which is also from the survey previously discussed. None of it is surprising—hypnotics are used most by the elderly, antianxiety agents by those in mid-life, and

TABLE 1-3 Percentages of ever used[a]/current[b] drug users in high school seniors in the spring of each year

Drug class (only nonmedical drug use reported)	Class						
	1975	1976	1977	1978	1979	1980	1981
Marijuana-hashish	47/27	53/32	56/35	59/37	60/37	60/34	60/32
Hallucinogens	16/5	15/3	14/4	14/4	19/6[c]	16/4[c]	16/3[c]
Cocaine	9/2	10/2	11/3	13/4	15/6	16/5	17/6
Heroin	2/0	2/0	2/0	2/0	1/0	1/0	1/0
Other opiates	9/2	10/2	10/3	10/2	10/2	10/2	10/2
Stimulants	22/9	23/8	23/9	23/9	24/10	26/12	32/16
Sedatives	18/5	18/5	17/5	16/4	15/4	15/5	15/5
Tranquilizers	17/4	17/4	18/5	17/3	16/4	15/3	15/3
Inhalants	—	10/1	11/1	12/2	19/3[d]	18/3[d]	18/2[d]
Alcohol	90/68	92/68	93/71	93/72	93/72	93/72	93/71
Cigarettes	74/37	75/39	76/38	75/37	74/34	71/31	71/29

From Highlights from student drug use in America 1975-1981, Washington, D.C., 1982, U.S. Department of Health and Human Services, National Institute on Drug Abuse.

a. Percentages rounded; 0 to 0.4 shown as 0.
b. Current users are those who used the drug in the month preceding the survey.
c. Includes PCP.
d. Includes amyl and butyl nitrites.

women at all ages and for all drug classes use more psychoactive medication. It's the old cup-is-filled-to-the-midpoint question: Is it half-full, or half-empty? Is it: "Goodness gracious! One out of 5 women and 1 of 9 men used some medically pre-scribed psychotherapeutic drug as a crutch" or "Hey, not bad—8 out of 9 guys and 4 out of 5 gals were able to fight off the stupidities, pressures, and hassles of this topsy-turvy world without having to see a doctor for a drug. Really good!"

Table 1-3 gives a good idea of nonmedical psychoactive drug use by teen-agers in America from the mid-seventies to the early eighties. The data are from high school seniors. This means those who have left school, who usually have a higher incidence of drug use, aren't included. Males and females are combined in the table. In general males engage in more drug use than females but the differences are declining every year. In each column there are two sets of figures: the first number is the percentage of seniors who have *ever used* the drug; the second number is the percentage of se-niors who *used it in the 30 days before the survey*. The increases, decreases, and leveling off that were mentioned earlier are easily seen. Note that there is no information in the table (nor is it available anywhere in detail) about the frequency of use. The most that is available is daily use—for marijuana that rose from 6% in 1975 to a high of 10.7% in 1978. In 1979, 1980, and 1981 daily use declined steadily: 10.3%, 9.1%, and 7.0%. There is, of course, no way to know what the potency is of the marijuana being smoked. The best bet is that it is now two to four times as great in THC (tetrahy-drocannabinol) concentration, the psychoactive in-gredient, as it was in the early and mid-1970s. One other important point: this is a well-done *national* survey and probably reflects the overall, national level of drug use in this age group. It is not possible to use these results as an indication of drug use in a particular state, city, or school.

A different perspective on psychoactive drug use is given in Table 1-4.[36] These are data from a dif-ferent survey; only two psychoactive drug catego-

TABLE 1-4 Percent of lifetime prevalence *(ever used)* trends in illegal psychoactive drug use by age group

Age (years)	Drug class	Years							
		1962*	**1967***	**1971**	**1972**	**1974**	**1976**	**1977**	**1979**
12-17	Marijuana	1	7	14	14	23	22	28	31
	Other†	0	3	NA	8	9	9	9	9
18-25	Marijuana	4	13	39	48	53	53	60	68
	Other	3	4	NA	17	22	25	27	33
25+	Marijuana	2	3	9	7	10	13	15	20
	Other	1	1	NA	2	3	4	4	6

From Drug abuse prevention, treatment, and rehabilitation in fiscal year 1980, Third Annual Report from the Secretary of DHHS to the President and Congress of the United States, Washington, D.C., 1981, U.S. Government Printing Office.
*Retrospective data, collected in 1977.
†Includes hallucinogens, inhalants, cocaine, heroin (except 1979), and other opiates.

ries are given: marijuana and other substances (this includes hallucinogens, inhalants, cocaine, heroin, and other opiates). Table 1-4 contains the percentages in the three age ranges of those who *ever used* the drugs. Few people begin their use of illegal drugs after age 25 but some continue using illegal drugs past this age. It is expected that the frequency of use and recency of use will continue to grow in the over-25 age group. No one knows what tomorrow will bring, but if you believe that predicting future patterns of drug abuse is going to be more successful than predicting tomorrow's weather, a 1981 publication is your cup of tea: *Demographic Trends and Drug Abuse, 1980-1995*.[37] In a nutshell, it says:

> Regular use of marijuana will be on the upswing but the percentage of occasional users should stabilize.
>
> Use of hallucinogens should not change dramatically.
>
> The percentage of cocaine users, particularly occasional users, will increase over the next decade.
>
> The percentage of young adults using heroin and other opiates should not change dramatically. (p. 67)

These almost sound like the type of predictions given at the Temple of Delphi: You will win the battle, if you fight hard enough!

Correlates and antecedents of drug use

alcohol and tobacco are the substances used most frequently by youth and the substances which in terms of social harm and social costs are the most damaging. . . .

the use of illegal drugs by youth is strongly related to the use of legal drugs . . . there would seem to be more cause for concern from the rising rates of alcohol consumption than the consumption of illicit drugs per se.[38]

You must understand that two of the major antecedent conditions for current patterns of drug use have already been discussed. The sections on pharmacological revolutions and cultural change spoke to the general background factors that make recreational drug use not unreasonable behavior. This section speaks more to the question of specific individuals using or not using drugs. We all live in the same general *zeitgeist*—why does one individual do drugs and not another? Appreciate that 15 years ago most of you would not have tried marijuana, 25 years ago probably none of you would have tried it, and 35 years in the past, if you had even heard of it, you couldn't spell it, but if you had heard of it, you would have *known* that it was a very dangerous thing. But today, why do some people, and not others, engage in drug-taking behavior?

There are many levels at which this question can

be answered. For some young people drug use in the sixties and/or early seventies was probably nothing more than a way to bug the system—especially parents. What better way to aggravate your parents than by doing drugs?

> Speak roughly to your little boy,
> And beat him when he sneezes:
> He only does it to annoy,
> Because he knows it teases.[39,p.54]

Drug taking was (and for the most part still is) an almost guaranteed way to upset parents, since there are many aspects of drug taking that can bother them: it's illegal, it may harm the user, it's a rejection of social standards and mores, and, most importantly, it's a denial of the value and the meaning of the parents' life and way of living. Since many parents live for the future only through their children, the threat of losing this link to posterity is particularly disruptive. This possibility was vividly phrased in 1969:

> Why, one wonders, is the older generation so perturbed at the spectacle of their children experimenting with mind-expanding drugs? It is not simply a realistic concern for their welfare. If this were all, the older people would be equally concerned to prevent their children from acquiring the habit of overindulgence in alcohol and in cigarette smoking. I suggest that the real cause for this exaggerated concern is recognition of the fact that young people are deliberately challenging, and in many cases repudiating, the values which their elders have lived by; and it is this which we of the older generation find so hard to tolerate.[40]

Some young people try some drugs, like marijuana, because it's a fad: "everyone is doing it," even though *not all* are doing it. That rationalization is reminiscent of the reason many people in earlier generations got introduced to alcohol in one of its many forms.

After all is said and done, illegal drug users take drugs, in part, for the same good and bad, right and wrong reasons as legal drug users: to reduce anxiety and tension, to remove fatigue and boredom, to blot out an unwanted world, to influence mood, to change activity level, to facilitate social interactions, or to feel good. Some motivations for illegal drug use are probably different from those for legal use: curiosity—I wonder what would happen if?

The remainder of this section deals primarily with the question of illegal psychoactive drug use, with the emphasis on marijuana. There are two reasons for this: one is that marijuana is the most widely used illegal drug, and it is possible to obtain enough users to ask questions and obtain meaningful results. The second reason is that marijuana is the entrée into the use of other illegal drugs. Most marijuana users do not become regular users of other illegal drugs, but those who do use other illegal drugs have usually tried marijuana first. The interaction of these factors was roughly summarized:

> While drug use by peers is the most important factor for initiation into marihuana use, progression to other, more serious drugs depends increasingly on intrapersonal factors and not as strongly on values and activities characterizing the peer group.[41]

The study of any behavior, including drug-taking behavior, usually proceeds through four questions. The first question asks, how prevalent is the behavior—what is its incidence? Tables 1-3 and 1-4 answer that question rather completely for drug use. The second question is, what are the correlates of drug use—what factors are associated with drug use? The emphasis here has generally been on studying the psychological, social, and demographic variables that relate to the presence or absence of drug-taking behavior. The third question asks, is there a standard or typical sequence of involvement with drugs? Does the use of a particular drug—always, usually, never—precede the use of another specific drug? Last, are there measurable antecedents to the start of drug use? Can individual, nondrug, psychosocial factors be identified that make it possible to predict future drug-taking behavior?

Correlates. Before commenting on some of the psychosocial variables that relate to drug use or nonuse, two other factors need to be mentioned. The availability of a drug is both antecedent to and correlated with the use of a drug. No one can use drugs that are not there. Law enforcement people frequently make this point. It's a good one. Chapter 2 speaks to the question of whether law enforcement is a good way to reduce drug availability. The second factor is opportunity to use a drug. Even if a drug is available in the general society, an individual cannot use a drug until given the opportunity.

Perhaps because this is a truism, there have been very few studies of factors that relate to having the opportunity to use a drug. Some investigators have asked individuals who are not marijuana users if they would use it if given the opportunity. As many as 17% of the nonusers say they might—if given the opportunity.

One comprehensive study of students of both sexes ages 9 to 20 in private high schools in Managua, Nicaragua, investigated "opportunity to use marijuana" as a variable in predicting use.[42] Of those who are *neither* regular drinkers nor smokers, 31% have had an opportunity to use marijuana, and, of those having the opportunity, about 1% have used marijuana more than once. Of those who are *either* regular drinkers *or* smokers, 63% have had the opportunity to use marijuana, and, of those, 10% have used it more than once. Of those who are *both* regular smokers and drinkers, 85% have usually had the opportunity to use marijuana, and, of those, 37% have used marijuana more than once. The pattern is clear: the use of legal alcohol or tobacco is associated with increased opportunity to use marijuana, and that, in turn, is associated with multiple use of marijuana, depending on the previous extent of alcohol/tobacco use. It is probably true that at the younger age levels, opportunity is a significant determinant of marijuana use. At college age and through the 18 to 29 age range, marijuana is more socially pervasive in the United States, and most sociable, party-going people are, at some time, given the opportunity to use it.

Once given the opportunity to use marijuana and other illegal drugs, what factors are associated with or influence the decision to use or not use? What are the correlates of marijuana use? A review[42] of 90 studies published from 1970 through 1976 evaluated the results of each study with respect to the variables listed in Table 1-5. All these studies concerned marijuana use in secondary schools. (Findings for university students are similar.) The table includes the actual number of studies that reported each variable's relationship to marijuana use and lists the percent of those studies in which the relationship was positive. For example, 74% of the studies found that the older the individual was, or the greater the number of years of schooling the individual had completed, the more likely it was that the individual was a marijuana user. That is, the number of marijuana users increases with age. When older (20 to 35) age groups are studied, there tends to be a progressive decline in marijuana use with age. It is important that the correlates shown in Table 1-5 not be overly interpreted or seen as chiseled in stone. Things do change, and several points need further comment.

Although males are still more likely to use marijuana than females, the difference in percent of users and frequency of use between the sexes decreases with age. This sex-based difference is diminishing as marijuana use becomes more prevalent. Another point is that the quality of the relationship between the individual and his parents is negatively related to marijuana use—the better the relationship the less likely the child is to use marijuana. This is a good example of the extreme care that is necessary in trying to understand many of these results. When both measures, relationship to parents and marijuana use, are taken at the same time, it is impossible to say which causes which. Do poor relationships with parents result in marijuana use? Or does marijuana use result in poor relationships with parents? Or are both true, or do both result only from increasing age? When the measures are taken at the same time, *all* you can say is that they are related. You cannot prove that one causes the other.

Of special interest to most of us is the variable labeled *personality problems*. This is a catch-all phrase that covers everything from high anxiety to low self-esteem, immaturity to depression. The data in Table 1-5 clearly show that there is no consistent relationship between marijuana use or non-

TABLE 1-5 Number of published studies (1970-1976) showing indicated relationship between psychosocial variables and marijuana use

Psychosocial variables	Direction of relationship with marijuana use		
	Positive	None or negative	Mixed*
Male sex	30 (75%)	10	0
Age or year in school	26 (74%)	7	2
Socioeconomic status	22 (79%)	6	0
Poor parent-child relations	36 (86%)	0	6
Drug use by parents	12 (75%)	1	2
Intense interaction with peers	13 (59%)	4	5
Personality problems	8 (36%)	7	7
Individual smokes	26 (93%)	2	0
Individual drinks	31 (94%)	2	0
Individual uses other drugs	25 (100%)	0	0
Peers use marijuana	27 (93%)	0	2
Nonconformity			
Religious	16 (89%)	0	2
Educational	24 (71%)	6	4
Political	12 (86%)	1	1
Legal	20 (100%)	0	0
Social	25 (83%)	1	4

*Classification as "mixed" usually refers to different relationships being found with different sexes or ages.

use and the presence or absence of personality problems. Mark well that this is as of the early to mid-1970s, and in high school students. Earlier users in the 1950s and early 1960s may have had more personality problems as a group because marijuana use was more deviant behavior in that period. Some reports[43,44] indicate that personality problems *are* related to marijuana use at the high school level, but that the same factors are not related to use among college students. It is true that marijuana use by high school students is more deviant than is use by college students.

Of course, some individuals at all ages begin to use marijuana because of personality problems, and it is also true that, in some, marijuana use results in personality problems. As a general rule, though, at the college level whether someone uses or does not use marijuana tells you nothing about his mental health. Take note that these comments only refer to use/nonuse. There are multiple reports that moderate to heavy use is related to an in-

creased number of personality problems—even among college students—and the problems generally precede use.[45] One other point: "The more out of keeping a pattern of drug abuse is from an individual's social background and cultural norms, the more likely he/she is to be suffering from serious mental illness."[46,p.295] This is a general rule that seems applicable in all cases. The more atypical a drug user is—from the group that usually uses the drug—the more likely it is that the atypical user will have serious emotional problems. A white male heroin user is atypical because most heroin users are black males. An alcoholic who is female is atypical because most alcoholics are male.[47] The white male heroin user and the female alcoholic are much more likely to have serious emotional problems than the black male heroin user and the male alcoholic.

The five variables listed under *nonconformity* are of particular importance. These factors are concerned with the extent to which the individual rejects conventional standards of morality and behavior. Thus a positive relationship indicates rejection of traditional cultural systems; for example, 89% of the studies showed that marijuana users, more often than nonusers, denied religious affiliation and beliefs and did not attend religious functions; 71% had low grades and rejected the value of education and school. It is legal and political nonconformity that many people associate with drug use—protests against the government, negative attitudes toward laws, actual arrests for violations—and that relationship is confirmed in these studies. Social conformity is a broad category that includes sexual permissiveness, rejection of the Protestant Ethic—work hard and achieve—and an absence of cooperation and participation in organized community activities.

A study in the late 1960s that looked at patterns of drug use in college students summarized much of the work in that period by reporting:

> Use of drugs was more likely to occur among those students whose behavior, attitudes or values, and self-image were indicative of opposition to the traditional, established order. Such differences occurred regardless of those demographic characteristics of the students also related to drug use, such as sex, socioeconomic status, and religion.[48]

Remember that times change. ". . . the middle-class drug use of the late 1970s was not the same as that of the 1960s and early 1970s. Unlike the drug use of 'hippies' and others who were trying to expand their consciousness and experience new levels of understanding and communication, contemporary middle-class drug use appears to be motivated by self-indulgence, boredom, and . . . the culture of narcissism."[49,p.18]

There are many papers that summarize the psychosocial correlates of drug use,[50,51] but only one final comment can be made. A frequent question is the extent to which marijuana use by adolescents is associated with the drug use patterns of parents and peers. The best study on this problem obtained independent reports on drug use from students, from their friends, and from their parents. The investigator concluded that

drug use by peers exerts a greater influence than drug use by parents. Friends are more similar in their use of marihuana than in any other activity or attitude. Parental use of psychotropic drugs has only a small influence, mostly related to maternal use. Peer and parental influences are synergistic; the highest rates of marihuana usage are observed among adolescents whose parents and friends are drug users.[52]

Sequence. Kandel and Faust[53] have outlined four sequential stages in the movement of a nondrug user to the use of illegal drugs other than marijuana. A summary of their major findings—which have been replicated on a second sample of students—is shown in Fig. 1-1. High school students 14 to 18 years of age in New York State were questioned on their drug use at two separate times 5 to 6 months apart.

Fig. 1-1 records the probability that an individual will move from one stage to the next over this period. For example, the figure shows that 28% of those who were nondrug users on the first survey had started using beer and/or wine by the time of the second survey. Of those who were using beer and/or wine (but not hard liquor or cigarettes) at the time of the first survey, 32% had started using hard liquor and 8% were using cigarettes when the second survey was taken. It is interesting that "a majority of the cigarette users eventually start drinking (68%), but only a minority of the liquor users start smoking (21%). Thus while drinking can proceed without smoking, smoking is almost always followed by drinking of hard liquor."

Some individuals moved more than one stage between surveys, but the same sequence of drug use holds true. Beer and wine are the primary entry drugs into the circle of drug users. Only 6% begin drug use with cigarettes, 3% with hard liquor, and 1% with an illegal drug. This sequential-stage model does not deal with nondrug factors that contribute to drug use, neither does it speak to the issue of the speed with which the progression moves. The first illicit drug is almost always marijuana, and, if an individual moves on to other drugs, the usual sequence is pills (stimulants, depressants, tranquilizers), psychedelics, cocaine, and heroin.

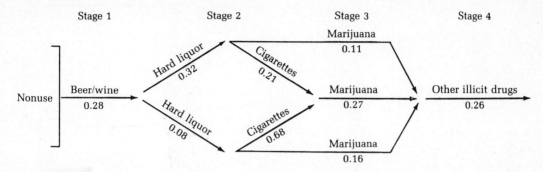

FIG. 1-1 Probabilities of moving from one step to another based on changes (5- to 6-month interval) between fall, 1971, and spring, 1972, in a cohort of New York State high school students 14 to 18 years old. (From Kandel, D., and Faust, R.: Archives of General Psychiatry **32**:923-932, 1975. Copyright 1975, American Medical Association.)

This sequence seemed to be the typical one for white students in the 1970s and was probably shaped by drug availability, as well as social, cognitive, and historical factors. There seems to be a different sequence for young, black, ghetto residents. After marijuana the drug sequence is cocaine, heroin, barbiturates, amphetamines, and psychedelics.[54] The difference in the typical sequence of drugs between blacks and whites may be due to many factors, such as age, drug availability, personality factors, and desired drug effects. The differences are diminishing yearly, and cocaine use occurs earlier in the sequence of drug use among whites in the 1980s. Remember also that in each of these sequences there are fewer and fewer individuals who reach the later stages. It needs to be mentioned again that these statements refer to the most probable or the typical sequence, but, as noted, there are exceptions.

Antecedents. The final stage in the study of the development of drug use has only recently been reached. This stage attempts to identify the antecedents of drug use. To do this requires a developmental, longitudinal approach. It is, of course, possible to study the antecedents of drug use at any stage in the sequence. You already know the antecedent-drug sequence. For most people the use of pills, psychedelics, or opiates is preceded by marijuana use, which is preceded by hard liquor and cigarette use, which is preceded by beer or wine use, which is preceded by . . .? Two ques-

tions arise: Is there other drug use that precedes the use of beer and wine? Are there psychosocial factors that can be identified as antecedent to any of these stages of drug use?

A 1975 report[55] spoke tangentially to the first question in a study of junior and senior high school students in California. Through interviews, the age at "first use" of a number of drugs was obtained; Fig. 1-2 plots the results. Little comment is needed, but it may help to know that the median ages for first use for each of the drugs listed was "coffee or tea = 7.8 years; wine or beer = 10.6 years; tobacco = 11.0 years; hard liquor = 13.1 years; marijuana = 13.8 years; and hallucinogens, stimulants, depressants, and narcotics = over 17 years but cannot be estimated."[55] The authors summarized their psychosocial findings:

the students with a predisposition to more rapidly ascend the hierarchy of drug use are not a random subsample of the student population. This group tends to be differentiated by their degree of social or peer orientation. Those who are higher in the drug hierarchy tend to date earlier and to spend much time with friends in raps or parties rather than in more organized activities, such as sports or homework. They tend to be more gregarious even when their friends are not ones they would prefer to have. . . . They are not active in religious activities, and they perceive the social aspects of school as more important than the intellectual as-

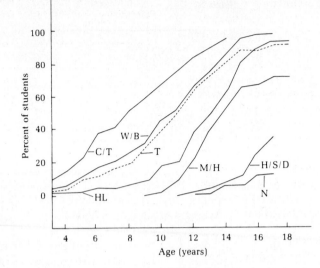

FIG. 1-2 Distribution of age at first use of drugs for 163 white junior and senior high school students. *C/T* = coffee or tea; *W/B* = wine or beer; *HL* = hard liquor; *T* = tobacco; *M/H* = marijuana or hashish; *H/S/D* = hallucinogens, stimulants, or depressants; and *N* = narcotics. (From Hamburg, B.H., Kraemer, H.C., and Jahnke, W.: American Journal of Psychiatry 132:1155-1163, 1975. Copyright 1975, the American Psychiatric Association. Reprinted by permission.)

pects. Finally, this group, for whom drug education programs would be most particularly pertinent, is very critical of existing drug education programs. At the same time, they are the most desirous of additional information.[55]

The question of psychosocial factors antecedent to drug use was answered in the affirmative by a 5-year study.[56] It started with students in the seventh and eighth grades of suburban Boston schools, and results from 23 variables in year one were related to drug use in the fifth year of the study. The 23 variables were grade-point average, cigarette smoking, 8 self-report and 5 peer-rated scales on personality, and 7 self-report scales on attitudes toward cigarette smoking. The drug-use data in the fifth year allowed the students to be placed in three groups: never used an illegal drug (208); used marijuana but no other illegal drugs (205); have used at least once opiates, hallucinogens, stimulants, or depressants (100). The results are both impressive and informative. The three drug-use groups of teenagers could be predicted from nondrug measures taken 4 years earlier. On the personality mea-

sures "the nonusers scored low on rebellious, untrustworthy, sociable, and impulsive, and scored high on hardworking, ambitious, self-reliant, orderly, likes school, feels accepted, feels capable, and feels confident academically.[56, p.282]

The researchers go on to say:

Four aspects of the results merit emphasis. First, the significant predictors are conceptually and methodologically diverse. . . . Second, for all but one of the 23 predictors, the mean scores for marihuana users were intermediate between the means for nonusers and hard drug users. Third, the self-report and peer rating measures of personality provided a reassuring degree of mutual support (e.g., rebellious and obedient, hardworking and works hard). Finally, the interval of four years . . . is long; and under such circumstances many influences operate to obscure . . . relationships.[56, p.280]

A study by one of the active researchers in this area started with students in the seventh, eighth, and ninth grades in a small Rocky Mountain town and measured drug use regularly for 4 years. He also found "substantial support for the relation of marijuana onset to a deviance . . . prone pattern of social-psychological attributes existing prior to onset."[57,p.287] The deviance-prone pattern

> includes lower value on achievement and greater value on independence, greater social criticism, more tolerance of deviance, and less religiosity . . . less parental control and support, greater friends' influence, and greater friends' models and approval for drug use . . . and more deviant behavior, less church attendance, and lower school achievement . . . The nonusers of marihuana tend to represent the opposite pattern, a pattern of relative conventionality or conformity.[57,p.297]

Everything interacts in each of our lives—nothing can be kept uniquely separate from everything else. Just as personality factors and attitudes influence behavior, including marijuana use, marijuana use is part of a behavior pattern that interacts and influences personality, attitudes, and values. One of the strong aspects of this research was that it was possible to study the impact of the beginning of marijuana use on behavioral and attitudinal changes in adolescence.

> It was quite clear that the course of adolescent development is significantly related to whether and to when marihuana onset occurs. Beginning to use marihuana leads to a developmental divergence from nonusers and a convergence upon the characteristics of those who are already users.
> Finally, it was shown that marihuana onset is related to the prevalence of other problem of transition-marking behaviors such as sexual intercourse experience, problem drinking, or participation in activist protest. The conclusion to be drawn is that deviance or transition proneness is not specific to a given behavior but constitutes a more general developmental notion.[57,p.297]

The last sentence of the quote is the key. Marijuana use by junior and senior high students in the 1970s *is* deviant behavior, that is, it is not the norm, the conventional. It is not surprising that marijuana use is associated with both prior deviant attitudes and behavior and a succeeding increase in other deviant behaviors. Will the coming decriminalization of marijuana make its use at the

TABLE 1-6 Risk factors related to drug use, misuse, and abuse in high school students

	Not scored	Scored
Grades	A, B, C	D, F
Religion	Yes	No
Independent use of alcohol before age 13	No	Yes
Psychological distress	Little	More
Self-esteem	High	Low
Perception of parental love	High	Low

Adapted from Bry, B.H., and others: Extent of drug use as a function of quantity of risk factors: an integrating concept. Prepublication Draft—Rutgers University, Piscataway, N.J.

high school level more of an acceptable, conventional behavior? It would certainly seem as if that would have to happen. Decriminalizing marijuana makes its use and possession less unacceptable and therefore less deviant. The developmental, long-term studies of the 1980s will probably reflect this to some extent. Remember, though, that social and/or recreational use of tobacco and alcohol and legal drugs, is not yet considered acceptable, conventional behavior for junior and senior high students. The world turns, things change, people predict—in fact, we will just have to wait and see.

One last study. If you have read, reviewed, and outlined the preceding material (as *my* students always do!) you will have a general feel for the antecedents and correlates of illegal drug use—even though they vary somewhat with the year, the population studied, the questions asked, and the geographical location. One attempt to bring it all together has been tested[58] and it seems to have some integrating value. This study focused on the *number* of risk factors as being predictive of drug use, not specific risk factors. The idea being that drug use may not be easily predicted by looking for specific psychosocial predictors but rather at how many stressors—risk factors—there are in a student's life. Although it needs to be replicated and expanded, it has been cross-checked. Of considerable importance is the finding that "no specific combinations of risk factors accounted for (extent of drug use) . . . subjects who exhibited four risk factors . . . proved to be 354% more likely to report very heavy drug use than would be expected. . . ." The risk factors and their scoring are shown in Table 1-6.

Maybe we *are* into a new era in which rebelliousness, nonconformity, and deviance hold true only for the very young drug users. Maybe the world is shifting even faster than I believe. I feel sure that future studies will show a decrease in the importance of these psychosocial factors, but the question for now is: Can drug education programs alter these patterns of drug-taking behavior?

DRUG EDUCATION

> I'm not sure education works. A lot of the programs are a little bit like telling a kid not to stick a string bean up his nose. . . .
>
> We have to motivate people to stay off drugs, especially when they're young. They've got to learn that there's no chemical solution to life.[59]

Probably everyone under the age of 30 has been exposed to some type of formal drug education. Many over 30 will have had varying amounts of information about drugs, drug use, and drug users thrust upon them—at a PTA meeting, at church, at a Kiwanis meeting. Drug education has been, is, and will continue to be everywhere. The question is—does it do any good? What do you mean by *good?* To decrease all drug use? To decrease harmful drug use? To decrease illegal drug use? To increase safe drug use? One of the reasons that educating about drugs has had so little measurable impact is that there has been ambiguity over goals. When there is no ambiguity about goals and concrete facts can be presented about harmful effects of using the drug, use decreases (Chapter 9).

Another problem is that very few drug education programs have been evaluated for effectiveness— no matter what effect is desired. Some programs, however, did include an evaluation of the effect. One study in Ann Arbor, Michigan, "found that 600 junior high school students who were exposed to a drug education program sharply increased their

experimentation with drugs."[60] That's hardly what most people had in mind, but there was a 22% to 36% increase in drug experimentation following a 10-week "fact-oriented" course on drugs. The course did increase the student's knowledge about drugs, and that probably resulted in a loss of fear about trying some drugs.

In 1981 "A Review of 127 Drug Abuse Prevention Program Evaluations,"[61] published between 1968 and 1977, yielded three relevant results: (1) "Overall, the 127 programs produced only minor effects on drug use behavior and attitudes" (p. 17), seven with negative effects, 46 with positive effects, and 74 with no effect; (2) of the 10 most intense (in terms of length and breadth) and best evaluated programs, one had a negative effect, eight had positive effects, and one had no effect. The only "information giving" program was the one with negative effects; the eight programs with positive effects used peer or process orientations and six of those eight had a positive effect only on attitudes, not on actual drug use; (3) ". . . the quality of evaluation data in primary prevention is still far from adequate for guiding policy formulation and program development" (p. 41).

In spite of government reports in the early seventies recommending the elimination of the prevention of drug use as the theme of educational programs,[62] and a national nongovernmental group concluding that drug abuse films "are doing more harm than good,"[63] the drug education business just kept rolling along.[64] Drug use and problems associated with drug use continued to rise. It seems essential that a drug education program—the same as any other education program—has to fit the age and social context of the user: "Drug taking does not go on in a vacuum, it goes on with sex experimentation, delinquency, alcohol . . . the decision to take drugs or not to take drugs is made in the context of a kid's life."[65] A White House report in the late 1970s was more oriented toward preventing personally and socially destructive drug use than toward eliminating casual experimentation and recreational use. Although the report avoided advocating the teaching of "responsible drug use," since that implies approval, the message comes through.

The best book available on drug education, which appeared in the mid 1970s, discusses all sides of the issues. Most important for us, though, is that it also reports the results of two well-designed drug education programs on students in grades 2 through 10. Much could be added to this discussion of drug education and many suggestions and precautions proposed. Two points from the book just mentioned must suffice to set the stage for the results of the study.

Drug education symbolizes the burden placed on the schools to prepare children, not simply to have skills and facts at their disposal, but to hold a given set of values and attitudes that are deemed to be in the service of their own health and adjustment and that conform to the community's view of propriety.

Drug education is one of the few interventions which society can employ which is both preventive and, on a per capita basis, cheap. Along with the family, the school is the only institution with a formative influence over children prior to the years when drugs became available to them and self-administered use begins. Education, unlike arrest or treatment, can be applied before either bad habits or bad outcomes have arisen.[66,p.2]

The study used two types of drug education programs. One was a *didactic*, or information-giving, approach, while the other was *process* oriented and involved value clarification and discussions of norm setting. A control group received no special drug education. Student self-reports on drug use were collected before the course and for the following 2 years. Two different impacts on drug use were found. Compared to the control group, students in both drug education groups were *more likely* to move to higher levels of drug use over the 2 years. That is, drug education increased drug use. In contrast to that, students in the two drug programs were *less likely* to show extreme increases in the amount and type of drug use compared to the control group. To put it another way, when control group students did increase their drug use, they were more irresponsible in their use. These two effects showed most strongly in students whose drug education occurred in the sixth grade, but the same trend was true at all grade levels.

The results of the didactic group seem clear and in line with what many people have predicted. If you give information about drugs, drug use will increase—but it will probably be safer drug use. The long-term effects will, of course, require a few years to obtain. It may be that the "controlled" drug use shown by the didactic group will persist. It may also be that what has been found in several other studies[66] will be found here: the earlier drug use starts, the longer it persists and the more intense it becomes.

Talk about a double-edged sword! No reason, though, to expect drug education to be different from other behaviors—very few things are all positive or all negative. Take care, though: just as one swallow doesn't make a summer, neither does one study make a firm conclusion. Similar studies in different areas of the country with different types of students and curricula are needed to make the preceding conclusions definite. The fact that these results fit in with other studies does, however, give this study a high level of credibility.

Of the "big three" in the socialization process—family, school, and peers—only the impact of the schools on drug abuse prevention has been well studied. The other two are coming up strong, though—a peer group program has been operating and expanding in New York City since 1977[67] and "Parent Power" is one of the themes the National Institute on Drug Abuse (NIDA) is emphasizing in its prevention programs.[68] Study of the family is probably the best direction in which to move. Research has identified the characteristics of families whose children are at low risk for drug misuse: religious involvement; traditional sex roles; love of country; emphasis on child rearing, discipline, and self-control and less allowance of freedom for children; emphasis on family togetherness and cohesion; an emphasis on, and a sense of, family tradition; some flexibility in child rearing but a basic firmness.[69,70] The ideal situation for the development of a nondrug misusing individual is to come from a solid, caring home and be exposed formally in school to accurate information about drugs and drug use.

Decisions will have to be made soon. Drug use is too frequent, too pervasive, and potentially too dangerous to let information be spread only casually. Perhaps educating for the safe and responsible use of drugs can be incorporated into the general health curriculum of the school system. It will be made clearer and clearer as you study different drugs: abstinence rarely succeeds, rehabilitation is at best marginally effective. The only choice is to teach safe drug use as well as alternatives to drug use.[71] Interestingly, parents want drug education to be given in the schools—no matter what the effect.[72]

TREATMENT AND REHABILITATION

A number of recent reports and studies indicate that despite claims for the effectiveness of particular treatment modalities or treatment programs . . . there is very little verified evidence in both the treatment of alcoholism and of drug dependence.[73]

Treatment and rehabilitation programs for users of specific drugs are discussed in the appropriate chapters. This brief section will provide an overall

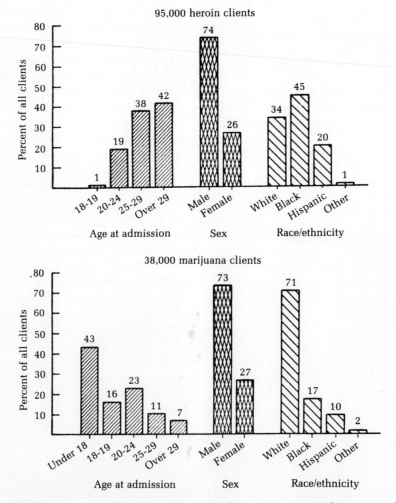

FIG. 1-3 Characteristics of individuals who entered treatment in 1979 by primary drug of concern. (From Statistical perspectives on drug abuse treatment, National Institute on Drug Abuse, Washington, D.C., 1981, U.S. Government Printing Office.)

view of the size of the drug treatment endeavor in America. Additionally, some general concerns and concepts relevant to all treatment programs are discussed.

In 1979 the United States spent $511 million to support the treatment of 235,414 individuals in 3600 treatment units; almost three fourths of these clients were in outpatient programs. Two out of three clients are in drug-free programs—the other usually being in a methadone maintenance program. Methadone is a long acting narcotic and is used only in the treatment of heroin users. Of those who enter these drug treatment programs, 80% do so voluntarily. Only about half of those entering stay for the entire treatment program. This is understandable since 55% of the entering clients had been using drugs daily and 95% had used their primary drug for over a year (70% for 3 or more

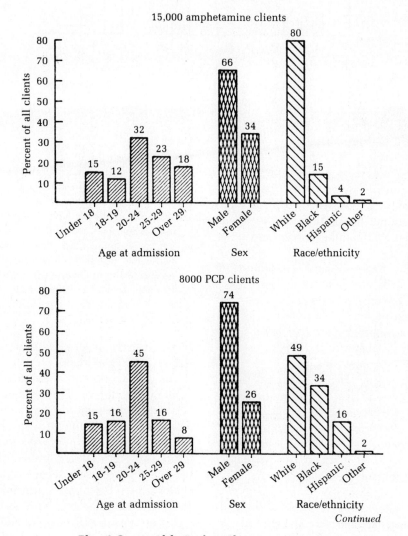

Fig. 1-3, cont'd. For legend see opposite page.

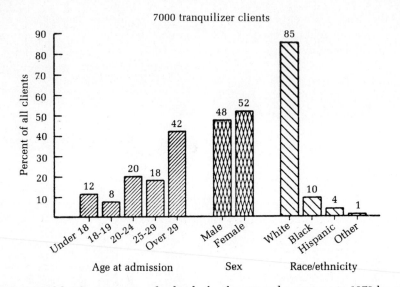

Fig. 1-3, cont'd. Characteristics of individuals who entered treatment in 1979 by primary drug of concern.

years). It is hard to give up a long-term acquaintance! Fig. 1-3 contains demographic characteristics for those entering treatment in 1979 because of problems resulting primarily from the use of heroin, marijuana, PCP, amphetamines, and minor tranquilizers.

In spite of this obviously large expenditure of time, employee skills, and money, there are serious questions about the effectiveness of any treatment and rehabilitation program. There are many reasons why treatment programs might fail to rehabilitate a drug abuser. Ignoring the very great problem of a lack of agreement on what it means to *rehabilitate* a drug user, there is still the reality problem that behavioral change techniques haven't been very successful in changing *any* type of asocial, antisocial, or personally distressing behavior.[74] It is naive to expect that a 4-week, a 4-month, or even a year's treatment program can frequently offset a life-style ingrained through 20 years of living.

Although the writer was referring to heroin addicts, the following statements are also true of most drug abusers, that is, individuals who center their lives around drugs to the extent that it causes a disruption of their interactions with others, their jobs, and/or themselves.

> Most heroin addicts have a large array of needs and inadequacies over and above their use of narcotics. (No money, no place to live, no readily marketable job skills, low frustration tolerance, low interest in or experience with the usual activities and pressures of the world . . . low motivation to solve any of these problems, and little trust in professional therapists.)[75]

In fact, treatment for many drug abusers is habilitation, not *re*habilitation.

The data support all of the points made. Unfortunately, it's all true. There are not many options, however. Since some programs help some people for some period of time, it seems best to continue while we search for new ways to solve old problems. And the problems are old. So are the basic treatment concepts, it seems. A 1970 article[76] includes a list of treatment principles published in 1804. The language is a bit archaic but the principles are the same as today. People problems don't change. Regrettably, neither do the proposed solutions.

It will become increasingly clear throughout the following chapters that solutions to the many existing drug problems do not reside only in the user. The environment and the surrounding society interact with the user's predispositions, background, and hopes. You never treat an individual in isolation—only in his sociocultural context. Even when all the social support systems are brought into play, it may not be enough. One staff member of the National Institute on Drug Abuse emphasized the importance of the individual's self-concept and competency when she said that

> the quantity of treatment research that I'm aware of indicates to me that the person being treated brings his probability of recovery with him. There's very little affected by what goes on in treatment . . . the variability in outcome is attributable more to subject variability at intake or baseline than it is to any variation in treatment or goals.[77,p.10]

ADVERSE DRUG REACTIONS

Much of the concern over the increasing use and misuse of legal and illegal drugs is related to their possible bad medical and psychological effects. No one can ever know the total number, or the frequency, of adverse drug reactions (ADR), but some indicators are available, and they provide valuable information. The Drug Abuse Warning Network (DAWN) system was established to obtain information in 24 metropolitan areas about the incidence, pattern, and trends of drug-related crises.

Reports of drug-crisis contacts are collected from over 800 hospital emergency rooms and 54 crisis centers, while 112 medical examiners (coroners) report drug-related deaths. Several factors need to be remembered about DAWN:

1. A report is made only when the user reports that his drug use is a problem requiring assistance.

2. Since no names are collected, one user may be counted more than once.

3. A user may report more than one drug (in fact, the average is about 1.6 drugs mentioned per contact).

4. No record is made of alcohol-only incidents, only of alcohol in combination with another drug.

5. The system gives a rough estimate of the pattern of drug crises *only* for the larger metropolitan areas, not for the entire United States.

There are about 175,000 drug mentions a year. This total has been fairly constant since the late 1970s. In the latest report, April 1980-March 1981 (Table 1-7), ten drug categories accounted for 44% of the drug mentions. Alcohol-in-combination and heroin/morphine mentions increased about 20% between 1978 and 1981, while diazepam mentions decreased a similar amount, and marijuana showed no change. Methaqualone mentions increased 127% and cocaine mentions increased 88% over the 3 years.

Table 1-8 gives some indication of the drugs that are related with drug abuse deaths in the larger American cities. Narcotics—heroin/morphine, methadone, propoxyphene, and codeine—are mentioned in 1 out of 4 drug-related deaths.

Some adverse drug reactions require hospitalization. One 3-year study, which excluded cases of drug abuse and suicide attempts, found that 3% of all admissions to a hospital medical unit resulted from a drug-induced illness. Of these admissions, 18% were due to legal, nonprescription drugs. Of these admitted patients, 6% died.[78]

Not all adverse drug reactions occur on the street, outside of hospitals, or in the absence of the medical profession. Drugs do so many things so well in modern medical practice that they are used with increasing frequency. There is a growing debate over whether physicians use too many drugs or use them wisely.

Several studies suggest that hospitalization has some risk. One report showed that of all the adverse events that occur on a medical ward, 62% were a result of drugs. Another study found that 36% of hospitalized medical-care patients had an adverse reaction to their treatment, and 42% of these adverse reactions were drug induced. A comprehensive survey of ten hospitals reported that 30% of hospitalized medical patients have at least one drug reaction while in the hospital.[79] Even if prescribed properly, drugs are frequently not ad-

TABLE 1-7 Most frequently mentioned drugs in the DAWN System (April 1980–March 1981)

Drug	Rank	Percent of total
Alcohol-in-combination	1	15
Diazepam	2	8
Heroin/morphine	3	5
Aspirin	4	3
Methaqualone	5	3
Marijuana	6	2
Flurazepam	7	2
Cocaine	8	2
PCP	9	2
Acetaminophen	10	2

From Statistical Series, Provisional Data, January-March 1981, Series G, Number 6, Washington, D.C., National Institute on Drug Abuse.

TABLE 1-8 Drug mentions* associated with drug abuse deaths in the DAWN system (January-December 1980)

Drug	Rank	Percent of total
Alcohol-in-combination	1	15
Heroin/morphine	2	11
Methadone	3	5
Amitriptyline	4	4
Diazepam	5	4
Propoxyphene	6	4
Codeine	7	4
Cocaine	8	3
Secobarbital	9	9
Phenobarbital	10	3

From Statistical series, Provisional Data, January-March 1981; Series G, Number 6, Washington, D.C., National Institute on Drug Abuse.
*Total mentions: 7677.

ministered in hospitals as prescribed. One survey showed that 2% of the time the wrong drug was given, in 5% the wrong dose, in 1% an extra dose, and in 4% the drug was not given at all! Overall there was a medication error in 13 of every 100 drug administrations by nurses in a hospital.[80,81] Keeping everything straight is not an easy job in the hustle and bustle of a busy ward, and the typical patient on a medical ward will receive 8 to 14 different drugs during hospitalization. Some receive none and others as many as 42! Usually older patients receive more than younger ones and females more than males.[82,83]

Drug interactions become more frequent and more severe as the use of drugs, on the street or prescribed, increases. One issue of the *Medical Letter on Drugs and Therapeutics* lists 196 "major adverse interactions that have been observed clinically."[84] The list is not exhaustive and includes only negative interactions that are frequent and severe enough to be of concern to the general practitioner.

Remember that drugs are potent chemicals selected because they have important effects on our biology. All reports confirm the adage that there are no safe drugs, only drugs used safely. Never forget, however, that the use of drugs which cause adverse reactions in a few have had therapeutic effects on many.

Some authorities[85,86] argue convincingly that many patients with emotional problems are undermedicated. This is even true with some drugs in medical patients. One study showed that 70% of hospitalized patients with pain received inadequate levels of a narcotic analgesic, usually because the physician "exaggerated the dangers of addiction. . . ."[87] The authors lament "undertreatment with narcotic analgesics, causing much needless suffering on medical inpatients."[87]

CONCLUDING COMMENT

The focus in this chapter has been on the general factors in our cultural and scientific history that have made us what we are today—a nation of drug users. Throughout the remainder of this book that fact will be documented, and there will be an attempt to illustrate similar patterns of behavior in other times and with other drugs. It is not that our present condition is just another repeat performance of what has happened before—it isn't. There are important differences this time in the kinds of drugs, the potency of the drugs, and the way the drugs are taken. Drug use today is having more influence on the entire society than ever before. A historical approach is not a search for answers in the past to present problems. Rather it is to gain a full understanding of the present problem so that effective solutions can be found. Winston Churchill said it best:

> The farther backward you can look, the farther forward you are likely to see.

REFERENCES

1. Handler, P.: Public doubts about science, Science **208**(4448):1093, 1980.
2. Lyons, R.D.: Refusal of many to heed government health advice is linked to growing distrust of authority, New York Times, June 12, 1977, p. 55.
3. Lees, H.: Farewell to benzedrine benders, Collier's **124**:32, 1949.
4. Huxley, A.: Brave new world, London, 1932, Chatto, Chatto, & Windus.
5. Mandell, A.J.: Neurobiological barriers to euphoria, American Scientist **61**:565-573, 1973.
6. Gattozzi, A.: Drugs and patients: evaluating chemicals that change human behavior. In Mental Health Reports 2, Public Health Service Publication No. 1743, Washington, D.C., 1968, U.S. Government Printing Office.
7. Klerman, G.L.: Drugs and social values, International Journal of Addictions **5**:313-321, 1970.
8. McGaugh, J.L.: Drug facilitation of memory and learning. In Efron, D., editor: Psychopharmacology: a review of progress 1957-1967, Public Health Service Publication No. 1968, Washington, D.C., 1968, U.S. Government Printing Office.
9. Evans, W., and Kline, N., editors: Psychotropic drugs in the year 2000: use by normal humans, New York, 1971, McGraw-Hill Book Co.
10. Reich, C.A.: Reflections (the greening of America), The New Yorker **46**:42-46, September 26, 1970.
11. Ruesch, J.: Technological civilization and human affairs, Journal of Nervous and Mental Disease **145**:193-205, 1967.
12. Rosayk, T.: The making of a counter culture, Garden City, N.Y., 1969, Anchor Books.
13. Schaar, J.H., and Wolin, S.S.: Education and the technological society, New York Review, p. 3, October 9, 1969. Reprinted with permission from the New York Review of Books.
14. King, S.H.: Youth in rebellion: an historical perspective, Drug Dependence **2**:5-9, 1969.
15. Yeats, W.B.: The land of heart's desire. In Buckley, J.H., and Woods, G.B., editors: Poetry of the Victorian period, ed. 3, Glenview, Ill., 1965, Scott, Foresman & Co.
16. Clymer, A.: Poll indicates turn toward optimism on nation's future, New York Times, July 1, 1981, p. A1.
17. Conservatism is found in top teen students, New York Times, December 3, 1981, p. C11.
18. Reinhold, R.: Leveling off of drug use found among students, New York Times, February 19, 1981, p. A1.
19. Quindlen, A.: Teen-agers call illicit drugs one of life's commonplaces, New York Times, July 19, 1981, p. 1.
20. Sullivan, R.: Surveys find youths regard illicit drugs as harmful, New York Times, July 20, 1981, p. B2.
21. Teen-age drug use declining, Congress told, American Medical News, p. 37, August 14, 1981.
22. Messolonghites, L.: Multicultural perspectives on drug abuse and its prevention, a resource book, DHEW Publication No. (ADM)78-671, Washington, D.C., 1979, U.S. Government Printing Office.
23. Spanier, G.B.: The changing profile of the American family, Journal of Family Practice **13**(1):61-69, 1981.
24. Dugan, G.: "Religious revival" forecast by Gallup, New York Times, June 19, 1977, p. L30.
25. Suchman, E.A.: The "hang-loose" ethic and the spirit of drug use, Journal of Health and Social Behavior **9**:146-155, 1968.
26. Maeroff, G.I.: The liberal arts degree and its real value, New York Times, June 12, 1977, p. E9.
27. White, D.: The challenge of change. In Biomedical communications: problems and resources, Annals of the New York Academy of Sciences **142**:405-414, 1967.
28. Nichols, J.R.: Addiction liability of albino rats: breeding for quantitative differences in morphine drinking, Science **157**:561-563, 1967.
29. Segovia-Riquelme, N., and others: Nutritional and genetic factors in the appetite for alcohol. In Popham, R.E., editor: Alcohol and alcoholism, Toronto, 1970, University of Toronto Press.
30. Goodwin, D.W., and others: Alcohol problems in adoptees raised apart from alcoholic biological parents, Archives of General Psychiatry **28**:238-243, 1973.
31. Science academy panel sees possible common factors in habitual behaviors, Washington Drug Review **2**(4):8-10, 1977.
32. Smith, H.: Do drugs have religious import? In Solomon, D., editor: LSD: the consciousness-expanding drug, New York, 1964, G.P. Putnam's Sons.
33. Larkin, J.K., and Wertheimer, A.I.: Old drugs at home (letter to the editor), New England Journal of Medicine **298**(15):857, 1978.
34. Mellinger, G.D., and Balter, M.B.: Prevalence and patterns of use of psychotherapeutic drugs: results from a 1979 national survey of American adults. In Epidemiological impact of psychotropic drugs: proceedings of International Seminar on Epidemiological Impact of Psychotropic Drugs, Milan, Italy, June 24-26, 1981, Amsterdam, 1981, Elsevier/North-Holland Biomedical Press.

35. Johnston, L.D., and others: Highlights from student drug use in America 1975-1980, DHHS Publication No. (ADM) 81-1006, Washington, D.C., 1980, U.S. Government Printing Office.

36. Drug abuse prevention, treatment, and rehabilitation in fiscal year 1980, Third Annual Report from the Secretary of DHHS to the President and Congress of the United States, Washington, D.C., 1981, U.S. Government Printing Office.

37. Demographic trends and drug abuse, 1980-1995, DHHS Publication No. (ADM)81-1069, Washington, D.C., 1981, U.S. Government Printing Office.

38. Kandel, D., Single, E., and Kessler, R.C.: The epidemiology of drug use among New York state high school students: distribution, trends, and changes in rates of use, American Journal of Public Health 66(1):43-53, 1976.

39. Carroll, L.: Alice in Wonderland, London, 1865, The Macmillan Co.

40. Carstairs, G.M.: A land of lotus-eaters? American Journal of Psychiatry 125:1576-1580, 1969.

41. Kandel, D.B., Treiman, D., Faust, R., and Singler, E.: Adolescent involvement in legal and illegal drug use: a multiple classification analysis, Social Forces 55(2):438-458, 1976.

42. Williams, H.: Progressive drug involvement: marihuana use among Nicaraguan private secondary school students, unpublished dissertation, Department of Sociology, Vanderbilt University, Nashville, Tenn., 1977.

43. Jessor, R., and Jessor, S.: Theory testing in longitudinal research. Presented at the Conference on Strategies of Longitudinal Research in Drug Use, San Juan, Puerto Rico, April 1976.

44. Jessor, R., Jessor, S., and Finney, J.: A social psychology of marijuana use: longitudinal studies of high school and college youth, Journal of Personality and Social Psychology 26:1-15, 1973.

45. Kandel, D.B.: Convergences in prospective longitudinal surveys of drug use in normal populations. Presented at the Society for Life History Research in Psychopathology, Fort Worth, Tex., October 1976.

46. Kaufman, E.: The abuse of multiple drugs. II. Psychological hypotheses, treatment considerations, American Journal of Drug and Alcohol Abuse 3(2):293-301, 1976.

47. Burt, M.R., and others: Psychosocial characteristics of drug-abusing women, DHEW Publication No. (ADM) 80-917, Washington, D.C., U.S. Government Printing Office.

48. Suchman, E.A.: The "hang-loose" ethic and the spirit of drug use, Journal of Health and Social Behavior 9:146-155, 1968.

49. Scarpitti, F.R., and Datesman, S.K., editors: Drugs and the youth culture, SAGE Annual Reviews of Drug and Alcohol Abuse, vol. 4, Beverly Hills, June, 1980, SAGE Publications.

50. Braucht, G.N., and others: Deviant drug use in adolescence: a review of psychosocial correlates, Psychological Bulletin 79(2):92-106, 1973.

51. Gorsuch, R., and Butler, M.: Initial drug abuse: a review of predisposing social psychological factors, Psychological Bulletin 83(1):120-137, 1976.

52. Kandel, D.: Adolescent marihuana use: role of parents and peers, Science 181:1067-1069, 1973.

53. Kandel, D., and Faust, R.: Sequence and stages in patterns of adolescent drug use, Archives of General Psychiatry 32:923-932, 1975.

54. Jessop, D., Kandel, D., and Lukoff, I.: Comparative analyses of stages of drug use in different ethnic groups: center cross study I. Mimeographed, Bedfort Stuyvesant and New York State Center for Socio-Cultural Research on Drug Use, June, 1976, New York, Columbia University.

55. Hamburg, B.H., Kraemer, H.C., and Jahnke, W.: A hierarchy of drug use in adolescence: behavioral and attitudinal correlates of substantial drug use, American Journal of Psychiatry 132(11):1155-1163, 1975. Copyright 1975, the American Psychiatric Association. Reprinted by permission.

56. Smith, G.M., and Fogg, C.P.: Teenage drug use: a search for causes and consequences. In Lettieri, D.J., editor: Predicting adolescent drug abuse: a review of issues, methods and correlates, Washington, D.C., December, 1975, U.S. Government Printing Office.

57. Jessor, R.: Predicting time of onset of marihuana use: a developmental study of high school youth. In Lettieri, D.J., editor: Predicting adolescent drug abuse: a review of issues, methods and correlates, Washington, D.C., December, 1975, U.S. Government Printing Office.

58. Bry, B.H., and others: Extent of drug use as a function of quantity of risk factors: an integrating concept. Prepublication draft, Rutgers University, Piscataway, N.J.

59. How U.S. is smashing "hard drug" rings: interview with John R. Bartels, Jr., Administrator of Drug Enforcement, Department of Justice, U.S. News and World Report, pp. 38-41, April 1, 1974.

60. Drug education is linked to use, New York Times, December 3, 1972.

61. Schaps, E., and others: a review of 127 drug abuse prevention program evaluations, Journal of Drug Issues 11(1):17, Winter 1981.

62. New federal regulations tightening confidentiality of drug patient information outlined by drug office, Drugs and Drug Abuse Education Newsletter 3(11):1,7-9, 1972.

63. Drug-abuse films termed harmful, New York Times, December 13, 1972.

64. Dobin, E.I.: Who cares about drug abuse, Apothecary, p. 20, July-August 1981.

65. Grafton, S.: The view from Washington (editorial), Addiction and Drug Abuse Reports 8(5):2, 1977.

66. Blum, R.H., Blum, E., and Garfield, E.: Drug education: results and recommendations, Lexington, Mass., 1976, D.C. Heath & Co.

67. Grafton, S., editor: How to use peer pressure constructively, Addiction and Substance Abuse Report 12(2):1-4, 1981.

68. Celebrating: parent power in Georgia, Prevention Resources, NIDA, 11(3,4):1, Winter, 1981, DHEW Publication No. (ADM) 79-827.
69. Gray, B., editor: Drug abuse from the family perspective: coping is a family affair, DHHS Publication No. (ADM) 80-910, Washington, D.C., 1980, U.S. Government Printing Office.
70. Glynn, T., editor: Drugs and the family, DHHS Publication No. (ADM) 81-1151, Washington, D.C., 1981, U.S. Government Printing Office.
71. Messolonghites, L., editor: Alternative pursuits for America's 3rd century, National Institute on Drug Abuse, Washington, D.C., 1974, U.S. Government Printing Office.
72. Children's drug use: educational and other correlates, Program in Drugs, Crime and Community Studies, Stanford, Calif., 1977, Stanford University.
73. Babow, I.: The treatment monopoly in alcoholism and drug dependence: a sociological critique, Journal of Drug Issues 5(2):120-128, 1975.
74. Ulrich, R., Stachnik, J., and Mabry, J., editors: Control of human behavior, vol. 2, Glenview, Ill., 1970, Scott, Foresman & Co.
75. Bewley, T.H.: Drug dependence in the U.S.A., U.N. Bulletin on Narcotics 21(2), 1969.
76. Edwards, G.: Place of treatment professions in society's response to chemical abuse, British Medical Journal 2:195-199, 1970.
77. Rittenhouse, J.D.: Selected themes of discussion. In Rittenhouse, J.D., editor: The epidemiology of heroin and other narcotics, Menlo Park, Calif., 1976, Stanford Research Institute.
78. Caranasos, G.J., Stewart, R.B., and Cluff, L.E.: Drug-induced illness leading to hospitalization, Journal of the American Medical Association 228(6):713-717, 1974.
79. Linkewich, J.A.: Adverse reaction reviews (ARR), Hospital Pharmacy 6:549, October 1981.
80. Study of health facilities construction costs, Report to the Congress by the Comptroller General of the United States, 1975.
81. Shaw, J.: Medication errors a 'great hidden problem,' American Medical News, p. 19-21, January 1-8, 1982.
82. Smith, J.W., Seidl, L.G., and Cluff, L.E.: Studies on the epidemiology of adverse drug reactions. V. Clinical factors influencing susceptibility, Annals of Internal Medicine 65:629-640, 1966.
83. Seidl, L.G., and others: Studies on the epidemiology of adverse drug reactions. III. Reactions in patients on a general medical service, Bulletin Johns Hopkins Hospital 119:299-315, 1966.
84. Abramowicz, M., editor: Adverse interactions of drugs, Medical Letter on Drugs and Therapeutics 19(2):5-12, 1977.
85. Kline, N.S.: The under-medicated patient, American Druggist, pp. 29-30, January 24, 1972.
86. Balter, M., and Levine, J.: Character and extent of psychotherapeutic drug usage in the United States. Presented at the Fifth World Congress on Psychiatry, Mexico City, November 30, 1971.
87. Marks, R.M., and Sachar, E.J.: Undertreatment of medical inpatients with narcotic analgesics, Annals of Internal Medicine 78:173-181, 1973.

CHAPTER 2

REGULATION OF NARCOTIC AND DANGEROUS DRUGS

ONCE UPON A TIME there weren't any regulations about drug use—at least there weren't any federal government regulations. That lasted for about 2 years. In 1791 Congress passed an excise tax on whiskey, which resulted in a disagreement that historians call the Whiskey Rebellion. West of the Appalachian Mountains, where most whiskey was made, the farmers refused to pay the tax and tarred and feathered revenue officers who tried to collect it. In 1794 President George Washington called in the militia, and they occupied counties in western Pennsylvania and sent prisoners to Philadelphia for trial. The militia and the federal government carried the day. The Whiskey Rebellion was an important test for the new government because it established clearly that the federal government had the power to enforce federal laws within a state.

Regulations are imposed either to bring money into the government, for the public good, or both. As the story of the laws and regulations about drugs and drug use unfolds and the number of laws and regulations increases, it will become clear that most of the debate centers on the question: What is the public good? Issues of fact, morality, health, personal choice, and social order are intertwined—and sometimes confused. In a democratic society the debate is usually open, but not necessarily rational. It should surprise no one that our laws about drug use are a patch-quilt that reflects the many different social changes and points of view this country encompasses.

In the United States, drug addiction became a major problem after the Civil War. There were three factors contributing to widespread narcotic addiction in the last third of the nineteenth century. One was the invention of the hypodermic syringe in 1853. Although Sir Christopher Wren as early as 1656 had injected through the skin, the procedure was quite crude and involved first making a slit in the skin with a knife and then using a dull quill.

The hypodermic syringe was introduced to the United States in 1856 and used on a large scale in the Civil War. Injecting morphine, the primary active ingredient in opium, gave near-immediate relief from pain. Morphine was used widely, and not always wisely, in the treatment of the two major afflictions in the Civil War—pain and dysentery. So many soldiers became addicted to morphine because of imprudent medical use that addiction was called the "soldier's disease" or the "army disease" in the years following the war.

The second development that contributed to narcotic addiction after the War Between the States was the importation of Chinese workers to help build the rapidly expanding railroads. The Chinese brought with them the habit of smoking opium. As always happens when a new pleasure is introduced into a society, the practice of opium smoking spread rapidly. A contemporary report in 1882 outlined the spread of opium smoking in San Francisco.

> The practice spread rapidly and quietly among this class of gamblers and prostitutes until the latter part of 1875, at which time the authorities became cognizant of the fact, and finding . . . that many women and young girls, as also young men of respectable family, were being induced to visit the dens, where they were ruined morally and otherwise, a city ordinance was passed forbidding the practice under penalty of a heavy fine or imprisonment, or both. Many arrests were made, and the punishment was prompt and thorough.[1,p.1]

This San Francisco act was the first ordinance in America forbidding opium smoking. In 1882 New York State passed a similar law aimed at opium use in New York City's expanding Chinatown.

The broadest impact on narcotic use in this country came from neither of these factors but instead from the widespread legal distribution of patent medicines. Patent medicines were dispensed by traveling peddlers and were readily available at local stores for self-medication. Sales of patent medicines increased from $3.5 million in 1859 to $74 million in 1904. The names of those well-advertised cure-alls are no longer familiar—for example, Dr. Pierce's Golden Medical Discovery and Mrs. Winslow's Soothing Syrup—but some of the general names for agents popular then are still in use. Paregoric (a Greek word meaning soothing) is an elixir containing 4 milligrams (mg) of opium per milliliter (ml) and is 44% alcohol; it was made a prescription drug only in June, 1972. Laudanum, which has had many formulas and dates from about the year 1500, is the miracle drug every doctor uses in western movies. It contains 100 mg of opium per milliliter and is about 20% alcohol.

As a result of these three factors—the hypodermic syringe, Chinese workers, and patent medicines—by the turn of the present century it was estimated that one individual out of every 500 in the United States was physically dependent on some form of opium or its derivatives.

EARLY REGULATIONS

Although alcohol had been taxed (and thus controlled) since the early years of the republic, opium was not taxed until 1842. The tax levied against crude opium brought into this country for medical purposes fluctuated considerably up to about 1900. In the 1850s it became clear that most of the opium being imported was not for medical purposes but for smoking. In 1864 smoking opium was identified for the first time as containing less than 9% morphine and was taxed separately. By 1890 the tax on smoking opium had increased to $12.00 a pound and the amount brought through customs decreased. When the tax was lowered in 1897, the amount of legally imported smoking opium increased again. Through all these tax changes the amount of smoking opium actually brought into this country gradually increased. When import taxes were low, a large percentage of smoking opium entered legally. As taxes increased it became worthwhile to smuggle opium, and the amount entering legally decreased. The 1890 act also, for the first time, permitted only American citizens to manufacture smoking opium.

Within the boundaries of the United States there was increasing conflict between the steady progress of medical science and the therapeutic claims of the patent medicine hucksters. The alcohol and/or narcotic content of the patent medicines was also a matter of concern. One medicine, Hostetter's Bitters, was 44% alcohol while another, Birney's Catarrh Cure, was 4% cocaine. In October, 1905, *Collier's* magazine culminated a prolonged attack on patent medicines with a well-documented, aggressive series, entitled "The Great American Fraud."[2]

Responding to pressure from scientists and physicians, President Theodore Roosevelt recommended in 1905 ". . . that a law be enacted to regulate interstate commerce in misbranded and adulterated foods, drinks, and drugs."[3] The 1906 publication of Upton Sinclair's *The Jungle*, exposing the horribly unsanitary conditions in the meat packing industry, shocked Congress and America. It was the necessary straw that 5 months later, on the thirtieth of June, 1906, led to the passage of the Pure Food and Drugs Act, which prohibited the interstate commerce of adulterated or misbranded foods and drugs.

In defining the word "drug," the act referred to those compounds listed in *The United States Pharmacopeia* (USP) and *The National Formulary* (NF) and designated their drug standards as the legal basis for enforcing the law on adulteration. *The United States Pharmacopeia*, started in 1820, and *The National Formulary*, begun in 1888, were continually revised, nongovernmental compilations of the best available drugs. (The two organizations combined in 1975 under *The United States Pharmacopeia* name.) They also listed established names and minimum standards for the listed drugs and their dosage forms. Beginning with the 1906 law, if a product used one of the USP or NF names, it had to contain the ingredients listed in the USP or NF, and no listing of the ingredients was required on the label. If a medicine failed to meet these standards, the label had to clearly indicate what the product did contain.

It was the 1906 act that began the decline of patent medicines because, in the section on misbranding, the act specifically referred to alcohol, morphine, opium, cocaine, heroin, *Cannabis indica* (marijuana), and several other agents. Each package was required to state how much (or what proportion) of these drugs was included in the preparation. This meant, for example, that the widely sold "cures" for morphine addiction had to indicate that they in fact contained another addicting drug.[4]

The 1906 Food and Drug Act did not regulate imports of addicting drugs. That remained for the Opium Exclusion Act of 1909 to do. This 1909 act prohibited the importing of opium or its derivatives except for medical purposes and was regulated by the Secretary of the Treasury. The act made it illegal only to import opium for nonmedical use; it was not illegal to use or manufacture opium for nonmedical purposes. Until the Opium Poppy Control Act of 1942 there was no basis for controlling cultivation of the opium poppy in the United States. This act required that opium poppy growers be licensed by the Secretary of the Treasury.

NARCOTIC RULES AND REGULATIONS, 1914 TO 1970

The basic narcotic control law in the United States until May of 1971 was the Harrison Act of 1914. In 1914 for the first time dealers and dispensers of narcotics (opium, cocaine, and their derivatives) had to register annually with the Treasury Department's Bureau of Internal Revenue, which was also charged with enforcement of the law. Physicians, dentists, and veterinary surgeons were named as potential lawful distributors if they registered. This was not a punitive act, penalties for violation were not severe, and the measure contained no reference to users of narcotics. The Harrison Act specifically supported the continued legality of the 1906 and 1909 laws and was primarily aimed at regulation and control of the narcotic drug traffic. In 1914 it was estimated that about 200,000 Americans—one in 400—were addicted to opium or its derivatives. The Harrison Act was the first step toward making it impossible for addicts to obtain their drugs legally. The result was the development of an illicit drug trade that charged users up to 50 times more than the legal retail drug price.

Two decisions in this period by the United States Supreme Court were important in making it more difficult for the addict to obtain drugs legally. In the Webb case, decided in 1919, the court declared that it was not legal for a physician to prescribe narcotic drugs to an addict for the purpose of maintaining his use and comfort. That is, narcotics could not be administered just to keep the user from developing withdrawal symptoms.[5] The 1922 Behrman case went one step further, declaring that a narcotic prescription for an addict was not legal even if the narcotic drugs were prescribed as part of a cure program.[6] In brief, these two Supreme Court decisions said there was no legal way for an addict to continue his habit at any level. The addict was forced to look for his drugs in the illegal market.

Partly in response to this growing illicit market,

Congress passed the Jones-Miller Act of 1922, which more than doubled the maximum penalites for dealing with illegally imported narcotics to $5,000 and 10 years' imprisonment. This act limited imports to *crude* opium and coca leaves for medical purposes and established the Federal Narcotics Control Board to initiate an active program against smugglers. Included also was the stipulation that the mere possession of illegally obtained narcotics was sufficient basis for conviction. In 1924 another act prohibited importing opium for the manufacture of heroin. (It should be mentioned that as a result of this law and an early amendment, it is illegal to possess heroin in the United States except for research purposes. Any heroin supply has thus been clearly obtained illegally.) In 1925 the Supreme Court reversed itself. In the Linder case it declared addiction an illness and said it was legal for a physician to prescribe narcotics for an addict if it was part of a curing program (that is, elimination of the addiction).[7]

Around 1930 several changes with lasting impact were made in the American handling of illegal narcotic use. Narcotic addiction in this period became a major problem for federal prisons. In 1928 individuals sentenced for narcotic drug–law offenses made up one third of the total prison population. Interestingly, since this was during prohibition, this was twice as many individuals as those imprisoned for liquor-law violations.[8] Responding to pressure for action, Congress established two narcotic farms in 1929 for the treatment of persons addicted to habit-forming drugs who had been convicted of breaking a federal law. Included among the habit-forming drugs, in addition to opium and its derivatives, were Indian hemp (marijuana) and peyote (of which mescaline is one active agent). A social definition of an addict was used in this Revenue Act of May 29, 1928:

> Any person who habitually uses any habit-forming narcotic drug as defined in this chapter (of this Act) so as to endanger the public morals, health, safety, or welfare, or who has been so far addicted to the use of such habit-forming narcotic drug as to have lost the power of self-control with reference to his addiction.

The farm in Lexington, Kentucky opened in 1935 and generally held about 1000 patients, two thirds of whom were prisoners. Although it was a Public Health Service Hospital, with an internationally famous narcotic research facility, the Lexington farm was primarily a prison. In 1967 the National Institute of Mental Health took over the hospital and developed a modern rehabilitation program. In February, 1974, the treatment units (but not the research facility) became part of the Bureau of Prisons to be used for federal prisoners with a history of drug abuse.[9]

In 1930 Congress took several actions that culminated in the formation of a separate Bureau of Narcotics in the Treasury Department. This bureau assumed all the duties that had previously been the responsibility of the Federal Narcotics Control Board and continued in operation until April, 1968, when it became part of a new group, the Bureau of Narcotics and Dangerous Drugs in the Department of Justice.

The Commissioner of Narcotics, the head of the Bureau of Narcotics, was appointed by the president. Harry Anslinger was the first commissioner and he remained in that position until 1962 when he retired. Mr. Anslinger had a background in foreign service and was regularly reappointed by new presidents just as was FBI Director, J. Edgar Hoover. As Hoover had great impact on federal criminal and espionage laws, Anslinger became a personality, nationally and internationally, who exerted considerable influence on nonmedical drug legislation for the period of his tenure. He was tough-minded in the area of drug use and early in his career led the fight that resulted in the passage of the Marijuana Tax Act of 1937. In 1956 Anslinger was one of the individuals responsible for the passage of the Narcotic Drug Control Act, which included the death penalty for anyone selling heroin to a person under 18. He commented on that particular provision by saying, "I'd like to throw the switch myself on drug peddlers who sell their poisons to minors."[10]

These laws, which were concerned with regulating the importation and manufacturing of drugs, were primarily aimed at the opiates and cocaine. In the 1930s another drug problem began to occupy the public eye—marijuana. Marijuana had been smoked in this country for many years and caused little excitement, but in the early 1930s its use increased and spread widely throughout the southwest and south central states. Originally carried into the United States by Mexican laborers, marijuana became common among the lower socioeconomic groups, and newspapers and police began to associate its use with crime. In the mid-1930s the use of marijuana moved to the eastern seaboard and up the Mississippi River. Supported by Anslinger, the police, and newspapers, public outcry reached such a level that in 1937 Congress passed the Marijuana Tax Act. By requiring payment of a tax on all marijuana transactions, it was hoped to regulate (that is, eliminate) the importation and use of marijuana. But, as was true with narcotic control laws, the law failed to be effective. In 1969 the Supreme court declared punishment for nonpayment of the tax unconstitutional. Marijuana was still controlled by the narcotic laws and was legally considered to be a narcotic until May, 1971.

World War II caused a decrease in the importation of both legal and illegal drugs. With the end of World War II and the resumption of easy international travel, the illegal narcotic trade resumed and increased in volume every year. In 1951 Congress passed the Boggs Amendment to the Harrison Act, which ushered in a hard-line attitude toward illegal drug use including marijuana. This amendment established minimum mandatory sentences for all narcotic and marijuana offenses. It also prohibited suspended sentences and probation for second offenses.

This more stringent enforcement attitude continued and was reflected in a report by a subcommittee of the Senate Judiciary Committee in 1955.[11] The subcommittee stated that drug addiction was responsible for 50% of crime in urban areas and 25% of all reported crimes and found drug addiction to be one of the ways Communist China planned to demoralize the United States. With this background it is easy to understand that the 1956 Narcotic Drug Control Act raised the mandatory minimum sentence for conviction of a violation of the narcotic laws. More importantly, this act prohibited

suspended sentences, probation, or parole for all narcotic offenses *except* a first conviction for possession. Under this law a convicted seller or distributor of illegal narcotics had to be jailed. In most federal cases an individual who possessed a "large amount" of narcotics or marijuana was presumed to be a seller and was treated as such.

It must be remembered that according to the Harrison Act and other federal narcotic laws it is not a crime to be an addict. Neither is the fact that someone is an addict with no legal source of narcotics adequate evidence for prosecution and conviction under federal laws. Several states did make addiction a crime, however, and instituted action to charge addicts under these laws and sometimes place them in treatment programs. In the 1962 Robinson case, in which an addict appealed his conviction, the Supreme Court declared it unconstitutional to call addiction a crime.

Partly in response to the developing World Health Organization program that was responsible for monitoring world production and medical needs of the opiates and partly to tighten internal controls on legal narcotics, the Narcotics Manufacturing Act was passed in 1960. This act licensed all medical narcotic drug manufacturers and made it illegal to manufacture or attempt to manufacture narcotic drugs unless registered. In addition annual quotas were established for the purchase and manufacture of these drugs.

To further increase controls the Bureau of Narcotics, in 1962, set up a four-part system for classifying drugs containing narcotics. Controls were tightened further in 1969, but this system was eliminated in the 1970 law when both narcotics and dangerous drugs were combined in a single five-part classification.

DRUG ABUSE CONTROL AMENDMENTS OF 1965

The early 1960s saw not only an increase in illegal drug use but also a shift in the type of drug being used illegally. The trend was for the new drug users to be better educated and to emphasize primarily drugs that alter mood and consciousness. In this period some university hospitals in large cities reported that up to 15% of their emergency room calls involved individuals with adverse reactions from illegal drugs. Responding to the need for better controls over the manufacturing and distribution of certain legal and illegal compounds (the so-called dangerous drugs), Congress passed the Drug Abuse Control Amendments of 1965.

These laws excluded narcotics and marijuana and brought three new classes of drugs under federal control.[12] The act specifically names the barbiturates and the amphetamines as being controlled and further states that derivatives of these drugs can be designated as controlled by the Secretary of Health, Education, and Welfare. The third group of compounds was broader and included any drug that the Secretary of HEW named as having *a potential for abuse because of its stimulant or depressant or hallucinogenic effects*.

In determining whether a drug is hallucinogenic, the FDA was to consider whether it causes hallucinations, illusions, delusions, or an alteration in:

1. Orientation with respect to time or place
2. Consciousness, as evidenced by confused states, dream-like revivals of past traumatic events, or childhood memories
3. Sensory perception, as evidenced by visual illusions, synesthesia, distortion of space and perspective
4. Motor coordination
5. Mood and affectivity, as evidenced by anxiety, euphoria, hypomania, ecstasy, autistic withdrawal
6. Ideation, as evidenced by flight of ideas, ideas of reference, impairment of concentration and intelligence
7. Personality, as evidenced by depersonalization and derealization, impairment of conscience and of acquired social and cultural customs[13]

It should be noted that through this act the FDA also brought under control the two chemicals lysergic acid and lysergic acid amide. These compounds are starting points for the manufacture of LSD and, beginning in 1964, methods of producing LSD from these compounds had been published in the underground press.

In the initial regulations implementing the 1965

amendments, the Native American Church, a religious organization of Indians of the Southwest, was exempted from certain parts of the act dealing with hallucinogens. The peyote cactus, which contains mescaline, a hallucinogen, is used in their religious ceremonies and has been for many years. This exemption was readily given because earlier California had restricted the use of peyote and in 1962 and 1963 had convicted members of the Native American Church for violation of the state law. The American Civil Liberties Union appealed the conviction on the grounds that it violated religious freedom. In 1964 the Supreme Court of California reversed the conviction on the basis that peyote was a major part of their religious ceremonies and a cornerstone of their religion.

The 1964 decision was not a blanket statement that any drug used in religious ceremonies would be exempt from regulation. In a 1967 court decision involving Dr. Timothy Leary, earlier judicial decisions in this country were cited in which it was clear that certain religious acts could be controlled if they posed a threat to public safety. In the Leary case the court decided that the use of hallucinogens constituted a threat to society and that marijuana was not essential to the practice of Hinduism![14]

COMPREHENSIVE DRUG ABUSE PREVENTION AND CONTROL ACT OF 1970

One of the last bills the Senate and the House of Representatives approved before adjourning for the 1970 election recess was H.R. 18583, the *Comprehensive Drug Abuse Prevention and Control Act of 1970*, signed on October 27, 1970, by President Richard M. Nixon. When first proposed the drug legislation was liberal and emphasized education, research, and rehabilitation. This was applauded by biomedical scientists, but the members of Congress, responding to the concerns of the nation's citizens, wanted to emphasize law and order.

The law became effective on the first of May, 1971, and since it is the present law of the land some of the provisions will be presented in detail. As is always true, the administrative regulations established to carry out the provisions of the act and the court decisions regarding the law have considerable influence on the actual implementation of the 1970 Drug Abuse Law. Appreciate also that laws are regularly amended.

The Comprehensive Drug Abuse Prevention and Control Act of 1970, usually referred to as *The Controlled Substance Act of 1970*, almost lives up to its title. It is comprehensive, since it repeals and replaces or updates all previous laws concerned with both the narcotic and dangerous drugs. The law specifically states that the drugs controlled by the act are under federal jurisdiction regardless of involvement in interstate commerce. The law does not eliminate state regulations; it just makes clear that federal enforcement and prosecution is possible in any illegal activity involving the controlled drugs.

The law dealt with prevention and treatment of drug abuse by appropriating funds for expanding the role of Community Mental Health Centers and Public Health Service Hospitals in the treatment of those who misuse drugs. It authorized the development of educational material and drug education workshops for professional workers as well as for the public schools.

The special status of marijuana and marijuana users is evident throughout the law. Of particular note is the fact that the law established a *Commission on Marijuana and Drug Abuse*. The Commission was instructed to complete a comprehensive summary on the medical, legal, and sociocultural aspects of marijuana and marijuana use and to submit a final report with "recommendations for legislative and administrative actions" within 2 years. The first report arrived in March, 1973, and was praised for its comprehensiveness.[15] (Perhaps it was a little too comprehensive, since one of the recommendations was the decriminalization of marijuana. There have been yearly reports since 1973, and they have ranged beyond marijuana.)

The control aspects of the bill were the most debated portions, and several basic philosophical, ethical, and legal issues are resolved (!) by the law. First is that this is a law to control drugs directly rather than through excise taxes. Enforcement authority was moved to the Department of Justice

from the Treasury Department. A second major issue is the separation of enforcement of the law from the scientific evaluation of the drugs considered for control. The Attorney General is responsible for the administration of the control aspects of the law, but the Secretary of Health and Human Services (HHS) now makes the final decision on which drugs should be controlled.[16] This separation of enforcement from the scientific and medical decision of what should be controlled was a major victory for those arguing for a sane drug law.

The Secretary of HHS has delegated to the Food and Drug Administration primary responsibility in determing whether a drug should be controlled. The FDA must consider the following factors:

1. Scientific evidence of its pharmacological effect, if known
2. The state of current scientific knowledge regarding the drug or other substance
3. What, if any, risk there is to the public health
4. Its psychic or physiological dependence liability
5. Whether the substance is an immediate precursor of a substance already controlled under this title

After specifically excluding "distilled spirits, wine, malt beverages, or tobacco" the law established five schedules of drugs that must be updated and published regularly. Table 2-1 summarizes the characteristics and penalties for illegally selling drugs in each of the five schedules. Remember that many prescription drugs are not included in these schedules, usually because they are not psychoactive—for example, antibiotics.

Several different aspects of control are contained in this law. This law reformulated some of the restrictions on drug prescriptions found in earlier acts. No prescription for a Schedule II compound can be refilled, but in an emergency a Schedule II drug can be dispensed on an oral prescription. Prescriptions for substances in Schedules III, IV, and V cannot be refilled more than five times and not at all more than 6 months after written. The label of a drug in Schedule II, III, or IV must contain this warning: CAUTION: FEDERAL LAW PROHIBITS THE TRANSFER OF THIS DRUG TO ANY PERSON OTHER THAN THE PATIENT FOR WHOM IT WAS PRESCRIBED.

TABLE 2-1 Summary of drug schedules and penalties for violation of the Comprehensive Drug Abuse Prevention and Control Act of 1970 (as of January 1, 1983)

Sched-ule	Potential for abuse	Medical use	Produc-tion con-trolled	Examples	Maximum penalties for illegal	
					Manufacturing distribution	Possession
I	High	None	Yes	Heroin, marijuana, THC (tetrahydrocan-nabinol), LSD, mes-caline; generally, op-iates, opium deriva-tives, and hallucino-genic substances	*Schedules I and II* Narcotics— 1st offense 15 yr/$25,000/3 yr* 2nd and more offen-ses 30 yr/$50,000/6 yr	
II	High	Yes	Yes	Morphine, cocaine, methadone, opium, codeine, secobarbital, amobarbital, pento-barbital, meperidine, methaqualone, all am-phetamine-type stim-ulants	Nonnarcotics— 1st offense 5 yr/$15,000/2 yr 2nd offense 10 yr/$30,000/4 yr	1st offense 1 yr/$5,000 2nd offense 2 yr/$10,000
III	Some, less than drugs in I and II	Yes	No	Nonamphetamine-type stimulants; some bar-biturates, some nar-cotic preparations, paregoric	1st offense 5 yr/$15,000/2 yr 2nd offense 10 yr/$30,000/4 yr	For first of-fense proba-tion may be given
IV	Low, less than drugs in III	Yes	No	Barbital, chloral hy-drate, meprobamate, phenobarbital, pro-poxyphene, diazepam, chlordiazepoxide, cer-tain nonamphetamine stimulants not listed in previous schedules	1st offense 3 yr/$10,000/1 yr 2nd offense 6 yr/$20,000/2 yr	Penalties for possession are the same for all schedules
V	Low, less than drugs in IV	Yes	No	Compounds, mixtures, and preparations with very low amounts of narcotics; dilute co-deine and opium compounds	1st offense 1 yr/$5,000/none 2nd offense 2 yr/$10,000/none	

*Maximum prison sentence/maximum fine/mandatory probation period after release from prison.

A statistic frequently appearing in the congressional debate on this law was that 8 billion doses of stimulant drugs were manufactured in this country each year and about half found their way into illegal distribution channels.[17] The best story about the looseness of the previous laws and the laxness of distributors concerned the regular large shipments of amphetamines to an address in Tijuana, Mexico. One problem: the address was nonexistent, and, if it had existed, it would have been the green of the eleventh hole of the Tijuana golf course!

To curtail this type of activity the law requires (as did the 1960 and 1965 laws) annual registration of everyone who manufactures, distributes, or dispenses any controlled substances. Researchers must also register. The law states that the Attorney General shall determine the quantity of substances in Schedules I and II needed for medical, scientific, research, and industrial use and then limit production of these compounds and assign quotas to the various companies manufacturing these drugs. All registrants must keep a complete record of all controlled substances—whence it came, whither it goest—and retain the record for at least 2 years. There is little doubt that these measures drastically decrease the amount of legitimately produced drugs which are funneled into the illegal market. The impact on the nonmedical use of these drugs has been minimal.

Use of drugs does not decrease just because one source is eliminated. The 1914 Harrison Act, which made it difficult for addicts, was responsible for the development of the illegal drug trade as we know it today. Probably the primary effect of the 1970 law was to shift drug users to illegally manufactured drugs and not to cause a decrease in drug use.

Another major change in the federal drug laws is apparent in the fact that there is now *no federal mandatory sentence for a first offense of illegal possession of any controlled drug*. A first offense of illegal possession of a controlled drug or "distributing a small amount of marijuana for no remuneration . . ." can be punished by a year's imprisonment and/or a fine of $5,000. In lieu of this the court can place the individual on probation for up to 1 year. If there is no probation violation the charge is dismissed, the conviction erased from the individual's record, and, for every legal purpose, the conviction never existed. This erasing of the conviction (and the return of rights that would be lost if the conviction were allowed to stand) can only occur once. Not only can the conviction be vaporized, but (a la *1984*) if the individual is not over 21 the court, if asked to, will have all public records relating to the arrest, trial, and conviction destroyed. From a legal point of view the individual is then restored to his prearrest status and can legally deny under oath that he was ever arrested on such a charge.

Obviously the law has become less stringent in its dealings with the possessor and user. Some have suggested that this is a result of the drug scene moving swiftly into white suburbia. "Since sons and daughters of prominent persons—including senators—started getting busted for crimes previously associated with lower-class blacks, compassion for marijuana criminals was sure to arise."[18] You can almost hear them saying, "The real pressure and penalties must be brought against the professional peddlers and pushers. Their operations must be shut down before they ruin all our children!" These are the same sentiments expressed in San Francisco in the late nineteenth century that resulted in the antiopium smoking laws.

Three classes of individuals have severe penalties placed on them by the 1970 law. One group consists of individuals over 18 who distribute a controlled drug to an individual under 21 years of age. If convicted the individual receives twice the usual penalty for a first offense and three times the penalty for a second or subsequent offense.

Aiming at the illegal drug entrepreneur, this law mentions specifically "continuing criminal enterprise" and "dangerous special drug offenders." An individual is engaged in *a continuing criminal enterprise* if he violates this law in conjunction with five or more other people to whom he is an organizer or holds ". . . other position of management . . ." and from whom he receives substantial income. Conviction under this section of the law has a first offense penalty of not less than 10 years and not more than $100,000, while a second offense is not less than 20 years and not more than $200,000. For either a first or second offense life imprisonment can be the sentence, and neither probation nor a suspended sentence can be given an individual under this category. The government can also confiscate all profits and property resulting from the enterprise. In 1981 the General Accounting Office (GAO) reported to Congress that the Justice Department wasn't doing this—they had collected only $2 million in the 1970-1980 period.

A United States attorney may identify an individual as *a dangerous special drug offender* if in violating this law an individual acted as a supervisor to three or more people, received a substantial portion of his income from dealing in controlled substances, or has been convicted on drug charges twice within a 5-year period and was imprisoned at least once. The information supporting this identification is above and beyond any used in a trial to prove guilt and is additional material to be used by the judge only in determining the appropriate sentence for the convicted individual. The law provides for a sentence of up to 25 years.

FEDERAL DRUG AGENCIES

Nowhere in the federal government is there better evidence of the adage, "If it doesn't work, reorganize," than in the area of drugs. Between the enactment of the 1970 Drug Abuse Control Act and mid-1971 there was a great increase in public and political awareness of illegal drug use. Most of the interest—and concern—was on the use of heroin by Americans in Vietnam. In response to this the President labeled drug abuse "Public Enemy Number One" and established a Special Action Office for Drug Abuse Prevention in the White House. Congress formalized the action in 1972 and amended that law in 1976 to establish the Office of Drug Abuse Policy (ODAP) in the Executive Office of the President. The 1972 Office had broad powers for "overall planning and policy"—the Director was essentially the czar of all actions taken by the federal government in the area of drug abuse, excluding the enforcement of laws. Under the 1976

amendment ODAP has much less authority. The critical issue, of course, is how strongly the President feels about drug abuse and how active he wants ODAP to be in the 1980s.

In July, 1973, all enforcement activities were consolidated into the Drug Enforcement Administration (DEA) of the Justice Department. The DEA incorporated the Bureau of Narcotics and Dangerous Drugs (BNDD) as well as several minor drug law enforcement groups. Also part of the DEA are the drug investigation and intelligence functions that were originally part of the Customs Bureau. In theory, the DEA was to coordinate all federal law enforcement activities dealing with drugs. Other agencies, such as the Internal Revenue Service and the Department of State, as well as the FBI and CIA, also expend money and time on enforcement, but their work was under the general overview of the DEA. Unfortunately, the theory never worked very well. A 1977 report of the Congressional Select Committee on Narcotics Abuse and Control concluded: "There continues to be a discouraging lack of coordination between the Federal agencies responsible for narcotics law enforcement."[19,p.65] That problem either became better, or worse, in 1982 when the FBI was given concurrent responsibility with the DEA to investigate violations of Federal criminal drug laws, The Director of the DEA now reports to the Director of the FBI![20]

The National Institute on Drug Abuse (NIDA) was established in 1973 to coordinate and direct the federal government's drug abuse policy and activity in prevention, treatment and rehabilitation, evaluation, training, and research. All these activities, except research, are partially carried out through the allocation of federal money to state governments, which develop programs that meet NIDA standards. In this way the federal government, to some extent, controlled and directed the thrust of most drug abuse activities in the country, but without becoming greatly involved in the day-to-day running of treatment or education programs. Beginning in 1981 NIDA started decreasing both its policy-setting and its funding activities.

Almost all federal agencies have their finger in

some part of the drug abuse pie—even if it only involves establishing alcohol and drug counseling and treatment programs for their employees. The Veterans Administration and the Department of Defense have each established large treatment programs for their special populations: veterans and military personnel. These efforts are very loosely coordinated at the national level, but each agency functions independently in most of its directions, goals, and types of activity.

The National Institute on Alcohol Abuse and Alcoholism (NIAAA) was organized and functional in 1971 but only became a separate institute in 1973. NIAAA's thrust has been much the same as NIDA's, except that alcohol is the specific and only drug of its concern. There have been proposals that the NIDA and the NIAAA be combined into a single Institute on Substance Abuse. There have also been proposals in the 1980s that these institutes be abolished and the federal government get out of the drug abuse treatment and education business. As of 1983 it is not clear which way the political winds will blow for the alcohol and drug agencies.

DRUG LAW ENFORCEMENT

The federal strategy on drugs, before the early 1980s, was to reduce the supply of drugs through law enforcement and reduce the demand through the availability of treatment programs.[21] As budgets were cut and philosophies changed, there was a decrease in funds available for both enforcement and treatment.

Being a federal narcotics agent must be very frustrating; of the nearly 2000 DEA agents in 1980, almost two thirds worked undercover. This means they had no public reputation or identity.[22] In addition to being an unsung hero, there are great personal risks involved and there's a chance you'll be a dead nobody. In areas of the country where drug crime flourishes—such as New York City and southern Florida—there is a large amount of violent crime related to drugs. In Miami the homicide rate increased 270% from 1978 to 1981—in 1981 there were about 12 homicides a week, and about half of these were drug related.[23] On top of having to hide your identity and being at great risk for life and limb—the pay is only moderate. When you're up against a $90 billion a year operation,[24] a single raid yields $10 million in cash, and $1 million bail is paid in a few hours, in cash—and the individual freed is never seen again—the temptations must be great. You have to really believe in what you're doing and that what you're doing is effective. A DEA spokesman suggested in 1981 that maybe 15% to 20% of the drugs being smuggled into this country are being stopped.[23] Most observers think it's closer to 10%.

A very big concern in the early 1980s—if you're a big drug dealer or courier of drugs—centered on the Fourth Amendment to the U.S. Constitution. That's the one that limits the ability of the police to stop and question an individual. Basically the amendment protects the individual from "unreasonable searches and seizures" and requires "probable cause" before a search can begin.

Over the years of working on drug trafficking, narcotic agents—individually and collectively—have developed a "drug courier profile." The profile consists of a number of ongoing behaviors or past actions that agents use to "screen" travelers—usually in airports—within the United States. The parts of the profile are not published, and each agent probably, in part, develops his own. Even you might be suspicious if someone pays for an expensive ticket with cash, changes planes more often than they have to, etc. . . . .[25]

The question is: If an individual "fits" the drug courier profile, is that a probable cause to stop and question the individual? In 1980 the U.S. Supreme Court said yes, well, probably yes.[26] No one, including the Supreme Court, liked that indefiniteness, so in 1982 they considered another case.[27] Note that this is an issue only for individuals traveling within the United States. When an individual returns from abroad the customs officials have the right to do a total search of anyone, except diplomats.

Things are getting tougher. A 1981 Court decision[28] said that trained animals—dogs—can be used to sniff luggage for odors associated with drugs and that agents have the right to open luggage selected by the dogs. Marijuana is the key subject here and the "canine cannabis connoisseurs" are fairly accurate. Man's best friend can also be readily trained to smell out heroin and cocaine (and for other purposes, explosives). It shouldn't be too hard to confuse the dogs—then the cops and robbers will have to move to a new level of sophistication.

The DEA rarely goes after users or street-level dealers but instead focuses on higher-level drug dealers. Dealing with the higher-level dealers automatically moves the situation into the realm of economics, wherein lies much of the problem. It is certainly true that if a drug is not available, it will not be used—but maybe some other more potent, more expensive, more dangerous drug will be used.

It is almost a truism that when enforcement activities increase, there is a shift by the consumer and the dealer to more potent, and more expensive, drugs. The money involved in illegal drug sales is great enough to make the risks worthwhile. Just how true this is can be seen from a 1974 DEA report. It studied narcotic dealers who had been arrested and then released on bail to await trial. While on bail 47% were implicated in selling narcotics, and 12% were rearrested for narcotic sales.[29]

The problem of bail and the kinds of sentences given second- and third-level narcotic dealers (not the dealer on the street) are additional factors that decrease the effectiveness of enforcement procedures. Most dealers are released on bail for the period between their arrest and their trial. One study of these individuals released on bail found that although 46% has prior drug arrest records and 64% had prior felony arrests, 77% were released on less than $10,000 bail. The head of the DEA lamented that individuals arrested for selling drugs are ". . . back on the street before the ink is dry on the paperwork."

Sentencing is an equally complex issue. One out of every 3 individuals convicted in federal courts of a heroin or cocaine charge is placed on probation. Of those sentenced to prison, 1 out of 3 receives a sentence of 3 years or less and is eligible for parole after 1 year of prison. It is known that one of the

factors that determines the effectiveness of a law is the probability of being arrested for breaking the law. At this time the odds seem overwhelmingly against being arrested.

Someone once said that locks on house doors are to keep honest people out, the criminals go in anyway. That must be true with drug laws—and maybe with all laws. At any rate it's difficult to get drug laws enacted that are enforceable, effective, and acceptable. A case in point is the 1973 drug law in New York State. Then Governor Nelson Rockefeller pushed hard for the enactment of the law because he was convinced that treatment and rehabilitation, his earlier hopes, did not work. It was a tough law, for example, if an individual sold any narcotic drug that individual could get a life sentence in jail. At least it was probation for life, if convicted.

College students showed that they were a bright group when a survey taken soon after the passage of the law found drug sales way down on college campuses in the state. Many students adopted a wait-and-see attitude, but very few expected the laws to have any effect in the long run.

Even street sales in New York City went underground for a period—one dealer described his attitude as "conservative"—and he was selling only to users he knew before the new laws went into effect. One report in the spring of 1974 mentioned several changes that had taken place—prices increased, more dealers and users carried guns, and the quality of heroin decreased. That's all. There was no rush by addicts to enter treatment programs, no increase in the difficulty of buying drugs, no great increase in arrests or convictions.

In 1976 the chairman of a Congressional Committee that had toured parts of New York City commented:

> As we drove along the streets in an unmarked police car, street pushers literally thrust themselves through our windows and offered to sell heroin, cocaine, marijuana, and a variety of drugs. . . . These pushers knew we were surrounded by police, and they didn't care. Their contempt for the consequences of the law is that great. However, it may be suggested that these

street pushers have learned their lesson: in reality, they risked little . . . they know that even if they are unlucky enough to get arrested for hard drugs, they will be released on bail, which has simply become one more bit of overhead, a couple of extra sales to be made.[30,p.2]

A January, 1977, report[31] of New York City judges and rehabilitation specialists found that over half said the tough New York State drug laws were ineffective in decreasing drug use or drug sales. Many believed the laws made things worse by introducing juveniles into the illegal drug business, since those under 16 can serve as couriers and if arrested are immune from harsh jail sentences.

You will have to judge that for yourself, but an article in the *New York Times*, titled "Thousands of Harlem Drug Runners, 9 to 16, Find the Rewards High, the Risks Low," started with the following paragraphs:

> [He] is 15 years old, has a $12,000 Mercedes, a woman on each arm and $500 in each pocket of his tailor-made suit, and refers to life as "nothing but a party."
>
> Call him Peter Brown. Central Harlem has been his promised land. A few years ago a friend, neighbor or acquaintance told Peter he could make a lot of money simply by giving a few glassine envelopes to the right people.
>
> Peter followed his orders well and was soon earning $500 a week. Thousands of dollars richer and years wiser. Peter plans to retire at 16—an age when he becomes liable to the full punishment of the law as an adult.[32]

There were other problems with the law. Juries didn't want to give someone a life sentence for the sale of a small amount of a narcotic. A federal evaluation a few years after the passage of the new law[33] said there were "fewer dispositions, convictions, and prison sentences for drug offenses" than under the old laws. It should be noted that the long prison sentences for small drug sales are constitutional.[34] The problem was they just didn't seem rational. A 1979 report to the governor of New York stated, "The sale of an eyedropper of cocaine by a first offender does not merit more punishment than forcible rape by a recidivist—yet such a tragic absurdity is precisely what the present law demands."[35] The drug laws in New York State were changed and brought more in line with other criminal laws.

After all this you might conclude that law enforcement and tough drug laws are ineffective in dealing with the realities of drug abuse and drug sales. Yes and no! It seems clear that in the present climate, the one which has evolved since about 1960, tough drug laws will not work and are not enforced because they are not supported psychologically, or fiscally, by the public or by many members of the law enforcement or criminal justice system. Philosophically it is true that tough drug laws have not been supported adequately and given a chance to have an impact on drug use and drug traffic. Pragmatically—yesterday, today, and tomorrow—enforcement of tough drug laws is not something most people will support, so it is senseless to look to the law as the primary way of reducing our current and future drug problems.

The general trend at both the national and state level is to decrease penalties for all but major drug dealers. State laws vary widely[36] and change frequently. Of special note, however, is the 1975 ruling of the Alaska Supreme Court which held that "possession of marijuana by adults at home for personal use" was protected by the right to privacy. That judicial point of view has not swept the nation. Although the U.S. Supreme Court has upheld the right to possess pornographic material for personal use in the home and has limited the authority of the state to interfere with a pregnant woman's decision to have an abortion, the Court does not agree that the right to personal privacy includes drug taking—even in one's own home.[37] The debate continues.

Drug paraphernalia

The topic of drug paraphernalia is not quite in the same league as those topics just discussed, yet it is important because it clearly points up some issues among drug users, nondrug users, the Constitution, capitalism, and law enforcement agencies. Drug paraphernalia is defined as:

". . . all equipment, products and materials of any kind which are used, intended for use, or designed for use, in planting, propagating, cultivating, growing, harvesting, manufacturing, compounding, converting, producing, processing, preparing, testing, analyzing, packaging, repackaging, storing, containing, concealing, injecting, ingesting, inhaling, or otherwise introducing into the human body a controlled substance . . ."[38,p.52]

This definition is from the model drug paraphernalia act, which the DEA hopes will be adopted by states and communities. The federal government does not have, nor does it want, any federal paraphernalia laws.

As drug use increased in the 1960s there was an increase in the demand for all the "things" that make drug use easier, more convenient, more pleasurable. The drugs of concern are usually marijuana and cocaine. By 1980 there were about 30,000 "head shops" in this country, and they sold $1.5 to $2 billion worth of "drug accessories." The business is so big that there are discount houses: "Our prices are lower so you can get higher." Parents, police, and others were horrified: How can they openly sell items that are clearly for use with illegal drugs? Many city ordinances and state laws were passed to close the shops down. Most of them have been declared unconstitutional, usually because they are too vague.

The owners of head shops protest: How can we know the intentions of our customers? "A scale can be used to measure gold as well as cocaine, a roach clip to hold a cigarette as well as a joint, and a bong for inhaling tobacco as well as hashish."[39] The other side wonders: "How can society encourage respect and adherence to laws if it allows merchants to flagrantly peddle instruments of crime?"[40] Civil libertarians worry about freedom of expression and freedom of trade. Customers don't wonder or worry—if it's not available openly, it'll be available covertly, only more expensive.

The federal model for state laws has six basic provisions:

- Provides a comprehensive definition of the term "drug paraphernalia" with specific descriptions of the most common forms of paraphernalia.
- Outlines the relevant factors a court or other authority should consider in determining whether an object comes within the definition.
- Makes the manufacture, advertisement, delivery, or use of drug paraphernalia a criminal offense.
- Makes the delivery of drug paraphernalia to a minor (a person under 18 years of age) a special offense.
- Defines clearly what conduct is prohibited regarding the manufacture, advertisement, delivery, or use of drug paraphernalia and specifies what criminal state of mind must accompany such conduct.
- Provides for the civil seizure and forfeiture of drug paraphernalia.[38,p.33]

It seems to be constitutional; as of 1982, 22 states had similar laws. Several federal courts have upheld different state and city versions of the federal model and in March 1982, the Supreme Court said they would not review those decisions—so they stand. In March of 1982 the Supreme Court did review and approve, in a 8 to 0 ruling, a city ordinance that did not ban paraphernalia shops but required them (1) to obtain a license to sell items "designed or marketed for use with illegal cannabis," (2) to record the names and addresses of purchasers, and (3) to allow the police to inspect these records. In the ruling Justice Marshall wrote, "If the promotion of illegal drug use is deemed 'speech,' then it is speech proposing an illegal transaction, which a government may regulate or ban entirely."

It looks as if the issue, and many of the head shops, are closed for a few years.

Criminal responsibility while under the influence of a drug

As a general rule, voluntary intoxication is not a defense for criminal behavior that will hold up in court. If the drug was taken willingly then the individual will most likely be tried for the crime, with the fact of drug use as accessory information for the judge and jury. The use of drug intoxication as a defense is most often limited to alcohol, LSD, or PCP. It's usually phrased as "temporary insanity as a result of drug use." There have not been a lot of cases, but almost always the defense loses in its attempt to have the criminal proceedings dropped. If the drug was not taken voluntarily, or knowingly, then the defense must show that the individual had "diminished capacity"—was not just intoxicated—because of the drug. In a court, diminished capacity centers on the ability of the individual to" . . . (a) deliberate, (b) premeditate, (c) maturely and meaningfully reflect upon his act, (d) harbor malice, (e) be able to form the necessary intent to commit the crime involved."[41,p.18]

INTERNATIONAL REGULATION OF NARCOTICS AND OTHER DANGEROUS DRUGS

Beginning with an 1833 treaty with Siam, the United States recognized the need for agreements with other countries on the opium trade. In 1887 Congress passed an act to execute an agreement between China and the United States that forbade importation of opium to the United States by Chinese nationalists and also forbade American citizens from engaging in the Chinese opium trade.

Awareness of the larger international nature of the narcotic problem increased slowly, and it was President Theodore Roosevelt who called the First International Opium Congress, which was held in Shanghai, China, in 1909. This Congress was attended by representatives of the United States, Great Britain, France, Germany, Austria-Hungary, The Netherlands, Persia, Portugal, Russia, Italy, Siam, Japan, and China. One of the results was the 1912 Hague Conference in the Netherlands where the 13 nations represented agreed, loosely, to regulate domestic sale and use of the opiates. Overall, however, the conferences did little more than focus world attention on the narcotic problem.

After World War I international control of the growth, manufacture, and distribution of the opiates was assumed by the League of Nations. From a preliminary meeting in 1921, several agreements developed, the most noteworthy being the 1931 convention in Geneva attended by representatives of 57 nations. This convention established rules for limiting production and regulating the distribution of narcotic drugs.

In 1948 the United Nations designated the World Health Organization as the agency responsible for the international control of narcotics. The World Health Organization has been quite active, and present international control is based on the 1961 Single Convention on Narcotic Drugs, which has been made a treaty obligation by over 60 countries. This 1961 agreement consolidated all eight previous international agreements on narcotics and became internationally effective in 1964. In 1967 it was ratified by the Senate and became a treaty obligation of the United States.

The operating arms of this agreement are two United Nations agencies with headquarters in Geneva. One, the Commission on Narcotic Drugs, is responsible for regularly updating and revising international agreements on narcotics. The most significant change made recently in international drug treaties came in 1971 when the Convention on Psychotropic Substances was developed. This treaty became effective in 1976 when it was ratified by a majority of the parliaments in the United Nations. The Convention requires government authorization for international shipments of hallucinogens and it brings under control the production and distribution of other dangerous drugs. This treaty has only recently applied to the United States; the Senate did not approve it until 1980. It had not been approved primarily because passing new drug laws in this country would first require amending the Convention—a big job. Failure of the United States to approve the Convention had hurt our relationships with other countries. They argued: Why should we respond to your requests for international help with the American drug problem if you're unwilling to make a commitment to help other countries with their drug problems?[42] That logic, and the increasing need of American law enforcement agencies for international cooperation, was enough to finally overcome the Senate's negative view of entangling alliances.

The second agency of the World Health Organization, the International Control Board, has the mandate to monitor and regulate the legal production, stores, and needs of narcotics for the world. It is not an enforcement agency and can only try to negotiate cutbacks in production when supply seems to outrun demand. The actual value of the

Board seems to be in keeping a reasonably good record of where legal narcotics come from and where they go.

A study group of the World Health Organization issued a report on youth and drugs in June, 1973, declaring that drug taking in itself should not be a crime. It called for efforts to "decriminalize drug-taking per se in those jurisdictions where such action is a crime."[43] That would be welcome news to some of the Americans now in foreign jails on drug charges. Most of them, however, were arrested at borders and charged and convicted for smuggling, not possession. In almost every case the drugs involved were marijuana or hashish.

The imprisonment in foreign jails of Americans on drug charges increased rapidly in the early 1970s. TV ads and posters were used to inform young Americans headed overseas that (1) most countries had stricter drug laws than the United States, (2) bail was not usually possible, (3) trial by jury was a rarity, and (4) the American embassies and government could do little more than offer sympathy. A 1972 report referred to the "many American youths languishing in foreign jails as a result of their ignorance of foreign drug laws" and offered a compilation of the drug laws of over 120 nations. There is wide variation. "For example, the death penalty is prescribed for possession of narcotics in Iran while the Federal Republic of Germany automatically issues suspended sentences for private use of narcotics."[44,p.1] Take care, things haven't gotten any better. As the Secretary of State said: "A passport is a travel document, not a license for a bad trip abroad."[45]

The international involvement of the United States does not end with its participation in these agreements. In his remarks to the International Narcotics Control Conference in 1972, President Nixon echoed President Theodore Roosevelt's sentiments of 1909 but phrased them more dramatically:

> The men and women who operate the global heroin trade are a menace not to Americans alone, but to all mankind. These people are literally the slave traders of our time. They are traffickers in living death. They must be hunted to the end of the earth. They must be left no base in any nation

for their operation. They must be permitted not a single hiding place or refuge from justice anywhere in the world and that is why we have established an aggressive international narcotics control program in cooperation with the governments in more than 50 countries around the world.[46]

Part of that international control program involves assigning narcotic agents to areas of the world where controlled drugs are grown, produced, and distributed. The pattern of overseas involvement shifts as the sources of illegal drugs move from continent to continent. There have long been agents in "drug centers" such as Istanbul, Marseilles, Bangkok, Mexico City, and Hong Kong.

In 1972, as the opium fields in Turkey were plowed under and the French Connection in Marseilles was broken, the action shifted to South America, Mexico, and then Southeast Asia. Agents in these areas cooperate closely with local enforcement groups but are primarily concerned with stopping shipments and disrupting organizations that are linked with illegal markets in America. Some shipments don't get stopped until they hit our borders.

The group that gets all the good publicity on the international enforcement scene is *Interpol*, the International Criminal Police Organization.[47] Started in 1923 and headquartered in Paris, Interpol has a membership of over 120 nations. About one third of its activities are devoted to drugs, and 20 persons work in the Drug Section in Paris. There are liaison agents on several continents, but the total drug force is not more than 30. The primary activity of Interpol is as a collator of intelligence reports collected by its member countries. It rarely participates in enforcement activities; instead its role is to expedite information exchange and cooperation by the various enforcement agencies around the world.

CONCLUDING COMMENT

Crystal balls are particularly cloudy about the future when questions involve the interacting forces of science, values, politicians, social change, and organized crime. These are the various factors that are continually pushing and pulling at the laws and regulations that govern the availability and use of drugs—legal and illegal. The 1970 Drug Abuse Law provides the best base this country has ever had for dealing with the users and dealers of illegal drugs. The actions and efficiency of the DEA are continually debated but considering its budget it does a pretty good job (2000 agents versus a $90 billion industry?). Whether being wedded to the FBI will help or hinder remains to be seen.

Drug laws and regulations are continually changing, just as are the social concerns about drug use and drug users.[48] Remember that whatever we do is a compromise. Some argue for the removal of criminal penalties (but not legalization) for all drug use.[49] Others argue that all drugs used for recreational purposes should be legalized and controlled the same as alcohol.[50] If you are concerned about the drug laws in this country—too harsh or too lax—you'd better speak up! Others are.

REFERENCES

1. Kane, H.H.: Opium-smoking in America and China, New York, 1882, G.P. Putnam's Sons.
2. Adams, S.H.: The great American fraud, Collier's, six segments from October 1905, to February 1906.
3. Congressional Record 40:102 (Part I), December 4, 1905, to January 12, 1906.
4. The best condensed reference to the federal drug laws is Handbook of Federal Narcotic and Dangerous Drug Laws, Superintendent of Documents, Washington, D.C., U.S. Government Printing Office. Ask for the latest edition. The only way to really appreciate and understand these laws is to read them as well as the Congressional hearings and debates prior to the enactment of the laws.
5. 249 U.S. 96, 99 (1919).
6. 258 U.S. 280 (1922).
7. 268 U.S. 5 (1925).
8. Schmeckebier, L.F.: The bureau of prohibition, Service Monograph No. 57, Institute for Government Research, 1929, Brookings Institute. Cited in Narcotic Drug Laws and Enforcement Policies, King, Rufus: Law & Contemporary Problems 22:122, 1957.
9. Walsh, J.: Lexington Narcotics Hospital: a special sort of alma mater, Science 182:1004-1008, 1973.
10. U.S. News and World Report 41:22, 1956.
11. Senate Committee on the Judiciary: The illicit narcotic traffic, Senate Report No. 1440, 84th Congress, 2nd Session, 1956.
12. Grapes, Z.T., and Brown, T.R.: Drugs with abuse potential: a 70-year history of increasing government control, Hospital Formulary, pp. 608-613, November 1976.
13. Depressant and stimulant drugs, Part 166, Title 21, Code of Federal Regulations, Washington, D.C., 1966, Food and Drug Administration.
14. Handbook of federal narcotic and dangerous drug laws (ref. 3), pp. 72-73.
15. Drug use in America: problem in perspective, second report of the National Commission on Marihuana and Drug Abuse, March 1973.
16. Falco, M., and Akins, C.: Federal drug abuse law enforcement, regulations, and control. The Drug Abuse Council, Inc., Washington, D.C., April 1975.
17. Congressional Record—House, September 24, 1970, p. H9170.
18. A little less illegal, New Republic 161:11, 1969.
19. Interim report, Select Committee on Narcotics Abuse and Control, Washington, D.C., February 1977, U.S. Government Printing Office.
20. Pound, E.T.: F.B.I. director to take over key role in narcotics cases, New York Times, January 22, 1982, p. A12.
21. Goldman, F.: Heroin and the federal strategy: a policy in search of evidence, Journal of Psychoactive Drugs 13:3, July-September 1981.
22. Pear, R.: Drug agency plays hard, but does it play smart? New York Times, August 24, 1980, p. 4E.
23. Jaynes, G.: Crime surges in Miami as illicit drugs pour in, New York Times, August 12, 1981, p. A10.
24. Director, National Institute on Drug Abuse: Personal communication, March 15, 1982.
25. Goodman, G., Jr.: A quiet suspicion: looking for drugs in airport crowds, New York Times, July 1, 1980, p. B3.
26. Profile for arrests of drug suspects at airports survives a test in court, New York Times, May 28, 1980.
27. Greenhouse, L.: Drug courier profile facing review, New York Times, December 1, 1981, p. A23.
28. Margolick, D.: Dogs can sniff for drugs in luggage, court says, New York Times, December 23, 1981, p. B2.
29. United Press International, May 20, 1974, Washington, D.C. In New York Times, May 21, 1974.
30. Second interim report, Select Commitee on Narcotics Abuse and Control, February 1977.
31. Raab, S.: Stiff antidrug laws held no deterrent, New York Times, January 2, 1977, p. 1.
32. Williams, L.: Thousands of Harlem drug runners, New York Times, April 21, 1977.
33. Drug law effectiveness questioned in U.S. study, New York Times, September 5, 1976, p. 1.
34. High court allows life sentences in drug offenses, New York Times, January 9, 1979, p. B16.
35. Goldstein, T.: The Rockefeller drug law, New York Times, May 14, 1979, p. B2.
36. Survey of state penal laws, National Commission on Marihuana and Drug Abuse, October 31, 1972.
37. Bogomolny, R.L.: Drug abuse and the criminal justice system, Journal of Drug Issues 6:380-389, Fall 1976.
38. Community and legal responses to drug paraphernalia, Ser-

vices Research Report, DHEW Publication No. (ADM) 80-963, Washington, D.C., 1980, U.S. Government Printing Office.

39. Smolowe, J.: Doubt clouding new state curb on head shops, New York Times, July 31, 1980, p. B12.

40. Barron, J.: Can drug paraphernalia be banned? New York Times, May 26, 1980.

41. Siegel, R.K.: Forensic psychopharmacology: the drug abuse expert in court, Drug Abuse and Alcoholism Review, vol. 1, no. 5/6, 1978.

42. The Convention on Psychotropic Substances: An analysis, Washington, D.C., May, 1973, The Drug Abuse Council, Inc.

43. Drug use no crime, W.H.O. unit believes, New York Times, June 10, 1973, p. 10.

44. Compilation of narcotic and dangerous drug laws of foreign nations, National Commission on Marihuana and Drug Abuse, October 25, 1972.

45. Schmidt, D.A.: Youths warned of drug laws abroad, New York Times, May 18, 1972, p. 5.

46. Nixon, R.M.: Remarks to the International Narcotics Control Conference, September 18, 1972.

47. Nepote, J.: The role of INTERPOL, Drug Enforcement 3(1):18-23, Winter 1975-1976.

48. A perspective on "get tough" drug laws, Washington, D.C., May, 1973, The Drug Abuse Council, Inc.

49. Stachnik, T.J.: The case against criminal penalties for illicit drug use, American Psychologist 27:637-642, 1972.

50. Szasz, T.S.: The ethics of addiction, Harper's Magazine, pp. 74-79, April 1972.

CHAPTER 3

REGULATION OF NONNARCOTIC AND NONDANGEROUS DRUGS

1982 REPORT[1] OF A GALLUP POLL that rated "things Americans value" put "physical health" neck-to-neck for first place with "a good family life." Over 80% of those polled responded that those two things were "very important" or "extremely important" to them—in contrast to 35% to 40% who said the same about income, material goods, and leisure time. Americans spend money to maintain that health, the dollar amount increases about 10% to 15% each year. In 1980 $220 billion was spent for personal health care—9.4% of the gross national product. Of that $220 billion, only 13%, $28 billion, was for drugs (hospital costs were $100 billion). Of that $28 billion, $6.2 billion was for over-the-counter (OTC) drugs. OTC drugs are those you can buy without a prescription. As you might expect, the cost of drugs is increasing—but not as fast as those things we buy. Using 1967 as the base (that is, 100), the price index of all commodities was 235 in 1980; the 1980 price index for pharmaceutical preparations was 154.

This chapter zeroes in on those who manufacture and sell these drugs and on the Food and Drug Agency (FDA), the federal government's regulation maker, evaluator, and watchdog. The focus is on the interactions among those who produce, sell, and regulate the legal drugs most of us regularly consume. Complex relationships exist between the science of drugs and the politics and economics of drugs. Public debate is increasing and everyone claims that their major concern is what is best for you and me—the consumer. We'll see.

A BRIEF HISTORY

In the last half of the nineteenth century there was considerable agitation at the state level for legislation to regulate the purity of drugs and to control the therapeutic claims made for medicines. Strongly supported by the American Medical Association, and the American Pharmaceutical Association, founded in 1848 and 1852 respectively, state laws spread, and 45 states had antiadulteration laws.

Federal regulation of nonnarcotic drugs progressed more hesitantly. In 1848 Congress passed the National Drug-Import Law in response to incoming shipments of drugs that were mislabeled, adulterated, and of general poor quality. The law authorized rejection of drugs that did not meet medical standards of quality and purity. Because unqualified political appointees were used as inspectors, the law was never effectively enforced.

The 1906 Pure Food and Drugs Act. This act brought the government full force into the drug marketplace, and subsequent modifications have built on it. This act defined a drug as "any substance or mixture of substances intended to be used for the cure, mitigation, or prevention of disease." Of particular importance, it developed, was the phrasing of the law with respect to misbranding. Misbranding referred *only to the label, not to general advertising*, and covered "any statement, design, or device regarding . . . [a drug], or the ingredients or substances contained therein, which shall be false or misleading in any particular." The law was used successfully to force some patent medicine labels to tone down their therapeutic claims. The first contested case under the law was won by the government against a headache remedy named Cuforhedake Brane-Fude!

In 1911 government action against a claimed cancer cure on the grounds that the claim was false and misleading was contested by arguing that the law applied only to the ingredients and not to therapeutic claims. After this position was upheld by the Supreme Court, Congress passed the 1912 Sherley Amendment that forbade therapeutic claims that were both "false and fraudulent." Even this was not enough because a 1922 case involving a tuberculosis cure was ruled not to be a fraudulent claim because it was truly believed to be effective by its manufacturer. Considering its ingredients of raw eggs, turpentine, ammonia, formaldehyde, and mustard and wintergreen oils, the claim was at least false, if not fraudulent.

As more and more cases were investigated, it seemed clear to the Food and Drug officials that many of the violations of the 1906 law were unintentional and caused primarily by poor manufacturing techniques and an absence of quality control measures. The Food and Drug Administration began developing assay techniques for various chemicals and products and collaborated extensively with the pharmaceutical industry to improve standards. The prosperous 1920s, coupled with a friendly Republican administration and increasing scientific knowhow, resulted in many voluntary changes by the drug industry that improved manufacturing and selling practices.

The depression of the 1930s and increased competition for business, plus the election of a Dem-

ocratic administration not overly friendly with big business, disrupted many of the working agreements between government and industry. FDA surveys in the mid-1930s showed that over 10% of the drug products studied did not meet the standards of *The United States Pharmacopeia* or *The National Formulary*. These findings contributed to the development of new regulations incorporated into the 1938 Food, Drug, and Cosmetic Act.

The 1938 Food, Drug, and Cosmetic Act. This act contained many provisions that changed the role of the FDA in drug control and is still the basic law in this area. One of the provisions resulted from the fact that in 1937, 107 people, primarily infants, died following treatment with the drug "Elixir of Sulfanilamide." The 1930s had seen an expansion in the use of sulfa drugs—agents potently effective against certain disease-causing microorganisms. Most sulfa products could not be used with infants because the dosage form was tablet or pill, but the prescription drug "Elixir of Sulfanilamide" was a palatable liquid widely used with infants. Following the death of these children it was shown that the liquid, diethylene glycol, in which the sulfanilamide was dissolved caused kidney poisoning. *There was no government requirement that a manufacturer show that a drug was safe before marketing a new product!* The concerns the government had up to this time were that a drug be properly labeled and/or meet *The United States Pharmacopeia* or *The National Formulary* standards. The only basis on which the government could stop the sale of "Elixir of Sulfanilamide" was that it was mislabeled—it contained no alcohol and a true elixir does.

Congress, appalled by the fact that a drug could kill but not be taken off the market for that reason, included in the 1938 amendments a requirement that manufacturers test a drug for toxicity. The safety of drugs was controlled by the requirement that before a new drug could be introduced in interstate commerce, a "new drug application" (NDA) had to be submitted by the company to the FDA. The FDA would determine whether the NDA met certain specifications in the regulations, and, if it did, the application was allowed to "become effective."

The specifications to be met included submission of "full reports of investigations which have been made to show whether or not such drug is safe for use." Note especially that the FDA does not *approve* the drug or make statements about its safety. The FDA only says that the new drug application has met certain requirements. Between 1938 and 1962, about 13,000 new drug applications were submitted to the FDA and about 70% were allowed to become effective.

The requirement that drug manufacturers present evidence showing a product to be safe is one of the three basic rules now governing the marketing of a new drug. In 1906 it was established that *a drug has to be pure and accurately labeled*. Since 1938 *a drug also has to be safe*. Only since 1962 is it a requirement that *a drug also has to be effective*. The 1938 amendments also stipulated that drug labels give adequate directions for use but added that the FDA could exempt drugs from that requirement on the basis that it was "not necessary for the protection of public health." If a drug was exempt from this direction-for-use requirement, it could be sold only on prescription and had then to carry the label: CAUTION: TO BE USED ONLY BY OR ON THE PRESCRIPTION OF A PHYSICIAN. The wording was later changed to CAUTION: FEDERAL LAW PROHIBITS DISPENSING WITHOUT PRESCRIPTION.

There was much confusion over what was to be termed a prescription drug until the Humphrey-Durham Amendment of 1951. It clarified the issue by setting up three classes of prescription drugs: (1) those that must be labeled, "Warning: may be habit forming" (the narcotic drugs); (2) those determined by the FDA to be unsafe because of toxicity unless administered by a physician; and (3) new drugs. Only then could the FDA effectively control which nonnarcotic drugs needed to be prescribed by a physician. The restriction seems only moderately successful, since one study found that retail pharmacists honored fake prescriptions 56% of the time![2]

The 1962 Amendments. In the late 1950s Senator Estes Kefauver began a series of hearings investigating high drug costs and marketing collaboration between drug companies. As the hearings progressed there was some involvement of the committee with the regulation and control of drugs, but it was the thalidomide disaster that gave the 1962 amendments their particular flavor and ensured their passage. It is clear that if thalidomide had been evaluated under the controls outlined in the 1962 amendments, its effects on fetuses would have been determined.

There are three important features in these 1962 amendments, including one that requires advertisements for prescription drugs to contain a summary of information about adverse reactions to the drug. Also, prior to marketing, every new drug has to be shown effective for the illnesses mentioned on the label or brochure accompanying the drug. Last, drugs marketed between 1938 and 1962 (that is, those which were safe but of unknown effectiveness) had to be evaluated by the FDA and removed from the marketplace if they were shown to be ineffective.

The requirement that there be an evaluation of the effectiveness of drugs introduced between 1938 and 1962 was a major task. In that 24-year period 237 companies had submitted NDAs for 4349 formulations of 2824 drugs for which they made over 16,000 therapeutic claims. It has been estimated that for each of these 4349 new formulations there were probably about five identical products on the market covered by each NDA. Thus, although only 4349 formulations were involved, there may have been over 20,000 new products between 1938 and 1962. Of these about 15% were over-the-counter compounds, the remainder being prescription drugs.[3]

In 1966 the Food and Drug Administration contracted the task of evaluating the formulations of prescription drugs to the National Academy of Sciences National Research Council (NAS/NRC). The Council established panels of medical and scientific experts in 30 areas to study the therapeutic claims of these drugs. In the fall of 1967 the panels began sending final reports to the Food and Drug Administration, with the last being forwarded in 1969.[4]

Overall, about 15% of the formulations were

found to be *ineffective* for their claimed therapeutic values. Since multiple claims are made for most drugs and each therapeutic claim is evaluated separately, some drugs will be approved for certain uses but not for all of their previous claims. To remain on the market these drugs will have to submit NDAs containing claims about effectiveness only for the approved uses. If they wish to extend the number of therapeutic uses, then additional information must be forwarded to the FDA.

The advisory panels also classed drugs as *"probably effective"* (7%) and as *"possibly effective"* (35%)—both classifications suggesting that there is some evidence of the compound's effectiveness but not enough for it to be finally approved. By the end of 1974 the FDA had taken action to remove from the market 6133 drug products manufactured by 2732 companies. These included 736 products covered by complete NDAs. The other products were "me-too" drugs, those marketed on the basis of their similarity to the approved items. The books are not yet closed. The early 1980s saw efforts to now have the pre-1938 drugs screened!

REGULATIONS CONTROLLING THE MARKETING OF A NEW DRUG

To translate the 1962 law on the safety and effectiveness of a new drug, the FDA has established certain regular procedures and standards that must be met by the pharmaceutical house that hopes to market a prescription drug. As does the consumer of legal drugs, the pharmaceutical industry has a considerable stake in these FDA requirements. Developing a compound to the point where it can be marketed is a long and expensive procedure for the drug company, maybe costing as much as $50 to $70 million.

In an average year, researchers in the pharmaceutical industry may screen 126,000 chemical compounds for possible utilization as drugs. About 1,000 of these will prove worthy of intense investigation. Years later, if the researchers are lucky, 16 compounds may eventually make it to pharmacies.[5,p.5]

It is not only new drugs that must be evaluated by the FDA but also a new use for an established drug. A drug may prove to be effective for a group of conditions and be passed by the FDA for sale as a treatment for those conditions. If the company finds the drug is also effective for a different group of conditions, it must submit the new information to the FDA and may not advertise the drug as effective for the new conditions until permitted by the FDA. A similar situation occurs when a new form of a drug is introduced, for example, a sustained-release form: the FDA requires that it be handled as a new drug.

The FDA formally enters the picture only when a drug company is ready to study the effects of a compound in humans. At that time the company supplies to the FDA a "Notice of Claimed Investigational Exemption for a New Drug" (IND). This IND must include the composition of the drug, its source if a biological preparation, and complete manufacturing information. At this time the manufacturer is required to submit all information from preclinical (before human) investigations, including the effects of the drug on animals. The principal purpose of this preclinical work is to establish the safety of the compound.

As minimum evidence of safety, the animal studies must include acute, one-time administration of several dose levels of the drug to different groups of animals of at least two species. There must also be studies where the drug is given regularly to animals for a period related to the proposed use of the drug in humans. For example, a drug to be used chronically requires 2-year toxicology studies in animals. Again two species are required. The method of drug administration and the form of the drug in these studies must be the same as that proposed for human use. (Requirements for new oral contraceptives are different from, and more stringent than, those presented here. See Chapter 12.)

In addition to these research results, the company must submit a detailed description of the proposed clinical studies of the drug in man. Information on the physicians who will conduct the clinical studies must also be submitted so that the FDA can evaluate their competency. In addition to the credentials on the clinical investigators, the FDA requires that it receive copies of *all* information given to the investigators about the drug.

The company must also certify that the human subjects will be told they are receiving an investigational compound and that the subjects will sign a form stating that they know they are to receive such a compound and that this is acceptable to them.[6] Finally, the company must agree to forward annually a comprehensive report and to inform the FDA immediately if any adverse reactions arise in either animals or humans receiving the investigational drug.

If the FDA authorizes the use of the drug in humans, the company can move into the first of three phases of clinical investigation.

> The first phase encompasses studies with very small amounts of the drug on a limited number of healthy people—company employees, medical school personnel, prisoners and others who volunteer for such trials. At this stage, the researchers are primarily interested in learning how their drug is absorbed and excreted in healthy people, and what side effects it may trigger.[5,p.12]

There has been increasing concern about the ethics, as well as the scientific validity, of using prisoners in Phase 1 studies. Can a prisoner freely volunteer? Is a group of prisoners similar enough to those individuals who will be taking the drug therapeutically? The federal government wanted to ban all biomedical research in prisons as of 1981. A lawsuit by prisoners stopped the regulation from being implemented and drug research in prisons continues. It will probably continue until the case reaches the United States Supreme Court.[7] In 1976 about 40% of Phase 1 testing was on prisoners.

> Phase 2 of the human studies involves patients who have the condition the candidate drug is designed to treat. These will probably involve as many as 100 hospital patients, who are chosen because the new agent may help them. . . . If all goes well with these trials, Phase 3 will follow. It can involve thousands of patients in and out of hospitals.[5,pp.12-13]

Phase 3 is quite extensive and involves administering the drug to individuals with the disease or symptom for which the drug is intended. If the compound proves effective in Phase 3, the FDA balances its possible dangers against the benefits for the patient before releasing it for sale to the public.

There is one big, continually debated issue surrounding the FDA "drug approval" system: Why does it take so long? This issue hits the media headlines frequently as the "drug lag"—the amount of time between the drug's submission to the FDA for approval and its approval for marketing. In the United States this is between 1½ and 2 years. In Great Britain it averages less than half a year.[8] This means that an effective drug was available to patients in Great Britain about 18 months before it could be marketed here.

In a 1980 report by the General Accounting Office (GAO), auditors for the federal government admitted that there were many reasons for the drug lag but put most of the blame on the bureaucratic rules and regulations of the FDA.[9] The FDA admitted to some responsibility, pointing to Congressional laws, but said it would try to do better. The issue is not just one of concern for the individual who is sick. Pharmaceutical manufacturers have only a 17-year patent on a new drug. They usually patent the chemical as soon as there is some evidence that it may be marketable. The manufacturers claim that by the time a drug is cleared for marketing, they only have about 7 years left on the patent—not long enough to reclaim costs and make a decent profit. The manufacturers have pushed for a 7-year patent extension to compensate for the FDA's slow approval process.

A 1982 report by the Congressional Office of Technical Assessment found that the time a drug spends ". . . in the regulatory process (at the FDA) was not a significant determinant of effective patent life."[10,p.D1] This report blames the manufacturers for the delay and says that if the manufacturers acted more expeditiously they would have 4 more years of patent life! Both reports may be right: the FDA does have some outmoded rules and procedures that slow the process (only now, in the mid-

1980s, has the FDA decided to review—and maybe revamp—its IND procedures, unchanged since 1962) and industry has been extremely careful in preparing an IND—both because of FDA rules (the average IND contains over 120,000 pages) and the great cost of marketing a drug that may not be profitable. The FDA said they would do better—and they did. A 1982 report showed that in 1981 the FDA approved 27 "totally new" drugs—in contrast to 12 approved in 1980.[10]

A Roper Survey in 1981 showed that 29% of the public didn't think the FDA went far enough in its regulations and that 14% thought it went too far.[11] In commenting on the drug lag the FDA Commissioner said:

> . . . compared to some countries, our standards are higher or if you will, more conservative or tighter or however you wish to call it. But on the other hand our people have very high expectations and the law is rather clear that drugs cannot be approved by the Food and Drug Administration unless they are safe and effective, and until and unless the law is changed, that's the overriding criterion.[12,p.22]

When the drug is marketed, the company must send reports on its use and effects to the FDA every 3 months for the first year, every 6 months for the second year, and every 12 months for the third and following years. Some members of Congress and pharmaceutical manufacturers believe that this evaluation of a newly marketed drug is not adequate and that a more formal Phase 4 is needed. In the 1980 final report to Congress, a government-industry commission recommended that this post-marketing surveillance (Phase 4) be carried out by a new agency independent of the FDA.[13]

REGULATORS, PRODUCERS, AND SELLERS
Regulators

The FDA is a David standing against the Goliaths of the pharmaceutical industry. Its total 1981 budget was $327 million, of which $77 million was spent on work related to human drugs, and it has over 7000 employees. This is not very large when you realize that the agency has about 3700 pages of regulations to enforce and that the products it regulates account for about 25% of all products bought by consumers. The fact that the FDA makes the rules evens things up a little with the multi-billion dollar food, drug, and cosmetic industries!

> The "age of consumerism" has thrust the Food and Drug Administration (FDA) into prominent public view, subjecting it to a barrage of criticism from the public and members of Congress.[14]

> In just a decade the Food and Drug Administration has evolved from amorphous obscurity deep within the capital bureaucracy into both the world's paramount regulator of consumer goods and the Federal Government's most criticized, demoralized and fractionalized agency.[15]

The Food and Drug Administration is in the undesirable position of always having to say they are sorry. When things go well, the pharmaceutical industry racks up its usual profits, consumers are not being deprived of anything they know about, and Congress has its attention directed elsewhere. Who thinks of the FDA? Let one problem arise, though, and it all hits the fan full force.

A good example of the problems the FDA confronts is the Delaney Amendment to the 1938 law. Congress said:

> . . . no additive shall be deemed safe if it is found to induce cancer when ingested by man or animal, or if it is found, after tests which are appropriate for the evaluation of the safety of food additives to induce cancer in man or animal.[16]

Representative Delaney went farther than most scientists approve: the law forbids any tolerance level being set for carcinogens. That may have been marginally acceptable when the law was passed in 1958—"zero" contamination was then about 50 parts per million. Technological advances have since increased sensitivity over one million times. As one Commissioner of the FDA phrased it: "Our scientific capacities to determine chemical residues have in many cases outstripped our scientific ability to interpret their meaning.[17]

The FDA has no choice but to ban *any* food additive that, in well-designed studies, causes *any* increase in *any* forms of cancer at *any* dose level in *any* animal. The same principle was extended to food coloring in 1960, and a few years later animal food was included if any residue could be found in products from the animals.

Saccharin provides a good example of how a law that was reasonable in the beginning has become a millstone around the neck of Congress, the FDA, industry, and the consumer. Because of the Delaney Amendment, the FDA started to ban saccharin, a noncaloric sweetener that has been around for 80 years and consumed at a rate of 5 million pounds per year in the United States (three fourths of which goes into diet soft drinks). One study had shown that some rats fed large amounts of saccharin developed cancer of the bladder. Saccharin has been a marginal chemical for many years, and a 1975 NAS/NRC evaluation concluded that the data were insufficient to call it a carcinogen. The relevance of the rat study to human levels of consumption is not readily apparent (you would have to drink 800 12-ounce bottles of diet soda a day to ingest an equivalent amount), and even the American Cancer Society wanted saccharin retained. Much lobbying and public outcry led to a note of sanity, and in November, 1977, Congress passed a law that prohibited, for 18 months, FDA from banning saccharin from foods. During this moratorium saccharin-containing food had to carry the label, USE OF THIS PRODUCT MAY BE HAZARDOUS TO YOUR HEALTH. THIS PRODUCT CONTAINS SACCHARIN WHICH HAS BEEN DETERMINED TO CAUSE CANCER IN LABORATORY ANIMALS.

In June 1979 the moratorium ran out and the FDA waited. Congress said: Do nothing for 2 more years, then we'll act! June 1981 came, the moratorium ran out, and the FDA waited. Nobody wants to act. If the FDA moves to ban saccharin Congress will surely stop them, but what Congressman wants to vote to approve the use of food additives that have been shown to cause cancer? A 1981 report by the American Medical Association[18] and other actions by scientists[19] may help eliminate the idiocy of a "zero risk" law—but who knows when it will occur. (In case you have a "sweet tooth": in mid-1981 the FDA approved a low-calorie sweetener—aspartame—that has one tenth the calories of sugar.)

Food additives are a part of FDAs work as of 1958 when the Food Additive Amendment to the 1938 law was passed by Congress. The amendment required proof that new additives were safe; it named 415 food ingredients, in use in 1958, as safe and acceptable without further evidence. In 1969 one of these accepted chemicals, cyclamate—an artificial sweetener—was linked to cancer and a review was later ordered of all food additives generally recognized as safe. The evaluation was completed[20] and 305 of the 415 were clearly safe. There were qualifiers for others—more research needed—but two are of special note: table salt and caffeine. The caffeine story appears in Chapters 4 and 10. Table salt (NaCl) is used much too extensively as an additive and probably contributes greatly to the large number of individuals with high blood pressure. The review committee urged laws restricting and reducing the use of salt in food processing.[21]

Just so you know that the FDA has enough to keep it busy: as of 1968 it is responsible for standards in radiation-emitting devices (from x-ray units to TV sets); since 1972 it has been responsible for biologicals (such as vaccines, blood banks, etc.); in 1976 the Medical Device Amendments said the FDA had to approve diagnostic and therapeutic devices for safety and effectiveness. The Food and Drug Administration is certainly a busy body—or is that busybody?[22]

Producers

The pharmaceutical industry is one of the largest and most profitable in the United States today. With sales well over $30 billion a year and the major companies reporting profits of about 13% based on their sales, the profits are more than double other American industries. The pharmaceutical companies point to four factors that they believe justify their activities and profits.

1. It is a high-risk, high-cost business. Development of a new drug may cost $70 million and then not be a marketable or profitable agent.

2. Drug costs have consistently increased at a much lower rate than the cost of other items.

3. The industry has always invested heavily in research and development of new products—about 10% of the total sales, compared to 1.5% in other industries. (Only about 1.5% is spent by drug companies on basic research, but this is still more than other industries.)

4. Drug costs now take less of the health care dollar than at any time in recent years. In 1964 drug costs accounted for 15 cents of each health care dollar, but only 13 cents in 1980. Such a defense proves valid, but it is still quite interesting that since 1953 the drug industry has been either the first or second most profitable industry in the United States.

With sales in the billions of dollars many people expect that there are zillions of drugs. Not so. Two of every three prescriptions are filled with only 200 different drugs. The 20 top-selling drugs account for almost 30% of retail sales. Psychoactive drugs are the basis for 14% of all prescriptions and throughout the 1970s the single number one seller was diazepam (Valium). (See Chapter 13.) By 1981 it had dropped to fourth place—being replaced by drugs effective against ulcers, heart attack, and arthritis. There are two opposing trends underway that make it difficult to predict growth patterns. One is that as the country becomes more health conscious and health knowledgeable, life-styles change and better health habits are established. Since many of today's diseases are a result of personal decisions—such as alcohol use, cigarette smoking, and nutritional factors—and not of a germ-laden poorly sanitized environment, it is likely that the incidence of most diseases will continue to fall. Fewer diseases, less need for drugs. The opposing trend is that we're all getting older—as a nation our average age is creeping up. With advanced age there is usually more illness—the body and the mind are no longer able to withstand the slings and arrows of the world. More disease, more

drug use. In 1981 10% of the population were over 65 years of age and used 28% of the prescription drugs. No matter what happens, no one expects the large pharmaceutical companies to go broke.

Products from the pharmaceutical industry are grouped in two major ways. One classification includes ethical and proprietary products. The term "ethical" means that the products are advertised only to professionals—physicians and pharmacists—and not to consumers. "Proprietary" refers to a company that advertises its products directly to the consumer. The other classification includes both prescription (legend) drugs, which can be dispensed to a consumer only with a physician's approval (a written prescription), and over-the-counter (OTC) drugs. Large drug companies will have both an ethical and a proprietary division. Sales of prescription drugs in the United States totaled $22 billion in 1980—and is rising about 10% a year. OTC expenditures in the United States in the same year were $6.2 billion, of which about $700 million were for vitamins.

It is understandable that the big issues confronting the drug industry have to do with profits. The drug lag mentioned earlier is a major concern. An equally, perhaps even more, important problem is that of the "me too" drugs: generic products jumping on the bandwagon that a brand name drug has built and brought to speed. This issue is discussed later in the chapter.

Sellers

At 60,000 locations in the United States, 150,000 pharmacists wait patiently for you and me to bring in one of the 750 million new or 650 million refill prescriptions written yearly by one of the 315,000 physicians in this country. We're not in a big hurry since the average prescription cost in 1982 was about $10.00. The pharmacist may be mixed up in his feelings. A 1981 survey[23] showed that Americans put pharmacists a close second to clergymen in honesty and ethical practice. That's good! On the other hand the Supreme Court Chief Justice noted that 95% of all prescriptions are filled with drugs already packaged by the manufacturers and in the other 5% " . . . the pharmacist performs three tasks: (1) he finds the correct bottle, (2) he counts out the correct number of tablets or measures the right amount of liquid, and (3) he accurately transfers the doctor's dosage instructions to the container."[24]

Oh for the good old days when pharmacy was pharmacy: "the art and science of preparing from natural and synthetic sources suitable and convenient materials for distribution and use in the treatment and prevention of disease."[25,p.1] That all started to change in 1843 when the first tablet was made; first gelatin capsule appeared in 1863. Today's pharmacist can and should do more than count pills. If John Q. Public buys all his drugs from a single store, the pharmacist should maintain a drug profile on each customer, which he *checks* and adds to each time he sells a drug. He should warn his customers of possible dangerous interactions between drugs prescribed by different physicians, advise on the selection of nonprescription drugs, and counsel on the proper use of prescription and nonprescription drugs. In brief, the local pharmacist should function as a knowledgeable advisor on the use of drugs and as an essential, independent monitor on prescribed drugs.

Prescriptions now account for over 50% of the income from all sales in the typical drugstore, although in the large drugstore chains—Walgreens being the largest—prescription sales may be less than 20% of total sales. The increasing cost of everything has moved the cost of a prescription up from the $5 average in 1975. About 60% of the average prescription cost is the cost of the drug. That may not seem like a lot but it is; profits in drugstores are less than 5% of sales.

The price of prescriptions is everybody's business—even if you don't have one filled, tax funds pay for 30% to 40% of all prescriptions (via Medicare, Medicaid, etc.). To hold down costs the federal government now reimburses the pharmacist a fixed fee for filling each prescription, plus a "reasonable" amount for the drug, even if the pharmacist paid more for the brand of drug used to fill the prescription. The brand of drug used to fill a prescription is a billion dollar issue that involves the government, the pharmacist, the manufacturer, and the physician. To understand this complex, important, and political issue we must leave our friendly pharmacist and enter the world of drug names.

DRUG NAMES

Commercially available compounds have several kinds of names: brand, generic, and chemical. The *chemical name of a compound* gives a *complete chemical description of the molecule* and is derived from the rules of organic chemistry for naming any compound. Chemical names of drugs are rarely used except in a laboratory situation where biochemists or pharmacologists are developing and testing new drugs. Chemical names of drugs are given here only when the structure of a chemical is shown. There are several sets of rules for naming chemical structures. The most commonly used rules in the United States are those of *Chemical Abstracts* and those of the International Union of Pure and Applied Chemistry (IUPAC). Structures shown in this book are generally named using the *Chemical Abstracts* system, although a few have been named by IUPAC where that system's name is more common.

Much more commonly used by scientists is the simpler generic (or nonproprietary) name of a drug. Generic names are the official (that is, legal) names of drugs and are listed in the USP. The generic, nonproprietary, names of chemicals are standardized by representatives of the American Medical Association, the American Pharmaceutical Association, the U.S. Pharmacopeial Convention, Inc., and the Food and Drug Administration. This group, known as the United States Adopted Name Council (USAN), has certain principles for assigning generic names to structures. Of primary importance in considering generic names are two facts: *a generic name specifies a specific chemical structure,* and *generic names are in the public domain.* The last point means they can be freely used by anyone and are not protected by trademark laws, clearly differentiating them from brand names.

The brand name of a drug specifies a particular formulation and manufacturer of a generic product. A brand name is usually quite simple and as meaningful (in terms of the indicated therapeutic use) as the company can make it. The over-the-counter compound Compōz and the prescription drug Vesprin, for example, certainly aren't stimulants. Vesprin is a tranquilizer, and the name alone almost makes you feel more relaxed, associating with it a quiet evening and vespers. Compōz, sold as a sleep aid and sedative, makes some people think of relaxation and smooth, easy experiences in life. However, brand names are controlled by the FDA, and overly suggestive ones are not approved.

BRAND-GENERIC NAME CONFLICT

When a new chemical structure, a new way of manufacturing a chemical, or a new use for a chemical is discovered, it can be patented. Patent laws in this country protect for 17 years, and, after that time, the finding is available for use by anyone. Brand names, however, are copyrighted and protected by trademark laws. These laws indefinitely restrict the use of the brand name to the original copyright holder.

For 17 years a company that has discovered and patented a product can manufacture and sell it without direct competition. If the product is a success in the marketplace, other companies will rush to discover equally effective agents with similar, but not identical, chemical structures. When the patent expires the discovery is free game for any manufacturer, and, if the drug has been a moneymaker, it is quite likely that new companies will develop the capability to produce the "same" drug. However, at this point a question arises—if the drug is chemically identical by FDA standards, is it the therapeutic equivalent?

A drug is initially released for sale by the FDA only after it has been shown to be safe and effective for the condition it is used to treat. This clearance is obtained by the original producer of the drug. The heart of the brand-generic conflict is whether it can be assumed that drugs manufactured to Food and Drug Administration standards by new companies do not have to go through the necessary preclinical and clinical trials to demonstrate safety and effectiveness.

A drug can be effective only if it is delivered to those cells where the drug acts. Almost all drugs reach the area where they are to act through the bloodstream, and any factors that influence a drug's ability to be absorbed by the bloodstream will influence its effectiveness. To separate out some of the factors involved in determining the equivalence of two drugs, three concepts have come into wide use.

The concept of *chemical equivalence* is fairly clear. Chemical equivalents are drugs that contain essentially identical amounts of the identical active ingredients in identical dosages and that thus meet present FDA physiochemical standards. *Biological equivalents* are drugs that, when administered in the same amounts, provide the same biological or physiological availability of the drug to the body tissues. The biological availability, or *bioavailability,* is usually assessed by determining the levels of the drug in the bloodstream.

Clinical equivalents are chemical equivalents that, when given in the same amounts, result in the same therapeutic effect. Thus, two drugs can be chemically equivalent but not be clinically equivalent. Whether biological equivalence is tantamount to clinical equivalence is not yet decided, but it seems probable. The primary factor involved in determining whether chemical equivalents have the same bioavailability is related to the way the drug is finally prepared for use. What would seem to be minor factors such as the hardness of the tablet of the drug and the solubility of the drug capsule become critical in determining the extent to which a drug can be absorbed into the bloodstream. If the drug does not reach the bloodstream, there is little chance it can have an effect. A study of two brands of chlorpromazine hydrochloride tablets reported the time it took for each tablet to release 60% of the active ingredient. One brand required over six times as long as the other.[26]

A case history of a brand-generic conflict involves Terramycin, the Charles Pfizer Company's brand of oxytetracycline. Terramycin was discovered by

Pfizer researchers in 1949 after screening over 100,000 samples of earth (hence the name "terra") and was a highly successful antibiotic. In 1967, when the patent ran out, several companies began producing oxytetracycline, which is the generic name for Terramycin and which was the chemical equivalent according to FDA tests. Considerable money was involved, since the cost to the patient for Terramycin was about 30 cents a capsule, whereas oxytetracycline was half that price. The Pfizer Company decided to study blood levels in groups of patients receiving Terramycin or the various brands of oxytetracycline.[27]

The FDA certified the chemical composition, amount, and purity of each of the generic brands and of Terramycin, and all were equivalent. After equal amounts of each drug, the blood levels of the drug in patients receiving the different brands were anything but equivalent. None of the generic brands gave blood levels (and thus "bioavailability") as high as Terramycin. The drugs produced by eight manufacturers resulted in blood levels too low to be acceptable, and the FDA called in 40 million capsules by those producers. The sales field was left to Terramycin and two generic forms of oxytetracycline that did yield adequate blood levels.

There is still no scientific resolution to the problem of therapeutic equivalence of brand name and chemically equivalent generic drugs. There are some political and economic attempts at "solving" the problem, but the plot continues to thicken. Since a patent permits manufacturing control for only 17 years, it is understandable that companies would seek other means to control the sale of the drug for a longer period of time. This is accomplished by advertising drugs under their brand names to physicians, not only through advertising in journals but also by direct contact of company representatives. According to some estimates, pharmaceutical houses spend about $2,400 a year per physician in this area of selling.

Since brand names are more familiar to physicians and easier to use, nearly all prescriptions are written using brand rather than generic names. In 1982 15% of prescriptions were written using generic names. In that same year the list of the 200 leading drugs included only 15 generic names. The name used on the prescription used to be really important—in the 1970s over 30 states still had antisubstitution laws. Those laws made it illegal for a pharmacist to substitute any drug for the one written on the prescription. If the physician wrote a brand name, that product had to be given to the consumer.

Laws change rapidly when Uncle Sam and state governments want to save money. As of 1982 it was legal in 48 states for a pharmacist to substitute a generic drug for the brand name drug written on the prescription, unless the physician had specified no substitutes. On top of that, since 1974 the United States has required, when possible, that all drugs bought with federal funds be generic rather than brand names.

In December 1980 the FDA decided that:

> Manufacturers will be permitted to sell generic versions of brand name drugs marketed since 1962 whose patents have expired, without repeating the costly testing done to show that the original version was safe and effective. . .
>
> Instead of repeating studies, manufacturers need only cite studies in the literature to show that the drug is safe and effective. . .[28,p.1]

These "paper" INDs (rather than the original research INDs) are the source of considerable debate.[29] Consumer groups, the FDA, and the manufacturers of generics think they're the best thing since night baseball. The manufacturers of brand name drugs are appalled and point to both administrative and scientific problems in ensuring effective, quality drugs for patients if the paper INDs are allowed to remain. They are also honest in saying that they'll lose a lot of money if things don't change. One pharmacologist said, "No amount of wishful thinking or administrative fiat can change the present state of affairs in which differences in drug bioavailability from different products are very common, and therapeutic inequivalence . . . is a potentially serious threat to patient welfare."[30,p.39] Even so, in 1980 the FDA published its first version of the *Therapeutics Equivalence List*, which is updated monthly. This list tells the pharmacist what generics they can substitute—with the FDA's approval—for a brand name drug. I'm sorry, maybe I'm more of a scientist than an administrator, but I'd like to see at least *one* study done on each different, accepted generic drug to show that there really is therapeutic equivalence,—not just chemical equivalence.

The question of whether a generic drug is as effective as a brand name drug has been overshadowed by a case before the U.S. Supreme Court: Is it an infringement of trademark or other laws if a generic drug is produced in the same distinctive color and size capsule as the brand name capsule, or if the generic drug uses the brand name in ads by saying it is the generic version of the brand name? I'd like to settle the therapeutic equivalence issue before worrying about packaging equivalence.

The use of brand names is a vital issue to the pharmaceutical companies, as well as to the consumer and the government. The high dollar sales of drug companies is partially a result of physicians using brand rather than generic names. Sometimes the price difference is considerable, several hundred percent, but a more realistic estimate of the average increased cost at the consumer level is 5% to 10%.

ADS, LABELS, INFORMATION, AND DRUG ABUSE

It's necessary to pause a moment to make clear the present status of the laws and regulations governing drug labels, drug advertising, drug safety, and drug effectiveness.[31] The 1906 federal law was concerned only with what the label said about the drug, not what was said in general advertising. A cancer cure could be advertised as such in newspapers and magazines and, as long as the label did not claim curative powers and did describe the ingredients accurately, no federal law was violated.

The 1938 act said that, henceforth, a manufacturer had to show that a drug was safe before it could be introduced into interstate commerce. The drugs already on the market at that time were presumed to be safe and were not required to prove

TABLE 3-1 Summary of major federal laws and actions regulating the marketing of legal drugs

1906	*Pure Food and Drugs Act.* Drugs marketed in interstate commerce had to meet professed minimal standards of purity and formulation.
1912	*Sherley Amendment.* A misbranded drug was one that made false and fraudulent claims about its therapeutic effect.
1938	*Food, Drug, and Cosmetic Act.* Before new drugs could be marketed, it had to be shown that they were safe when used as labeled.
1962	*Kefauver-Harris Amendment.* All new drugs, and those marketed since 1938, had to be proved effective (as well as safe) for the use indicated on their labels.
1966	FDA had the National Academy of Sciences begin a review and evaluation of the effectiveness of prescription drugs.
1972	FDA used nongovernmental advisory panels to review and determine the safety, effectiveness, and appropriate labeling of the active ingredients in nonprescription, over-the-counter drugs.

their safety. The 1962 act clearly stated that a drug had to be shown to be both safe and effective before introduction to the public. It also required the 1938-1962 drugs to be evaluated for effectiveness. Nothing was said about drugs already on sale before 1938.

Furthermore, these laws are concerned only with interstate commerce. A drug manufactured and sold within a single state does not come under these laws but is subject to the individual state regulations. Recently there have been attempts to include these drugs on the basis that *the ingredients* moved in interstate commerce. Table 3-1 summarizes the major changes and actions in the federal regulation of legal drugs.

The FDA and the Federal Trade Commission (FTC) have been working since 1962 to decide who will do what about advertising claims and statements and how it will be done. The FDA has responsibility for the labels of all drugs—prescription and OTC. The FDA also has responsibility for the advertising of prescription drugs and, as of 1971, requires that their ads contain any adverse conclusions reached by the NAS/NRC. Remember that prescription drugs are advertised only to professionals.

The FTC was established in 1914 to guard against any unfair business practices. The burden of proof is on the FTC. OTC drug ads can continue until the FTC proves in court that the ad makes claims that are not legitimate. In 1977 the FTC started to move toward the idea: If the FDA won't let you say it on the label, you can't say it in an ad. This idea fell through in 1981 because the FDA had not finished its review of nonprescription drugs.[32] There were some problems with using material approved by the FDA for the label in ads to consumers. One comment was: "If you advertise an 'antiflatulent' some people will think you are advertising a bust developer instead of something for gas."

The FTC actually has several ways of regulating advertising. One is the Advertising Substantiation Program, begun in 1971. An example of the type of question permissible under this truth-in-advertising law was their request for a substantiation of the claim that Queen Helena Skin and Beauty Treatment "rinses away blackheads and whiteheads in a matter of minutes." Statements of this type coupled with a general suspicion of Madison Avenue and the continuing concern of increasing illegal drug use and abuse, has make many people very concerned about OTC advertising.

> It is advertising . . . which mounts so graphically the message that pills turn rain to sunshine, gloom to joy, depression to euphoria and solve problems and dispel doubts.[33]

Reaching a conclusion about drugs and advertising has more similarities with the task of Hercules cleaning the stables at Elis than just the enormous size of the job. There are two major issues: (1) Is advertising in magazines and on television honest about the effects of drugs? (2) Does the large amount of television advertising increase the misuse and abuse of drugs? There are no easy answers.

The questions are important, however. Drug advertising on TV in 1975 cost $350 million. Four of the top five network advertisers are drug companies, and one of every eight TV ads are for drugs and remedies. No wonder I never feel well!

In 1961 the FTC wondered if Bufferin, Excedrin, Bayer Aspirin, and Anacin could all really be "faster" or "more effective." It is relatively easy to show that even a placebo is "faster" and "more effective," so there was no trouble for each of the three manufacturers involved to support their claims for their products. (Faster and more effective than what? Quiet, don't ask!) Unable to really press its case in court, the FTC withdrew.

In 1972 the FTC rebounded, accusing the Bufferin, Excedrin, Bayer Aspirin, and Anacin manufacturers of deceptive advertising. The FTC cited an FDA report that nonprescription analgesics are equally effective when the products contain equivalent quantities of analgesics. The FTC also claimed that it is deceptive advertising to suggest that analgesics are effective in reducing stress and tension.

Many good examples of the type of advertising the FTC is unhappy about were included in a series of articles on advertising and drugs. The most interesting one was titled "Are Magazine Ads for O-T-C Drugs based on Fact?"[34] One example shows a man holding a package of Excedrin. The printed part of the ad was:

> You don't have to take my word that Excedrin has worked better than regular aspirin. Doctors said it did in two medical studies.
>
> In two research studies on pain, one at a major hospital and another at an important university medical center, the doctors reported Excedrin worked significantly better than the regular aspirin tablet. So the next time you get a headache, try Excedrin. See if it doesn't work better for you.

The author of the journal article comments that only one of the studies was actually published in a medical journal, and this study also reported that Excedrin "was more likely to cause gastric upset than the other analgesics tested." The other study never was published, probably because, as *Consumer Reports* found, the study was "worthless."

It also needs to be pointed out that "the pain mentioned in the advertisement is not headache pain as one might imagine, but post-partum pain." One more thing: the ad neglected to mention that Excedrin contains aspirin. Oh, well, all's fair in love and war and advertising.

The dilemma of drugs being suggested as panaceas for the problems of living has been repeatedly considered. A particularly clear statement about the possible connection between the expanding illegal use of drugs and television commercials for OTC compounds was made by New York City's Mayor John Lindsay:

> In a sense, the impulses driving our children to this [drug addiction] are beyond our effective control. How can any institution, for example, compare with the force of television on the mind of a child? We are told that the average family watches television 5½ hours a day. Thus if a city child begins serious watching when he is 2, then by the time he comes into your schools, he has seen some 8,000 hours of TV.
>
> And what has he been taught? He has been taught to relax minor tensions with a pill; to take off weight with a pill; to win status and sophistication with a cigaret; to wake up, slow down, be happy, relieve tension with pills—that is, with drugs.[35]

Is it true? Do OTC ads push, lead, or point the way so people move into drug abuse? The gut reaction of most people is that it probably does, or at the most it does not do anything to diminish the drug abuse problem.

In December, 1976, the Federal Communications Commission (FCC) responded to a petition from the attorney generals of states who had asked that

> the Commission prohibit the broadcast of "over-the-counter" . . . drug advertisements from early morning until mid-evening (6 a.m. to 9 p.m.) because of their belief that such advertisements have an unhealthy influence, particularly on the young.[36]

The FCC and the FTC sponsored a series of panel discussions with authorities and decided that:

> Existing studies suggest that the correlation between exposure to advertising and drug abuse is neutral—or even negative.[37]

Maybe that's true. Common sense used to tell us the world was flat. Perhaps the problem is that the entire drug scene and drug ads are just too pervasive to make it possible to separate their effect from other changes in society. Probably long before the question is answered, the issue will have disappeared. Changes in ads and rules governing the ads are now making them more conservative and honest. Hopes should not rise too much, however. There was no significant decline in cigarette use when cigarette ads were removed from TV.

CONCLUDING COMMENT

Drugs are usually most effective when they are taken by the patient! "Much time, effort and expense is spent in the study of the effects of drugs, but little attention is devoted to whether or not patients take them as directed. . . . A recent review of over 50 studies found that complete failure to take medication often occurred in between ¼ and over ½ of all patients."[38] Only recently have investigators begun to worry about whether patients take the drugs which have been prescribed for the illness that took them to the doctor's office.[39] Drugs do little sitting in the medicine cabinet or on a bedside table. They can also cause problems if they fall into the wrong hands or are used for other conditions.

The problems and solutions associated with *patient compliance*, that is, the patient complying with the physician's instructions about treatment, are discussed at length in the sources referred to in these paragraphs.

A review of over 800 studies on compliance showed that neither demographic characteristics, disease condition, nor severity had much relationship to compliance. The more difficult the treatment regimen (number of daily doses, cost, duration, etc.), the less likely the patient is to comply. Some factors related to better compliance are good physician-patient relationship, support of the family, and the patient's belief that he—as an individual—is susceptible to the ill effects of the disease.[40]

Pay attention! After the manufacturers, the FDA, and the pharmacist have gone through all the hassle just mentioned to provide you with safe, effective drugs, the least you can do is take them as prescribed!

REFERENCES

1. Kerr, P.: Rating the things Americans value, New York Times, January 28, 1982, p. C3.
2. Glass, A.A., Goodman, K.G., and Hinkley, S.W.: Project script: a study of prescription fraud vulnerability, Bureau of Narcotic and Dangerous Drugs, U.S. Department of Justice, 1973.
3. Biomedical News, p. 8, January 1971.
4. Hampshire, G.D.: The NAS-NRC drug efficacy study: a peer review, FDA Papers 3:4-7, 1969.
5. A prognosis for America, Washington, D.C., 1977, Pharmaceutical Manufacturers Association.
6. Adams, A., and Cowan, G.: The human guinea pig: how we test new drugs, World, pp. 20-24, December 5, 1972.
7. Sue, M.: Inmates sue to keep research in prisons, Science 212:650-651, May 8, 1981.
8. The GAO drug lag report: new perspective on an old controversy, Drug Therapy September 1980.
9. Legislation, regulation, drug lag, and new drugs, The Drug Year, vol. 241(13), March 30, 1979.
10. Hinds, M.I.C.: Industry cited for drug delay, New York Times, February 4, 1982, p. D1.
11. Public backs stronger role for FDA, survey says, American Medical News, p. 11, November 20, 1981.
12. Rockwell, L.H.: Prescribing science and safety for the 1980's, Private Practice, p. 22, September 1981.
13. Postmarketing surveillance vs phase III, Medical News, Journal of the American Medical Association, vol. 245(24), June 1981.
14. FDA: future of consumer protection agency in doubt, Congressional Quarterly Inc., pp. 1908-1911, September 11, 1971.
15. Lyons, R.D.: Demoralization plaguing F.D.A.; some top jobs remain unfilled, New York Times, March 14, 1977, pp. 1, 49.
16. Wade, N.: Delaney anti-cancer clause: scientists debate on article of faith, Science 177:588-591, 1972.
17. Lyons, R.D.: F.D.A. is caught between demand for new goods and public safety, New York Times, March 13, 1977, pp. 1, 57.
18. Carcinogen regulation: Council on Scientific Affairs, Journal of the American Medical Association, 245(3):253-256, July 17, 1981.
19. Frawley, J.P.: The 1980's—a decade of change, Regulatory Toxicology and Pharmacology 1:3-7, 1981.
20. HHS News, P80-64, December 30, 1980.
21. Yesterday's additives—generally safe, FDA Consumer, pp. 14-15, March 1981.
22. Hayes, A.H.: Food and drug regulation after 75 years, Journal of American Medical Association, 246(11):1223-1226, September 11, 1981.
23. Gallop Poll: Stat-O-Grams, Pharmacy Times, p. 1, November 1981.
24. Garcha, B.S., editor: Is the justice blind? Pharmacists answer Burger, Drug Topics, pp. 55-59, October 15, 1976.
25. Deno, R.A., and others: The profession of pharmacy, ed. 2, Philadelphia, 1966, J.B. Lippincott Co.
26. Desta, B., and Pernarowski, M.: The dissolution characteristics of two clinically different brands of chlorpromazine HCl tablets, Drug Intelligence and Clinical Pharmacy 7:408-412, 1973.
27. Biodecision Laboratories Second Annual International Symposium, Pittsburgh, September 1975.
28. HHS News: U.S. Department of Health and Human Services, P80-59, December 8, 1980.
29. Kolata, G.B.: Large drug firms fight generic substitution, Science 206:1054-1056, November 30, 1979.
30. Schwartz, L.L.: Generic drug rules: science or politics, Medical Tribune p. 39, August 26, 1981.
31. Janssen, W.F.: The story of the laws behind the labels, FDA Consumer p. 32, June 1981.
32. DeWitt, K.: Trade panel ends effort to make rules for drug ads, New York Times, February 12, 1981, p. A15.
33. Advertising: the darkening drug mood, Time, p. 60, August, 10, 1970.
34. Hodes, B.: Are magazine ads for O-T-C drugs based on fact? Journal of the American Pharmaceutical Association NS16:513-515, 1976.
35. Lindsay, J. Quoted in Goddard, J.L.: Tax drugs to fight abuse, American Druggist, p. 34, March 9, 1970.
36. FCC News, December 14, 1976, Report No. 14754, p. 1.
37. Memorandum Opinion and Order, FCC 76-1135, pp. 4-5, December 8, 1976.
38. Blackwell, B.: Drug therapy: patient compliance, New England Journal of Medicine 289:249-251, 1973.
39. Komaroff, A.L., The practitioner and the compliant patient, American Journal of Public Health 66:833-835, 1976.
40. Blackwell, B.: What do we really know about noncompliance? Consultant, p. 259, January 1981.

CHAPTER 4

DRUGS AND. . . .
DRIVING
CRIME AND VIOLENCE
SPORTS
SEXUAL BEHAVIOR
PREGNANCY
BAD TRIPS

MANY OF THE THEMES AND FACTS in this book will have, or seem to have, only indirect effects on the reader. That may be true. Some of what you read here will only gradually influence your life. In sharp contrast, the topics in this chapter have been selected because they involve drug use effects that are now—or soon will be—directly affecting your life. These here-and-now topics are: drugs and driving; drugs and crime and violence; drugs and sports; drugs and sexual behavior; drugs and pregnancy; drugs and bad trips. These sections are filled with "what happens" but do not emphasize "why and how" the effects occur. At times you may want to know more about a drug or drug effect than is mentioned here. If that happens, turn to and read the relevant chapter in this book.

DRIVING

A 1980 report on drugs and highway safety by the U.S. Department of Transportation concluded:

- With the exception of alcohol, no drug has been established to be a high priority highway safety concern.
- The frequency with which drug-impaired drivers drive, are arrested, or are involved in crashes is not known.
- Drugs which may impair driving, which are used by drivers, include prescription and over-the-counter drugs as well as illicit drugs.
- The information on marijuana and driving is incomplete and does not support arguments either for or against establishing marijuana as a high priority highway safety concern.[1,p.2]

Even though much is not known, some is—particularly with respect to alcohol blood levels and traffic accidents. The blood alcohol level (BAL), which can be estimated with a Breathalyzer, gives a good index of the extent of impairment in judgment and behavior caused by alcohol. (See Chapter 8.)

There are 20 million traffic accidents a year in the United States, and four out of five involve no injury to people. Ever since the classic Grand Rapids study,[2] there has been good evidence that the probability of being involved in a traffic accident increases directly with an increase in BAL. Most authorities agree that a BAL of 0.05% to 0.1% is enough to indicate that the individual is "high," or intoxicated. A BAL of 0.1% is reached by drinking at least four or five beers or mixed drinks in 1 hour. Closer analysis of the Grand Rapids and other data points out the interesting result that when the driver who is *responsible* is compared to the *innocent* driver, the relative risk of an accident increases rapidly only for the responsible driver when BALs rise above 0.06% and may be six to seven times as great as normal at a BAL of 0.1%. The fact that low levels of alcohol do not cause a significant increase in traffic accidents but that impairment-producing BALs do increase the risk of the individual causing an accident strongly supports the idea that *alcohol impairment is a causative factor in accidents* and is not just casually related to accidents.[3]

That's important because in 5% to 10% of all accidents there is some alcohol in one of the drivers, while in about 1% of all accidents, alcohol-induced impairment is a factor. As you probably know from personal experience, a lot of people out there are driving around with alcohol in their bodies. Although fatal accidents are a small percentage of all accidents (there are about 50,000 traffic fatalities a year), a very high percentage, 35% to 50%, are caused by drivers with BALs greater than zero.[4] Most significantly, 45% of all fatally injured drivers have a BAL over 0.1%. In two out of every three single-car fatalities, the driver has a BAL of 0.1% or more. Amazingly, today one third of the pedestrians who are fatally injured have a BAL of 0.1% or more. One final fact: when you see on TV that a driver was killed in a single-vehicle crash between 9 P.M. and 1 or 2 A.M., the odds are 8 to 1 that the driver had been drinking heavily.

As the man said, alcohol clearly contributes significantly to traffic accidents—and high BALs are most closely related to serious accidents involving fatalities. What does one do about it? There are two approaches. One has been to try to identify the psychomotor and cognitive factors that are impaired by alcohol to see if automobile and highway designs can be modified or law enforcement changed to reduce the impact of the impairment. The other approach takes note of the fact that most of the serious alcohol-related accidents are not caused by social drinkers but by problem drinkers and alcoholics. Anyone who takes five drinks in 1 hour is hardly a social drinker! Each of these approaches needs comment.

Alcohol-induced impairment

Many studies have been aimed at identifying the specific abilities and skills that are most disrupted by BALs in the 0% to 0.15% range. One problem is that although laboratory tests can be done and driving simulators used, there is no evidence that the results obtained with simulators are directly and closely related to driving ability in the real world. The laboratory and simulator results do give some strong suggestions of the impact of alcohol on driving. The effect of the antianxiety agents, such as diazepam, chlordiazepoxide, and meprobamate, is very similar to those of alcohol. One of the most significant results of laboratory and simulator work is that there is a dose-related impairment in performance when the individual is forced to divide his attention between driving and another activity. When the individual had only to concentrate on driving a simulator car,[5] BALs up to 0.085% did not impair performance. The addition of another task—moving levers when lights located near the rearview mirror were turned on or when auditory stimuli were presented—decreased performance considerably, up to 30%.

The same type of decrement was found in the effect of alcohol on "simple" and "complex" reaction times. When attention can be focused and decisions are easy—as in simple reaction time tasks where you either respond or do not respond—performance is relatively resistant to the effects of alcohol. Many people probably drive home from a bar or party without an accident even though their BAL is over 0.1%. The problem arises when the unusual occurs, attention is divided, and decisions have to be made rapidly. In complex reaction time experiments, the individual has to decide which of two or three things to do depending on what signal is given. Performance deteriorates in this task as BALs increase. Similarly, if the person driving home from a party is confronted with the need to shift his attention, recognize a new situation, and decide what to do, he may very well be involved in an accident.[6]

Alcohol use has been shown to have two other effects that seem relevant. Alcohol increases the variability in performance of all tasks in a dose-related way. Increased variability increases the likelihood of error, even if no error is made under no-stress conditions. One author[7] has suggested that the better drivers are more consistent in their performance and that variability is a signal of poor control of the driving situation. The last effect to be mentioned is that alcohol-impaired individuals do not recognize their impairment and, in fact, may see their performance as improving. This belief that performance is better than normal may be the basis for increased risk taking under the influence of alcohol, which is reported by some, but not all, investigators.

If you want to boil all of the preceding down to its fundamentals, it is probably

> that human limits of attention and memory are the prime source of limitations in man-machine control situations . . . it appears that accidents occur in those circumstances where the amount of information required to be processed to control a vehicle is beyond the capacity of the driver.[5,p.1]

Clearly, alcohol and similar drugs increase information-processing capacity.

Problem-drinker drivers

Different facets of driving are important causes of accidents for different groups of individuals. An excellent survey and on-location investigation of the causes of traffic accidents[8] was done in such a way that its information is probably representative of national statistics. They found that in 57% of all accidents *only* human factors were involved. Additionally, human factors were definitely involved in 84% and probably involved in all but 1% of all accidents. Vehicle (for example, bad brakes) and environmental conditions (like wet roads) were much less important as causes of accidents.

Excessive speed is a major factor in 10% of all accidents, and the only age group in which it is disproportionately high is the less-than-20 group. Of all the accident causes identified by these researchers, excessive speed is the only factor that is highest in this age group. This means that these individuals do not have bad driving habits in general—they just drive too fast. And with deadly results: excessive speed is the biggest factor in fatal accidents for males in this age range.

Drivers in the age range from 45 to 54 drive slower but are probably sloppy and casual drivers, since inattention (attending to things other than driving) and improper lookout (pulling away from a stop sign into the path of another vehicle) are highest in this age group as causes of accidents. You should also know that these two accident causes, inattention and improper lookout, increase with educational level—the absent-minded teacher may be a danger on the highway!

These researchers also found that alcohol impairment was a significant factor in almost 4% of the accidents and other drug impairment in over 2%. Alcohol-related accidents are very different from those which do not involve alcohol.[9] They are not distributed equally throughout the day or week but cluster in the late night and early morning and on Fridays and Saturdays (in one study, half of all accidents occurred on these two days). Most alcohol-related accidents involve a single vehicle and single occupant, and in over half the vehicle runs into a fixed object. (It should be mentioned that speed at impact is less than 30 miles per hour for 50% of these accidents.)

The point of all this is that alcohol-related accidents are not just like all other accidents except that they occur to people with alcohol in their systems. Accidents that are alcohol related are quite different from other accidents, and the drivers of these cars are also different.[10] The major difference is the amount of alcohol consumed and the frequency with which it is used. In one typical study,[11] more than half of the first-offender individuals arrested for driving while intoxicated (DWI) had drinking habits that were clearly indicative of a problem with drinking. High levels of alcohol intake, memory lapses and blackouts, starting the day with a drink, and similar behaviors obviously separate this individual from the social drinker who "had one too many."

This poses real problems for efforts to reduce alcohol-related accidents. Problem drinking and alcoholism are not behaviors that can be eliminated by 10 to 20 hours in a DWI school. A very large project by the U.S. Department of Transportation has studied the effect of putting drunk drivers through driver safety programs. The final report in 1976 was not very encouraging. "In general, it would appear fair to conclude that the individual analytic studies submitted in 1973 and 1974 provided no overwhelming evidence of program effectiveness as measured by reductions in crash or arrest recidivism."[12,p.51] Much good information was collected, however. Recidivists usually showed higher BALs at the time of their arrest than did the nonrecidivists, and this supports again the contention that problem drinkers account for a high percentage of alcohol-related, and serious, accidents.[13]

Not all drivers arrested under DWI charges are problem drinkers. On a 3-year follow-up about 70% of these "nonproblem" drinkers were not arrested again on a DWI charge even if DWI school was not attended. Attendance at a DWI school improved that rate so that 80% were not rearrested. Results over the same period for problem drinkers were 60% not arrested for those who did not attend DWI school and 64% of those who did attend. There are reports of effective treatment programs for DWI individuals[14] but there is not yet any evidence that these programs will work in other cities.

In fact, nothing has yet worked well for any pe-riod of time. But maybe every little bit helps. Britain passed a laws in 1967 that mandated a 1-year license suspension for drivers found with a BAL of 0.08% or more. The immediate effect was dramatic: a 66% drop in fatalities and serious injuries on weekends during the first month. Probably everyone was scared! Slowly, however, the fatality and serious accident rate returned so that 3 years later it was at the level where it would have been even without the law.[15] Still, 3 years is better than nothing.

As a driver who may sometimes drink, you should know that since 1972 all states have laws stating that if you obtain a license from the state, you automatically consent to be willing to take a chemical test to determine alcohol concentration in the body. However, in only 12 states are the laws phrased so that the implied consent also holds for other drugs.[16] In every state but one the BAL for legal intoxication is 0.1%; in Utah it is 0.08%.

One other thing to remember is that when the Twenty-Sixth Amendment was ratified in 1971 giving 18-year-olds the right to vote, many states argued that if you're old enough to vote, you're old enough to drink! Twenty-nine states lowered their legal drinking age—usually to age 18. In the mid-seventies studies showing large increases in alcohol-related auto accidents in the 18 to 21 age range led 15 of those states to reverse their decision and raise their minimum drinking age. A 1981 report showed that when Maine and Michigan raised the minimum age for drinking there was a 17% drop in traffic accidents in the age group affected.[17] When a drug is more available, more people use it. When more people use a drug, more people abuse it.

The motto "If you drive, don't drink. If you drink, don't drive" is true for all of us, even though it is the problem drinker, not the social drinker, who is most involved in traffic fatalities. When the police stop you at a New Year's Eve roadblock, it's for real—not just to let you know they are working. They know, and now you should, that the drunk driver is not usually dead drunk but has a good chance of becoming one.

Marijuana

The effect of a marijuana high on simple behaviors is minimal or nonexistent. As the task becomes more complex, as speed becomes more important, and as accurate time and distance estimates are involved, there is an increasing impairment of behavior from a single-joint marijuana high. You know that if you drink you shouldn't drive, but what about marijuana? Many studies have reported on the relationship between marijuana and driving ability.[16]

We are still in the early stages of data collection on the effects of marijuana and driving in the real world.

A recent study of 300 drivers responsible for fatal accidents in Boston showed that 39 percent were intoxicated on alcohol, and 16 percent were under the influence of marijuana at the time of the fatal crash. Although it cannot be definitely attributed to an increase in marijuana use while driving, California reported a 46 percent increase for adults and a 71 percent increase for juveniles in driving under the influence of a drug, following the recent change in their marijuana law.[18,p.2]

There is still no simple, easy way to monitor levels of THC (tetrahydrocannabinol, the active agent in marijuana) in the field—as is done with the Breathalyzer and alcohol. This poses major problems.

One of the best studies done in this area looked at the effects on college-age drivers of varying dose levels of the active ingredient in marijuana. The individuals were tested under both restricted driving conditions and on city streets. The authors concluded:

It is evident that the smoking of marijuana by human subjects does have a detrimental effect on their driving skills and performance in a restricted driving area, and that this effect is even greater under normal conditions of driving on city streets. The effect of marijuana on driving is not uniform for all subjects. . . .

What are the recommendations that emerge from this study? Driving under the influence of marijuana should be avoided as much as should driving under the influence of alcohol.[19]

That's probably very good advice, since college-student marijuana users were found to have twice the usual number of traffic accidents in the 6- to 12-month period preceding their conviction on marijuana charges.[20] Another report indicated that marijuana users had as many accidents under the influence of alcohol as they did under the influence of marijuana.

There is no question, however, about the differences between the effects of marijuana and alcohol, in general and on the various components of driving. A brief summary of the laboratory work in this area is still valid: "alcohol impairment is related to division of attention and information processing rate; the effect of marihuana is not. Marihuana may affect perceptual performance in situations where alcohol would not, but the impairment of marihuana appears not to be determined by the demands for information processing from a divided attention task, a factor of prime significance in driving. . . . It is possible . . . that marihuana causes brief dropouts of attention."[5,p.6] And, of course, it may be those lapses of attention which are the relevant factor in marijuana-related accidents, but more work needs to be done—especially out in the real world on the highways.

Concluding comment

Evidence slowly accumulates proving that drugs other than alcohol and marijuana play a role in some auto accidents, including therapeutic drugs prescribed and taken under ideal conditions.[21] The sedatives, the hypnotics, and the minor tranquilizers can all slow down response time and the integration of information that is necessary to drive—and stay alive. As always, with drugs extra precaution is required. Best of all—if you take any drug: have a friend and leave the driving to them.

DRIVING REFERENCES

1. Marijuana, other drugs, and their relation to highway safety; a report to Congress, DOT HS 805 229, February 1980, U.S. Department of Transportation.
2. Borkenstein, R.F., and others: The role of the drinking driver in traffic accidents, Blutalkohol 11(suppl. 1), 1974.

3. Voas, R.B.: Roadside surveys, demographics and BACs of drivers. In Israelstam, S., and Lambert, S., editors: Alcohol, drugs, and traffic safety, Toronto, 1975, Addiction Research Foundation of Ontario.

4. Alcohol and health: new knowledge, National Institute on Alcohol Abuse and Alcoholism, Publication No. (ADM) 75-212, U.S. Department of Health, Education, and Welfare, Washington, D.C., 1975, U.S. Government Printing Office.

5. Moskowitz, H.: Alcohol and drug impairment of the driver, 1973, Society of Automotive Engineers.

6. Shinar, D.: Psychology on the road, the human factor in traffic safety, New York, 1978, John Wiley & Sons.

7. Lewis, R.E.: Consistency and car driving skill, British Journal of Industrial Medicine **13**:131-141, 1956.

8. Tri-level study of the causes of traffic accidents, Bloomington, Ind., 1974, Indiana University, Institute for Research in Public Safety.

9. May, G.W., and Baker, W.E.: Human and environmental factors in alcohol-related traffic accidents. In Israelstam, S., and Lambert, S., editors: Alcohol, drugs, and traffic safety, Toronto, 1975, Addiction Research Foundation of Ontario.

10. Donelson, A.C., and others: Drug research methodology, Vol. 1: The alcohol-highway safety experience and its applicability to other drugs; Final Report, DOT HS 805 374, March, 1980, U.S. Department of Transportation.

11. Fine, E.W., and other: Alcohol abuse in first offenders arrested for driving while intoxicated. In Israelstam, S., and Lambert, S., editors: Alcohol, drugs, and traffic safety, Toronto, 1975, Addiction Research Foundation of Ontario.

12. Program level evaluation of ASAP diagnosis, referral and rehabilitation efforts, Vol. 3, Final Report, September 1976, U.S. Department of Transportation.

13. McGuire, F.L.: "Heavy" and "light" drinking drivers as separate target groups for treatment, American Journal of Drug and Alcohol Abuse, vol. 7, no. 1, 1980.

14. McGuire, F.L.: The effectiveness of a treatment program for the alcohol-involved driver, American Journal of Drug and Alcohol Abuse **5**:517-525, 1978.

15. Ross, H.L.: Law, science, and accidents: the British road safety act of 1967, Journal of Legal Studies **2**(1), 1973.

16. Joscelyn, K.B., and others: Drugs and highway safety 1980, Final Report, DOT HS 805 461, May 1980, U.S. Department of Transportation.

17. Peterson, I.: Drinking age tied to fall in crashes, New York Times, November 4, 1981, p. A18.

18. DuPont, R.L.: Science, values, and the marihuana issue, Paper presented to the Committee on Problems of Drug Dependence, Cambridge, Massachusetts, July 7, 1977.

19. Klonoff, H.: Marijuana and driving in real-life situations, Science **186**:317-324, 1974.

20. Smart, R.G.: Marijuana and driving risk among college students, Journal of Safety Research **6**:155-158, 1974.

21. Joscelyn, K.B., and Donelson, A.C.: Drug research methodology, Vol. 2: the idenfification of drugs of interest in highway safety, Final Report, DOT HS 805 299, March 1980, U.S. Department of Transportation.

CRIME AND VIOLENCE

There is a widespread popular belief that narcotic-drug addiction has in recent years been responsible for much violent crime . . . implanted . . . through the medium of popular articles in newspapers and magazines . . . by the publication of statistics as to the number of addicts in various prisons in the last few years.[1]

Even though that was written in 1925, it has a very contemporary sound. Some things seem to never change when actually they go in cycles. One article[2] studied the "dope fiend mythology" from 1890 to 1970 in the popular, law enforcement, and scientific literature. Myths in popular literature about narcotic users increased from 1915 to 1956 and by 1970 had returned to the lower level that existed at the turn of the century. As you well know from your own reading, there are still a number of myths around. The 1925 article stated that

there is probably no more absurd fallacy extant than the notion that murders are committed and daylight robberies and hold-ups are carried out by men stimulated by large doses of heroin or cocaine which have temporarily distorted them into self-imagined heroes incapable of fear.[1]

We know that was a fallacy in 1925. Is it still?

The belief that there is a close and causal relationship between many forms of drug use and criminality and violent behavior probably forms the basis for many of our laws concerning drug use and drug users. The relationship between crime and illegal drug use or abuse is complex, and only recently have data-based statements become possible. Facts are necessary because political actions are taken and laws are enacted on what we believe to be true.

Harsher criminal penalties for drug users were put into law in New York State on the basis of data collected by the New York Narcotic Addiction Control Commission. The study claimed that "drug addiction costs New York State about $6.5 billion a year in thefts." There is a slight problem: New York City, which has over 80% of the state's heroin addicts, only had $238 million of reported stolen property! It is unlikely that addicts steal more than

25 times the amount of all property reported stolen.

It is true that narcotic addicts engage in a disproportionately high percentage of robberies in which arrests are made. On top of that, probably "less than 1% of the crimes committed by addicts resulted in arrests by the police."[4] The icing on *that* is that in New York City, of all arrests made for drug felonies, only 13% ever served any jail sentence![5] A classic study[6] about the street life of heroin users reported data from New York City in which 16% of the arrests of narcotic addicts were for robbery, while only 13% of *all* arrests (addict and nonaddict) were for robbery. Robbery is one of the few borderline crimes: it can either involve or not involve confrontation of a victim—and thus pose potential physical danger. On the question of the addict and violence, the study commented that heroin users " . . . avoid crimes not involving financial gain . . . where financial gain is involved, as in robbery, the risk of violence is taken by heroin users in a higher percentage of cases than with nonaddicts.[6]

A comprehensive 1971 study of six metropolitan areas by the U.S. Department of Justice reached a similar conclusion in finding that "there is strong evidence that robberies account for a large proportion of arrest charges among 'Current Drug Users' (18.3%), a considerably higher proportion than among arrestees for which there is no evidence of drug usage at any time (11.3%)."[7,p.385] They did reaffirm the relationship between narcotic users and robbery but they also reported:

> For all drug substances considered, i.e., heroin, cocaine, morphine, methadone, marijuana, hashish, amphetamines, barbiturates, tranquilizers, psychedelics, and special substances such as glue, ether, etc., the distributions of arrest charges for "Users" of these substances versus "Nonusers" are either essentially the same (no significant differences) or significantly different in that "Drug Users" are *less often involved* in crimes of violence including homicide, rape, kidnapping, and aggravated assault.[7,p.383]

That may have been true in the 1960s, but the world is continually changing. Remember that individuals who use drugs, including those addicted to narcotics, are cut from the same pattern and cast in the same mold as you and I. Our society is becoming more violent—violent crimes have increased at a faster rate than nonviolent crimes since 1960—and it should be expected that drug users would become more involved in violent crimes. And they have. A summary of much research and many interviews by one of the major researchers in this field stated in 1977[8] that "the most disturbing of all our most recent findings, the contemporary addict is much more likely to commit crimes against persons than his counterpart in earlier years." The report continued:

> Probably as many as two-thirds of all addicts now engage in crimes against persons (usually muggings and armed robberies) and as many as one-third of all addicts commit these crimes as their primary means of support.[8]

This group has reported regularly on the evolving relationship between narcotic use and criminal activity and has suggested that one reason for the change is that "the younger narcotic addicts appear to be criminal opportunists—whatever criminal opportunity presents itself attracts this contemporary addict."[9,p.140] The younger addict, as with most young people, is less skilled, more impulsive, and more active than the older addict, and this may contribute to the changing pattern of criminal behavior.

That may not be true only of narcotic addicts. A 1979 study of delinquent boys, aged 12 to 18, who had been committed to a training school compared those who had committed an offense against a person to those who had committed an offense against property. The study found that ". . . person-offenders were significantly older, came from larger communities, abused a greater number of drugs, had higher asocial index scores, and had lower full-scale IQ scores than property-only offenders."[10,p.1444] The *number* of different drugs abused was the best simple factor separating person- and property-offenders.

One perennial concern is the relationship between the street price of heroin and the amount of crime committed. Higher heroin prices could increase crime, or they could drive addicts into treatment programs and, thus, decrease crime. The results of several studies on the relationship between crime and the price of heroin are ambiguous. Nine cities were studied, and "both positive and negative effects (in some cases significant) are estimated."[11] In New York City a strong relationship was found: only crimes associated with revenue raising—robbery, larceny, and auto theft—increased with increases in heroin prices. An excellent study in Detroit by these same investigators

> has shown that the level of property crime in Detroit is in part affected by the price of heroin. When the price rises, crime rises. When the price falls, crime falls. This finding supports the general hypothesis that criminal heroin users as a class try to maintain their level of consumption in the face of price increases, and that they rely partly on property crime for the additional funds. The level of personal crime is little affected by the price of heroin.[12]

There is one final question on the relationship of narcotic use and criminal behavior: Which usually comes first?

> In England, where addicts do not have to steal in order to buy their drugs but steal anyway, people conclude that addict-thieves are thieves first and addicts second; in America where addicts steal and drugs are expensive, people conclude that addict-thieves are addicts first and thieves second.[13,p.62]

The Department of Justice study[7] spoke to this question and gave a mixed answer. From the data they presented it seems that for those who began drug use in the 1960-1963 period, there was a significant increase in conviction rate following onset of drug use from the predrug-use period. Those who started in the 1964-1967 period also showed an increase in convictions after the start of drug use, but it was no greater than that of the nondrug group.

Beginning in the mid-seventies, however, there is no ambiguity. Several good studies point in the same direction: a positive relationship exists between beginning narcotic drug use and profit-producing crime that may or may not involve the threat

of violence. A 1976 study[14] in Washington, D.C., of heroin addicts in a treatment program reported that only one fourth of the heroin addicts interviewed showed no change in level or type of criminal activity following onset of drug use. About 40% of the addicts reported an increase in the level of criminal activity but no change in the type, which was usually robbery. Of those interviewed, 30% had no preaddiction criminal behavior but learned it following addiction. One very detailed study of the criminal behavior of self-admitted narcotic addicts jailed in Denver reported confirming results. These were mostly males (84%) under the age of 30 (70%):

> In summary, the onset of addiction is highly associated with substantial increases in property acquisitive crime and dramatic increases in violent and drug offense crimes. The data lead to the conclusion that the onset of addiction realizes an increase in all criminal activity.[15]

A final comment, as of the late seventies:

> Addicts today are much more likely to be criminally involved *prior* to using drugs than they were in the past. My work would indicate almost all contemporary addicts engaged in criminal acts prior to becoming addicted and from ⅓ to ⅔ had been arrested prior to the onset of narcotic use . . . most of these persons were criminals long before the onset of drug use.[8]

This is probably true. However, a 1981 report suggests just how much criminal activity increases during periods of addiction. "When addicts were not dependent on heroin, their crime rate was 84% lower than when they were regularly using the drug."[16,p.22] Put another way, when using heroin their crime rate increased 600%! Reducing addiction will certainly result in lower crime rates.

The emphasis thus far has been on narcotic users and addicts, and a brief summary may tie the ends together. Some individuals begin criminal behavior only after the start of addiction, but the majority of addicts are criminals first and addicts second. Of addicts who were previously engaged in crime, perhaps more than half increase their criminal activity after the onset of addiction. The emphasis in addict crime is on money: if confrontation or violence is necessary to produce revenue, then addicts will engage in it. The developing trends are for an increase in the relationship of narcotic addiction and criminal activity, including the threat of, or actual, physical harm to the victim. There are multiple reports that criminal activity decreases—sometimes to zero—when an addict is in a treatment program.[17,18] Many return to their previous lifestyles when they leave the program. It needs to be reaffirmed that there is, to this time, no evidence that nonaddictive illegal drug use results in an increase in criminal behavior.[19,20,21] Additional comment needs to be made on the relationship between violence and aggression and certain specific drugs.

Alcohol and barbiturates

The angry, fighting drunk is a well-known stereotype. It is not completely false. A 1972 review of the literature concluded that "a large number of studies indicate that alcohol, the most widely used drug in the world, is clearly linked with violent crime. In many assaultive and sexually assaultive situations alcohol is present in both assailant and victim."[22,pp.75-76] You may not appreciate that most homicides are among people who know each other—and alcohol use is associated with over three fifths of all murders. Of all reported assaults, 40% involve alcohol, as do one third of forcible rape and child-molesting cases.[19,23] One study of adolescents in prison for assault reported in 1981 that alcohol was involved in 61% of their assaults resulting in tissue damage and in 67% of assaults resulting in death.[24]

One report[25] of individuals arrested for violent crimes looked at their blood alcohol levels. Table 4-1 shows a good relationship: there are fewer individuals with very high or low blood alcohol levels. Note well that these are apprehended individuals; the overall relationship between violent crime and alcohol level may be higher or lower.

A longitudinal study of males born between 1944 and 1954 reported in 1976 that "those who had used alcohol were more likely to report fights as a consequence than were users of the other drugs. When

TABLE 4-1 Blood alcohol level in arrestees for violent crimes

Blood alcohol level	Percentage of arrestees
0	12
0-0.09	9
0.1-0.19	26
0.2-0.29	30
0.3-0.39	18
0.4 and over	3

From Shupe, L.M.: Alcohol and crime, Criminal Law, Criminology, and Police Science 44(5):661-664, 1954.

only the heavy and heaviest users of alcohol were examined, some 38 percent reported fights resulting from their use of alcohol."[26,p.78]

A 1980 review of the world literature—although critical of many studies on its topic of Alcohol, Violence and Aggression—concluded: "It is quite clear that consumption of alcohol is associated with a wide range of violent acts which include accident, suicide, sexual assault, violence within the family, felony and homicide."[27,p.114]

A report on barbiturate users concluded:

Intoxication with barbiturates is similar to alcohol, and is usually accompanied by a sense of well being or "disinhibition euphoria." Like alcohol intoxication, a barbiturate "high" produces a reduction in the ability to make accurate judgments and decreased control of voluntary body movements.[28]

Since the barbiturates and alcohol are cut from the same pharmacological cloth, it should not be too surprising that the behavioral effects are similar. Of particualr note may be the relationship between secobarbital and aggression. It may be that other barbiturates in the same general class would have similar effects, but one group of assaultive youthful offenders reported that they expected to be more aggressive when they used secobarbital, and they were.[24] They had to work at staying awake and moving—literally, they were "fighting to stay awake." To counter the depressant effects, they needed much stimulation—and aggression is one way to increase stimulation!

Amphetamine

Amphetamine, and other stimulants to some extent, has two effects that suggest a relationship to violent behavior. Even low doses increase activity level, and, as the dose increases, there is an increase in feelings of power and capability. Large doses used chronically or an abrupt increase in the amount of amphetamine used frequently causes a paranoid, psychotic reaction. This latter behavior is primarily associated with the injection of amphetamine—speed freaks.

One authority has stated:

> From all evidence, amphetamines do tend to set up conditions in which violent behavior is more likely to occur than would be the case had the individual not used it. Suspiciousness and hyperactivity may combine to induce precipitous and unwarranted assaultative behavior. Under the influence of amphetamines, lability of mood is common, the user abruptly shifting from warmly congenial to furiously hostile moods for the most trivial of reasons.[29,p.16]

There were multiple reports of the association of amphetamine use and violence and aggression in the late 1960s and early 1970s. In almost every case large amounts of amphetamines were used, which resulted in suspicious ideas and hostile behavior. This type of emotional arousal can easily explode into violence and homicide if the appropriate conditions are met. Users of large amounts of amphetamine (especially if taken by injection) are good people to stay away from. (See Chapter 14.)

One study[30] of 13 amphetamine abusers who committed murder while under the influence of amphetamine reported that seven were paranoid at the time of the killing, three were impulsive, and two panicked during a robbery. This triad of paranoid ideas, impulsive behavior, and hypersensitivity is directly related to the pharmacological actions of the amphetamines, no matter what the personality of the user is in the absence of the drug.

In interviews with assaultive and nonassaultive adolescents,[24] amphetamine was not very much related to assaultive behavior in these males. Mark well, though, that these individuals were primarily using moderate doses of amphetamine taken orally; they were not injecting the drug.

A review of the world literature on amphetamine use and crime and/or violence de-emphasized the large-dose users and the resulting paranoia predisposing to hostility and violence. It was then possible for the author to generalize and conclude, truthfully, that "the use of amphetamine per se is not particularly conducive to violence. The outbreak of violence in association with amphetamine use must be approached from a multivariate perspective. . . ."[31] There is clear evidence, though, that high doses of amphetamine result in paranoid suspiciousness, and that, coupled with hyperactivity and hypersensitivity, makes aggressive behavior very probable.

Cannabis

Most of the research has been concerned with marijuana use rather than with the more potent forms of *Cannabis*. Very little discussion is needed. The stories in the popular press in the 1930s (prior to the passage of the Marijuana Tax Act) that related marijuana use with crimes of great violence were just that—stories made up by those who wanted to outlaw marijuana. (See Chapter 19.) The general relationship between marijuana use and violence was summarized in 1972:

> During the past seventy-five years several distinguished commissions have investigated evidence of the possible role of marihuana in criminal behavior and reached strikingly similar conclusions: the behavioral effects of marihuana do not usually incite violent or sexual crimes; rather, the use of marihuana may reduce the possibility of aggression in most people. Recent laboratory and clinical studies support these conclusions. . . .[32]

A review article[33] looked at the available information and stated, "The main impression from the available evidence is that in general, use of marijuana is not a major cause of aggression." This article also points out that there are individuals with "a prior history of violent behavior associated with poor impulse control, and the use of drugs such as marijuana may reduce inhibitory control even further." That is always a possibility with not only marijuana but most other drugs and serves to emphasize one of our recurring themes: there are no safe drugs, only drugs used safely.

One further specific precaution is that in some social situations *Cannabis* may increase irritability and aggression. There is good evidence in animal studies "that in combination with stress, cannabis can induce aggressive behavior."[33] The evidence is much less clear with respect to human behavior, and the possibility is still being studied.

Concluding comment

A superb article,[34] which contains more useful and important information than many books, looked at many relationships between drugs and crime and violence; two are important here. In thinking about the data in Tables 4-2 and 4-3 there are three major points to remember: (1) the results on drug use and the results on involvement with the criminal justice system are self-reports of the individuals; (2) the groups are not exclusive, users are grouped by their primary drug of abuse; and (3) these individuals are regular users of the drug or, at least, well beyond the experimental-user level.

The data in Table 4-3 should not surprise anyone—but it's nice to see the information in black and white, the result of a reasonable study. The two surprises in Table 4-2 may be the high involvement of inhalant abusers and the low involvement of alcohol abusers in criminal activity and the criminal justice system. These results may in part result from the fact that inhalant users are among the youngest at first involvement with the police and alcohol abusers are among the oldest at first involvement.

This section has avoided almost all mention of drug offenses—obviously drug users will have more than nondrug users. Most addicts are sellers as well as users, so they frequently have multiple drug charges placed against them.[35] If the predic-

TABLE 4-2 Criminal activity and involvement with criminal justice system of regular drug users* (1 is highest, 11 is lowest)

Drug used	Index number
Inhalants	3.0
Heroin	3.6
Cocaine	3.9
Other opiates	4.1
Illegal methadone	4.8
Barbiturates	5.6
Amphetamines	6.0
Hallucinogens	6.8
Minor tranquilizers	8.3
Marijuana	9.9
Alcohol	10.0

*Involvement: includes young age at start, severity of offense, number of offenses, sentences, etc.

TABLE 4-3 Commission of crime for the support of a substance abuse habit (percent of regular users of the substance)

Drug used	Percent
Illegal methadone	55
Heroin	44
Cocaine	41
Other opiates	40
Barbiturates	29
Amphetamines	26
Inhalants	23
Minor tranquilizers	22
Marijuana	22
Alcohol	20
Hallucinogens	19

tions are right, the relationship between crime and illegal narcotic use will continue to increase into the mid-1980s. One possible bright spot is the declining number of young people; with fewer individuals available to misuse and abuse drugs, the magnitude of the problem will at least decrease. That may be a frail straw to grasp at, but . . .

CRIME AND VIOLENCE REFERENCES

1. Kolb, L.: Drug addiction in its relation to crime, Mental Hygiene 9(1):74-89, 1925.
2. Reasons, C.E.: Images of crime and the criminal: the dope fiend mythology, Journal of Research in Crime and Delinquency 13(2):133-143, 1976.
3. Fellows of the Drug Abuse Council: Disabusing drug abuse, Social Policy 4(5):43-45, 1974.
4. Ball, J.C., and others: The impact of heroin addiction upon criminality. In Harris, L.S., editor: Problems of drug dependence, NIDA Research monograph 27, Washington, D.C., 1979, U.S. Government Printing Office.
5. Grizzle, G.A.: Law enforcement policies directed toward illicit drug selling and usage, Journal of Psychoactive Drugs 13(3):227-234, 1981.
6. Preble, E., and Casey, J.J.: Taking care of business—the heroin user's life on the street, International Journal of the Addictions 4(1):1-14, 1969.
7. Eckerman, W.C., and others: Drug usage and arrest charges, Bureau of Narcotics and Dangerous Drugs, Department of Justice, December, 1971.
8. Chambers, C.D.: A review of recent sociological and epidemiological studies in substance abuse. Text of paper presented at the Neurobiology Seminar, Vanderbilt University, Nashville, Tenn., May 6, 1977.
9. Chambers, C.D.: Narcotic addiction and crime: an empirical review. In Incoiardi, J.A., and Chambers, C.D., editors: Drugs and the criminal justice system, Beverly Hills, Calif., 1974, Sage Publications, Inc.
10. Simonds, J.F., and Kashani, J.: Drug abuse and criminal behavior in delinquent boys committed to a training school, American Journal of Psychiatry 136(11):1444, 1979.
11. Brown, G.F., and Silvermon, L.P.: The retail price of heroin: estimations and applications, Journal of the American Statistical Association (Applications Section) 69(347):595-606, 1974.
12. Silverman, L.P., and Spruill, N.L.: Urban crime and the price of heroin, Journal of Urban Economics 4:80-103, 1977.
13. Gould, L.C.: Crime and the addict: beyond common sense. In Incoiardi, J.A., and Chambers, C.D., editors: Drugs and the criminal justice system, Beverly Hills, Calif., 1974, Sage Publications, Inc.
14. Baridon, P.: Addiction, crime and social policy, Lexington, Mass., 1976, Lexington Books (D.C. Heath & Co.).
15. Weissman, J.C., and others: Addiction and criminal behavior: a continuing examination of criminal addicts, Journal of Drug Issues 6:153-165, 1976.
16. Ball, J.C., and others: cited in Study stresses link between heroin dependence and incidence of crime, New York Times, March 22, 1981, p. 22.
17. Dupont, R.L.: Heroin addiction treatment and crime reduction, American Journal of Psychiatry 128:7, 90-94, 1972.
18. Newman, R.G., and others: Arrest histories before and after admission to a methadone maintenance treatment program, Contemporary Drug Problems 2(3):417-430, 1973.
19. Alcohol and health: new knowledge, National Institute on Alcohol Abuse and Alcoholism, 1974, Publication No. (ADM) 75-212, U.S. Department of Health, Education, and Welfare, Washington, D.C., 1975, U.S. Government Printing Office.
20. Greenberg, S.W., and Adler, F.: Crime and addiction: an empirical analysis of the literature, 1920-1973, Contemporary Drug Problems, pp. 221-270, 1975.
21. Kandel, D.: Convergence in perspective longitudinal surveys in drug use in normal populations, research in psychopathology. Presented at the Society for Life History, Fort Worth, Tex., October 1976.
22. Tinklenberg, J.R.: Drugs and crime. Consultant's report for the National Commission on Marihuana and Drug Abuse, October 1972.
23. Tinklenberg, J.R.: Alcohol and violence. In Alcoholism, progress in research and treatment, New York, 1973, Academic Press, Inc.
24. Tinklenberg, J.R., and others: Drugs and criminal assaults by adolescents: a replication study, Journal of Psychoactive Drugs 13(3):277-288, 1981.
25. Shupe, L.M.: Alcohol and crime, Criminal Law, Criminology, and Police Science 44:661-664, 1954.
26. O'Donnell, J.A., and others: Young men and drugs—a nationwide survey, National Institute of Drug Abuse Research Monograph 5, February 1976.
27. Evans, C.M.: Alcohol, violence and aggression, British Journal on Alcohol and Alcoholism 15(3):104-115, 1980.
28. Wesson, D.R., and Smith, D.E.: Barbiturate use as an intoxicant: a San Francisco perspective. Testimony given to the Subcommittee to Investigate Juvenile Delinquency, December 15, 1971.
29. Kramer, J.C. In Amphetamines, Fourth report by the Select Committee on Crime, House Report No. 91-1807, Washington, D.C., 1971, U.S. Government Printing Office.
30. Ellinwood, E.H.: Assault and homicide associated with amphetamine abuse, American Journal of Psychiatry 127(9):90-95, 1971.
31. Greenberg, S.W.: The relationship between crime and amphetamine abuse: an empirical review of the literature, Contemporary Drug Problems pp. 101-130, Summer 1976.
32. Tinklenberg, J.R., and Murphy, P.: Marijuana and crime: a survey report, Journal of Psychedelic Drugs 5:183-191, 1972.
33. Abel, E.L.: The relationship between cannabis and violence: a review, Psychological Bulletin 84:193-211, 1977.
34. Incinard, J.A.: Crime and alternative patterns of substance abuse. In Gardner, S.E., editor: Drug and alcohol abuse: implications for treatment, HHS No. 80-958, National Institute on Drug Abuse, Washington, D.C., 1981, U.S. Government Printing Office.
35. Drug use and crime: report of Panel on Drug Use and Criminal Behavior, prepared for National Institute on Drug Abuse, September 1976.

SPORTS

Forty or more years ago the only discussion that would have included both the use of drugs and a sporting event involved horse racing. Everyone knew that drugs were sometimes used to decrease the pain of an injury or to imporve the performance of a healthy animal. Not that drugs were approved of—there just wasn't any way to really determine their use, and besides, not too many people cared all that much. The disqualification of the winner of the 1968 Kentucky Derby, Dancer's Image, because of the presence of an anti-inflammatory agent (phenylbutazone, "bute") in the urine didn't bother many people—by 1975 it or similar drugs were approved for use before races in 23 racing states.

Many changes have since occurred, some coming in only the early eighties. Most states now ban the administration of "any foreign substance" to a horse in the 24 hours preceding a race. Appropriate testing is also mandated.[1]

Before discussing the use of drugs by humans participating in athletic events it is necessary to give some basic information about athletic activity. Different events require different muscle capabilities and combinations of capabilities, but there seem to be five primary factors: (1) strength, (2) endurance, (3) speed, (4) coordination, and (5) flexibility. There are, of course, many other factors that contribute to the final performance, such as motivation, training, compatibility of the sport with the individual's personality,[2] and genetically fixed factors.[3]

Strength is most closely linked to muscle mass; muscle mass is increased only by muscle work. Endurance is dependent on the delivery of oxygen to the working muscles and on the availability of glycogen stored in the working muscles. Speed has a large genetic component but in most sports is related to endurance, strength, and training. Coordination, which depends on the interaction of the nervous system and muscles, seems to have some clear genetic limits, but training can move individuals closer to their limits. Flexibility seems to be limited primarily by the type and amount of exercise.[4,5]

Drugs and other procedures are used to influence and improve any and all of these factors. Some work, some don't. Before commenting on specific drugs some nondrug approaches will be mentioned. Most people know that if you train at a high altitude and compete at sea level, your endurance should be improved—the rationale being that higher altitudes—and thus a lower level of oxygen in the air—will cause an increase in the oxygen-carrying capability of the blood. Competing at lower altitudes with greater oxygen-delivery capability should increase endurance.

A more efficient way to increase the oxygen-carrying capacity of the blood is *blood doping*. This process consists of withdrawing about 1 liter of an athlete's blood, holding it for 9 to 12 weeks while hemoglobin levels return to normal, and then reintroducing the withdrawn blood into the athlete's body just before competition. A 1981 review found that ". . . the majority of 13 new studies support the physiological rationale and efficacy of the use of blood doping to increase endurance capacity."[6,p.59] For example: there has been reported an average decrease of 45 seconds in the time it takes to run 5 miles on a treadmill!

All manipulations of the number of red blood cells—and their hemoglobin carrying oxygen—presuppose an adequate level of iron. For most of the readers of this book this is not a problem. Women are at a higher risk for anemia, because of the loss of blood during menstruation, even in well-fed middle-class America.[4]

Increased nutritional and physiological information has resulted in an eating regimen called "carbohydrate loading." This *doubles* the amount of glycogen stored in the muscles, thereby increasing endurance. It works. In the week prior to competition, for the first 3 to 4 days it is necessary to vigorously use the muscles involved in the competition and cut back drastically on carbohydrate intake; for the next 3 to 4 days a very high, residue-free, carbohydrate intake and a very low level of training is required. The worst thing an athlete can do is eat protein before competition.[4]

One of the waste products from the use of muscle glycogen for energy is lactic acid. Its accumulation is associated with both fatigue and the development of pain. Some athletes use vitamin B_{15}, pangamic acid, to increase endurance. Although the chemical formula of the substance used may vary, the active agent is probably dimethylglycine (DMG), a normal intermediate in choline metabolism. The Food and Drug Administration (FDA) calls vitamin B_{15} a food additive (not a vitamin) that has no value and is attempting to remove it from the marketplace. There have been some reports that vitamin B_{15} lowers blood lactic acid and that it increases oxygen utilization by muscle. Other reports are negative on all counts. Until more is known about its effects and its safety, vitamin B_{15} is a good chemical not to use.[7]

Another interesting study showed that competitive athletes are not any less sensitive to the pain that accompanies fatiguing muscles than are noncompetitive athletes. What separates these two groups is that the competitive athlete learns to accept and tolerate the pain. Competitive athletes feel the pain but they persist because they know they must if they are to be successful.[8]

One last preliminary topic: the use of drugs in amateur sporting events has been a matter of great concern.[9] Urine tests for drugs were introduced in the Winter Olympic Games at Grenoble in 1968 and have been expanded and sophisticated for each of the Olympic Games since. Rule 27 of the Olympic Medical Code states that a competitor who refuses ". . . to take a doping test or who is found guilty of doping shall be eliminated." In the 1972 Olympics at Munich, 12 of 2049 samples contained banned drugs; over 200 drugs are currently banned. As of 1976 testing was automated and computerized.[10] In May 1982 the International Olympic Committee (IOC) prohibited the use of caffeine and testosterone by Olympic athletes. Random urine tests for these two substances during the 1980 Moscow Games showed that the majority of specimens had significant levels of one or both of these substances.

Professional organizations have been more casual about drug use by the players. The National Football League banned amphetamines in 1971 but decided against urine screens because they were an "invasion of privacy." Their first effort on player education was a 1973 locker room sign that read in part: "It is League policy that the use by NFL players of any nonprescribed drugs . . . is not in your interest. . . ."[11] The National Basketball Association didn't even have a committee on drug education until 1980.[12] Things probably won't change unless there is a major scandal or serious injuries related to drug use.

Stimulants

> There seems to be no public condemnation of the use of coffee by athletes, either before an athletic contest, or in ordinary living. Nevertheless, caffeine produces the same general sort of central stimulation and reduction of fatigue that is characteristic of the amphetamines, the only difference being that the effects of caffeine are commonly less than those of the amphetamines. . . . In contrast to public indignation at the use of amphetamines to increase physical performance, the situation regarding caffeine is an interesting commentary on what constitutes social acceptability. It seems that what has long been used, what is well established in social custom, and about which people think they know the facts generally, are sufficient to assure social acceptability.[13,pp.126-127]

As just noted, that statement from 1958 may no longer hold.

Amphetamine and caffeine are the only two stimulants in wide use in sports. Three effects of caffeine are of primary interest: (1) delay in the decline of performance over time; (2) decrease in the feeling of exertion during activity; and (3) increased speed of gastric emptying. In one study trained cyclists were given 250 mg of caffeine before and then another 250 mg divided over a 2-hour cycling period. Three results are clear, straightforward, and of special interest: (1) work productivity increased 7%; (2) the cyclists did not feel they were working harder; and (3) fat oxidation increased 31% during the last hour of work, thus sparing the muscle glycogen and increasing the capacity for endurance.[14]

An excellent 1981 review of the effects of am-

TABLE 4-4 Three dose ranges of amphetamine administration

Dose, mg	Life role	NFL position	Rationale
5-10	Author	Quarterback	Creative performance
	Composer	Wide receiver	Energy
	Housewife	Defensive back	
	Executive		
	Artist		
	Musician		
15-45	Soldier	Special team	Fearlessness[a]
	Hyperactive child	Linebacker	Stability
	Anxious depressive	Offensive lineman	
50-200	Speed freak	Defensive end	Manic high
		Defensive tackle	Paranoid rage

From Mandell, A.J., Stewart, K.D., and Russo, P.V.: The Sunday Syndrome: from Kinetics to altered consciousness, Federation Proceedings **40**:2693-2698, 1971.

phetamine on athletic performance concludes: ". . . there is indeed an amphetamine margin in sports. It is small but important."[15,p.2689] The most extensive study was published in 1959[16] and looked at amphetamine effects on the performance of swimmers, runners, and weight throwers. It concluded, "This study has shown that the performance of highly trained athletes, of the classes studied, can be significantly improved in the majority of cases (about 75%) by the administration of amphetamine." There are a few other studies, but not many. Most of the experimenting is carried out on the playing field, not in the laboratory. Success in the laboratory results in published papers and the spread of knowledge. Success on the playing field results in greater secrecy, higher salaries, or greater glory. "There is an amphetamine margin. It is usually small, amounting to a few percent under most circumstances. But even when that tiny, it can surely spell the difference between a gold medal and sixth place."[15,p.2691]

Not all athletes use amphetamines to increase strength and/or endurance. Very interesting commentaries on amphetamine use by professional football players appear in several places.[2,17] Table 4-4 shows some of the relationships among user, drug dose, and desired effect. The probable basis

for these effects of amphetamine are discussed in Chapter 14.

Anabolic steroids

Testosterone, the male sex hormone, has two primary types of action: androgenic and anabolic. The androgenic effects are those that are masculinizing, causing the growth of the accessory sex glands and the larynx, changing the amount and distribution of body hair, etc. The anabolic effects stimulate the growth of muscle. Anabolic steroids are synthetic modifications of testerone that are designed to enhance the anabolic actions and decrease the androgenic effects. As one writer put it—compared to testosterone that anabolic steroids should give "more muscle per whisker."

The supposed basis for the positive effects of anabolic steroids is that they increase muscle size and strength. Not all groups of athletes want or need greater bulk or strength, but those that do—football players, weight lifters—are reported to use the anabolic steroids extensively. Urine testing, which was possible beginning in 1973, confirms some use: in the Montreal Olympic games seven male weight lifters (from six nations) had positive tests and were disqualified, resulting in the return of two gold medals and one silver medal!

The big questions are: Do the anabolic steroids work? Are they safe? These questions have answers that few coaches accept.

> . . . in spite of claims made by some of the investigators that the use of anabolic steroids by male athletes in conjunction with progressive weight resistance training will afford a greater increase in lean muscle bulk, and greater strength than by weight resistance training alone, there is, in fact, no substantial evidence that this is so. On the contrary, there is a substantial body of evidence . . . to indicate that anabolic steroids will not contribute to gains in lean muscle bulk or muscle strength in healthy young adults males.[18,p.2684]

> Administration of androgenic-anabolic steroids to healthy adult males reduces their output of testosterone and gonadotrophins and reduces spermatogenesis.[18,p.2685]

Not only don't the anabolic steroids make guys big and strong, they decrease fertility and the production of the masculinizing hormones. Long-term effects are unknown. Remember that these agents have some androgenic effects—their use by females will result in masculinization, for example, the growth of facial hair.

In all honesty, two things are not yet known. One is the effect of the high doses used by the competing athletes. It is clear, though, that the doses are not safe. The second unknown is the effect of anabolic steroids on the still growing male. It is unlikely that controlled studies will be done, but probable effects are accelerated bone growth and muscle growth in response to work, as well as an accelerated overall rate of maturation. The result of rapid maturation would be a decrease in maximum height.[4,p.96]

Female sex hormones have been used to feminize males so that they can compete in women's events. The woman's gold medal sprinter in the 1964 Olympics was shown by chromosome testing to be a male; she/he had to return the medal! Cyproterone, an antiandrogenic agent, has probably been used to delay puberty in females. This is particularly important in gymnasts since puberty shifts the center of gravity lower in the body and changes body proportions in ways that adversely affect ability. In gymnastics, small is good: the top three Soviet gymnasts in 1978 international competition were 17 or 18 years old but their height and weight were: 53 inches, 63 pounds; 60 inches, 92 pounds; and 57 inches, 79 pounds.

The final whistle

Athletic events are another arena in which we can expect the use of drugs to increase. Winning may not be everything, but if winning means fame or fortune then everything possible will be used to increase the likelihood of winning. The U.S. Olympic Committee organized a sports medicine committee in 1977 to study world class and other athletes to determine optimal training programs. It's hard to believe that they will not evaluate the effects of drugs on performance.[19] Whether they do or not, we all know that coaches and trainers will evaluate drug effects on performance—not *here*, of course, but they will at that other school!

SPORTS REFERENCES

1. Crist, S.: Federal threat spurs thoroughbred drug reform, New York Times, September 10, 1980, p. B8.
2. Mandell, A.J.: The nightmare season, New York, 1976, Random House.
3. Dunn, K.: Twin studies and sports: estimating the future? The Physician And Sports Medicine 9(5):131-136, 1981.
4. Smith, N.J.: Nutrition and athletic performance, Medical Times, p. 92, August 1981.
5. Mead, W.F., and Hartwig, R.: Fitness evaluation and exercise prescription; The Journal of Family Practice 13(7):1039-1050, 1981.
6. Williams, M.H.: Blood doping: an update, The Physician and Sports Medicine 9(7):59, 1981.
7. Gray, M.E., and Titlow, L.W.: B15: myth or miracle, The Physician and Sports Medicine 10(1):107, 1982.
8. Scott, V., and Gijsbers, K.: Pain perception in competitive swimmers, British Medical Journal 283:91-93, July 11, 1981.
9. Burks, T.F.: Drug use in athletics, Federation Proceedings 40:2680-2681, 1981.
10. Elaborate drug control set for Montreal Olympics, Science 193:306, 1976.

11. Keese, P.: People in sports: drug tests are for cows, New York Times, June 28, 1973, p. C62.
12. Goldaper, S.: N.B.A. sets meeting on drug abuse amid reports of cocaine use, New York Times, August 21, 1980, p. B14.
13. Leake, C.D.: The amphetamines: their actions and uses, Springfield, Ill., 1958, Charles C Thomas, Publisher.
14. Ivy, J.L., and others: Influence of caffeine and carbohydrate feedings on endurance performance, Medicine and Science in Sports 11(1):6-11, 1979.
15. Laites, V.G., and Weiss, B.: The amphetamine margin in sports, Federation Proceedings 40:2689-2692, 1981.
16. Smith, G.M., and Beecher, H.K.: Amphetamine sulfate and athletic performance, Journal of the American Medical Association 170:542-557, 1959.
17. Mandell, A.J., Stewart, K.D., and Russo, P.V.: The Sunday syndrome: from kinetics to altered consciousness, Federation Proceedings 40:2693-2698, 1981.
18. Ryan, A.J.: Anabolic steroids are fool's gold, Federation proceedings 40:2682-2688, 1981.
19. Amdur, N.: Wider Olympic drug abuse is seen, New York Times, January 22, 1977, pp. E1, 3.

SEXUAL BEHAVIOR

Much is still unknown about the "chemistry" of sexuality . . . In human sexual expression, the brain and mind are far more important than the penis or vagina.[1,p.16]

Sexual behavior in humans is very different from sexual behavior in other animals. Human sexual behavior (HSB) is not determined solely, or even primarily, by the endocrine system or the presence of certain specific "releasing" stimuli in the environment. HSB is not instinctive or reflexive; it is voluntary behavior that is to some extent dependent on a physiological and a hormonal base. Cognitive factors seem to be the major determinant of human sexual motivation, arousal, and behavior. Since psychoactive agents have their primary effect on cognitive processes, it is reasonable that these drugs would alter many aspects of sexual desire and activity.

Even voluntary behavior has a neurophysiological basis. The two phases of sexual behavior—vasocongestion and orgasm—are controlled by different parts of the nervous system. Vasocongestion, resulting in erection in the male and lubrication and swelling of the vagina in the female, is controlled by the parasympathetic nervous system, a cholinergic system. Orgasm, reflex muscular contraction and ejaculation in the male and reflex muscular contraction in the female, is controlled by the sympathetic nervous system, an adrenergic system. Any drug that has anticholinergic activity, thus blocking the cholinergic, parasympathetic system, has the potential to interfere with vasocongestion. Antiadrenergic drugs have the potential to block or disrupt orgasm.

Underlying all of this is the fact that there is considerable evidence that sexual capabilities are to some degree determined by genetic makeup and that essential to any degree of arousal is an adequate level of testosterone in the male and androgen in the female. One final introductory comment is necessary. A convenient way to approach the analysis of sexual behavior is to start with the formula:

$$SA = (O \times C \times M) - I$$

In this equation SA is sexual activity, O is opportunity, C is capability, M is motivation, and I is inhibition. Capability includes both the ability to attain an adequate amount of vasocongestion and to achieve orgasm. Motivation—drive, libido—is most closely related to testosterone and androgen levels although experience certainly plays a part. Opportunity seems to have only socially defined limits and those limits seem to change with each passing year. Inhibitory factors include socially learned prohibitions, fatigue, distracting stimuli, and anxiety. Where possible, the actions and effects of the various drugs will be related to these factors. It should be noted that if opportunity, capability, or motivation are zero—no sexual activity will occur.

Alcohol

Candy
Is dandy
But liquor
Is quicker[2]

Lechery, sir, it provokes, and unprovokes; it provokes the desire, but it takes away the performance.[3]

The first quote summarizes what most of us grew up believing is true about women and the second quote what we grew up believing about men. Alcohol, since it is a depressant drug, decreases inhibitions and at least makes the thought of sexual activity more likely. It may be that the amount of HSB increases following moderate alcohol intake but there is considerable anecdotal evidence that the quality decreases. A little knowledge is not only dangerous, it also makes it difficult to predict the effect of alcohol on HSB. Alcohol is a depressant and thus might/should decrease capability. Alcohol also has antianxiety characteristics that might/should decrease inhibitions. A priori then, it is possible to support either prediction—that alcohol increases, or decreases, sexual behavior.

A 1970 survey of *Psychology Today* readers found that men were equally divided as to whether alcohol use increased or decreased sexual pleasure. Women reported that alcohol use increased sexual pleasure by a 3 to 1 margin. A 1974 survey of male business executives found a positive relationship between reported frequency of alcohol use and whether the respondent said that alcohol acted as a sexual stimulant. It was also true that those who drank less also engaged in less sexual activity.[4] In the absence of other data these findings are explained more parsimoniously as a result of different life-styles rather than supporting the idea that alcohol is a sexual stimulant.

A sophisticated and well-designed study[5] using college females as subjects explored the relationships among the dose of alcohol ingested (0.05, 0.25, 0.50, 0.75 g/kg), self-reports of sexual arousal, and vaginal vasocongestion. There were two experimental conditions—watching an erotic-pornographic film and watching a nonerotic film of a tour of a computer facility—and two sets of instructions—one suggesting that alcohol would increase sexual arousal and the other suggesting that alcohol would decrease sexual arousal. The subjects were tested about 40 minutes after alcohol intake. Each subject was tested under each alcohol dose and in each session both the erotic and nonerotic films were viewed.

Several results are worthy of note. The instructional set did not generally alter the *expected* effect of alcohol: most of the college females expected alcohol to increase sexual arousal. There was a good relationship between the dose of alcohol and the percentage of subjects who reported that alcohol increased their sexual arousal to the erotic film: 0.05—25%; 0.25—44%; 0.50—69%; and 0.75—75%. On the self-report measure: (1) sexual arousal increased with alcohol intake and (2) the percent of subjects reporting arousal to the erotic film increased as the amount of alcohol ingested increased.

The erotic film elicited much greater vaginal vasocongestion than the computer film—providing some validity to vaginal vasocongestion as a measure of sexual arousal. Importantly, the amount of increase in vaginal vasocongestion decreased as the dose of alcohol increased. As the authors put it, "The data clearly demonstrate a negative linear relation between increasing levels of alcohol consumption and sexual arousal as measured by vaginal [vasocongestion]."[5,p.495] For women increased alcohol intake results in self-reports of increased sexual arousal along with a decrease in a physiological measure of arousal.

A similar study[6] was carried out on college males by the same research team. The physiological measure of arousal was also vasocongestion—speed, amount, and duration of penile erection. The doses of alcohol ingested were: 0.08, 0.4, 0.8, and 1.2 g/kg. The instructional set had no effect on physiological arousal in these males. All three measures of penile vasocongestion decreased as the dose of alcohol was increased. Self-reports of degree of arousal were highly correlated with the extent of vasocongestion.

One study,[7] which used a lower dose of alcohol, reported a slight increase in penile vasocongestion at the lower dose level. In general, however, increasing levels of alcohol result in less physiological arousal (as measured by vasocongestion) in both males and females.

In the infrequent, social user of alcohol the body returns to normal as the alcohol is metabolized and leaves the body. The alcoholic is not as fortunate. It has long been known that heavy alcohol users and alcoholics suffer from a variety of sexual problems and show atrophy of the testicles and impaired sperm production. One report found that 8% of male alcoholics were impotent, and in half of those the condition persisted during years of sobriety.[8] There may be, of course, a large psychological factor in impotence, so it is of some interest that there seems now to be a physiological basis for it in alcoholism. One biochemical study in humans required volunteers to drink about 3 g of alcohol per kilogram of body weight a day for 4 weeks.[9] A twofold to fivefold increase was found in the activity of the liver enzyme that metabolizes testosterone. There was not an increased production of testosterone, and reduced levels of this male sex hormone could, over time, result in the physical and behavioral changes mentioned earlier. Don't panic, guys—to achieve the level of alcohol intake used in the experiment would require you to drink about a quart of distilled spirits a day. Note, however, that a dose-response curve was not done, and no information is available about the effects on testosterone of prolonged low-level alcohol intake.

A January 1982 report in *Medical World News* told of the reversal of alcoholic impotence with daily doses of oral androgen—even though the pre-drug testosterone levels of these nondrinking ex-alcoholic men were normal. Further work is needed but this finding may be a major breakthrough. It may also be a useful adjunct to alcoholic rehabilitation programs. As motivation to keep the ex-alcoholic from drinking, the discoverer of this approach said, "If you tell someone you're going to fix his liver, he'll just shrug his shoulders. But if you tell him you're going to fix his gonads, he'll pay attention."

Tranquilizers and antidepressant drugs

Perhaps the greatest effect of tranquilizers and antidepressant drugs on sexual behavior results from their therapeutic results—the less depressed individual will be more responsive to and interested in all aspects of the world, including sexual activity. The less anxious or less disturbed individual may become interested in sex as he begins to

relate to his environment in a more normal way. One effect of the major tranquilizers is a decreased responsiveness to the environment—this may reduce sexual motivation. The outcome, an increase or decrease in sexual activity, will depend on the particular individual, the specific drug, dose, duration of use, etc.

Those same issues enter in when specific neurochemical effects are considered. The major tranquilizers—the antipsychotic agents (see Chapter 13)—vary greatly in their anticholinergic activity. As the potency of the anticholinergic effect increases, so does the probability of disruption of vasocongestion.[10] The tricyclic antidepressant drugs are potent anticholinergic agents and the possibility of impotence in males is always present when these drugs are used. It should be noted that OTC drugs (such as cold remedies) that contain anticholinergic drugs, such as atropine, scopolamine, belladonna alkaloids, and antihistamines, may also disrupt vasocongestion—but probably only if taken at above the recommended doses.

One side effect of the antipsychotic agents is the increased production of prolactin in both sexes. This may result in enlargement of the breasts and secretion of milk.[11]

The effects of the "minor" tranquilizers—antianxiety agents such as the benzodiazepines—are very similar to the effect of alcohol and equally dose dependent. No studies on sexual behavior have been reported but low doses of these drugs have been used clinically to decrease inhibitions. Higher doses lead to greater sedation and a reduction of all behavior, including sexual behavior.

Hallucinogens

None of the better known hallucinogens, such as LSD, mescaline, psilocybin, PCP, has potent effects on the cholinergic or adrenergic systems. However, they all induce considerable changes in the user's sensitivity to, and experience of, their inner and outer world, which could have an effect on sexual experiences. Since responses to these drugs are very individual and partly based on the user's expectations, some individuals may find the combination of a hallucinogen and sex better than either by itself. In 1967 *Playboy Magazine* gave visibility to Leary's view of LSD as the world's greatest aphrodisiac with an article titled, "Sex, Ecstasy, and the Psychedelic Drugs."[12] Unfortunately there are no hard data to support Leary's claim—but there is some evidence to refute it. After using hallucinogens some individuals report that sexual activity no longer interests them.[13]

Marijuana and sex have a long history but the actual effect of marijuana on sexual activity—frequency or pleasure—is still not clear. Perhaps the effect is clear—we just need more information to understand it. In some surveys many individuals, but not all, report an increase in sexual pleasure while using marijuana.[14,15] One brief review lists nine effects of marijuana use that are possibly relevant to sexual behavior.[16] The most likely basis for the enhancement of pleasure is the decrease in inhibitions and the general euphoric state caused by marijuana, as well as the distortion of the perception of time.

Stimulants and depressants

If you're going to have an orgy what better class of drugs to use than one that produces euphoria, decreases fatigue, and increases alertness: stimulants.[17] Amphetamines and cocaine do all of these things. There are some people who consider these drugs as aphrodisiacs.[18] A group of young multi-drug-using individuals in the Haight-Ashbury area in the early 1970s chose cocaine as the drug that did most for sexual functioning.[15] Prolonged vasocongestion and delayed orgasm have been reported following the use of cocaine and high levels of intravenous amphetamine. Most reports of a positive relationship between oral amphetamine use and enhanced sexual activity are probably based on the factors in the first sentence of this paragraph! In fact there are reports of impaired sexual activity in both males and females after oral amphetamine use.

Those same Haight-Ashbury folk also put depressant drugs—barbiturates and methaqualone—near the bottom of the list when it came to enhancing sexual activity. Although methaqualone has a street reputation as a "love drug," it is no different from other depressant drugs. In low doses depressant drugs function the same as alcohol; they lower inhibitions and produce a mild high. As the dose increases, so does the depressant effect. As the depressant effect increases, sexual interest and activity decrease.

Narcotics

"The general impression, based on almost all possible evidence, is that opiates seriously impair sexual functions."[17,p.87] One effect of heroin use and high-dose methadone maintenance is a decrease in the testosterone level.[19] This may be the basis for the high level of impotence, the low level of desire, and the greatly increased ejaculation time that has been reported.[20] The increased ejaculation time is probably why there are reports of opiates being considered as aphrodisiacs.[21]

Withdrawal from heroin or movement into a low-dose methadone maintenance treatment program is almost always followed by increases in sexual desire and capability, as well as an improvement of the quality of the sexual experience.[22]

Amyl nitrite

Amyl nitrite, a volatile, highly flammable substance, has been used therapeutically since 1867 for the treatment of angina (a heart pain associated with an inadequate supply of oxygen to the heart). It has now been almost completely replaced for this purpose by nitroglycerin. Amyl nitrite is sold in thin, glass, cloth-mesh-covered ampules. When an angina attack occurs the individual crushes the ampule and inhales the amyl nitrite. When crushed the ampules pop—hence the street name *poppers*. In seconds a decrease in blood pressure of about 40 mm of mercury and bodywide vasodilation result. This decreases the work of the heart and thus the need for oxygen. In about 90 seconds everything is back to normal.[23]

Amyl nitrite causes a relaxation of the smooth muscles of the body. One possible reason for its early and extensive use by male homosexuals was the relaxation of the anal sphincter muscle.[24] The use of amyl nitrite has spread beyond its association with sexual activity[25] but its reputation as an aphrodisiac is what keeps most users "popping and sniffing."

The reported effects on sexual pleasure are at the least nonspecific; they may be a result of the dizziness that accompanies the drop in blood pressure. A frequent aftereffect is headache—probably from the dilation of blood vessels in the brain. These effects on the circulatory system make it unwise for someone with a heart or respiratory condition to use amyl nitrite,[26] but there have been no deaths reported as a result of its use.

Probably more commonly used than the prescription drug, amyl nitrite, is its first cousin: isobutyl nitrite. An intermediate step in the manufacture of amyl nitrite, butyl nitrite is sold in several commercial products as a room odorizer. It's legal, but ridiculous—unless you want your room to smell like old, dirty, sweaty gym socks! Even though it has the smell of a locker room at the end of a busy July day, butyl nitrite has essentially the same effects as amyl nitrite.

Aphrodisiacs and anaphrodisiacs

Whether you define an aphrodisiac as a substance that increases sexual desire, capability, or pleasure (or all three)—the evidence is clear: the only agent that has been reported to always be effective in every user is an elixir of powdered unicorn horn. Of course many claims have been made for other substances. Some of the drugs already mentioned might be considered aphrodisiacs by some individuals. Usually, though, we talk of aphrodisiacs as a substance having only sexual effects. To now, no such drug exists, but it may in the future. One preliminary comment: testosterone, the male sex hormone, is not usually effective as an enhancer of sexual performance or pleasure—unless testosterone levels have decreased considerably from normal. In elderly males testosterone can restore some of the sexual vigor lost because of declining testosterone levels. Positive effects have not been shown in normal, healthy, young males.

Yohimbine, originally from the bark of the African yohimb tree but now available as a synthesized chemical, is an agent with a long history of native use as an aphrodisiac. Some years ago the FDA had a drug, Afrodex, which was used to treat male impotence, removed from the market because there were no controlled studies showing that two of its three ingredients were useful in improving erection capability. The ingredients were yohimbine, nux vomica, and methyltestosterone.[27] In the early 1980s scientific reports began to support the belief that yohimbine is a cure for certain kinds of organically caused impotence![28] Yohimbine seems to act by increasing noradrenaline levels. Much work is needed to determine mechanisms, safety, side effects, etc.—but it is interesting that the witch doctors may have been correct about yohimbine.[29]

Drugs are given to women to increase their production of ova, and thus the chance of becoming pregnant. Use of this class of drugs is the reason why there are so many multiple births today. These drugs cause an increase in the production of FSH and LH (see Chapter 12) and stimulate the ovaries. In males they have the same effect on FSH and LH—but these hormones act on the testes to increase the production of testosterone and sperm. Increased production of testosterone probably will not effect the sexual motivation or capability of healthy males with normal levels of testosterone. In 1982 the FDA approved the use of one of these drugs in the treatment of infertility in males.[30]

Cantharidin (Spanish fly) is an extract containing dried and powdered blister beetles. In human use the material is actually quite dangerous and sometimes deadly.[31] Spanish fly has a reputation as an aphrodisiac because it is an irritant to the urethra. The irritation sometimes causes the penis to become swollen and semirigid—as well as causing painful and bloody urination.

Ginseng has a reputation thousands of years old as a remedy for every sexual problem. That's all it has—a reputation. Even today ginseng is one of the principal ingredients in herbal concoctions to increase "sexual energy."

Nothing would be gained by detailing chapter and verse to show that there is no evidence for the effectiveness of the many reported aphrodisiacs.[29] You must remember two things: most of the reported aphrodisiacs have not been well studied and, most importantly, sexual desire and performance are in part dependent on what an individual expects and wants to happen. Even placebos are effective 30% to 40% of the time—if the individual expects them to work.[32]

Anaphrodisiacs are not chemicals that interest most people. Anaphrodisiacs act to decrease sexual desire and capability. The only chemical most people believe to have this effect is saltpeter—potassium nitrate. ("They put it in your soup in prep schools!") There is *no* evidence that it is effective—but remember, placebos work here too!

There is one effective anaphrodisiac: cyproterone. Cyproterone acts by blocking the effect of the testosterone molecule—the body responds as if no testosterone was present. Actually, cyproterone use results in a pharmacological castration—the advantage being that normal effects of testosterone recur when cyproterone use stops. The drug has been used experimentally in Europe as a way of decreasing and eliminating the sex motivation in sexual assault cases.[33]

A final shot

Sex and drugs. Drugs and sex. It is obvious that there are many more drugs that interfere with sexual activity than there are that enhance it. The side effects on sexual desire and capability should always be remembered when drugs are administered therapeutically.[34] The use of drugs taken to enhance sexual desire, capability, or pleasure is more often than not doomed to fail. Research suggests that the best bets are probably very low doses of alcohol or marijuana. Being of the Woody Allen generation I

have to agree with him. Talking about sex, he commented, "The worst I ever had was great!" And that's without drugs.

SEXUAL BEHAVIOR REFERENCES

1. Renshaw, D.C.: Drugs and sex, Nursing Care, pp. 16-19, February 1978.
2. Nash, O.: Reflections on ice breaking. In Bartlett, J., editor: Familiar quotations, ed. 14, p. 1051, Garden City Publishing Co., Inc.
3. Shakespeare, W.: Macbeth, Act II, Scene 1.
4. Wilson, G.T.: Alcohol and human sexual behavior, Behavior Research and Therapy 15:239-252, 1977.
5. Wilson, G.T., and Lawson, D.M.: Effects of alcohol on sexual arousal in women, Journal of Abnormal Psychology 85(5):489-497, 1976.
6. Briddell, D.W., and Wilson, G.T.: Effects of alcohol and expectancy set on male sexual arousal, Journal of Abnormal Psychology 85(2):225-234, 1976.
7. Farkas, G.M., and Rosen, R.C.: Effect of alcohol on elicited male sexual response, Journal of Studies on Alcohol 37(3):265-272, 1976.
8. Lemere, F., and Smith, J.W.: Alcohol-induced sexual impotence, American Journal of Psychiatry 130(2):212-213, 1973.
9. Rubin, E., and others: Prolonged ethanol consumption increases testosterone metabolism in the liver, Science 191:563-564, 1976.
10. Segraves, R.T.: Male sexual dysfunction and psychoactive drug use, Post Graduate Medicine 71(1):227-233, 1982.
11. Dotti, A., and Reda, M.: Major tranquilizers and sexual function. In Sandler, M., and Gesso, G.L.: editors: Sexual behavior: pharmacology and biochemistry, pp. 193-195, New York, 1975, Raven Press.
12. Masters, R.E.L.: Sex, ecstasy, and the psychedelic drug, Playboy 14(11):94, 1967.
13. Cohen, S.: Drugs and sexuality, Drug Abuse and Alcoholism Newsletter, vol. 7, no. 10, 1978.
14. Dawley, H.H., Winstead, D.K., Baxter, A.S., and Gay, J.R.: An attitude survey of the effects of marijuana on sexual enjoyment, Journal of Clinical Psychology 35(1):212-217, 1979.
15. Gay, G.R., Newmeyer, J.A., Elion, R.A., and Wieder, S.: Drug-sex practice in the Haight-Ashbury or "the sensuous hippie." In Sandler, M., and Gessa, G.L., editors: Sexual behavior: pharmacology and biochemistry, pp. 63-79, New York, 1975, Raven Press.
16. Nowles, V.: Categories of interest in the scientific search for relationships (ie., interaction, associations, comparisons) in human sexual behavior and drug use. In Sandler, M., and Gessa, G.L., editors: Sexual behavior: pharmacology and biochemistry, pp. 93-96, New York, 1975, Raven Press.

17. Hollister, L.E.: The mystique of social drugs and sex. In Sandler, M., and Gessa, G.L., editors: Sex behavior: pharmacology and biochemistry, pp. 85-92, New York, 1975, Raven Press.

18. Gay, G.R., and Sheppard, C.W.: "Sex-crazed dope fiends"—myth or reality? Drug Forum 2(2):125-140, Winter 1973.

19. Mendelson, J.H.: Plasma testosterone levels in heroin addiction and during methadone maintenance, The Journal of Pharmacology and Experimental Therapeutics 192(1):211-217, 1975.

20. Parr, D.: Sexual aspects of drug abuse in narcotic addicts, British Journal of Addiction 71:261-268, 1976.

21. Jarvik, M.E.: Drugs and sexual functioning. In Jarvik, M., editor: Psychopharmacology in the practice of medicine, New York, 1976, Appleton-Century-Crofts.

22. DeLeon, G., and Wexler, H.K.: Heroin addiction: its relation to sexual behavior and sexual experience, Journal of Abnormal Psychology 81(1):36-38, 1973.

23. Lowry, T.P.: Neurophysiological aspects of amyl nitrite, Journal of Psychedelic Drugs 12(1):73-74, 1980.

24. Everett, G.: Amyl nitrite ("poppers") as in aphrodisiac. In Sandler, M., and Gessa, G.L., editors: Sexual behavior: pharmacology and biochemistry, New York, 1975, Raven Press.

25. Bennetts, L.: Butyl nitrite, a popular mind altering drug, is legal and proliferating, The New York Times, November 21, 1978, p. C7.

26. Israflstam, S., and others: Poppers, a new recreational drug craze, Canadian Psychiatric Association Journal 23:493-495, 1978.

27. Bush, P.J.: Drugs, alcohol and sex, New York, 1980, Richard Marek Pub.

28. Scorned African aphrodisiac scores against organic impotence, Medical World News, p. 115, January 18, 1982.

29. Gottlieb, A.: Sex drugs and aphrodisiacs, 1974, High Times/Level Press.

30. Brozan, N.: U.S. approves men's use of drug to help fertility, New York Times, January 21, 1982, p. A15.

31. Till, J.S., and Majmudar, B.N.: Cantharidin poisoning, Southern Medical Journal 74:444-447, April 1981.

32. Gawin, F.H.: Drugs and eros: reflections on aphrodisiacs, Journal of Psychedelic Drugs 10(3):227-236, 1978.

33. Saba, P., Salvadorini, F., Galeone, F., Pellicano, C., and Rainer, E.: Antiandrogen treatment in sexually abnormal subjects with neuropsychiatric disorders. In Sandler, M., and Gessa, G.L., editors: Sexual behavior: pharmacology and biochemistry, pp. 197-204, New York, 1975, Raven Press.

34. Drugs that cause sexual dysfunction, The Medical Letter 22(25):108-110, 1980.

PREGNANCY

Drugs used by a pregnant woman pass via the placenta to the circulation of the developing embryo and fetus; drugs used by a nursing mother are passed through her milk to the nursing child. This section discusses what is, and is not, known about the effects of certain psychoactive drugs on prenatal development and the nursing child. One thing is certain: this is already a major problem and the surface has just been scratched. One study considered all types of drugs and found that almost every pregnant woman used at least two different drugs— 93% used five or more drugs during their pregnancy![1]

Teratogens are chemicals that tend to cause developmental malformations. Sometimes the malformation is an obvious morphological one—as is true with the effects of thalidomide. Increasing concern has been focused on the not-so-obvious teratogenic effects on the nervous system, effects that are manifested only in behavior at a later stage of development. Identification of teratogens is not easy—drug dosage is an obvious consideration, as is the species of animal in which the drug is tested. Thalidomide, for example, is teratogenic only in primates and rabbits—not in rats, dogs, or guinea pigs. The incidence of the effect is also important because 7% of all children are born with some type of malformation or neurobehavioral impairment.[2]

The stage of the pregnancy is a critical variable. The fetus is most susceptible during the first 2 months of pregnancy—a period when the woman may not even know she's pregnant. The high risk at this time comes from several factors: ". . . the embryo contains few cells . . . [and they have] rapid rates of proliferation and a higher proportion of undifferentiated cells . . . normal development during this period requires precise temporal-spatial sequencing which may be affected by toxins. The unique metabolism of the embryonic cells includes immature repair and detoxification mechanisms."[3,p.164] This early period is when most morphological effects occur. Note: *the central nervous system (CNS) remains vulnerable to drugs until birth.* These CNS effects can cause functional and behavioral actions in the absence of obvious malformations.

Alcohol

The unfortunate condition of infants born to alcoholic mothers was noted in an 1834 report to the British Parliament: They have "a starved, shriveled, and imperfect look." In 1899 it was reported that the stillborn and infant mortality rate of children of heavy alcohol users was twice that of children born to their sober relatives.[4] Until recently most scientists and physicians believed that any effects on the offspring of heavy alcohol users were the result of poor nutrition and/or poor prenatal care. On June 9, 1973, an article appeared in a prestigious journal that summarized its report:

> Eight unrelated children of three different ethnic groups, all born to mothers who were chronic alcoholics, have a similar pattern of craniofacial, limb, and cardiovascular defects associated with prenatal-onset growth deficiency and developmental delay. This seems to be the first reported association between maternal alcoholism and aberrant morphogenesis in the offspring.[5,p.1267]

With that publication *fetal alcohol syndrome,* FAS, started on its way to being a household word, the object of much research, the center of many cocktail party discussions, the basis for governmental rules and regulations, and a topic that would eventually elicit great disagreement among knowledgeable scientists.

In 1981 a review article[6] would refer to the over 800 studies that appeared since the 1973 report and spell out the main characteristics of FAS:

> . . . prenatal and postnatal growth retardation, especially microcephaly (small heads); facial anomalies, for example, short palpebral fissures (eye slits); indistinctive philtrums (the groove between nose and mouth); low set and unparallel ears; limb, joint, and organ disorders; the behavioral or cognitive impairment such as subnormal intelligence, fine motor dysfunction, and hyperactivity.[6,p.564]

The bottom line was that although there is still much we do not know, ". . . there is considerable evidence . . . that prenatal alcohol exposure adversely affects fetal development, as reflected by behavioral deficits in the offspring . . . [even] . . . in the absence of observable physical anomalies."[6,p.578]

The important questions are: How much alcohol—and when—is necessary to cause FAS? A 1980 report found that 1 ounce of alcohol (two drinks) a day is linked to decreased birthweight, and that 2 ounces a week is linked to increased spontaneous abortions.[7] In 1981 the Surgeon General, via the FDA, advised physicians that, "Pregnant women should drink absolutely no alcohol because they may be endangering the health of their unborn children."[8,p.7] It really hit the fan. Most researchers in this area could agree that 2 to 3 ounces of alcohol a day resulted in clear effects and that 4 or 5 ounces a day (8 to 10 drinks) caused severe effects, as those mentioned previously. But 1 ounce a week? Many believed the complete abstention rule went too far beyond the data—it is a lively and ongoing debate![9] But then again, who is willing to say that there is *no* risk from an occasional drink? Not me—there may be an increased risk to the fetus with any alcohol use by the mother. We just do not know if there is a safe level of use. As the mechanisms underlying the effects of alcohol become clear,[10,11] so will the guidelines for use by pregnant women.

Smoking

This section will be brief—the data are clear and there is no debate. Most of the research has been done on cigarette smoking but this section is only labeled "Smoking." The negative effects on the fetus from the mother smoking do not come from the nicotine in cigarettes; the negative effects are from the blood carbon monoxide that results from smoking. This includes smoking marijuana, tobacco, and anything else that results in the inhalation of the gaseous waste product of a burning substance.

Carbon monoxide (the chemical that is the cause of death from poor auto exhaust systems and poorly vented gas heaters) combines with the hemoglobin in the red cells of the blood and decreases their ability to carry oxygen. The smoking mother-to-be can literally suffocate the fetus she is carrying. The Surgeon General is less blunt, but more specific:

> Mothers who smoke cigarettes during the last two trimesters of their pregnancy have been found to have babies with a lower average birth weight than nonsmoking mothers. In addition cigarette smoking mothers had a higher risk of having a stillborn child, and their infants had higher late fetal and neonatal death rates. . . . These effects may occur because carbon monoxide passes freely across the placenta and is readily bound by fetal hemoglobin, thereby decreasing the oxygen carrying capacity of fetal blood.[12]

Other work has shown that "Drinking and smoking are independent risk factors for spontaneous abortions; and the effect of drinking is greater. . . ."[13,p.175]

The British Perinatal Mortality Survey reported that mothers who smoked after the fourth month of pregnancy, compared to nonsmoking mothers, delivered babies that were on the average 170 grams lighter and ½ inch shorter.[14] It should also be noted that babies born to smoking mothers had blood carboxyhemoglobin levels up to ten times as high as babies born to nonsmoking mothers. As if that were not enough:

> Several studies have shown that the children of parents who smoke are more liable to chest illnesses than the children of parents who do not smoke. A recent study has shown that after correction for parents' liability to respiratory infections, a twofold increase in the incidence of bronchitis and pneumonia occurred in the first year of life.[15,p.17]

A 1981 study[16] used information collected from over 8100 pregnancies at 12 medical school hospitals and concluded: "Results of the study exclude undernutrition, genetic factors, and placental underperfusion as major contributing factors to the fetal growth retardation associated with cigarette smoking."[16,p.18] There aren't many other choices: it's the carbon monoxide that is associated with smoking, and not just with cigarette smoking.

Other drugs

In July, 1976, the FDA issued a warning that all minor tranquilizers, meprobamate and the benzodiazepines, should be avoided by women in the first 3 months of pregnancy. "Three recent studies indicate there may be an association between use of the tranquilizers in early pregnancy, and malformations such as cleft lip in babies."[17] You should take special note that this warning was first issued 21 years after meprobamate was placed on the market—how many more surprises are in store for us? The evidence is overwhelming; it sometimes takes a long time to clearly establish a danger from the use of a drug.

Since caffeine is everywhere in our society there has been much concern over its use by pregnant women. There have long been reports that there may be some slight effect of caffeine as a mutagen in nonmammals but an extensive review and report to the FDA in 1976 could not show that this was of concern in humans.[18] Scientists work, papers get published, things change. In 1980 the FDA advised pregnant women to avoid caffeine, or at least to use it in very small amounts! More scientists work, more papers get published, more things change. In the spring of 1982 a comprehensive study was published that concluded:

> After controlling for smoking, other habits, demographic characteristics, and medical history . . . we found no relation between low birth weight and heavy coffee consumption. Furthermore, there was no excess of malformations among coffee drinkers. These negative results suggest that coffee consumption has a minimal effect, if any, on the outcome of pregnancy.[19,p.141]

Next year?

An excellent study in the early 1980s[20] compared drug use in mothers whose children had congenital malformations to matched mothers whose newborns did not have defects. Only a sketch of the results is possible here. Three groups of drugs used in the first trimester had high odds of being associated with a malformed child: (1) antidepressants, (2) narcotics, and (3) minor tranquilizers. In children with defects, the odds that their mother had used antidepressants, compared to no drugs, was 7.6 to 1. For narcotic analgesics and the tranquilizers the odds were 3.6 and 2.3 to 1. In the second trimester the only significant effect was with tranquilizers. A final point: tranquilizer use by smoking mothers increased the risk of a malformed child 3.7-fold over the risk of smoking without tranquilizer use. That combination has powerful negative effects on the fetus and should be avoided at all costs.

In 1978 the contents of a draft report were leaked to the world about the long-term effects of drugs used in conjunction with childbirth. The report said that there were negative effects from some drugs on the child that lasted at least up to age 7. The inhalant anesthetics seemed to be the worst offenders. The report was released reluctantly in 1979 but was not given much attention. Presentations at national meetings by the authors of the government-supported study confirm and repeat what is written above. There is a great need for more information on the long-term behavioral and neurological effects of drugs used in the delivery process.

Breast feeding

Even though we make a big deal out of birth, there is no super big change in the developmental process as a result of birth. Two items are of importance here. The first is that the newborn does not have the opportunity to transfer toxins via the placenta to the mother for detoxification and excretion. Since the regulatory systems in the neonate are not well developed it sometimes means that once drugs are taken into the child they act and persist for longer periods of time than in the fetus or adult. The second item is that the only drugs that are transmitted from mother to child are those in the milk. There is still very incomplete information, but

> . . . diffusion from the maternal circulation appears to be the principal pathway by which drugs appear in milk; un-ionized drugs, which bind minimally to maternal plasma protein and are lipid-soluble, diffuse most readily; and generally no more than 1-2 percent of a maternal dose is ultimately excreted in milk.[21,p.75]

Alcohol is one drug in which the breast milk level has been shown to be almost always about the same as the blood level. One case is of note because the mother's milk was assayed and it had an alcohol content equivalent to a blood level of 0.1/100 ml—the level at which you are legally drunk. The nursing child showed large weight gains but a slowed rate of growth. When the mother stopped her alcohol intake, the child's normal growth resumed.[22]

What would seem to be very low levels of a drug in breast milk may act as very high levels in the nursing child because of both slow metabolism and the fact that drugs in the very young do not attach to blood proteins—thus, all of the drug is active. There are some drugs, such as meprobamate, that appear to concentrate in the mother's milk. One review article[23] stated that research is just beginning and caution is the watchword. Better fewer drugs and healthier babies.

> With our present inadequate knowledge, it is difficult to prepare a list of drugs that are safe or are harmful to the breastfed infant. However, we do know that drugs such as diazepam, lithium, bromides, reserpine, and opium alkaloids are to be avoided and that barbiturates, haloperidol . . . should be administered with caution.[23,p.804]

Two reports appeared in 1980. One listed drugs and classes of drugs that appear in breast milk following use by the mother, including those that appear only in clinically unimportant amounts.[24] The other report lists only those drugs and classes of drugs known to be of concern.[25] The important thing is to realize that new information comes along almost every month. Your physician will know.

At term

This section has been devoted to drugs—chemicals that people take voluntarily. There are also many chemicals that we take into our system without wanting to or thinking about it. These are the chemicals in the environment.[3] As of now there is very inadequate information—we'll have to wait, perhaps many years, to know their effects.

Chemicals that most people do not consider as

drugs need to be thought about by the pregnant individual, such as aspirin, vitamins, and all of the nonprescription drugs that can be bought over-the-counter. Most of these chemicals used in moderation will not have negative effects on the fetus. Even so they need to be used judiciously. Some authorities recommend acetaminophen rather than aspirin for the pregnant female. They caution against very high levels of the fat-soluble vitamins, such as A and D, because of known negative effects on the fetus.[2]

Three final items. All of the rules and regulations and quality checks will not prevent a thalidomide-type disaster[26] from occurring as a result of using illegal, and thus unstudied, drugs. Second, there is an accumulating body of information from non-primate research that suggests that drug use *by the father* may be linked to birth defects.[27] Last, but by no means least, is the fact that the field of behavioral teratology is becoming an important area of research. One article calls this area the study of "Birth Defects of the Mind"[28] because the teratological effects are not visible to the naked eye—they are in the structure and function of the brain areas that are necessary for thinking and doing. This is a difficult area to study since the effects may not show up for many years.[29]

We'll have to wait and see on these last two factors. But while we wait, let's be cautious. Your life *is* your life—but your child's life should belong to the child. Don't do things that decrease your child's options.

PREGNANCY REFERENCES

1. Doering, P.L., and Stewart, R.B.: The extent and character of drug consumption during pregnancy, Journal of the American Medical Association **239**:843-846, 1978.
2. Berlin, C.M., and others: Assessing effects of maternal drug use, Patient Care, **14**(1):68, May 30, 1980.
3. Pries, C.N.: Reproductive effects of occupational exposures, American Family Physician, **24**(2):161-165, 1981.
4. Little, R.E.: Drinking during pregnancy: implications for public health, Alcohol Health and Research World **4**(1):36-42, Fall 1979.
5. Jones, K.L., and others: Pattern of malformation in offspring of chronic alcoholic mothers, Lancet, **1**(7815):1267-1271, June 9, 1973.
6. Abel, E.L.: Behavioral teratology of alcohol, Psychological Bulletin **90**(3):564-581, 1981.
7. MD's put on spot by federal no-drink-pregnancy edict, Medical World News, p. 39-40, August 17, 1981.
8. Greenberg, J.: Pregnant women warned on alcohol, New York Times, July 18, 1981, p. 7.
9. Kolata, G.B.: Fetal alcohol advisory debated, Science **214**:642, November 6, 1981.
10. Sulik, K.K., Johnston, M.C., and Webb, M.A.: Fetal alcohol syndrome: embryogenesis in a mouse model, Science **214**:936-938, November 20, 1981.
11. Henderson, G.I., and others: Inhibition of placental valine uptake after acute and chronic maternal ethanol consumption, Journal of Pharmacology and Experimental Therapeutics **216**:465-472, 1981.
12. The health consequences of smoking, 1975, Public Health Service Publication No. (CDC) 76-8704, U.S. Department of Health, Education, and Welfare, Washington D.C., 1976, U.S. Government Printing Office.
13. Harlap, S., and Shiono, P.H.: Alcohol, smoking, and incidence of spontaneous abortions in the first and second trimesters, Lancet **1**(8187):173-176, July 26, 1980.
14. British Perinatal Mortality Survey. Cited in Steinfeld, J.L.: The health consequences of smoking, Proceedings of the Third World Conference on Smoking and Health, vol. 1, Publication No. (NIH) 76-1221, U.S. Department of Health, Education, and Welfare, Washington, D.C., 1976, U.S. Government Printing Office.
15. Smoking and its effects on health, report of a WHO Expert Committee, World Health Organization Technical Report Series No. 568, Geneva, 1975.
16. Naege, R.L.: Influence of maternal cigarette smoking during pregnancy on fetal and childhood growth, Obstetrics and Gynecology **57**(1):18-21, 1981.
17. HEW News, U.S. Department of Health, Education, and Welfare, 76-20, July 22, 1976.
18. Select Committee Report to the FDA: Tentative evaluation of the health aspects of caffeine as a food ingredient, Bethesda, Md., 1976, Life Sciences Research Office, Federation of American Societies for Experimental Biology.
19. Linn, S., and others: No association between coffee consumption and adverse outcomes of pregnancy, New England Journal of Medicine **306**(3):141, 1982.
20. Bracken, M.B., and Holford, T.R.: Exposure to prescribed drugs in pregnancy and association with congenital malformations, Obstetrics and Gynecology **58**(3):336-344, 1981.
21. Petrie, R.H., and others: Drugs and pregnancy, The Female Patient **5**:68-78, June 1980.
22. Binkiewiez, A., and others: Pseudo-Cushing syndrome caused by alcohol in breast milk, Journal of Pediatrics **93**(6):965-967, December 1978.
23. Ananth, J.: Side effects in the neonate from psychotropic agents excreted through breast-feeding, American Journal of Psychiatry **135**(7):801-805, 1978.

24. Blake, J.P.: Drugs excreted in mother's milk, Patient Care, June 30, 1980, p. 87.
25. Lipman, A.G.: Effects of drugs in breast milk; Modern Medicine, **48**(1):71, June 30, 1980.
26. Insight Team: Suffer the children, the story of thalidomide. New York, 1978, Viking Press.
27. Marks, R.G.: Maternal *and* paternal drug use now linked to birth defects, Current Prescribing, p. 21, July 1979.
28. Kolata, G.B.: Behavioral teratology: birth defects of the mind, Science **202**:732-734, November 17, 1978.
29. Vorhees, C.V., and others: Psychotropic drugs as behavioral teratogens, Science **205**:1220, September 21, 1979.

BAD TRIPS

There have always been individuals with drug-related emergencies appearing at hospitals. With the arrival of widespread, heavy, and indiscriminate drug use in the middle and late 1960s the number of drug emergencies began to increase. In 1967 several large city hospitals reported that 15% to 20% of their emergency room business involved the treatment of drug problems. This was also the period when rap houses, crisis call centers, and other nonmedical groups and agencies began to develop for several reasons. One reason was that people with drug problems had, for the most part, engaged in illegal activity—to get or use the drugs—and these users were reluctant to expose themselves to the scrutiny of and identification by the establishment. Also, when appearing at a medical setting for help they were frequently given second-class treatment because of their long hair, strange dress, etc.[1] A final reason for not going to hospital emergency rooms for treatment was also quite realistic; the physicians and nurses usually did not know what to do about the medical-pharmacological problems. It was a completely new area of treatment.

Things have changed drastically since the flower children and the hippies first suggested different life-styles and different values. Both the establishment and the drug-using populations have changed. The doctor in the emergency room and the person walking or being carried through the door are probably no different from you and me in speech, dress, and education. Medicine has also learned a lot about both the short- and long-term management of drug problems.[2,3] The law changed in 1975 when the federal government established very strict rules about the confidentiality of patient information and records whenever drug or alcohol abuse is involved. The rules apply to hospitals as well as alcohol and drug treatment programs and "state that any records of the identity, diagnosis, prognosis, or treatment of any drug abuse patient are required to be kept confidential . . . nor may such records be divulged in any civil, criminal, administrative, or legislative proceedings conducted by a federal, state or local authority. . . ."[4,p.267] Release of information except when authorized by the individual or in a life-threatening medical emergency is punishable by a fine. The federal regulations do not say whether parents must be informed about alcohol or drug treatment given to a minor child. Each state may issue its own rules on this point.

Dealing with emergency drug problems will continue to be distributed among various social and medical facilities. As the use of drugs increases and more people try more drugs more times, there will be an increase in the possibility of drug-related emergencies. At the same time, however, users become more sophisticated and more knowledgeable about the effects of drugs and are less likely to overreact to a new, different, or unexpected drug experience. There are some things, though, that everyone should know about the negative physiological and psychological reactions to drugs. Whether you "do" drugs or not, it seems more likely every year that each of us will be called on to help someone who is in a drug-related crisis. You will do yourself, and others, a favor if you take time to learn cardiopulmonary resuscitation (CPR).

Street drugs, *caveat emptor*

The problem with street drugs (those you buy illegally) is that there is no FDA or FTC to protect the consumer. Without the FDA to monitor quality, purity, and quantity, buying drugs on the street is

TABLE 4-5 Street drugs: a comparison of what they were sold as and what they were analyzed to be (percentages)

| Analyzed as | Sold as | | | | | | |
	LSD	Mescaline	Psilocybin	Amphet-amines	Cocaine	THC	Heroin
LSD	87	63	47				
Mescaline		14					
Psilocybin			14				
Amphetamines				3			
Amphetamines and other drugs				24			
Cocaine					58		
Cocaine and other drugs					36		
Heroin							70
Phencyclidine						87	

Calculated and summarized from Brown, J.K., and Malone, M.H.: Pacific information service on street drugs 6(1-2):22, 1978.

like playing Russian roulette—you never know what you're going to get. But one thing is sure: most often you probably will *not* get what you think you're getting.

There are several organizations around the country that analyze the chemical makeup of drugs bought on the street. Their findings are interesting, and a summary of some of the results from the mid-1970s is shown in Table 4-5.[5] Marijuana is almost always marijuana, although sometimes it has various additions.

Table 4-5 shows that LSD *was* LSD 87% of the time. However, the amount of LSD in each dose ranged from 10 to 500 micrograms (μg). Using 10 μg would not cause any effect, but 500 μg is about four times the usual amount taken for an LSD experience! What sold as mescaline or psilocybin was usually LSD alone. Amphetamine availability decreased from the early seventies but 55% contained some amphetamine. Cocaine was pure cocaine 58% of the time, but 36% of the time it was combined with a local anesthetic.

The foregoing points up quite clearly that frequently even the user doesn't know what was tak-

en. That makes dealing with a drug-related emergency even more complicated.

There are a few basic facts to remember when buying from your friendly neighborhood dealer. Take note that society stopped calling those who sell drugs *pushers* when it was appreciated that rarely did anyone push the sale of drugs. The consumer sought out the seller. One thing to keep in mind is that THC has *never* been identified in any street drug anywhere in the world. The synthesis of THC, the psychoactive ingredient in marijuana, is too complicated and too expensive to manufacture for illicit distribution. That means that anyone who bought "THC," didn't. Another basic rule of thumb in street buys concerns LSD. If the one dose—a hit—offered is a pill or powder big enough for you to see, there is a lot of excess material, filler, mixed in with the drug. LSD is very potent—50 to 150 μg is the usual quantity taken, barely enough to cover the head of a pin. The rest of what is bought is filler, adulterants of unknown chemistry. Sometimes these adulterants cause big problems and bad trips.

Table 4-6 is a brief summary of the primary ef-

TABLE 4-6 Symptoms and signs of drug abuse*

Drug of abuse	Acute intoxication and overdose	Withdrawal syndrome
Hallucinogens		
LSD; psilocybin; mescaline; PCP	*Pupils* dilated (normal or small with PCP); *BP* elevated; *HR* increased; *tendon reflexes* hyperactive; *temperature* elevated; face flushed; euphoria, anxiety or panic; paranoid thought disorder; sensorium often clear; affect inappropriate; illusions; time and visual distortions; visual hallucinations; depersonalization; with PCP: cyclic coma or extreme hyperactivity, amnesia, analgesia, gait ataxia, muscle rigidity.	None
Cannabis group		
Marijuana; hashish; THC; hash oil	*Pupils* unchanged; *BP* decreased on standing; *HR* increased; increased appetite; euphoria, anxiety; sensorium often clear; dreamy, fantasy state; time-space distortions; hallucinations rare.	Nonspecific symptoms including anorexia, nausea, insomnia; restlessness, irritability
Narcotics		
Heroin; morphine; codeine; meperidine; methadone; hydromorphone; opium; pentazocine; propoxyphene	*Pupils* constricted (may be dilated with meperidine or extreme hypoxia); *respiration* depressed to absent with cyanosis; *BP* decreased, sometimes shock; *temperature* reduced; *reflexes* diminished to absent; stupor or coma; pulmonary edema; constipation; convulsions with propoxyphene or meperidine.	*Pupils* dilated; *pulse* rapid; goose-flesh; muscle jerks; "flu" syndrome; vomiting; diarrhea; tremulousness, yawning

Adapted from Diagnosis and management of reactions to drug abuse, The Medical Letter **22**:73-76, September 5, 1980.
*Mixed intoxications produce complex combinations of signs and symptoms; BP: blood pressure, HR: heart rate.

fects that result from the use and the withdrawal from use of pure forms of certain classes of drugs.

What to do until the doctor comes

There are some things a nonprofessional can do with a person in drug distress, but the first thing everyone should learn is when they need to send for medical assistance. The signs and symptoms discussed here are indicative of a serious problem that requires a physician as soon as possible. Never hesitate to call. It's better to make a call you didn't need to, than not make one and lose a friend—permanently.

Medicine refers to *respiration rate, heart rate, temperature,* and *blood pressure* as the *vital signs,* since these characteristics are extremely sensitive to any changes from normal functioning of the body. You cannot readily measure blood pressure, but the other three signs can and should be monitored frequently in someone who is having a drug-related problem. When you monitor respiration rate, heart rate, and temperature, *write down* what you find and record the time.

Breathing difficulty. Sometimes a conscious user will show slower and slower respiration. Usually we breathe in and out about 16 to 20 times a minute. If the rate drops below 12 per minute, then

TABLE 4-6 Symptoms and signs of drug abuse—cont'd

Drug of abuse	Acute intoxication and overdose	Withdrawal syndrome
CNS sedatives		
Barbiturates; chlordiazepoxide; diazepam; flurazepam; glutethimide; meprobamate; methaqualone; others	*Pupils* usually unchanged or small (but dilated with glutethimide or in severe poisoning); *BP* decreased, sometimes shock; *respiration* depressed; *tendon reflexes* depressed; drowsiness or coma; confusion; ataxia, slurred speech, delirium; convulsions or hyperirritability with methaqualone overdosage; serious poisoning rare with benzodiazepines alone.	Tremulousness; insomnia; sweating; fever; agitation; delirium; hallucinations; disorientation; late convulsions; fever; shock
CNS stimulants		
Amphetamines; most antiobesity drugs; cocaine; methylphenidate; phenmetrazine	*Pupils* dilated and reactive; *respiration* shallow; *BP* elevated; *HR* increased; *tendon reflexes* hyperactive; *temperature* elevated; cardiac arrhythmias; dry mouth; sweating; tremors; sensorium hyperacute or confused; paranoid ideation; impulsivity; hyperactivity; stereotypy; convulsions; exhaustion.	Muscular aches; abdominal pain, voracious hunger; prolonged sleep, lack of energy; profound psychological depression, sometimes suicidal
Anticholinergics		
Atropine; belladonna; henbane; scopolamine; trihexyphenidyl; benztropine mesylate	*Pupils* dilated and fixed; *HR* increased; *temperature* elevated; drowsiness or coma; flushed, dry skin and mucous membranes; sensorium clouded; amnesia; disorientation, visual hallucinations; body image alterations.	None

the respiratory centers in the medulla are seriously depressed, and the individual may be heading toward respiratory arrest—stoppage of breathing. Usually overdose of a narcotic, a barbiturate, or a solvent inhalation is the drug involved. As less and less oxygen is delivered to the cells of the body, the individual may develop *cyanosis*—a blue tinge at the mouth and fingernails that indicates an inadequate supply of oxygen. Begin mouth-to-mouth breathing immediately after you've sent for help. Table 4-7 gives you some appreciation of how important time is when breathing stops—every second counts.

Sometimes an increase in respiration rate occurs with the use of stimulants. In rare cases the individual will hyperventilate—breathe very rapidly with deep breaths. This can lead to unconsciousness, and breathing may stop for 30 to 40 seconds before starting again.

Pulse rate irregular or less than 50 or more than 140 a minute. If the pulse is not steady—thump, thump, thump—call a doctor no matter what the average rate is per minute. Irregular heart rate is quite common following inhalation of a volatile substance. High heart rates, tachycardia, may result from high-level marijuana or stimulant use, but rates above 140 are unusual with marijuana alone. Decreasing or low-level heart rate, bradycardia, is

TABLE 4-7 Relationship between time without breathing and probability of recovery

Time without breathing (minutes)	Probability of recovery (percent)
1	98
2	92
3	72
4	50
5	25
6	11
7	8
8	5
9	2
10	1

usually associated with an overdose of depressant drugs, and the danger is a decrease in oxygen supply.

High temperature. An individual who has a temperature—oral or in the armpit—of 102° F or more always requires medical attention. In a drug-use situation, high fever is most commonly due to high doses of central nervous system (CNS) stimulants (such as amphetamine) or to anticholinergic agents, such as atropine, scopolamine, jimsonweed, and belladonna alkaloids. These drugs decrease the activity of the parasympathetic nervous system and with their effects on the CNS give rise to the saying that the person with a high dose of anticholinergic agents is

> hot as a hare
> blind as a bat
> dry as a bone
> red as a beet
> mad as a hatter
> limp as a wet noodle

The temperature results from several things: a failure of the sweat glands to function and vasodilation of the peripheral blood vessels, which make the person feel hot, as well as hot to touch. The flow of blood to the surface of the skin also gives the individual a flushed, red appearance. Anticholinergic drugs are what the doctor puts in your eyes

when he examines them because these drugs cause extreme dilation of the pupils. This impairs vision, and bright lights cause only a brief flick of a response, not constriction as is normal. The salivary glands are also blocked by these drugs, and the mouth and other tissues dry out to an uncomfortable degree. The central nervous system effects of these agents cause severe confusion and delirium: the user is disoriented and will probably have amnesia for the entire episode. Finally, these drugs make it difficult for males to obtain erections. The primary medical dangers of these drugs are malfunction of the heart or paralysis of the respiratory muscles—and death.

Unconsciousness. If the individual is unconscious and cannot readily be awakened or kept awake, it may be that he is moving toward coma and death. If the individual has stopped breathing, first call a doctor, and then immediately give mouth-to-mouth resuscitation and continue until the ambulance or physician arrives. The same is true with heart massage if you are unable to detect a heartbeat. If breathing is satisfactory, it is important that the individual be placed on his side, or his head be turned, so that he will not aspirate vomit. Many drug-related deaths are caused by unconscious users lying on their backs and vomiting and then either suffocating in their own vomit or breathing some of the material into their lungs. There it may cause an infection and a particularly deadly form of pneumonia.

Suicidal statements or gestures, or a continually aggressive attitude. This behavior may result from the use of many different drugs, but the important thing is that you call a physician to protect both yourself and the drug user. The physician can take appropriate legal *and* medical action when the user is a threat to himself or others. You cannot do either of these. If the drug user is a serious immediate threat to those around him, do not hesitate: call the police.

Lack of bilateral symmetry in physical or physiological symptoms. If one pupil is dilated and one constricted, or if there is a loss of strength in one hand, arm, or side of the body, it is suggestive of some form of brain trauma, not a neat, new drug.

A concussion and/or internal bleeding in the brain can cause an alteration in only one side of the body, whereas a drug cannot. It is not unusual for a person using high doses of depressant drugs to fall down and hurt his head and *not be aware* of doing so. At any rate, call a doctor.

Doing the right thing, *primum non nocere*

There are many actions related to bad drug experiences that you can take without medical training. Some of them are responses to the medical crises just mentioned, while others involve situations where medical help is not usually required. If you have not been involved in the drug-using situation but have come or been called only when things went bad, there are a few things you should do after you've called for medical help.

You should first try to find out what has been taken, either from the user or others who were there. Write it all down and attempt to determine how much, what they think it was, what it looked like, how long ago it was taken, what drugs are usually used by the individual, and what effects these drugs usually cause in the individual. Perhaps of primary importance, what happened to other individuals who used the same drug? You should also try to obtain as much medical information about the user as possible: Is the person using any prescription or nonprescription medication? Do they have any illnesses that may cause a coma, such as diabetes or epilepsy? Many users and their friends will be more likely to talk with a nonthreatening age and social peer than with the white coats, so the more information you can obtain the better.

In talking with the users and/or their friends, remember that they are under the influence of one or more drugs. Their comprehension will be slow, their anxiety and suspiciousness may be high, their memories not too accurate. Keep repeating questions, ask for specifics, get as many details as you can. Be sympathetic, be nonthreatening, be nonjudgmental. Your job is to obtain information and reduce the problem, not to give a lecture on how stupid it is to take a drug you don't know anything

about. When you don't understand, do *not* say: "You didn't explain that very well, tell me again." Instead, say something like: "*I* didn't understand that, try me again, say it a different way, I'm not picking up on it." Throughout all this pay attention to the emotions that underlie what they say—not just the content. Almost everything we say conveys both a feeling and a fact. Make sure you do not ignore the feeling or you will not get any more facts.

If you have the opportunity, collect a urine sample from the user. Cover it and put it in the refrigerator; it may help later if it becomes necessary to know what the individual has really taken. It is legal to collect the urine and give it to medical personnel to assist in the treatment. It is illegal to collect it and give it to the police—that's self-incrimination and cannot be voluntarily done by an individual while in a drugged condition. Another thing you should do is prevent, if at all possible, the user from eating or drinking anything. It is imperative not to try and treat the problem with more drugs. The less the user has in his system, the easier it is for the medical people to do their thing.

Sometimes there is no need to seek medical assistance. A bad trip can frequently be handled without professional help if none of the physiological signs mentioned earlier are present.[6] A bad trip, a bummer, is a drug experience that the user defines as depressing, frightening, anxiety arousing, or in some other way as bad, bad, bad! Usually one of the phantasticants—LSD, the anticholinergics, or marijuana—is involved. These bad experiences are best handled without the use of medication, since it permits the individual to work through the experience, rather than have it stopped pharmacologically without any resolution of the feelings and problems raised by the experience. The technique used is called "talking down" from the high. In general terms, talking down consists of continual verbal reassurances and defining of reality.

The many reasons for a bad drug experience include a drug that was not what the user expected it to be, a new (to the user) combination of drugs, a negative attitude that existed before the drug was taken, or a new, different, or nonsupportive group of people in the drug-using situation. When you are trying to help someone through a bad drug experience, none of the reasons for the bad trip is important. Instead, focus on the experience and reduce the discomfort the individual is feeling.

One of the more common feelings that makes a trip bad is a panic reaction. The user may not be able to control and/or accept the changing sensory or perceptual experiences—he feels that he is losing control of his mind, and, most commonly, that he is going crazy. Reassurance is the key element here; you do it in two ways. One is by your actions and attitudes. Stay calm, warm, friendly. The other is in what you say. Keep reminding the individual that the drug is causing the feelings and the sensory and perceptual changes. His brain and his mind are the same as they were before; when the drug gets out of his system, he'll be like he was before. The drug is causing the changes; when it goes, so will the disturbing effects. You can reinforce this attitude by regularly orienting the individual to reality and the control he still has over himself. Some report good success in this by having the individual control his rate and depth of breathing. Another technique that should reduce some of the panic and anxiety is to tell the person not to fight the sensory and perceptual images, but let them flow and look at them as he would movies on a screen. This usually helps the person put some psychological distance between himself and the experience and that makes it less threatening.

A second type of bad "head trip" (panic being the first type) is being confused or completely disoriented. This is due more commonly to the use of PCP or the anticholinergics. Not infrequently the user will have no memory of the episode once the drug has been metabolized. The only aid possible in this situation is to emphasize and reemphasize the here-and-now reality: tie the person in with real-world people, events, and things as much as possible. Whenever it can be done, use the delusional content as points of contact with reality. If the individual mentions an automobile in his ramblings, ask what make, what color, what year the car is.

The last type of bad head trip is perhaps the most difficult with which to deal—the desire to problem solve. The phantasticants have many different pharmacological actions, but they all reduce the strength of the contacts with the nondrug world we usually live in. Thus we lose some of our psychological stability and our defenses against things we have denied or repressed and do not want to think about. Sometimes under drugs an individual will realize, or at least believe, something about himself that he cannot accept. As an example, a person may become aware of homosexual leanings and want to talk about that, becoming more anxious and depressed. The only option for help here is to assume the role of a good friend, not a professional. Do not try to resolve the problem. Instead, continually point out that the drug magnifies and distorts our feelings and that it's better to wait until the drug effect has gone away before dealing with the problem. Throughout, be accepting and nonjudgmental and try to avoid digging into and uncovering thoughts and ideas that will only threaten the individual even more.

Bad head trips as just mentioned are best handled without the use of drugs. By talking a person down from the high, there is the chance to resolve the anxieties and conflicts that made the trip a bummer. The bad body trips mentioned earlier do require medical assistance; they can be very dangerous and, obviously, life threatening. When in doubt, call a doctor.

With the needle

Some individuals use some drugs by injecting them into the skin or into a vein. The advantage is that the drug is delivered in high concentration into the bloodstream (*mainlining*) or just under the skin where the blood vessels rapidly absorb the drug (*skin popping*). Both these methods give a faster onset of drug action and a greater maximum drug effect than oral intake. There are very serious dangers associated with the injection of street drugs. Three things are involved in injecting a drug through the skin: the needle, the drug, and the skin.[7]

Most of us who have had an injection or given blood probably wondered why such a big deal was made about cleaning the skin, after all we showered last night. The skin contains many bacteria, and usually we have had the same colonies since birth. They have been with us through thick and thin, and through antibiotics and penicillin. Usually they are resistant to antibiotics and penicillin, and that is the problem. When you push a needle through skin containing these bacteria, the bacteria will be pushed into lower levels of the skin, or into the body tissue, where they will be nourished and grow—and laugh at the antibiotics used in an attempt to get rid of the abscess that develops. A skin abscess you can usually live with. If these bacteria are injected into the blood, you talk about blood poisoning—but that just means the bacteria are growing. And they lodge and grow in some bad places. Abscesses develop especially in the lungs, and infections are common in the valves of the heart. The valves become scarred, and sometimes it is fatal; it is always to some extent disabling.

Everyone knows you need to have clean needles or you might get *hepatitis* or *tetanus*. Unsterile injections are unlikely to cause tetanus (lockjaw) in most young people because they have received inoculations against tetanus early in life. The inoculations do not provide lifetime protection, so tetanus is possible—and it is a bad scene: only 10% survive. Hepatitis is a viral infection of the liver and is often transferred by sharing needles—even needles that look clean may not be. In a normally healthy individual hepatitis is not too dangerous. With rest and good food, few carbohydrates, and no alcohol, full recovery usually occurs in 4 to 12 weeks. If there are repeated infections, or a chronic infection, then serious liver damage will occur.

Perhaps the worst problem is still to come. Most street drugs contain contaminants or dilutants that do not dissolve. Two of the filler substances commonly used in making tablets are talc and cornstarch. When tablets are crushed so the drug can be used for injections, these fillers become part of the material injected.[8] Most drug users know this

and filter their solution by drawing it through cotton into the syringe or medicine dropper. They still inject some talc or starch and usually add some cotton fibers to the solution. There are two problems with this type of injection. One is that neither the solution nor the solids are sterile, so blood poisoning can result.

The other problem is that the nondissolving inert materials will become lodged in small capillaries. One of the most common places for this to occur is in the alveoli (air sacs) in the lung.[9] The immediate, obvious effect is that this reduces the area available for oxygenation. With repeated injections over time this can be a significant amount, and the individual may have trouble breathing. Lung abscesses are common as a result of the nonsterile particles lodging there. A secondary effect of the partial or total blocking of many capillaries in the lungs is the need for an increase in the force necessary to push the blood through the lungs. This not only increases the strain on the heart but can lead to edema. Neither the reduction in the air exchange area nor the chronic pulmonary hypertension is reversible. They persist because the little particles sit undissolved in the alveoli.

The person who injects drugs adds considerably to the risks of drug use. Drugs not meant to be injected, used with nonsterile needles and other paraphernalia, really compound the problem. All of us suffer from the delusion that such bad things "can't happen to me." The evidence is otherwise.

Concluding comment

The use of street drugs will always be with us as long as there are illegal drugs that people want to use. It is also true that the more stable, the more mature, the more psychologically secure a young adult is, the less likelihood there is of a bad drug experience. Along the same lines, the more you read about drugs and drug effects, know who you are buying drugs from, who you are doing drugs with, and what negative effects can occur, the better the chance of minimizing bad drug experiences.[10]

BAD TRIP REFERENCES

1. Jacobs, P.E.: Emergency room drug abuse treatment, Journal of Psychedelic Drugs 7(1):43-48, 1975.
2. Diagnosis and management of reactions to drug abuse, The Medical Letter 22:73-76, September 5, 1980.
3. Bourne, P.G., editor: Acute drug abuse emergencies, New York, 1976, Academic Press, Inc.
4. Dormer, R.A.: Confidentiality and the drug abuse patient. In Bourne, P.G., editor: Acute drug abuse emergencies, New York, 1976, Academic Press, Inc.
5. Brown, J.K., and Malone, M.H.: Pacific Information Service on Street Drugs 6(1-2):22, 1978.
6. Goldschmidt, R.H., and Beforado, J.M.: Emergency procedure for bad trips, Stash Capsules 2(2):1-2, 1970.
7. Smith, R.F., and Smith, S.L.: Overdose aid, Ann Arbor, Mich., 1972, Michigan Department of Social Services.
8. Hahn, H.H., and others: Complications of injecting dissolved methylphenidate tablets, Archives of Internal Medicine 123:656-659, 1969.
9. Hopkins, G.B., and Taylor, D.G.: Pulmonary talc granulomatosis, Annual Review of Respiratory Disease 101:101-104, 1970.
10. Schonberg, S.K., and others: Somatic consequences of drug abuse among adolescents, Pediatric Annals, pp. 22-41, February, 1973.

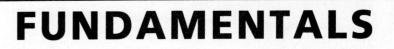

UNIT **2**

FUNDAMENTALS

CHAPTER 5

NERVOUS SYSTEM

PSYCHOACTIVE DRUGS HAVE many actions. Some we experience as pleasant, some as unpleasant, some as bizarre, some as natural as warm apple pie. Whatever the experience, it results from an action on the information-processing systems of the body. A detailed analysis of these systems is not necessary, but an overview is essential to appreciate where drugs act and why and to begin to understand how they can influence consciousness, mood, and feeling.

Complex organisms such as human beings can survive only if they continually adapt and adjust themselves to the changing environment. Both the internal (inside the body) and the external (outside the body) environments have important effects on the well-being of the individual. It is necessary to maintain the physiology and biochemistry of the body within certain limits, and human beings are equipped with many self-adjusting systems to keep body functions within these limits. The term for these self-adjusting characteristics is *homeostasis*.

To maintain homeostasis the body needs to carry out three types of functions. First, it must be able to monitor the activity of the internal and external environments, that is, to sense changes and constancies in those environments. Second, information about the environments must be integrated with memories of previous features of the environ-

ment. Third, when the processing of old and new information is complete, there must be a way for the necessary adjustments of the body to be carried out.

In humans there are two information-processing systems, each with certain characteristics, capabilities, and qualities that make it uniquely suited for its particular role in maintaining homeostasis. These two systems are the *nervous system* and the *endocrine system*.

The nervous system is a combination electrical-chemical system with several distinctive functions. It is designed to monitor relatively specific changes in the environments, to carry information about these changes along distinct routes to a specific processing center, and to do these things rapidly. Communications in the nervous system are both specific and fast, reaching a speed of 200 miles per hour at times.

The endocrine system is a chemical system and has a role that complements and, in part, underlies the nervous system. In contrast to the nervous system, it is slower and more diffuse in terms of both what elicits a response and how the response occurs. The endocrine system is responsive to a wide range of not clearly defined changes in both environments. Much of the output from this system has effects on all cells of the body, and as such it has a pervasive effect. Some parts of this system, though, are sensitive only to restricted changes in the internal environment and have quite discrete effects. The endocrine system does not have a pathway used only for the transmission of its information, since the complex molecules that carry the information of the endocrine system are secreted into the bloodstream to be carried to the places where they are to have their primary effect. Speed of information transmission is slow in the endocrine system (blood circulation time is about 60 seconds in humans) when compared to the nervous system.

It is accurate to say that the endocrine system is more involved in setting base levels from which the nervous system functions, but it is not a complete statement, since these two systems are interrelated and affecting one affects the other. Because they primarily play different roles and are quite different anatomically and physiologically, they are usually studied separately. Since our concern is with the psychoactive drugs, which primarily have their effects through actions on the nervous system, only the nervous system will be outlined here.

FUNDAMENTALS

The basic unit in the nervous system is a specialized cell called a *neuron*. There are about 14 billion separate neurons in humans, and since the end of the nineteenth century it has been clear that the nervous system is not continuous like the circulatory system. Information moves from one neuron to another only across a specialized gap of 0.00002 mm, called a *synapse*.

A neuron has three parts that are important in information transmission. *Dendrites* receive information that is then carried along the threadlike *axon* to the *terminals*. The length of a neuron is almost completely determined by the axon, which may vary in humans from much less than a millimeter in the brain to a few feet when connecting the spinal cord to the toe. The diameter of axons varies some but is rarely larger than 20 micrometers (μm). There are many dendrites collecting information and many terminals, but a neuron has only

a single axon. The terminals of one neuron end close to dendrites of other neurons, and this terminal-dendrite area is the synapse. Information movement in a neuron is from dendrite to axon to terminals. From the terminals of one neuron information moves via the synapse to the dendrite of the next neuron. Dendrites may also receive information from specialized cells called *receptors*, which are the windows to the inside and outside world for the nervous system. Receptors change one form of information—light, sound, carbon dioxide concentration, and the like—into electrical activity, which is the way information is carried in neurons.

The nervous system is electrical in that information is carried from dendrites along axons to terminals as an electrical pulse. Usually, this information is actually a series of pulses, with each pulse lasting about $\frac{1}{500}$ of a second and having an amplitude of $\frac{1}{10}$ volt. The electrical pulses are little affected by most drugs. However, the pulse is generated because of certain characteristics of the neuron's cell wall, and some drugs do influence information processing by acting on and changing the cell wall.

At the synapse information is *not* transmitted electrically. It was only in the 1940s that the evidence became overwhelming that electrical pulses did not jump the synaptic gap but instead caused a release of chemicals from the terminals. These chemicals move across the synapse and cause electrical changes in the dendrite of the next neuron. The dendrites of a single neuron may have many synapses, up to 100,000, with terminals of many neurons. If enough synapses in a dendrite are active at about the same time, an electrical pulse is initiated in the axon, which then travels to its terminals. The sequence of information movement in the nervous system is summarized in Fig. 5-1.

The chemicals released from the terminals are called *neurotransmitters*, and the best evidence now is that only one kind of chemical is released from each cell. There are four chemicals almost all authorities accept as neurotransmitters: acetylcholine, noradrenaline, dopamine, and serotonin. There is still controversy over the exact number of

Electrical pulse in axon	→	Electrical pulse in terminals	→	Chemicals released from terminals	→	Chemicals attach to receptor site	→	Chemicals in receptor sites cause changes in electrical activity of dendrite	→	Initiates electrical impulse in axon

FIG. 5-1 Sequence and mode of information movement in the nervous system.

neurotransmitters. Most psychoactive drugs exert their actions through their effects on these neurotransmitters.

The exact way in which neurotransmitters bring about changes in the dendrite is not yet known, but the place on a dendrite where a transmitter has its effect is called a *receptor site*. It is established that both the electrical characteristics and the structural configuration of the neurotransmitter must conform to those of the receptor if the electrical activity of the dendrite is to be affected. The standard analogy is to a lock and key. The receptor, the lock, is such that various chemicals, keys, may occupy it, but only one—the specific neurotransmitter—normally unlocks it, that is, causes a change in the electrical activity of the dendrite.

The receptor site is still hypothetical, but much research attempts to specify the characteristics it must have for the nervous system to function as it does. Appreciate the fact that a synapse in the brain is only about 0.5 μm^2 in area—a square inch could contain 63 billion. Within this 0.5 μm^2 there must be many receptor sites, since each electrical impulse may release thousands of molecules of the transmitter. These molecules must move across the gap, occupy a molecular-sized receptor site, and have their effect in a few milliseconds. It may be helpful to realize that the acetylcholine molecule is only about 10 square angstroms; a square inch could contain 62.5 trillion of the molecules.

Within the nervous system integration of information occurs in the dendrite. If certain conditions are met, an impulse is initiated and travels down the axon. Functionally, this is one of two types of synapses and is called an *excitatory synapse*, since the neurotransmitter acting at the receptor sites makes it likely that an electrical impulse will travel along the axon. There are also inhibitory synapses,

which are similar except that the chemicals released affect the dendrite to make it less likely that an impulse will be initiated in the axon.

The final output from a dendrite, pulse or no pulse in the axon, will depend on what type of synapses are active, how many of each type, and how frequently they are active in a brief period of time. Phrased a little differently, the dendrite acts as a gate at each step of information processing. No matter how many neurons carry information to a dendrite, there are only two possible outputs: an electrical pulse in the axon or no electrical pulse.

Therefore, no matter what effect a drug has on synaptic transmission, it should be clear that at the level of the neuron there are basically only three things that can happen to a neuron. It can be made more excitable (that is, easier to elicit an electrical impulse in the axon), less excitable, or it can be made more variable in its normal action. It is a combination of what a drug does to these synaptic processes, where it does it, and for how long that determines what effects a drug will have.

Many psychoactive agents have their action by affecting the production, storage, or deactivation of the neurotransmitters. Normal functioning of the nervous system depends on the regular manufacturing of neurotransmitters in neurons, their release as a result of an electrical impulse, and their breakdown or deactivation after they have had their effect on the dendrite. By changing one of these processes, information transmission is modified or blocked.

The receptor site is the place where drugs act that mimic or block the neurotransmitters. Some drugs have electrical and spatial characteristics similar to the transmitters so that they can occupy the receptor and activate it—they open the lock! Other agents prevent transmitters from having an effect because they occupy but do not activate the receptor site.

NEUROTRANSMITTERS

Although it is only probable that *acetylcholine*, *noradrenaline*, *dopamine*, and *serotonin* are neurotransmitters in the brain, it is well established that acetylcholine and noradrenaline are neurotransmitters in other parts of the body. These chemicals are manufactured and stored in the neurons that release them. To understand how drugs disrupt these processes, it is necessary to know something about the manufacturing and storing process.

Manufacturing complex molecules in the body is frequently accomplished in several steps, with each

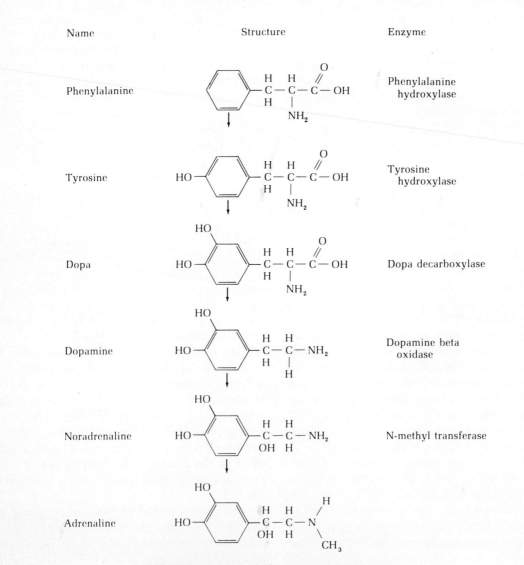

Name	Structure	Enzyme
Phenylalanine		Phenylalanine hydroxylase
Tyrosine		Tyrosine hydroxylase
Dopa		Dopa decarboxylase
Dopamine		Dopamine beta oxidase
Noradrenaline		N-methyl transferase
Adrenaline		

FIG. 5-2 Synthesis of adrenergic neurotransmitters.

step adding to or taking away some part of the existing molecule. The particular action at each step is accomplished by a molecule called an *enzyme*. An enzyme acts as a catalyst, that is, a substance which makes possible a chemical reaction but does not itself get used in the reaction. If one of the enzymes involved in building a neurotransmitter is destroyed or prevented in some way from having its effect, then the supply of the neurotransmitter will eventually decrease and drop below the amount necessary for normal functioning of the neuron. The same process is employed in the deactivation of a neurotransmitter. Specific enzymes change the transmitter to a molecule that is no longer active at the receptor site. In some cases the enzymes further modify the molecule so that it can readily be excreted. Blocking the activity of a deactivating enzyme may result in a prolongation or intensification of the action of the neurotransmitter.

The manufacture of noradrenaline is a four-step process and begins with the amino acid phenylal-

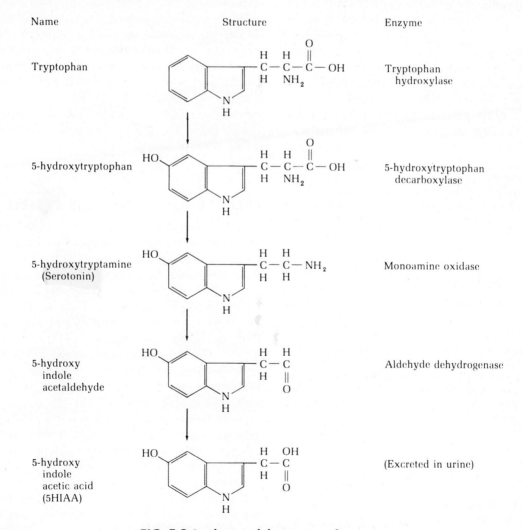

Name	Structure	Enzyme
Tryptophan		Tryptophan hydroxylase
5-hydroxytryptophan		5-hydroxytryptophan decarboxylase
5-hydroxytryptamine (Serotonin)		Monoamine oxidase
5-hydroxy indole acetaldehyde		Aldehyde dehydrogenase
5-hydroxy indole acetic acid (5HIAA)		(Excreted in urine)

FIG. 5-3 Synthesis and deactivation of serotonin.

anine. Fig. 5-2 shows the chemical structure,* name of the molecule, and the name of the active enzyme at each step. Note especially that dopamine is the step just before noradrenaline, so this series of biochemical transformations manufactures two neurotransmitters.

The step changing noradrenaline to adrenaline has been included because, under some conditions, the chemical adrenaline is released from the adrenal gland into the bloodstream, and it then acts at the same receptor sites as noradrenaline. The deactivation processes of dopamine, noradrenaline, and adrenaline are quite complex and will not be detailed here. It must be mentioned that there are two primary enzymes involved, monoamine oxidase (MAO), and catechol-O-methyl transferase (COMT), but in normal functioning the adrenergic transmitters leave the receptor site and are taken up again in the terminals to be reused.

The synthesis of serotonin is simpler than that of noradrenaline. Beginning with the essential ami-

no acid tryptophan, it takes only two steps to build serotonin. Fig. 5-3 shows the synthesis of serotonin as well as its deactivation. Deactivation is not complex, and excretion in the urine of the end product provides an easy way to monitor the deactivation of serotonin.

Acetylcholine formation and breakdown is the simplest of them all. Starting from choline and acetic acid, acetylcholine is formed directly, and its deactivation is readily accomplished as shown in Fig. 5-4.

Neurons that release acetylcholine are termed *cholinergic* and noradrenaline-, dopamine-, and serotonin-releasing neurons are called, respectively, *adrenergic*, *dopaminergic*, and *serotonergic*. Most frequently, a system of neurons that serves a specific function is made up of one type of neuron. Usually acetylcholine acts as an excitatory neurotransmitter, serotonin is probably an inhibitory transmitter, whereas noradrenaline and dopamine can be either excitatory or inhibitory, depending on the place of action.

---

*Throughout this book the standard convention will be used in showing chemical structures of ring-shaped (closed) molecules. Although the atoms joined together are carbon atoms (C) and each has a hydrogen (H) atom attached to it, neither the carbon nor the hydrogen atoms are indicated. Thus

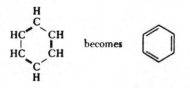

This is a benzene ring. When a hydrogen atom is replaced with another atom or atoms, then the new atoms are shown. When only one hydrogen in a benzene ring is replaced with any atom or group of atoms, then the unit is called a *phenyl*. When two hydroxyl groups (OH) are substituted on a benzene ring, the structure is called a *catechol*:

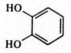

It should be noted that both dopamine and noradrenaline are catechols, and, since they have an amine group, NH2, attached, they are frequently referred to as *catecholamines*.

PRELUDE TO THE NERVOUS SYSTEM

The combination of individual neurons into a smoothly functioning mechanism that carries information from the environment to the brain and then, sometimes, back out to muscles or glands is a remarkable achievement. To simplify the task of understanding the way in which the nervous system works, it is usually divided into two parts. Protectively enclosed in the skull and vertebral column are the brain and spinal cord, which together are called the *central nervous system* (CNS) and which form the major integrating system of the body. A second integrating system is the *autonomic nervous system* (ANS), which forms a ladderlike network of nerves along each side of the vertebral column. This ladder with clusters of terminals and dendrites connects with the spinal cord at each vertebra.

Dividing the entire nervous system of the body into the CNS and the ANS is a convenience, but it is not completely honest, since part of the ANS

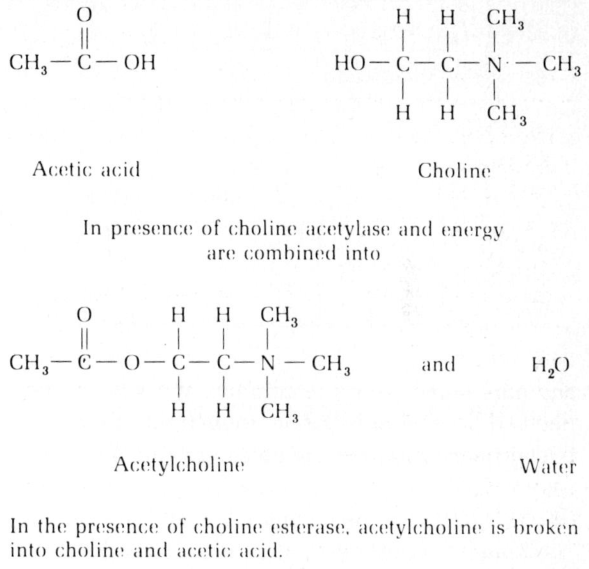

$$CH_3 - \overset{\overset{\displaystyle O}{\|}}{C} - OH$$

Acetic acid

$$HO - \overset{\overset{\displaystyle H}{|}}{\underset{\underset{\displaystyle H}{|}}{C}} - \overset{\overset{\displaystyle H}{|}}{\underset{\underset{\displaystyle H}{|}}{C}} - \overset{\overset{\displaystyle CH_3}{|}}{\underset{\underset{\displaystyle CH_3}{|}}{N}} \cdot - CH_3$$

Choline

In presence of choline acetylase and energy
are combined into

$$CH_3 - \overset{\overset{\displaystyle O}{\|}}{C} - O - \overset{\overset{\displaystyle H}{|}}{\underset{\underset{\displaystyle H}{|}}{C}} - \overset{\overset{\displaystyle H}{|}}{\underset{\underset{\displaystyle H}{|}}{C}} - \overset{\overset{\displaystyle CH_3}{|}}{\underset{\underset{\displaystyle CH_3}{|}}{N}} - CH_3 \qquad and \qquad H_2O$$

Acetylcholine   Water

In the presence of choline esterase, acetylcholine is broken
into choline and acetic acid.

FIG. 5-4 Acetylcholine formation and breakdown.

is in the CNS and some of the outputs from the CNS travel via the ANS to muscles and glands. The two systems have characteristics unique enough to make separation of them meaningful for the purpose of discussion, but it must be realized that the systems are intimately related in many of their functions. Briefly, the ANS is primarily concerned with the regulation of visceral functions and the maintenance of a stable internal environment, whereas the CNS functions to integrate incoming information from the internal and external environments and then sends out information to muscles and glands.

AUTONOMIC NERVOUS SYSTEM

The ANS is primarily a motor or output system and has most of its synapses outside the CNS. This point is important, since there are many chemicals that cannot enter the CNS and thus have effects only on the ANS. The ANS is meaningfully divided into two units, the *sympathetic* and the *parasympathetic systems*, which have generally opposite effects on an organ or function. Both systems send neurons to most visceral organs as well as to smooth muscles, glands, and blood vessels.

Since the control of most visceral functions and the circulatory and glandular systems is through the ANS, there are many examples that could be given of opposing sympathetic and parasympathetic effects. A few of the most relevant are given in Table 5-1. The sympathetic system is quite diffuse and undifferentiated in its actions compared to the parasympathetic system. The sympathetic division of the ANS functions principally to mobilize the organism for action, whereas the parasympathetic system generally operates to maintain ongoing production of necessary materials by the digestive system.

Of particular interest is the fact that in the parasympathetic system synapses at each structure being affected are cholinergic, while the sympathetic synapses at the same structure are adrenergic. When blood levels of adrenaline rise or when drugs are given that mimic the action of noradrenaline, the result is the same as if the sympathetic nervous system had been activated. These sympathomimetic effects are important in considering the actions of many drugs, since most drugs do have an effect on the ANS. Sometimes these are more important than the effects on the CNS.

TABLE 5-1 Sympathetic and parasympathetic effects on selected structures

Structure or function	Sympathetic reaction	Parasympathetic reaction
Pupil of eye	Dilation	Constriction
Heart rate	Increase	Decrease
Breathing rate	Fast and shallow	Slow and deep
Stomach and intestinal glands	Inhibited	Activated
Stomach and intestinal wall	No motility	Motility
Sweat glands	Secretion	No effect
Skin blood vessels	Constriction	Dilation

CENTRAL NERVOUS SYSTEM

The brain and spinal cord make up the CNS, but since the spinal cord functions primarily to carry information to and from the brain, it will not be mentioned further. The human brain is a wondrous structure that contains about 11 billion neurons and weighs 3 pounds. It is an integrating and storage device that is not yet equaled by the largest computers. Even though the brain is much slower than a computer in its operations and in processing each bit of information, the brain has the advantage of being able to handle more channels of information simultaneously.

The functions of some parts of the brain will be detailed because they have particular importance for the study of drug actions and for understanding the effects of drugs on behavior. The *reticular activating system* is in the area where the spinal cord connects with the brain. It modulates incoming sensory information and outgoing motor impulses and regulates the degree of arousal and alertness an individual shows. The *hypothalamus* is located near the bottom of the brain and is the integrator of information from many sources as well as being the control center for the autonomic nervous system. The hypothalamus is also the primary point of contact between the nervous system and the endocrine system. The *medial forebrain bundle* is a collection of axons of neurons coursing along both sides of the hypothalamus and is the anatomical focus of pleasure. The *periventricular system* is another collection of nerve fibers. These fibers interact with the medial forebrain bundle; this fiber

system seems to be the substrate for punishment. Several clusters of neurons above and to the sides of the hypothalamus form the *basal ganglia*, which are the primary control centers for involuntary motor movements such as those involved in posture.

The *cerebral cortex* is the most complex structure in the animal kingdom and is the part of the brain that gives humans their special uniqueness among animals. It almost completely surrounds the rest of the brain and lies just inside the skull. It is responsible for the analysis of incoming information and for the initiation of voluntary motor behavior. In the cortex the center for speech has been identified as well as areas for sensation and movement. These six parts of the brain will be briefly discussed, some general rules about brain functioning will be mentioned, and, finally, some possible mechanisms for drug actions will be suggested.

Reticular activating system

The reticular activating system (RAS) is very old phylogenetically and is characterized as being an area that receives inputs from all the sensory systems as well as from the cerebral cortex. The RAS is multisynaptic and sends many axons throughout the brain. Being multisynaptic means that information moving through this structure must cross many synapses, and thus it is particularly susceptible to influence by drugs.

One of the primary functions of the RAS is to control the arousal level of the brain, especially the cerebral cortex. The RAS is stimulated following input to any sensory system and sends impulses to many parts of the cortex. The RAS initiates impulses in the neurons there and thus prepares the cortex to receive further information through the sensory pathways. When the cortex has been activated by the RAS, the organism is behaviorally aroused, and the nervous system is active and alert to environmental stimuli.

The RAS receives electrical impulses from the sensory systems through *collaterals*, which are branches of the sensory neurons. Input into a sensory system, then, sends impulses directly to the appropriate receiving area of the cortex and also to the RAS. Both paths are essential if the individual is to be aware of the stimulus. Information arriving at an unaroused cortex is equivalent to no information, and arousal without sensory input to the cortex results in an alert person without anything to be alert about!

The RAS seems to be predominantly adrenergic. High blood levels of adrenaline or noradrenaline result in its activation and thus activation of the cerebral cortex. Compounds that are sympathomimetic activate the RAS, whereas compounds that disrupt adrenergic synapses decrease the responsiveness of the RAS to sensory input.

Hypothalamus

The hypothalamus is probably best described as the structure that primarily controls the autonomic nervous system and therefore functions to integrate information from the body that is relevant to the maintenance of the organism. The hypothalamus is composed of pairs (one in each side of the brain) of nuclei, which are clusters of the dendrites of neurons serving a common function. Some of these nuclei monitor blood levels of various chemicals, and if the blood level goes outside the normal range, the hypothalamic neurons send impulses to appropriate control centers to restore normal levels. The hypothalamus is also the interface between the nervous system and the endocrine system and acts to adjust the release of hormones to the homeostatic needs of the body.

The hypothalamus is an area with a rich blood supply, and because of this fact many drugs first enter the brain in high concentrations at this structure. The initial effects of these drugs are frequently autonomic ones, with changes in consciousness and mood developing more slowly as drug levels increase in the areas of the brain controlling these experiences.

Medial forebrain bundle

For years hedonists have talked about and sought the locus of pleasure, but it was not until 1954 that the specific brain systems were discovered that seem to form the physiological substrate of pleasure and reward. The details of this system, the medial forebrain bundle (MFB), are only slowly being uncovered, but two things are clear. First, animals and humans will perform work to have the neurons in this system activated electrically by a permanently implanted electrode. Electrical activity in the system seems, then, to act as a reward. Second, humans report that activation of this band of neurons is experienced as pleasurable, and there is evidence that stimulation in this area will counteract feelings of depression.

The function of this system in humans is not well understood, and its relationship to natural stimuli that result in pleasurable feelings, such as food and sex, is not known. The suggestion has been made that psychosis is related to abnormal functioning of the MFB. This has not been shown directly, but drugs that calm the agitated psychotic person also decrease the reward value of electrical stimulation of the MFB. Another hypothesis is that the level of electrical activity of the MFB is the decisive factor in determining general mood level and clinical depression. Again, most drugs that affect clinical depression also affect the reward value of electrical stimulation in this area, with agents that reduce depression making the MFB more sensitive to direct stimulation.

Periventricular system

One of the long-standing questions in philosophy has been whether negative feelings and unhappiness are only the absence of good feelings or whether there is an active process involved. A question moves into the scientific realm when techniques become available for answering it. Paralleling the discovery and explanation of the characteristics of the medial forebrain bundle has been investigation of the punishment or aversive collection of fibers called the periventricular system (PV).

In both the reward and the punishment systems are two kinds of effects that must be kept clear, although they may have the same physiological basis. One effect is the experience, the feeling that accompanies electrical stimulation of these systems. A second effect is that which these neural paths have on the other aspects of behavior. There have not been many studies in which humans have been electrically stimulated in these brain areas. The procedure is obviously very experimental, so caution must be used in accepting the results. It does seem clear, however, that the feelings and emotions an individual experiences are drastically different when these two systems are electrically stimulated.

Stimulating the reward system brings forth expressions of pleasure and satisfaction, whereas periventricular stimulation is followed by strong verbalization of discomfort. Similarly, MFB stimulation increases behavioral activity, while a slowing or stopping of behavior seems related to PV activation. Pharmacologically, the best evidence is that adrenergic synapses dominate the reward system, while the inhibitory PV system seems to be mostly serotonergic. The two systems may be related functionally so that activation of the MFB inhibits the inhibitory PV system. Inhibition of an inhibitory system results in a release of the neural fibers normally inhibited, and this results in activation.

Basal ganglia

The basal ganglia consist of a group of nuclei that form a secondary motor system. The primary motor system originates in the motor area of the cerebral cortex and controls voluntary movements. It is in the cortical motor area that electrical impulses orig-

inate when an individual decides to make a behavioral response. The basal ganglia are concerned with the nonvoluntary, nonconscious adjustments of the skeletal muscles that maintain posture and muscle tone.

The basal ganglia are mentioned here for two reasons. One is that damage to this secondary motor system sometimes results in a syndrome called *Parkinson's disease*. This disorder is characterized by postural rigidity, tremors, and a decrease in facial expressiveness. Recent work suggests strongly that dopamine is the neurotransmitter in this area, and some cases of Parkinson's disease have been successfully treated by the administration of the drug L-dopa, which is the precursor to dopamine.

The second reason for identifying these ganglia and their functions is that one of the undesirable effects of the phenothiazine drugs used in the treatment of psychotics is the appearance of Parkinson-like symptoms. Frequently these symptoms are so severe that they must be controlled by the administration of an additional drug.

Cerebral cortex

The cerebral cortex is a structure weighing about 1 pound. It contains the dendrites and axon terminals of 9 billion neurons, their supporting cells, and blood vessels. The cerebral cortex is the brain structure that has changed most from other animals to humans; a much higher percentage of the brain is devoted to the cortex in humans. The human cerebral cortex has become so large that it folds over on itself in many places and almost completely covers the other parts of the brain. A side view of the brain would show only the cortex and few of the other brain centers.

The cerebral cortex can be divided into receiving areas, output areas, and association areas. The receiving areas, those to which neurons from the various senses send information, and the output areas are clearly affected by some psychoactive agents. The sensory areas and their sense organs are connected in very specific ways so that receptors responding to a particular stimulus characteristic always terminate in the same general area of the cortex. Any drugs that affect the electrical activity in the receptors or the connecting neurons or synapses in the pathway from receptor to cortex will thus affect that specific stimulus quality.

The part of the cortex that has changed most in the evolutionary process is the area called the association cortex. In large part, the proportion of the cerebral cortex that is association cortex is a good index of the extent to which an animal is not under the direct influence of the environment. The association areas neither directly receive inputs from the environment nor directly initiate outputs to muscles or glands. These association areas may function, for example, to store memories or control complex behaviors; much is unknown, but it is clear that some of the psychoactive drugs disrupt the normal functioning of these areas.

A QUICK REVIEW

The nervous system is the primary site of action for psychoactive drugs. Individual neurons are the building blocks that are functionally but not structurally joined to transmit information. Information is carried within a neuron as an electrical impulse, and this intraneuronal activity is little affected by most drugs.

The functional connection between neurons is the synapse. Complex molecules called neurotransmitters carry information from one neuron to another. Most psychoactive drugs influence the functioning of the nervous system by modifying the production, release, action, or breakdown of these neurotransmitters. The type of effect a drug will have depends on the neurotransmitter with which it interacts, the form of such interactions, where in the nervous system that neurotransmitter is found, and what function that area of the nervous system serves.

It is possible to spend a lifetime worrying about the bits and pieces that go to make up the nervous system and still have almost no idea about how the brain works. The capabilities that neurons have set limitations on what the brain can do and how it can function, but these limitations are so broad as to be almost meaningless. The true, fantastic potential of the brain becomes clear only as its processes and operations, not just its parts, become known.

TOWARD AN UNDERSTANDING OF DRUG EFFECTS ON COMPLEX PROCESSES

The autonomic effects of drugs can be fairly readily understood, since much knowledge exists about the anatomy and biochemistry of the autonomic nervous system. Similarly, when a drug acts on a sensory system input, there is at least a partially acceptable neural basis for the drug experiences. With more complex behaviors and experiences, a complete physiological explanation of a drug's effects becomes impossible, since neither the neuroanatomical locus nor the biochemical processes involved are known.

One approach to understanding psychoactive drug effects on complex behaviors is to study the general ways in which the cerebral cortex functions. Another method is to analyze aspects of behavior that in part determine the effects of drugs. Briefly, some modes of central nervous system functioning are consistent no matter what drug is being used. Similarly, some aspects of behavior influence the effects of all drugs.

Principles of nervous system functioning

To understand the role of the cerebral cortex in determining psychoactive drug effects, four rules must be remembered. One is that the cortex varies continually in its state of arousal, that is, its receptivity and sensitivity to incoming information. Sleep is a condition of low arousal, alertness, and responsiveness to environmental changes. In conditions of intellectual activity and emotional stress the cortex is "activated," alert and responsive to electrical pulses coming to it. The level of arousal is primarily controlled by the reticular activating system, and inputs from the senses go both to the reticular system and to the cerebral cortex.

A second rule is that any electrical activity in a

sensory area is experienced and interpreted by the individual as coming from the receptors which normally feed into that sensory area. For example, electrically stimulating the visual cortex directly with an electrode is experienced as flashes of light or "seeing" geometric figures. The experience of a sensation does not depend on where the electrical activity comes from but rather on the part of the cerebral cortex that receives the electrical pulses. To go one step further, *all experience, thoughts, and feelings are nothing more than electrical activity in some part of the brain*. By modifying the electrical activity of neurons in the central nervous system, psychoactive drugs influence and modify experience, thoughts, and feelings.

The third rule is that once information arrives at a sensory receiving area, it then goes to memory areas. The incoming information has meaning only if it coincides with some information in the memory storage area. For incoming impulses to be understood, they must not only arrive at the correct sensory area but also be transmitted to the correct memory area. Location of the memory areas is not well known, but probably both cortical and subcortical portions of the brain are involved. Since impulses from a sensory area must travel to a memory area, it may be that this type of organization is the basis for certain drug effects. With some drugs there seems to be interaction between the senses, and inputs to the visual system may be experienced as both a visual and an auditory experience. This could occur if impulses leaving the visual cortex are incorrectly processed (because of the drug) and sent to both the visual and auditory memory areas.

A fourth rule is that many of the functions of the cerebral cortex are carried out by inhibiting or suppressing other parts of the brain or of the cortex itself. In the process of maturing, both physically and psychologically, one role of the cortex seems to be to inhibit some behaviors and thoughts. The inhibition seems to be an active process, so that when the inhibition is removed, the ideas and behaviors reappear. This occurs in some kinds of organic brain damage where the cortex is physically incapable of functioning normally, the inhibited behaviors, thoughts, and emotions appear. The same

phenomenon occurs with some drugs when the functioning of the cortex is disrupted so that it temporarily ceases its inhibitory role. This fact is one of the reasons for the wide range of effects reported with some psychoactive drugs—what appears depends in part on what was inhibited originally.

Behavioral determinants of drug effects

Behavior is the final output of a complex and incompletely understood nervous system. It results from both past and present inputs to that system. Even though the underlying processes are not clear, it is possible to relate the actions of drugs to at least five dimensions of behavior.

Three behavioral dimensions that are clearly different, but perhaps highly related, are level of abstraction, level of complexity, and level of learning. The more abstract and the more complex the behavior, the more likely it is to be changed following ingestion of a drug. Abstract ideas and complex motor or thought patterns probably are more susceptible in part because they are less well learned than simpler or more concrete behaviors. With a particular task the probability of disrupting it with a given dose of a drug decreases with an increase in the degree of learning. Some behaviors are probably such well-learned habits that very little this side of a coma will disrupt them.

One way of viewing these dimensions is to consider what the neural basis might be. For complex behaviors there must be a lengthy sequence of neural events, all of which must be correct if the behavior is to be intact. In abstract ideas there may be a large number of essential associations (neural connections) if the level of abstraction is to be constant. When there are many elements in a situation, all of which are necessary for complete functioning, a greater probability exists of a drug disrupting at least one step of the neural activity than if there were only a few component parts. In the same vein, an increase in level of learning may improve synaptic functioning or increase the redundancy of the neural patterns that underlie the behavior. Either of these changes would result in a decrease in the ease with which a given drug dose could modify the behavior.

The other two behavioral dimensions relating to the actions of drugs are concerned with motivational aspects of the behavior. Motivation may vary with respect to both type and level. Motivation for a particular behavior might be positive or negative. That is, the behavior may primarily be moving toward or approaching a particular kind of stimulus. It is expected that this behavior would be physiologically based in a normally functioning medial forebrain bundle. Or the behavior may be oriented toward avoiding or escaping from some event. The periventricular system is the physiological substrate underlying this negatively motivated behavior. Some drugs do have different behavioral effects, depending on the type of motivation governing the behavior.

Motivation level seems also to be an important factor in predicting the effect of a drug on behavior. It seems likely that as the motivational level increases, there will be an increase in the amount of electrical activity in the motivational systems. This may be the result of more frequent pulses in the same neurons or of the same frequency of pulses in more neurons. In either case, the predicted effect would be increased electrical activity in the motivational systems, and the data support the prediction: as the motivation level of a behavior increases, it becomes more difficult to disrupt the behavior with drugs.

CONCLUDING COMMENT

The preceding factors point out very well the difficulty involved in talking about specific drug effects when the drugs do not act on parts of the nervous system that have built-in functions. All of these behavioral factors refer in some way to the history of the individual. As the history changes, so will the behavioral effects of the drug.

Psychoactive drugs act on the nervous system. To the extent that the actions are on the parts and processes of the nervous system that have built-in, specific functions, the effects of a drug can be predicted. As the behaviors studied become more dependent on factors in the individual's personal history, the exact effects of a drug become less predictable.

CHAPTER 6

PRELUDE TO
PHARMACOLOGY

IN CONSIDERING THE WAYS in which a drug can act and the numerous factors that influence the effectiveness of a drug, it is necessary to push headlong into the complex science of pharmacology. The field of pharmacology has a long past, but, as a science, it has a short history. Although the earliest clear record of a compendium of drugs is about 1500 BC, according to some authorities the modern era of pharmacology did not begin until the work of Francois Magendie (1783-1855). American pharmacology began even later, with John J. Abel (1857-1938) as the father.

An early connotation of the Greek word "pharmakon" was of a harmful substance—something to be eliminated. However, pharmacology is now defined as the study of the interaction of chemical agents with living material. Interactions whose effects are harmful are generally relegated to the specialty area called *toxicology*. Another specialty area, the most active field in pharmacology and one that cuts across all its research areas, is pharmacodynamics. *Pharmacodynamics is concerned with studying the mechanism of action of drugs*. It deals with the problem of how a drug has its effect on the living organism. Chapter 7 is in large part a discussion of pharmacodynamics.

The word *drug* comes from the French *drogue*, meaning dry substance. It reflects well the con-dition of many of the early herbs used for the treatment of various illnesses. The classic story of a plant making the transition from folk remedies to the mainstream of science and therapeutic usefulness is illustrated by digitalis. A folk remedy for the treatment of dropsy was a combination of many herbs plus an extract from the purple foxglove plant (*Digitalis purpurea*, purple finger, because of its shape and color). William Withering studied the remedy and reported in 1785 that the purple foxglove was effective in reducing the excessive body fluids in some types of dropsy.[1] In 1799 J. Ferrior pointed out that the primary action of digitalis was on the heart; it is still a basic therapeutic agent in cases of congestive heart failure. Drugs of natural origin are still found in about 50% of prescription drugs and about 40% of OTC preparations.

In the science of pharmacology, *a drug is any substance, other than food, that by its chemical or physical nature alters structure or function in the living organism*. Drugs can be classified in many ways ranging from their chemical structure, to their effects on biochemical, physiological, or behavioral systems, to their social uses. The drugs in this book have been primarily categorized into socially meaningful clusters of compounds and then subgrouped on the basis of their chemical structure.

CATEGORIZING DRUGS

Physicians, pharmacologists, chemists, lawyers, psychologists, and users all have drug classification schemes that best serve their own purposes. A compound such as amphetamine might be categorized as an antiappetite agent by many physicians, since it reduced food intake for a period of time. It might be classed as a phenylethylamine by a pharmacologist, since its basic structure is a phenyl ring with an ethyl group and an amine attached. The chemist wastes no time and says flat-out that amphetamine is 2-amino-1-phenylpropane. To the lawyer amphetamine may only be a drug of abuse falling in Schedule II of the 1970 federal drug law, while the psychologist may say simply that it is a stimulant. The user may call it a diet pill or an upper. The important thing to remember is that any scheme for categorizing drugs has meaning only if it serves the purpose for which the classification is being made.

Hopefully, some appreciation of the social meaning of the uses of drugs can be conveyed here as well as an understanding of the scientific basis of their use. Toward that end, socially and scientifically meaningful groupings are used in this book. A listing of the major classes of compounds in this scheme can be seen by looking at the Table of Contents. A brief survey of these classes and the rationale behind the classification may be helpful in following the unfolding story of drugs. It should be clear that this classification is only for psychoactive drugs, chemicals that alter experiences and mood.

There are some drugs—chemicals affecting living organisms—that few people think of as drugs. These nondrug drugs include alcohol and caffeine (a depressant and a stimulant), as well as compounds that can be picked up at the friendly supermarket—aspirin, antihistamines, and antacids. Although the oral contraceptive is a prescription drug, it is not taken to reduce a symptom or to control a disease. Unfortunately many women use them daily with no more concern than if they were vitamins. The single most important factor about all these compounds is that they are widely used and readily available. Since most can be purchased without a prescription and *everyone* uses them, they are not usually considered to be drugs—but they are.

The general grouping of *psychotherapeutic agents* seems to be widely accepted—these are the drugs used in psychiatric medicine. These compounds are prescribed when the symptom of illness is a disruption of the interaction between an individual and his environment. The drugs that reduce either the disruption or the reaction to the disruption are discussed together. At least two social characteristics distinguish these agents: they are used therapeutically to treat "mental disturbances," and they rarely fall into the category of abused drugs. Other therapeutically useful drugs are widely known and grouped together because they frequently are abused, and their medical use is for the treatment of minor problems (For example, obesity and insomnia).

Although nearly everyone knows that the *opiates*, morphine and heroin, can have considerable therapeutic value, these drugs are generally not viewed as therapeutic. Rather, these narcotics are seen as the hard drugs, the drugs used by addicts and the ones peddled on the street by low-level members of organized and disorganized crime. In a very real sense these drugs are unique both socially and scientifically.

The *hallucinogens* form a separate class in our social thinking. To group drugs such as LSD and marijuana together and still clearly separate them does justice to the scientific data as well as the social scene.

Clearly, as time changes, so may the rational way to categorize drugs. The biochemical actions and the physiological effects do not change, but the relevance and implications for society of these effects may change considerably from one generation to another. Over 40 years ago a now-classic categorization of drugs was accomplished by Lewin primarily on the basis of social, behavioral, and experienced effects.[2] This is still a useful scheme, and contrasting it to the one used in this book will help provide a glimpse of the broad picture of drug classification. Lewin combines some drug groups dif-

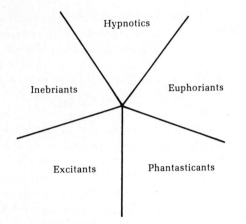

FIG. 6-1 Lewin's classification of centrally acting drugs.

ferently than is done here, and tranquilizers and mood modifiers were unknown in 1931.

Lewin divided the centrally acting drugs into five groups and placed them in a circle (Fig. 6-1). By arranging them this way, he brought home the fact that many drugs have multiple effects and fit into more than one group.

The *excitants* are compounds that cause behavioral and central nervous system stimulation. A naturally occurring agent in this group is caffeine, which is found in coffee and kola nuts. The amphetamines are good examples of synthetic excitants. All drugs in this group have as their primary effect an activation of the central nervous system that results in behavioral arousal and stimulation.

The *inebriants* are drugs that cause intoxication, in the social sense. The initial effect of these compounds is behavioral excitement, but it is soon followed by distortions in perception and thought that accompany behavioral depression. Alcohol, a natural product of fermentation, is included in this class, as is the synthetic compound ether.

The *hypnotics* are divided into two major categories, but all are agents that cause amnesia and/or confusion and result in a state of consciousness that eliminates reality. Sedatives and anesthetics are included here, with the barbiturates perhaps the best example. In Lewin's classification this group also contains the delusional agents such as atropine.

The *euphoriants* are drugs that act to eliminate perception of the present world by replacing it with one in which the individual experiences no problems. Opium and its derivatives are naturally occurring substances that have just such effects, and a number of synthetic opiates such as methadone can act similarly.

The *phantasticants* are not an off-Broadway group but rather those drugs which replace the present world with an alternative world—one that is equally real, but different. Lewin separates these agents from the delusional hypnotics on the basis that with these drugs there is an awareness of "both realities." Both the drug-induced and the nondrug world can be attended to at the same time, and there is memory for the drug-induced reality after the drug effect diminishes. Peyote, a cactus of southwestern United States, is a naturally occurring phantasticant, while LSD is a well-known synthetic drug in this group.

NONSPECIFIC FACTORS IN DRUG EFFECTS

Most of the discussion on generic and brand name drugs (see Chapter 3) involved the issue of bioavailability: the availability of the biologically active molecules to the cells of the body where the drug must act to have a therapeutic effect. The assumption was made that the level of a drug in the circulatory system would have a high positive relationship with the therapeutic effect of the drug. Drug blood level monitoring has become an important part of decision making in treatment for many drugs.

Would that life were so simple that the effect of psychoactive drugs could be predicted by their level in the blood. With compounds such as the antibiotics, there is good evidence that blood levels are highly related to therapeutic effectiveness. This is readily understood, since these drugs have very clear specific effects on the invading microorganisms responsible for the disease. If the drug is delivered to the area of the infection, it acts so that the body can reduce the disease process. Since the critical problem is getting the drug to the infected area, monitoring blood levels of the drug gives good evidence of the effectiveness of the product.

As will be discussed in a later chapter, there is no evidence that a similar causative agent exists for the mental disturbances. The psychoactive drugs appear to have their effect by altering patterns of neural functioning. Since these drugs act by altering function, it follows that the effects will in part depend on the activity that is already present. Another consideration in understanding the actions of these drugs is that they are frequently used to affect moods, feelings, and the individual's reaction to changes in environment. These kinds of changes can also be brought about by nonchemical means, and this fact must be always considered when evaluating the effects of psychoactive drugs.

The bases for the effects of a psychoactive drug are usually divided into two groups. One group consists of molecular, physiological, and biochemical changes that result from specific chemical characteristics of the drug and the cells or chemicals with which it interacts. Thus a basis for the effects of atropine in the body is the occupation of the acetylcholine receptor site by atropine. One specific effect resulting from this is the cessation of the flow of saliva and a drying of the mouth and throat. This effect will occur regardless of whether the patient believes it will happen, whether he knows he is receiving a drug, whether he likes his doctor, or whatever. *The specific effects of drugs are caused by physiobiochemical actions of the drug,* which depend only on the drug's reaching the site of action and a normal body chemistry.

The second group of causes for a drug's effect has only recently been widely studied and is termed nonspecific factors; "nonspecific" *means merely that these effects of the drug are not based on its chemical activity.* These nonspecific factors are those which reside in an individual with a unique background and a particular perception of the world. In brief, the nonspecific factors can include anything except the chemical activity of the drug and the direct effects of this activity. For example, a good trip or a bad trip from pure LSD seems to be dependent in part on the personality and mood of the user prior to taking the drug. In part, the kind of trip experienced depends on what the user expects to experience. The expectation is a nonspecific factor with respect to drug actions, since it influences the experienced effect of the drug but not the chemical activity of the drug.

Since the expectation of a drug effect can influence the effect that is experienced by the user or seen by an observer, most of the acceptable drug research with humans is carried out under *double-blind* conditions. In a double-blind experiment, neither the physician nor the patient knows whether the patient is receiving a drug or an inert substance—a *placebo*. When neither the patient nor his doctor knows if a drug is being used, a better evaluation can be made of the drug's specific effect on the symptoms. Another factor is necessary for a study to be considered adequately controlled. The patients should be assigned randomly to the drug and the placebo groups. A meaningful study of the effects of a drug can best be accomplished if patients are randomly assigned to groups and double-blind conditions are met.

However, even a double-blind study does not provide a pure evaluation. One investigator[3] studied the differential effects of two mild tranquilizers on anxiety in a group of patients of general practitioners. Neither the patient nor the physician knew which drug was being used, and, *prior to the start of medication,* both the physician and patient had to indicate whether they were optimistic, indifferent, or pessimistic about the outcome of treatment. After 2 months, regardless of the drug used, patients for whom the doctors were optimistic showed a 50% reduction in symptoms, whereas those patients for whom the physician had been pessimistic showed only a 20% decrease. Optimistic patients showed a 45% reduction in their anxiety symptoms, while the patients pessimistic about outcome showed a symptom drop of only 35%.

It may simply be that the physicians were good predictors of treatment outcome, but other studies have also shown that the effectiveness of drug treatment compared to placebo varies in part with the attitudes of the physician. In general, authoritarian, extroverted physicians who believe in the effectiveness of drug treatment have higher patient improvement rates than do physicians with contrasting characteristics, regardless of whether the study is double-blind.[4]

Perhaps more impressive are studies relating patient variables to improvement under drug and/or placebo administration.[5] One report[6] compared the responses of neurotic outpatients receiving either minor tranquilizers or placebos during a 4-week treatment period. Several patient characteristics were related to clinical improvement following drug or placebo treatment. Of the patients with high intelligence, 77% improved with drug treatment, whereas only 44% improved with placebo. With low-intelligence patients improvement was the same whether they had received drug or placebo—about 70%. In the same vein more patients with high initial anxiety improved under drug (69%) than with placebo (39%), but with initial low anxiety 79% improved with placebo and 65% with drug. The amount of improvement was greatest for those patients who reported high feelings of adequacy irrespective of whether they received drug or placebo. Other studies have suggested the importance of additional patient personality characteristics as determinants of response to psychoactive drugs and placebos.[7] Although many studies have tried to show a consistent relationship between particular personality traits and response to placebo, there is no convincing evidence. Two characteristics appear regularly as predictors of response to placebo: a high level of anxiety and extroversion.[8,9]

Several interesting results come from a large, federally funded research program[10] designed to evaluate the effectiveness of several potent antipsychotic agents in reducing symptoms of hospitalized schizophrenic patients. In this nationwide study it was found that drugs were consistently more effective than placebo in reducing symptoms. Studies also indicated that female patients showed more improvement to drug treatment than did males, but less improvement to placebo than did males. Another differential response was that blacks and whites responded equally to drug therapy, but blacks responded more to the placebo than did whites.

Perhaps the major implication in this study was that, when using potent antipsychotic phenothiazines in acutely psychotic patients, there were *no*

treatment effects that could be attributed to the many existing differences among the hospitals were the study was conducted. From this and other studies it seems that

> the non-specific effects are important for *small treatments* and *small illnesses*. . . .
> If we have effective treatments, non-specific effects cease to be a practical problem . . ., In the milder illnesses the personality of the patient, his environment, and his problems are factors which play a part not only in the treatment but also in the illness as well. . . .[11,p.134]

This seems to be the consensus of the work done in this area. When there is a relatively ineffective treatment, or if the illness is one reflecting nonorganic abnormal patterns of neural functioning rather than an illness resulting from an organic change, then nonspecific placebo effects may be important in determining the course of the illness. When the illness has an organic basis and when the drug's chemical actions result in specific effects on the organic basis, then nondrug factors become less important.

Nowhere has it been said that the psychoactive drugs do not have very specific physiochemical actions. This might be inferred from the preceding section, but it would not be true and represents incomplete understanding. Psychoactive drugs do have specific effects. Because the underlying brain mechanisms are not known, no one is certain which drug effects are important for certain changes in mood and thinking to occur.

As one researcher stated succinctly:

> The more the response system being measured involves cortical processes such as awareness, consciousness, and subjective feelings, the greater will be the role of nonspecific factors influencing drug response.[12,p.35]

A nice transition from "nonspecific effects" of drugs and placebos to the "specific effects" of biologically active drugs has been developing since the late 1970s. When the term "nonspecific" is used, it just means that we don't know what factors are operating, or how they are operating, to give the effect. No one here, I hope, believes in magic or ghosts so we must agree that there are real, biophysiochemical mechanisms underlying the "nonspecific" and placebo effects—we just don't know what they are. However, the evidence is slowly building. There is now good reliable research that tells us some of the steps involved in the reduction of pain by placebos.

In a dental study[13] some patients receiving a placebo reported a reduction in pain. When they were given a drug whose only effect is to block the opiate receptor in the brain, pain increased (just as it would have if the pain reduction were the result of morphine rather than a placebo). It's known (see Chapter 16) that the body manufactures chemicals—endorphins—very similar to morphine and that these endorphins play an important role in the normal control of pain. The results of the dental study suggest that the placebo (that is, the belief that the individual was taking a drug that would reduce pain) resulted in an increase in the production of endorphins and thus a decrease in pain. "Nonspecific" effects will eventually become "specific," that is, effects with an unknown basis will become effects with a known mechanism.[14-16]

General mechanisms of drug actions in neural systems

There are three general kinds of interactions a drug can have with a neuron that change the functioning of the neuron. A drug may interact with specific receptors at a synapse and thus alter synaptic functioning. Another possibility is that a drug may interact with one of the enzyme systems involved in the production or deactivation of a neurotransmitter. A final mechanism of action, and the one most poorly understood, is that a drug may act on the entire neuron membrane in such a way as to alter its normal functioning. In every case, however, the drug has an action that modifies neural functioning and thus disturbs the normal communication of information in the nervous system.

The way in which transmitters and receptors interact to cause electrical changes in the dendrite is not fully understood. That an agent must have particular structural and electrical characteristics in order to occupy the receptor has been established. One theory of receptor action suggests that the electrical change that occurs lasts as long as the transmitter occupies the receptor. The analogy is to an organ in which a tone is emitted as long as the note is held down. More likely, though, is the belief that the electrical changes occur only when the receptor is first occupied, that is, there is action only as a result of the combining, not of the occupation. Analogously, a piano key must be struck repeatedly if the tone is to persist.

There are then two characteristics of a drug molecule that influence its action at the receptor. One is its electrical and structural characteristics: Can it occupy the site at all and will it excite the receptor or just occupy it? The second characteristic is the affinity of the drug for the receptor. That is, does the molecule occupy the receptor and remain there, or does it exit and permit another molecule or itself again to reoccupy it?

Even a minor discussion of the question of a drug fitting a receptor would take us far afield. The area of structure-activity relationships is large, and no overall generalizations have emerged. It is clear, though, that some agents mimic the postsynaptic action of a transmitter very well, while others are effective in blocking the action of transmitters by occupying the receptor site but not activating it.

Between these two extremes of drug actions are many degrees of activity: Some relate to the matter of a drug's affinity for a receptor site. Nicotine can be mentioned as an example. It clearly mimics acetylcholine at first, causing stimulation of some cholinergic fibers, but later causes a depression of activity in the same fibers. It has been proposed that this biphasic effect of nicotine results from its occupying the acetylcholine receptor and thus exciting it, but then continuing to occupy the site and preventing other molecules from combining, thus blocking any further stimulation of the neuron. Nicotine, some evidence shows, has a much stronger affinity for the site than the normal transmitter and also is not deactivated as rapidly as the normal transmitter.

One comment must be made about a particular aspect of structure-activity relationships, namely, the direction in which molecules will rotate polarized light. Some molecules exist in two forms, chemically identical but differing in whether they rotate polarized light to the right (dextro) or left (levo). The magnitude of the rotation is the same, only the direction differs. These two forms have been found to be mirror images (optical isomers) of each other, and this is the basis for the difference in direction of the rotation of polarized light.

Of relevance here is the fact that one of the isomers is usually much more active physiologically than the other. Probably only when the chemical structure has a specific form can the drug occupy a receptor site. Usually the left (levo) rotating, or *l*, isomers are more active than the *d* (right, dextro) forms. This characteristic of a drug is indicated by using the letter *d* or *l* before its generic name.

The second mechanism by which a drug can have its effect is through interacting with one of the enzyme systems involved in information processing. These are usually enzymes involved in building neurotransmitters or in deactivating them. To understand the possible ways in which these enzyme-drug interactions can occur, it is necessary to appreciate what enzymes do.

Enzymes are necessary catalysts for manufacturing, dividing, or altering complex molecules. They are usually quite singular in their actions, and some function by combining certain atoms and molecules into new specific molecules having definite roles in the overall metabolism of the cell. Other enzymes act by breaking down molecules either into their more usable component parts or at least into molecules that are physiologically less active. The molecules on which an enzyme normally acts are called the *substrate* for that enzyme. The outcome of the substrate-enzyme interaction is the *end product*. A drug can clearly change the end product by affecting either the substrate or the enzyme.

In some cases the drug forms a better substrate for the enzyme than the usual substrate and in this way impairs the normal manufacturing of transmitter substances. Sometimes a drug acts by forming a bond with an enzyme, thus preventing the enzyme from acting. No matter which interaction occurs, normal neural functioning is impaired.

Drugs that act on neural membranes at other than receptor sites exert effects in one of several ways. They may act on one of the transport systems in the membrane or directly on the general physicochemical makeup of the membrane. Alcohol is a good example of a drug that exerts its action by altering the structure and permeability of the entire membrane. Changing cell membrane permeability changes the electrical difference across the membrane and thus affects the overall excitability of the neuron. The most familiar agent that acts on a transport system in the cell membrane is the naturally occurring hormone *insulin*. The presence of insulin is necessary for glucose to be transported into body cells so it can be used for energy. In the absence of insulin, as in a diabetic person, the glucose remains outside the cell, and the body starves in spite of an adequate diet. Some drugs act on the presynaptic axon terminals and cause a release of the neurotransmitter. The physiologically active amphetamines act in this way. Other drugs affect the same area to prevent the reuptake of the adrenergic transmitter. Both cocaine and amphetamine seem to have this effect.

Dose-response relationships

Perhaps the most fundamental concept in understanding drug actions is the dose-response curve and phenomena associated with it. In simple terms the *dose-response curve*, mentioned in Chapter 1, *refers to the fact that as the amount of the drug administered is varied, there may be a change in a monitored behavior*. A basic point is that since the effects of a drug can be studied on many behaviors or responses, there are many different dose-response curves for the same drug.

Drug effects arise from the collective effects of many molecular interactions. The more drug molecules there are at the site of action, the more interactions there can be, and the greater their collective effects may be. A minimum number of molecular interactions is always required before the result of their collective effects can be measured. When an effect is seen, it is called a threshold response, and the dose of the drug administered is called the threshold dose.

With an increase in the amount of drug given,

there is an increase in the collective effect of the molecular interactions and thus of the response being monitored. At some point molecular interactions are occurring at the most rapid rate possible; the addition of more drug does not then increase the response. This, in essence, is what a dose-response curve is. At some low dose (few drug molecules) there is an observable effect on the response system being monitored. This dose is the threshold, and, as the dose of the drug is increased, there are more molecular interactions and a greater effect on the response system. At the point where the system shows maximal response, further additions of the drug have no effect.

In some drug-response interactions, the effect of the drug is all-or-none, so that when the system does respond, it responds maximally. There may, however, be variability in the dosage at which individual organisms respond, and, as the dose increases, there is an increase in the percentage of individuals who show the response. The relationship between the change in the response system

and the dose of the drug is shown in Fig. 6-2. Each of the graphs is a dose-response curve and indicates the relationship between the amount of drug administered and a particular measure of the response being monitored. Three different types of measures are used, and they all indicate the same basic relationship.

Previously, mention was made that, as the drug dose increased, sometimes new response systems are affected by the drug. This fact suggests that some response systems have higher drug thresholds than others or that they are less accessible to the drug. Fig. 6-3 shows a dose-response curve that is reasonably accurate in indicating the relationship between the dose of LSD an individual takes and the changing response systems affected or (and it's impossible to know now which is correct) the increasing effect on a single response system.[17]

In the rational use of drugs there are four questions about drug dosage that must be answered. First, what is the effective dose of the drug for a desired goal? For example, what dose of morphine

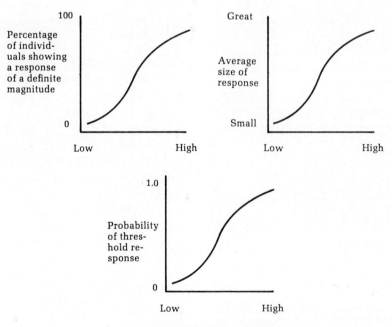

FIG. 6-2 Relationships between drug dose and a single-response system.

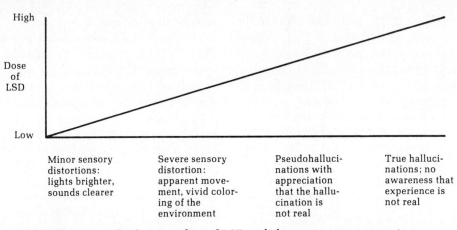

High

Dose
of
LSD

Low

| Minor sensory distortions: lights brighter, sounds clearer | Severe sensory distortion: apparent movement, vivid coloring of the environment | Pseudohallucinations with appreciation that the hallucination is not real | True hallucinations; no awareness that experience is not real |

FIG. 6-3 Relationship between dose of LSD and changes in sensory experiences.

is necessary to reduce pain 50%? What amount of marijuana is necessary for an individual to feel euphoric? How much aspirin will make the headache go away? The second question is, what dose of the drug will be lethal to the individual? How much of the drug is necessary to kill a person? Combining those two, what is the safety margin—how different are the effective dose and the lethal dose? Finally, at the effective dose level, what other effects, particularly adverse reactions, might develop? Leaving aside for now this last question, a discussion of the first three deals with basic concepts in understanding drug actions.

In any biological system there is considerable variability; response to drugs is no different. Some individuals will be very sensitive to a drug and show the desired effect at low dose levels. Others will be quite resistant, and the desired effect of the drug will be reached only after high doses are administered. Between these sensitive and resistant individuals is usually an increasing percentage of effective responses as the dose of the drug is increased. This relationship is shown in Fig. 6-2, upper left.

The basis for this variability is partially understood and is the object of much research. Many factors about the individual contribute to drug effect variability. These include body weight, sex, and age—infants and children are usually more sensitive to drugs than adults, whereas the elderly frequently show unique responses to drugs—rate of absorption from the digestive tract, activity of the drug metabolizing enzymes in the liver, diet, etc. Genetic factors are of considerable interest and importance in determining the rate of drug metabolism.[18,19] Factors that determine how long a drug remains in the body—"such as drug absorption, metabolism, distribution, and excretion—all tend to be more similar in those who are genetically close (identical twins) than in those who are genetically more disparate (fraternal twins). There is a tendency for blood levels in response to drugs to be similar for members of a family in spite of the multiple factors which determine these levels."[20]

The *effective dose* (the dose that is effective in causing a particular effect) is abbreviated *ED*, and a number is attached to indicate the percentage of individuals who show the desired effects at a particular dose level. The term ED 50 means that at the indicated dose level, 50% of the people or animals showed the desired response. The ED 1 is a dose level at which the effect is observed in only 1% of the individuals, while the ED 99 is the dose at which 99% of the individuals showed the effect.

The *lethal dose, LD,* is determined in the same way; what percentage of the animals at each dose level die within a specified period of time? The *safety margin* refers to the dose difference between

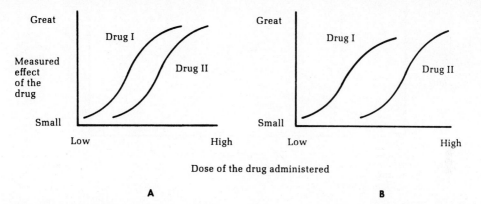

FIG. 6-4 Relationship between the measured effect of two drugs at varying dose levels. In **A,** drug I is more potent than drug II; that is, less of drug I than of drug II is needed to obtain a given effect, but both drugs have the same maximum effect. In **B,** drug I is more potent, but drug II can give greater effects.

an acceptable level of effectiveness (ED 50? ED 90?) and the LD 1. For most psychoactive drugs there is a considerable range between the dose giving the desired effect and a lethal dose. For some experimental anticancer compounds there is a small margin of safety.

Since most of the psychoactive compounds have an LD 1 well above the ED 95 level, the practical limitation on whether or not, or at what dose, a drug is used is the occurrence of side effects. With increasing doses there is usually an increase in the number and severity of side effects, those effects of the drug not relevant to the treatment. If the number of side effects becomes too great and the individual begins to suffer from them, the use of the drug will be discontinued or the dose lowered, even though the drug may be very effective in controlling the original symptoms. The selection of a drug for therapeutic use involves both these concepts. Drug choice should be made on the basis of specificity of action on the symptom with minimal side effects.

Potency

The potency of a drug is one of the most misunderstood concepts in the area of drug use. *Potency refers only to the amount of drug that must be given to obtain a particular response.* The less the amount needed to get a particular effect, the more potent the drug. Potency has nothing to do with the effectiveness of the drug. Neither is potency related to maximum effect of a drug. These relationships are indicated in Fig. 6-4. If drug A is one half as potent as drug B, then you can get the same effect by using twice the dose of drug A as of drug B. Potency refers only to relative effective dose; the ED 50 of a potent drug is lower than the ED 50 of a less potent drug. Rarely is it true that two drugs will differ only in their potency.

Time-dependent factors in drug actions

Fig. 6-5 roughly describes one type of relationship between the administration of a drug and its effect over time. Between points A and B there is no observed effect, although the concentration of drug in the blood is increasing. At point B the threshold concentration is reached, and from B to C the observed drug effect increases as drug concentration increases. At point C the maximal effect of the drug is reached, but its concentration continues increasing to point D. Although deactivation of the drug probably begins as soon as the drug enters the body, from A to D the rate of absorption is greater than the rate of deactivation. Beginning

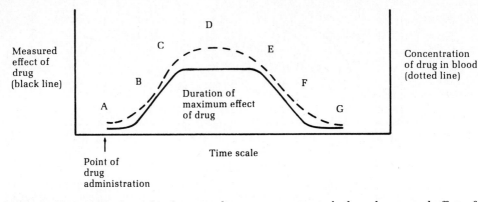

FIG. 6-5 Possible relationship between drug concentration in body and measured effect of the drug.

at point *D* the deactivation proceeds more rapidly than absorption, and the concentration of the drug decreases. When the amount of drug in the body reaches *E*, the maximal effect is over. The action diminishes from *E* to *F*, at which point the level of the drug is below the threshold for effect, although there is still drug in the body up to point *G*.

It should be clear that if the relationship described in Fig. 6-5 is true for a particular drug, then increasing the dose of the drug will not increase the magnitude of its effect. Aspirin is probably the most misused drug in this respect—if two are good, four should be better, and six will really stop this headache. No way! When the maximum possible therapeutic effect has been reached, increasing the dose *may* prolong the effect, but such an increase primarily serves to add to the number of side effects. If a high dose is used originally, there may be some shortening of the time of onset (the amount of time between taking the drug and the experiencing of effects), but in the case of aspirin there will also be an increase in gastric irritation.

A different type of relationship between a drug and its effect is presented in Fig. 6-6, *A*. In this case the effect of the drug parallels the concentration of the drug in the body. In Fig. 6-5 the situation was shown where a drug's maximum effect was in some way limited—perhaps all available re-

ceptor sites were occupied, or perhaps the system on which the drug was acting had reached its limit for change. Alcohol is one of the drugs where as the concentration in the blood increases, the effects on the central nervous system increase. And with alcohol the drug effect can continue to increase until loss of consciousness or death occurs.

Alcohol is also a good example for the relationship shown in Fig. 6-6, *B*. This graph shows how drugs can have a cumulative effect so that, with repeated doses of a drug, you get increasing effects. Usually *cumulative effects* occur when a second dose is given before the first dose has been deactivated. Similar to cumulative effects are those called *additive*, which refer to the fact that different drugs can act on the same system. Even though low doses may be taken of each drug, together the effect may be the same as a high dose of a single drug. Alcohol and the barbiturates are drugs that show additive effects—sometimes their combined depressant effects are lethal.

One of the important changes in manufacturing drugs related to the temporal aspects of drug effectiveness is the development of time-release preparations. These compounds are prepared so that following oral use the active ingredient is released into the body over a 6- to 10-hour period. With a preparation of ths type a large amount of the drug is initially made available for absorption, and then smaller amounts are released continu-

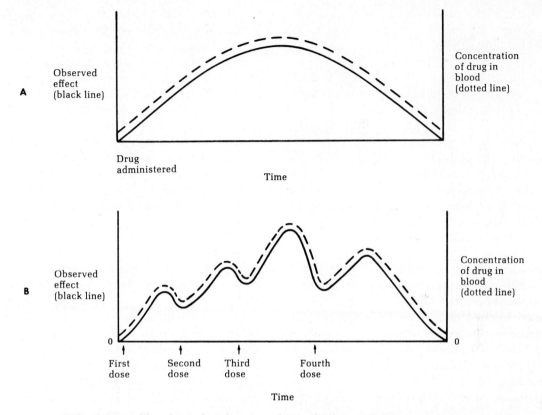

FIG. 6-6 Possible relationships between observed effects and drug concentration.

ously for a long period. The initial amount of the drug is expected to be adequate to obtain the response desired and the gradual release thereafter is designed to maintain the same effective dose of the drug even though the drug is being continually deactivated. In terms of Fig. 6-5, a time-release preparation would aim at eliminating the unnecessarily high drug level at *C-D-E* while lengthening the *C-E* time interval. Unfortunately, up to this time there is no way to manufacture orally active drug products so that drugs can be retained in the gut and reliably released over more than 8 to 10 hours.

Tolerance and addiction

Another drug phenomenon that is temporally related is tolerance. *Tolerance* refers to a situation in

which repeated administration of the same dose of a drug results in gradually diminishing effects. That is, the second dose does not give as great an effect as the first dose. If the same dose is repeated a number of times, eventually the drug has no effect. Some effects of a drug may show tolerance while others do not, since a drug may have multiple effects that may occur by different mechanisms.

With some drugs, LSD for example, tolerance develops relatively rapidly. If LSD is taken once each day for a week, a dose that gave a good effect the first day would probably give little if any effect on the fifth or sixth day. When tolerance develops rapidly, it also diminishes rapidly. In the case of LSD, if the user does not ingest any LSD for a week, the full effect of the dose will again be experienced.

Other agents show a slower onset and decrease of tolerance. The barbiturates and the opiates are good examples of the situation where repeated use of a drug gradually requires larger and larger doses of the drug to maintain the level of effect. A rapidly occurring decrease in response to repeated administration of some drugs (within minutes or, at the most, hours) is given a special name—*tachyphylaxis*. Tachyphylaxis is believed to result from the activation of compensatory mechanisms that prevent the recurrence of the initial drug effect or to the persistent occupation of receptors by earlier doses, but again, much more information is needed.

Three types of tolerance merit comment (see also Chapters 8 and 16). *Behavioral tolerance* is the state in which an individual learns to compensate for an effect of the drug. In this type of tolerance the drug may continue to have the same chemical effect but with fewer behavioral responses. The drug user has learned to counteract or diminish the behavioral effects. Behavioral tolerance is a factor in the greater resistance of some alcoholics to the intoxicating effects of alcohol.

Tolerance can also develop because the drug is deactivated and/or excreted more rapidly on repeated administration. This is *drug disposition tolerance*. At least two mechanisms may be involved with this tolerance. Most drugs are deactivated by special enzymes in the liver. Some drugs, including alcohol, act to increase the number and activity of these enzymes. The greater the activity of the enzymes, the more rapidly drugs are deactivated. To maintain the same effect, more drug is needed, since the duration of action is briefer. But additional amounts of the drug increase the activity of the enzymes even further, and the circle continues. Some drugs are excreted unchanged in the urine. The rate at which excretion occurs varies with the acidity of the urine, as in the classic case of amphetamine. Here, too, intake of the drug is responsible for increasing the rate at which the drug is excreted, which requires even more drug intake to offset the more rapid loss—and so it goes. With a normal diet and moderate amphetamine intake, the urine stays slightly alkaline, so very little am-

phetamine is excreted unchanged. As the use of amphetamine increases and food intake goes down, the urine becomes more acid, and amphetamine is excreted more rapidly. More amphetamine is used, less food is eaten, the urine becomes more acid, and so on. Amphetamine is excreted 20 times as rapidly in urine with a pH of 5 as compared to a pH of 8.

Pharmacodynamic tolerance refers to the adjustment of the nervous tissue to the drug. Acting homeostatically, the nervous tissue counters the effect of the drug. As the drug is metabolized, additional drug is required, more is needed than originally, since now the drug must not only alter the normal activities of the nervous tissue but also the compensatory mechanisms used to counter the original effect of the drug. Ever-increasing amounts of the drug are thus necessary to maintain the status quo.

An understanding of one mechanism of physical dependency and the withdrawal symptoms provides a better understanding of this form of tolerance. Tolerance can occur with either stimulant or depressant drugs. When pharmacodynamic tolerance develops to a compound, it is accompanied by physical dependence on the drug. Physical dependence is said to have occurred when stopping the administration of the drug results in "withdrawal symptoms." The actual symptoms observed vary from drug to drug but are based on the drug-induced changes in the activity of the cells involved.

The mechanisms underlying physical dependence are not well understood. One simple, and certainly incomplete, explanation is that when a depressant drug is administered, it sometimes has its effects by slowing the metabolic processes of cells. To offset this decrease in metabolic activity, the cells initiate processes that return cellular activity to normal even though the drug continues to have a depressant effect on the metabolism. Under this condition, to continue to affect the output of the cells, the amount of drug must be increased, since it now must depress not only the normal activity but also the compensation that homeostatic mechanisms brought into play. This necessary increase in drug dose to obtain the same effect is pharmacodynamic tolerance.

When administration of the drug is abruptly stopped, its depressant effect on cellular mechanisms disappears over a period of hours as the drug is deactivated. The compensatory mechanisms that were initiated in an attempt to maintain normal cellular functioning continue to act. Without the drug-induced depression to counteract them, the compensatory systems increase the activity of the cells above normal, and this cellular hyperactivity and hypersensitivity cause the withdrawal symptoms. Homeostatic processes again come into action, and, as the compensatory systems decrease their activity, the withdrawal symptoms subside.

Still debated is the question of physical dependency on stimulant drugs. When stimulant use stops, overactive compensatory mechanisms may continue to operate and decrease body functions below normal. This may be withdrawal in the case of stimulants. Over time, homeostatic processes return the body to its predrug baseline.

To recapitulate briefly, tolerance can occur with both stimulants and depressants and refers to the observable fact that repeated administration of the same dose of a drug results in fewer and fewer effects. Conversely, when tolerance to a drug develops, the amount of the drug given each time must increase in order to obtain the same effect with repeated administration. Physical dependence refers to the situation where compensatory mechanisms in the body counteract the effect of the drug and continue to act when the drug is no longer given.

Mention must again be made of the phrase *psychological dependence*, which occurs frequently in the literature. It usually refers to the fact that some individuals will be highly motivated to obtain and use a drug because of its pleasurable effects and not just to avoid the occurrence of withdrawal symptoms. Since the same behavior occurs toward other objects and experiences, not just toward drugs, the use of a special term to denote drug-seeking behavior seems unnecessary and suggests incorrectly that this behavior is unique (see Chapter 1).

CONCLUDING COMMENT

We are cautiously moving into the final phase of understanding how drugs can act on the body and nervous system to give the effects we experience. This chapter has provided some of the guidelines that determine the magnitude, speed, duration, and repeatability of an effect following the use of a drug. Every one of the terms learned in this chapter will help in the chapters dealing with specific classes of drugs. Dose-response, LD, potency, tolerance, and all the rest are labels for important concepts. Learn them well. The classification of drugs is fairly straightforward and should not pose any problems. The idea of specific and nonspecific effects of drugs may not be something you've thought about, but every 4 or 5 year old who falls and skins a knee and goes running to mother to "make it better" has experienced a nonspecific effect. Of particular importance is the increasing knowledge about the specific mechanisms responsible for the nonspecific effects. As they become clearer our ability to use drugs efficiently and effectively will increase. Forward, to The Actions of Drugs!

REFERENCES

1. Age of reason, MD, pp. 21-22, 27-28, 32, February, 1977.
2. Lewin, L.: Phantastica narcotic and stimulating drugs: their use and abuse, New York, 1931, E.P. Dutton & Co.
3. Wheatley, D.: Effects of doctors' and patients' attitudes and other factors on response to drugs. In Rickels, K., editor: Non-specific factors in drug therapy, Springfield, Ill., 1968, Charles C Thomas, Publisher.
4. Rickels, K., and Cattell, R.B.: Drug and placebo response as a function of doctor and patient type. In May, P.R.A., and Wittenborn, J.R., editors: Psychotropic drug response, Springfield, Ill., 1969, Charles C Thomas, Publisher.
5. Benson, H., and Epstein, M.E.: The placebo effect; a neglected asset in the care of patients, Journal of the American Medical Association **232**:1225-1227, 1975.
6. Rickels, K.: Non-specific factors in drug therapy of neurotic patients. In Rickels, K., editor: Non-specific factors in drug therapy, Springfield, Ill., 1968, Charles C Thomas, Publisher.
7. McNair, D.M., and others: Patient acquiescence and drug effects. In Rickels, K., editor: Non-specific factors in drug therapy, Springfield, Ill., 1968, Charles C Thomas, Publisher.

8. Shapiro, A.K.: Placebo effects in medicine: psychotherapy and psychoanalysis. In Bergin, A.E., and Garfield, S.L., editors: Handbook of psychotherapy and behavior change: an empirical analysis, New York, 1971, John Wiley & Sons.

9. Gerald, M.C.: Factors modifying drug response. VI. The placebo and other nonspecific factors, Pharmacy World 3(6):13-15, 1976.

10. Cole, J.O., Bonato, R., and Goldberg, S.C.: Nonspecific factors in the drug therapy of schizophrenic patients. In Rickels, K., editor: Non-specific factors in drug therapy, Springfield, Ill., 1968, Charles C Thomas, Publisher.

11. Hamilton, M: Discussion of the meeting. In Rickels, K., editor: Non-specific factors in drug therapy, Springfield, Ill., 1968, Charles C Thomas, Publisher.

12. Fisher, S.: Nonspecific factors as determinants of behavioral response to drugs. In DiMascio, A., and Shader, R.I., editors: Clinical handbook of psychopharmacology, New York, 1970, Science House, Inc.

13. Levine, J.D., and others: The mechanism of placebo analgesia, Lancet, p. 654, September 23, 1978.

14. Fields, H.L., and Levine, J.D.: Biology of placebo analgesia, American Journal of Medicine 70(4):745, 1981.

15. Evans, F.J.: The placebo response in pain control, Psychopharmacology Bulletin 17(2):72-76, 1981.

16. Ross, M., and Olson, J.M.: An expectancy-attribution model of the effects of placebos, Psychological Review 88(1):408-437, 1981.

17. Gorodetzky, C.W.: Marihuana, LSD, and amphetamines, Drug Dependence, National Clearinghouse for Mental Health Information, No. 5, October, 1970.

18. Vesell, E.S.: Introduction: genetic and environmental factors affecting drug response in man, Federation Proceedings 31(4):1253-1269, 1972.

19. Mendlewicz, J.: Recent advances in genetics and psychopharmacology, Current Developments in Psychopharmacology 4:113, 1977.

20. Goldman, P.: Patient variables and drug response, Drug Therapy, pp. 24-30, April 1976.

CHAPTER 7

THE ACTIONS OF DRUGS

THE BASIC FACT IN understanding the actions of drugs is that the drug molecule must form a physicochemical bond with a cell or a constituent of a cell. This interaction is necessary for a drug to have its effect, and of concern here are cases where a drug interacts with neurons. Such interaction can occur either on the surface (the membrane) of the cell or inside the cell. Acting at the membrane, a drug may have a physicochemical effect in one of three ways. It may combine with a specialized area of the membrane, a receptor; it may act on the membrane structure itself; and, finally, it may act on one of the mechanisms in the membrane that transports material in and out of the cell. The effects a drug has inside a cell are usually on enzymes, molecules necessary for the production and deactivation of the neurotransmitter. Drugs sometimes act inside cells by affecting neurotransmitter release or reuptake mechanisms.

Three very important and perhaps very obvious general concepts will be used repeatedly in talking about drug action. First is that the action of a drug is always mediated by a naturally occurring process of the body. A drug either mimics, facilitates, or antagonizes a normally occurring phenomenon in order to have its effect. Second, a drug can have only one of three effects on a cell. It can increase or decrease a cell's normal activity or sensitivity, or it can disrupt the cell so that normal activity is sporadic. The third concept is that the magnitude of the effect obtained with a drug depends on the concentration of the drug at the place of action, that is, the place where the drug forms a physicochemical bond with a part of the cell.

One must appreciate that a drug does have very specific biochemical actions, and failure at times to detail these actions indicates a lack of knowledge. Because of the very specific ways in which drugs act, only minute amounts of pharmacologically active agents are needed at the site of action. Some indications of this specificity is suggested by the fact that 0.00001 mg of the antidiuretic hormone administered to a man results in the retention of body fluid by the kidneys. Similarly, the action of a potent phenothiazine drug is obtained with the delivery of only 10^{12} molecules to a rat, which means 10^{-9} g of the drug in the entire brain is enough to cause observable changes in the behavior of a rat. If these molecules were put in a monomolecular layer, the total area would be only 0.1 cm^2!

The specificity of action of drugs was first suggested by some work of Claude Bernard (1856) on the peripheral nervous system. He was using the drug curare as a tool to study the interaction between the nervous system and the skeletal muscles. Curare is the poison in which South American natives dip their arrow tips. An animal wounded by one of these arrows collapses within seconds, since the effect of curare is to paralyze the animal. The question was, how does this poison work?

Bernard used a preparation in which he could isolate nerves that carry impulses to skeletal muscles. In the absence of curare, electrically stimulating the nerve caused the muscle to contract. Following curare, nerve stimulation had no effect on the muscle. If the muscle were *directly* stimulated, it would contract, showing that it could function normally. Similarly, stimulating the nerve and recording at the point where the nerve joined the muscle showed that the nerve functioned properly. The only possibility left was that curare in some way prevents the nerve from activating the muscle. It is now well established that curare is a specific blocker for the skeletal neuromuscular junction and does so by occupying the acetylcholine receptor. Acetylcholine is the neurotransmitter normally released by the neuron that causes skeletal muscle contraction when it combines with the receptor.

Drugs are, then, quite specific in their actions when they are at the site of action. No matter whether they act on the cell membrane or inside the cell, they either increase, decrease, or disrupt the normal functioning of the cell. This means that a drug does not introduce a new quality of nerve action; it only modifies the normal one. First and foremost, though, the drug must be delivered to the cells with which it interacts.

DRUG ACTION
Overview of events prior to drug action

Tracing the path of drug molecules from their entry into the body to their site of action will sketch some of the factors that must then be detailed. Even though oral intake may be the simplest way to "take a drug," absorption from the gastrointestinal tract is the most complicated way to enter the bloodstream. Here the drug must first be taken up

(absorbed), either by diffusion or by an active transport system, by cells lining the gastrointestinal tract. To be absorbed, the drug must have certain characteristics. It must be in solution, be lipid soluble, and be in a suitably high concentration. Not all drugs can fulfill these requirements.

Ease of movement of a drug across cell membranes is important in determining its activity. Since cell membranes have a substantial amount of lipid, drugs that are lipid soluble readily enter cells and move through capillary walls. Lipid solubility can be fairly well predicted from the chemical structure of the compound; one of the crucial factors is the degree of its ionization. As ionization goes up, lipid solubility goes down. Water solubility is increased with ionization, and this acts to keep the drug outside of cells. Because of this, ionized, water-soluble drugs, if absorbed at all, will remain extracellular, be *poorly* metabolized, and be readily filtered out by the kidneys and excreted. Physiologically active drugs and hormones that are not lipid soluble need a special transport system to cross cell membranes.

To move into the blood system clearly requires a series of complex steps in most cases. When a drug is delivered by injection directly into a vein, then it is in the circulation. When an intramuscular or subcutaneous injection is used, the drug enters the bloodstream by diffusion from one intercellular space where it was deposited. If taken orally, a drug must diffuse into capillaries from cells lining the stomach and intestines. Such movement occurs for some agents that move from an area of higher concentration into one of lower concentration. Other compounds cannot so easily cross the cell membrane, and an active transport system, which requires energy, is necessary. The active transport systems can move a compound from an area of low concentration to one of high concentration.

The circulatory system is the mode of transportation for drugs from the place where they entered the body to the site of action. As the blood moves through the filtering system in the kidneys, the possibility exists that the drug will be removed from circulation and excreted. In the liver, which is the primary place of deactivation, the compound may be removed from circulation and metabolized (deactivated).

To reach the extracellular fluid space outside the cell, drug molecules have to move from the blood through capillary walls by diffusion. Before the drug can leave the circulatory system, though, it must be separated from the proteins in the blood with which it may have formed a bond. If a drug acts inside a cell, its last barrier to cross is the cell membrane. Neuron membranes are complex structures that are primarily lipid material built on a protein latticework. The membrane contains some pores or openings that permit quite small molecules to enter and leave the cell by diffusion without energy being expended by the cell. Lipid-soluble agents too large to enter through the pores move directly through the cell membrane. Moving a drug into the bloodstream by absorption through the skin is not very effective, since the skin poorly absorbs most material applied to it. Suppositories are rarely used but are an effective drug delivery system that makes possible rapid movement of drugs into the body. They are sometimes necessary in the very young and very old. Direct delivery of a drug into the brain is possible with available techniques and is used at times in animal research.

Only three primary drug delivery methods are used with humans: oral, injection, and inhalation. Inhalation is used with volatile anesthetics and is also the drug delivery system used for nicotine in smoking. It is a very efficient way to deliver some drugs. Onset of drug effects is quite rapid because the capillary walls are very accessible in the lungs, and the drug thus enters the blood quickly. Aerosol dispensers have been used to deliver some drugs via the lungs, but three considerations make inhalation of limited value. First, the material must not be irritating to the mucous membranes and lungs. Second, control of dose is more difficult than with the other drug delivery systems. Last, and perhaps the prime advantage for some drugs and disadvantage for others, there is no depot of drug in the body. This means that the drug must be given as long as the effect is desired, and also that when drug administration is stopped, the effect rapidly decreases.

Injection

Chemicals can be delivered with the hypodermic syringe directly into the bloodstream, deposited in a muscle mass, or under the upper layers of skin. With the intravenous (IV) injection, the drug starts in the bloodstream and does not have to be absorbed first, so the onset of action is faster than with any other means of administering drugs. Another advantage is that very irritating material can be injected this way, since blood vessel walls are relatively insensitive. A major advantage frequently is that the material injected, the bolus, can deliver a high concentration of the drug to the brain tissues. The major disadvantage to IV injections is that the vein wall loses some of its strength and elasticity in the area around the injection site. If there are many injections into a small segment of a vein, as with an addict who must inject where he can see, the wall of that vein eventually collapses, and blood no longer moves through it, necessitating the use of another injection site.

Subcutaneous and intramuscular injections have similar characteristics, except that absorption is more rapid from intramuscular injection. Muscles have a better blood supply, and thus more area over which absorption can occur, than the underlying layers of the skin. Absorption is most rapid when the injection is into the deltoid muscle of the arm and least rapid when the injection is in the buttock. Intermediate between these two areas in speed of drug absorption is injection into the thigh. The rate of absorption can be varied in both subcutaneous and intramuscular injections by adding a vasodilator or vasoconstrictor to increase or decrease the area of absorption. When slow absorption is desired, a less soluble salt of the drug is frequently put in a suspension rather than a solution. Since only material in solution can be absorbed, the suspended material has to first go into solution. An additional factor influencing the rate of absorption is that movement into the blood depends on the concentration of the drug. As more drug enters the bloodstream, the concentration outside decreases, and so does the rate of absorption. One disadvantage to subcutaneous injection is that if the material injected is extremely irritating to the tissue, the skin around the site of injection may die and be shed. This method of injection is not very common in medical practice but has long been the kind of injection used by beginning narcotic users. Colloquially this is called "skin popping."

There is less chance of irritation if the injection is *intramuscular* because of the better blood supply and faster absorption. Another advantage is that larger volumes of material can be deposited in a muscle than can be injected subcutaneously. Most of the shots given by a physician are intramuscular injections, and anyone who has had a series of tetanus shots may question the fact that this is one of the less irritating ways of injecting a drug.

Oral administration

Most drugs begin their grand adventure in the body by entering through the mouth. Taking biologically active agents orally is unquestionably the oldest route of administration and probably the easiest. It is not necessarily the most effective, since a chemical in the digesive tract has to withstand the actions of the acid of the stomach and the digestive enzymes and not be deactivated by food before it is absorbed. As long as the drug remains in the digestive tract, it can be considered to be outside the body. The process of drug absorption from the stomach and intestines is a special area in and of itself.

A good example of the dangers in the gut for a drug is that which develops with tetracycline. This antibiotic readily combines with calcium and aluminum ions to form a compound that is poorly absorbed. If tetracycline is taken with milk (calcium ions) or with antacids (aluminum ions), blood levels will never be as high as if it were taken in the absence of these or similar agents.

Many factors compete in getting the drug through the cells lining the wall of the gastrointestinal tract on into the capillaries in the area. If taken in capsule or tablet form, the drug must first dissolve and, as a liquid, mix in the contents of the stomach and intestines. However, since as concentration goes down so does rate of absorption, the drug will be less rapidly absorbed when it is diluted by other material in the stomach.

Drugs are frequently prepared as salts, and they are weak electrolytes, since this ionization increases their water solubility, which is necessary for the compound to spread throughout the stomach. Once distributed, though, absorption is primarily of the nonionized form of the drug. If organic molecules are too strongly ionized, they will be poorly absorbed and pass through the intestines to be excreted in the feces. Lipid-soluble and very small water-soluble molecules are readily absorbed into capillaries and go into the general circulation. There is very little drug absorption during the first 5 minutes, even on an empty stomach, but by 30 minutes most has been absorbed. After 6 to 8 hours, essentially all the drug will have been absorbed.

Once in the bloodstream the dangers of entering through the oral route are not over. The veins from the gut go first to the liver. If the drug is the type that is rapidly taken up and metabolized by the liver, very little may get into the general circulation. A drug may thus be ineffective by the oral route but very effective if given by injection.

The brain has a high lipid content and thus is a target organ for drugs with high lipid solubility. Drugs that act on the central nervous system are usually active when given orally because the lipid solubility of these agents increases their absorption from the gastrointestinal tract. Similarly, because of the high lipid solubility and low water solubility, these agents are usually not excreted but are reabsorbed in the kidneys and thus show cumulative effects.

As with all generalizations, there are exceptions. If a lipid-soluble drug is taken with a fatty meal, the drug will to some extent be taken up and remain in the fat. Since fat is only slowly digested and the drug released, the rate of drug absorption is slowed. A slow absorption rate could possibly lower the drug concentration in the blood to an ineffective level.

Transport in blood

When a drug enters the bloodstream, usually its molecules will attach to one of the protein molecules in the blood, albumin being the most common protein involved. The degree to which there is binding of drug molecules to plasma proteins is important in determining drug effects. As long as there is a protein-drug complex, the drug is inactive and also cannot leave the blood. In this condition, the drug is protected from inactivation by enzymes.

An equilibrium is established between the free (unbound) drug and the protein-bound forms of the drug in the bloodstream. As the unbound drug moves across capillary walls to sites of action, there is a release of protein-bound drug in order to maintain the bound-free equilibrium. Considerable variation exists among drugs in the affinity that the drug molecules have for establishing a bond with plasma proteins. Alcohol has a low affinity and thus exists in the bloodstream primarily as the ethyl alcohol molecule. The salicylate ion has a high affinity, and about 80% is bound to blood proteins. Acetylsalicylic acid, in contrast, has a low affinity. Differences in blood protein binding are reflected in their effects. Acetylsalicylic acid (aspirin) has a more rapid onset of action but a shorter duration than the salicylates.

Since differences exist in the affinity of drugs for the plasma proteins, one might expect that drugs with high affinity would displace drugs with weak protein bonds. And they do. This fact is important because it forms the basis for one kind of drug interaction. When a high-affinity drug is added to a situation where there is a weak-affinity drug already largely bound to the plasma proteins, the weak-affinity drug is displaced and will exist primarily as the unbound form. The increase in the unbound drug concentration helps move the drug out of the bloodstream to the sites of action faster and may be an important influence on the effect the drug has. At the very least, there will be a shortening of the duration of action.

Taking into consideration that only the free drug can leave the circulatory system, the same rules apply for leaving the bloodstream and entering cells as for leaving the stomach and moving into blood. Small, lipid-soluble, nonionized molecules diffuse through these cell membranes very easily, whereas larger lipid-insoluble, ionized molecules move more slowly, if at all, without an active transport system.

Blood-brain barrier

The brain is very different from the other parts of the body in terms of the ability of drugs to leave the blood and move to sites of action. A barrier acts to keep certain classes of compounds in the blood and away from brain neurons and glial cells. Thus some drugs act only on neurons outside the central nervous system, that is, those in the peripheral nervous system, whereas others may affect all neurons.

The blood-brain barrier is not well developed in infants; it reaches complete development only after 1 or 2 years of age in humans. Although the nature of this barrier is not well understood, several factors are known to contribute to the blood-brain barrier. One is the makeup of the capillaries in the brain. They are different from other capillaries in the body, since they contain no pores at all. Even small, water-soluble molecules cannot leave the capillaries in the brain; only lipid-soluble substances can pass the lipid capillary wall.

If a substance can move through the capillary wall, another barrier unique to the brain is met. About 85% of the capillaries are completely covered with glial cells—there is little extracellular space next to the blood vessel walls. With no pores and close contact between capillary walls and glial cells, almost certainly an active transport system is needed to move chemicals in and out of the brain. In fact, known transport systems exist for some naturally occurring agents.

A final note on the mystery of the blood-brain barrier is that cerebral trauma can disrupt the barrier and permit agents to enter that normally would be excluded. Concussion or cerebral infections frequently cause enough trauma to impair the effectiveness of this screen, which normally permits only selected chemicals to enter the brain.

Possible mechanisms of drug actions

Many different types of actions will be suggested as ways in which drugs can affect physiochemical processes, neuron functioning, and ultimately thoughts, feelings, and other behaviors. It is possible for drugs to affect all neurons, but many exert actions only on certain presynaptic or postsynaptic processes in some neurons or only on presynaptic neurons. Since the action of a drug is usually quite specific—that is, it affects one phase of the information-processing systems—it is unusual to find a drug that has more than one of the actions to be discussed.

Effects on all neurons. Chemicals that have an effect on all neurons must do it by influencing some characteristic common to all neurons. One general characteristic of all neurons is the cell membrane. It is semipermeable, meaning that some agents can readily move in and out of the cell, but other chemicals are held inside or kept out under normal conditions. The semipermeable characteristic of the cell membrane is essential for the maintenance of an electric potential across the membrane. It is on this membrane that some drugs seem to act and, by influencing the permeability, alter the electrical characteristics of the neuron. Some drugs do affect the transport systems involved in maintaining the neuron, but usually the effect is a more general one.

The anesthetics, including alcohol, are chemicals that have their effects on the central nervous system by a general influence on the cell membrane. Note that the agents which act in this way are depressants and that there are no drugs that increase the cell's activity level by affecting general membrane characteristics.

Postsynaptic effects. Alteration in the information-processing system is usually accomplished by affecting synaptic functioning. A tremendous increase in possible selectivity of action results from action at the synapse because different synapses involve different types of neurohumors. By using a drug that operates only by mimicking or blocking one kind of neurotransmitter, a much greater precision of action occurs than when using a compound that acts on all neuron membranes.

Drugs that act postsynaptically can only make contact with the electrical system through the receptor itself or the enzymes that deactivate the neurotransmitters. When a drug acts at the receptor, it can have one of two possible effects. It may mimic the normal transmitter and thus cause either an increase or a decrease in the excitability of the postsynaptic neuron similar to that produced by the normal transmitter. Carbachol, which mimics the action of acetylcholine at many places in the nervous system, is a good example. It activates cholinergic fibers, but, unlike acetylcholine, it is not readily deactivated by cholinesterase. As a result, it continues to have its effect on the receptor for a longer period of time than would acetylcholine. Nicotine, at places where carbachol is ineffective, also mimics the action of acetylcholine but initially activates and then depresses activity of the postsynaptic neuron.

Some drugs act at the postsynaptic receptor by occupying the site but are unable to influence the electrical characteristics of the neuron. These agents are called "blockers," since by occupying the site, they prevent the normal neurotransmitters from having an effect postsynaptically. Atropine and scopolamine are well-known compounds that can occupy some cholinergic receptors and thus prevent acetylcholine from having an effect. These drugs act on both the central and the peripheral nervous systems, but if a methyl group is added to their chemical structure to form methylatropine and methylscopolamine, the effects are restricted to the peripheral nervous system. The addition of a methyl group prevents the chemical from crossing the blood-brain barrier and provides a valuable tool for research. By comparing the effects of atropine and methylatropine, important clues can be obtained to indicate which actions of the drug are mediated by the central and which by the peripheral nervous systems.

In cholinergic systems the enzyme responsible for deactivating acetylcholine is located postsynaptically. Any drug that prevents this deactivating enzyme, cholinesterase, from acting increases the duration of effect that acetylcholine can have. Cholinesterase inhibitors, then, prolong the effect of acetylcholine, which is released under normal physiological stimulation. Some drugs are short-acting, reversible inhibitors (such as physostigmine), whereas others (such as diisopropyl fluorophosphate, DFP), because of the nature of their effect, are called nonreversible and may alter cholinesterase functioning for days.

Thus drugs acting postsynaptically can have major effects on the information-processing system. Emphasis here has been on the cholinergic system, since alteration of function in the adrenergic system is most readily accomplished presynaptically. It is quite difficult to do this with the cholinergic system.

Presynaptic effects. Drugs affect synaptic processes by acting on the presynaptic neuron in several major ways. One of these, blocking the release of the neurotransmitter, is of importance only in the peripheral nervous system and will not be discussed. The other ways of altering the effectiveness of the neurotransmitter are concerned with modifications of its synthesis, storage, uptake, and deactivation processes.

Synthesis of the endogenous neurotransmitters can be blocked by inhibiting one or more of the enzyme systems involved in the construction of the transmitter. Preventing or slowing new synthesis results in a depletion of the transmitter under normal functioning and thus a cessation, or at least an impairment, of synaptic transmission. Interestingly, one of the important enzymes involved in the synthesis of noradrenaline plays a similar role in building serotonin, so that inhibition of that enzyme causes a decrease in the level of both these neurotransmitters.

Some drugs effectively decrease the synthesis of the normal transmitters because they are better substrates for the synthesizing enzymes than the endogenous material. The synthesizing enzymes thus act on these drugs rather than on the normal substrate. Because the manufacturing system is not disrupted, complex molecules are built and stored in synaptic vesicles. Since these are not the same as the normal transmitters but are released in the same way as the real transmitters, these synthesized compounds are called *false transmitters*. The false transmitters are usually only moderately, if at all, effective in activating the receptor postsynaptically, so information processing is disrupted by their presence.

When a transmitter is manufactured, it must be stored in a vesicle to prevent its deactivation. Some drugs, such as reserpine, prevent the transmitter from being taken up into vesicles. The transmitter is then open to deactivation by the deactivating enzymes, but, more importantly, the vesicles are unable to collect and release the transmitter when the neuron fires. Obviously, without transmitter release, the synapse will cease to function normally.

An important distinction must be made between the cholinergic and the adrenergic systems of neurotransmission. The cholinergic system is relatively straightforward. Acetylcholine is synthesized presynaptically, bound in vesicles, released, bound to the postsynaptic receptor site (thereby changing the electrical characteristics of the dendrite), and deactivated postsynaptically. In adrenergic neurons there are a few differences. First, two classes of noradrenaline are accumulated presynaptically: a functional store, released in neural firing, and a bound (reserve) form of noradrenaline that is not used in synaptic functioning.

A second difference is that after the transmitter molecule has had its effect at the receptor, it is not usually deactivated but instead is released into the synaptic gap, where it is taken up by the presynaptic neuron and stored again in the vesicles of the functional pool of transmitter substance. Some clinically important drugs impair this reuptake, thereby increasing the noradrenaline level at the receptor. Cocaine and imipramine are drugs that have their primary action in this way.

Two enzymes are important in the breakdown of the adrenergic transmitters. One of these enzymes, monoamine oxidase (MAO), is also important for the deactivation of serotonin, so use of an MAO inhibitor results in an increase in brain levels of both noradrenaline and serotonin. The increase in noradrenaline, however, is not an increase in the transmitter used in neurotransmission (the functional form) but rather an increase in the reserve form. Therefore there is no increase in the activity of the adrenergic transmitters after administration of an MAO inhibitor.

There are available inhibitors of the second deactivating enzyme, catechol-O-methyl transferase (COMT), but these have not been used clinically because COMT is relatively unimportant in deactivating noradrenaline. This COMT system seems to function both pre- and postsynaptically, although the postsynaptic site seems to be of primary importance.

A final presynaptic mechanism of drug action causes a continuous slow release of newly synthesized noradrenaline. Amphetamine, a stimulant, has this effect. This action (along with a second action of amphetamine, blocking noradrenaline reuptake) increases the activity of the adrenergic system and forms the biochemical basis for amphetamine's behavioral and experienced effects.

Summary of drug actions. Psychoactive drugs have their central effects only by changing the effectiveness and sensitivity of neurons and thus their information-processing characteristics. There are many ways in which this can be accomplished, however, and a brief survey of these methods gives only a hint of the total complexity. Some drugs act on cell membranes. Those compounds are usually nonspecific depressants, since they act similarly on all neurons. (Unique are the opiates, which have their effect through the special opiate receptor.) By interfering with the synthesis, storage, release, or reuptake of a neurotransmitter or its combination with receptors, the efficiency of the synapse is modified and information transmission changed. By mimicking the transmitter at the receptor or preventing its normal deactivation, the postsynaptic neuron is changed electrically more than under normal conditions, and integrated functioning is also then impaired.

DRUG DEACTIVATION

Before a drug can cease to have an effect, one of two things must happen to it. It may be removed unchanged from the body, or it may be chemically changed so that it no longer has the same effect on the body and then is excreted from the body. Few drugs are eliminated unchanged from the body, although this is true of the volatile anesthetics. They are eliminated in the same way they enter the body—through the lungs. Alcohol, if taken in large amounts, may be partially eliminated unchanged through the lungs or sweat glands. Some drugs are excreted unchanged in the urine because they are filtered out, but not reabsorbed, in the kidneys. Even drugs that are primarily deactivated biochemically in the body are occasionally found unchanged in the urine.

Most drugs, though, are metabolized in some way in the body and the end products excreted in the urine. Drug metabolism aims primarily at two ends: inactivation of the agent and increasing the water solubility so that it can be excreted by way of the kidneys. Ionized, nonlipid-soluble substances are filtered out of the blood plasma in the kidneys and, instead of being reabsorbed, pass on to the urine for excretion. In part, the rate of excretion of ionizable substances depends on the pH of the urine, and this reflects to some extent an individual's diet.

Drug metabolism is not an incidental part of the study of drugs and drug actions. Since a drug continues to act until it is changed or excreted, the duration and intensity of a drug's action are determined to a great extent by the speed of its metabolism. Most drug metabolism is accomplished by special detoxification enzymes in the liver. The liver is *the* organ of drug metabolism; anything that interferes with the normal functioning of the liver will impair the drug-metabolizing capability of the body.

The enzymes in the liver that metabolize drugs are quite different from the enzymes in the body. These liver microsomal enzymes are unique in that they can use oxygen directly for metabolism, whereas most enzymes cannot. Another peculiar quality is that they are almost specific for foreign compounds. They do not act on normally occurring chemicals (except steroids), but the reason for this specificity is still not clear. Interestingly, although these microsomal enzymes are specific for foreign chemicals, they are relatively nonspecific within that group of compounds. Therefore, they metabolize a number of very different drugs.

The activity of these microsomal enzymes can be affected by drugs. Over 200 drugs have been shown to increase the activity of these drug-metabolizing enzymes; meprobamate, phenobarbital, and DDT all have this effect in common. When the enzymes are stimulated, drug metabolism speeds up, and the duration of action of the drugs in the body is decreased. Some drug interactions may occur so that one drug may inhibit the metabolism of a second and thus increase the second's effects. Alcohol given after meprobamate decreases meprobamate's metabolism, thereby increasing the effects of meprobamate (perhaps sedation).

Some drugs are deactivated at their site of action and, in fact, some are altered in the process of having an action. Furthermore, some drugs are not active in the form in which they are administered but become quite active after they have been altered by the metabolizing process. Marijuana may be one example of this situation where the metabolite is just as active as the original compound.

SOME GENERAL RULES ABOUT DRUGS IN THE BODY

As mentioned in the preceding section, anything that interferes with liver functions will retard the metabolism of drugs. Such retardation will increase the magnitude and the duration of effect following administration of a drug. The most familiar examples of interference with the liver are illness and damage to the liver such as cirrhosis. However, also important is an adequate diet, since near starvation will result in a reduction of the amount of detoxification enzymes.

In the same line, advanced age may be accompanied by reduced blood flow to the liver and thus a decrease in the rate of drug detoxification. Older people frequently have a lower metabolic rate than the young, and this also acts to prolong drug activity. Impaired kidney function for any reason would clearly impair excretion of the drug metabolites. In the elderly there is also a higher percentage of body fat than in the young adult. Because of the accumulation of drugs in body fat, this also tends to prolong the duration of a drug's effect.

This last point must be expanded by a further comment on some unique characteristics of fat in the body. Lipid-soluble drugs are slowly taken up by the fat cells. Since fat cells generally have a relatively poor blood supply, they release the drug more slowly than other cells. This slow release may mean that 3 to 4 hours after a drug has been administered there may be higher levels in the system of a fat person than of a lean individual. Since women have more body fat, they may require less of a very lipid-soluble drug after the initial administration because the drug settles in the fat cells and is then released over a longer period of time than is the case with men. As a familiar example, this seems to be the situation with the barbiturates.

SUMMARY AND CONCLUSIONS

To understand how drug taking is related to the experienced effects of a drug, some appreciation is necessary of each of the steps involved in getting the drug to the site of action, the kind of action it has, and the ways in which the action is stopped.

Since a drug must travel through the circulatory system to reach the area where it is to have an effect, some of the time between taking a drug and experiencing its effect is caused by the problem of getting the drug into the bloodstream. Compounds that are only slightly ionized and quite lipid soluble should have a shorter time to onset of action if everything else is equal.

Usually, though, everything else is not equal. Some drugs never do get past the combination of factors that are referred to as the blood-brain barrier. If a drug readily enters the brain, it may be that its mechanism of action is by blocking the receptor for a neurotransmitter. The resulting effects may be experienced as depressing or stimulating, but the onset should be fairly rapid, since synaptic functioning is impaired as soon as the drug acts. With other agents and other mechanisms of action there may be only a gradual onset of effects, since the impact of decreased synthesis, or decreased storage, of transmitter substances is realized more slowly in synaptic functioning.

Overriding all this is the rate of metabolism of the drug. As the activity of the microsomal enzymes in the liver increases, so does the rate at which drugs are metabolized and thus deactivated. These enzymes act in a variety of ways to make the drug easier to excrete (that is, less lipid soluble and more water soluble). However, their specific actions need not concern the reader. Suffice it to say that the ability to metabolize drugs is related to the amount of liver microsomes that contains the detoxifying enzymes.

The processes and concepts outlined in this chapter will be used repeatedly in explaining differences in drug actions. Note especially that drugs can only increase, decrease, or disrupt the activity of neurons and that the differential effects result from where the drug acts in the nervous system. By incorporating these principles of pharmacology, new dimensions will be added to the understanding of drug effects.

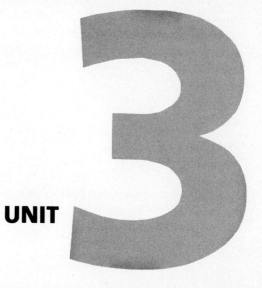

UNIT

THE NONDRUG DRUGS

CHAPTER 8

ALCOHOL

SOMEDAY I WANT TO write a sentence like: Battle bubbles in beer business as brewers bite bullet. It's true; in 1970 the Phillip Morris Company bought the Miller Brewing Company and things began to hop. Using lots of money from Marlboro profits and a new approach to marketing beer, Miller was able to spring Coors loose from the number four slot in 1975, edge Pabst from its blue-ribbon number three position in 1976, and in 1977 with gusto took the bull by the horns to move into the number two position ahead of Schlitz. Anheuser-Busch, who makes the "King of Beers," Budweiser, has been clippety-clopping along as the number one brewer ever since it rolled over Schlitz in the 1950s.

Table 8-1 contains the market share of the major breweries in 1981. Schlitz, Heileman, Pabst, and Coors are so close in sales that there will be much shifting for a few years and arguing about the number three, four, five, and six positions. Who's Heileman? A company that buys lots of breweries and continues selling their beers under the original labels (now about 30), for example, Blatz, Old Style, Carling Black Label, and National Bohemien. "Others" also includes imported beers—less than 3% of the market, and Heineken accounts for 45% of imports.

Table 8-2 lists the top ten brands in 1981. Of the total market of 180 million barrels about 14% is low-calorie beer—and Lite has about 60% of that market. The successful introduction of low-calorie beer in 1975 by Miller was a major innovation. Most low-calorie beer has about one third fewer than the 150 calories in a regular 12-ounce serving. Some brewers produce beers with half the normal calories. When you remove calories you also remove alcohol—most low-calorie brands have an alcohol content between 2.5% and 3.5%. If you see a similarity to the cigarette business—you're right. One of the trends Phillip Morris started with Miller was to increase the number of choices available to the user: bottle size, calories involved, premium-standard-economy beers. It's done two things: increased sales and provided the buyer with the opportunity to buy the specific type of product that they want. There hadn't been too many great ideas in the beer business before this: cans in 1935; throw-away bottles in 1959; and the snap-top can opening in 1962. Before we move on to distilled spirits and wine, we'd better detour and learn some fundamentals—then we'll come back to alcohol as a consumer item. Just to set the scene, however, in 1979 Americans age 18 and over spent $34.2 billion so that each could drink, on the average: 34

TABLE 8-1 Beer brewers' market share and production (1981)

Brewer	Barrels*	Percent of market
Anheuser-Busch	54.5	30.3
Miller	40.3	22.4
Schlitz	14.3	7.9
Heileman	14.0	7.8
Pabst	13.5	7.5
Coors	13.3	7.4
Strohs	9.2	5.1
Others	20.9	11.6

*Millions of barrels; a barrel contains 31 gallons—enough for 330 12-ounce servings.

TABLE 8-2 Largest selling beer brands, 1981

Brand	Brewer	Sales*
Budweiser	Anheuser-Busch	38.2
Miller High Life	Miller	23.6
Miller Lite	Miller	15.0
Coors Premium	Adolph Coors	10.4
Pabst Blue Ribbon	Pabst	9.9
Michelob	Anheuser-Busch	8.3
Schlitz	Schlitz	6.5
Stroh's	Stroh Brewing	5.7
Old Style	Heileman	5.2
Old Milwaukee	Schlitz	5.1

*Millions of barrels.

gallons of beer; 2.7 gallons of distilled spirits; 2.6 gallons of still wine; and ⅙ gallon of bubbly wine.

FERMENTATION AND FERMENTATION PRODUCTS

Many thousands of years before the World Health Organization declared ethyl alcohol a drug intermediate in kind and degree between habit-forming and addicting drugs, Neolithic man had discovered booze. Beer and berry wine were known and used about 6400 BC, while grape wine dates from 300 or 400 BC. Mead, which is made from honey, may be the oldest alcoholic beverage; some authorities suggest it appeared in the Paleolithic Age, about 8000 BC. Early use of alcohol seems to have been worldwide: beer was drunk by the American Indians whom Columbus met.

Fermentation forms the basis for all alcoholic beverages. Certain yeasts act on sugar in the presence of water, and this chemical action is fermentation. Yeast recombines the carbon, hydrogen, and oxygen of sugar and water into ethyl alcohol and carbon dioxide. Chemically, $C_6H_{12}O_6$ (glucose) + H_2O (water) is transformed to C_2H_6O (ethyl alcohol) + CO_2 (carbon dioxide).

Most fruits, including grapes, contain sugar, and addition of the appropriate yeast (which is perva-sive in the air wherever plants grow) to a mixture of crushed grapes and water will begin the fermentation process. The yeast has only a limited tolerance for alcohol, so that when the concentration reaches 15%, the yeast dies, and fermentation ceases. If white grapes are used, or red grapes with the skins removed, a white wine results. Red wines come from red grapes in which the grape skins are retained in the fermenting mixture. A rosé results if the red grape skins are allowed to remain in the mix for only 1 or 2 days. Champagne is produced by bottling the wine before the fermentation is complete, thus retaining the carbon dioxide.

Cereal grains can also be used to produce alcoholic beverages. However, cereal grains contain starch rather than sugar, and, before fermentation can begin, the starch must be converted to sugar. This is accomplished by means of enzymes formed during a process called *malting*. In American beer, the primary grain is barley, which is malted by steeping it in water and allowing it to sprout. The sprouted grain is then slowly dried to kill the sprout but preserve the enzymes formed during the growth. This dried, sprouted barley is called malt, and, when crushed and mixed with water, the enzymes convert the starch to sugar. Only yeast is needed then to start fermentation. Usually ground corn is added to the malt to increase the amount of starch available, and all solids are filtered out before the yeast is added to the mash for fermentation. Hops (dried blossoms from only the female hop plant) are added with the yeast to give beer its distinctive, pungent flavor. One-fourth pound of hops is enough to flavor a 31-gallon barrel of beer. In most commercial beers today, alcoholic content is about 4.5%.

Other cultures use other plants as the starting place for fermentation. Cortez, in his expedition to Mexico in 1518, commented on the native alcoholic beverage, pulque, which is made from the agave cactus and has an alcoholic content of about 6%. In home brewing of pulque, a cavity is sometimes made in the body of the cactus and the fermentation carried out there, yielding 5 to 6 quarts of pulque a day until the cactus dies. Mead has an alcoholic content of about 10% and is still available in parts of Great Britain and Denmark. Sake, the traditional rice beer of Japan, is between 12% and 16% alcohol. Apple cider allowed to ferment may develop an alcohol content as great as 14%.

DISTILLED PRODUCTS

To obtain alcohol concentrations above those which can be reached by fermentation, distillation must be used. Distillation is a process in which the solution containing alcohol is heated and the vapors collected and condensed into liquid form again. Since alcohol has a lower boiling point than water, there is a higher percentage of alcohol in the distillate (the condensed liquid) then there was in the original solution.

There is still debate over who discovered the distillation process and when the discovery was made, but many authorities place it in Arabia around 800 AD. The term *alcohol* is from an Arabic word meaning "finely divided spirit" and originally referred to that part of the wine collected through distillation—the essence of the wine! Only fermented beverages were used in Europe until the tenth century, when the Italians first distilled wine, thereby introducing "spirits" to the western world. These new products were formally and informally studied and used in the treatment of many illness-

es, including senility. The prevalent feeling about their medicinal value is best seen in the name given these condensed vapors by a thirteenth century Professor of Medicine at the French University of Montpellier: *aqua vitae*, the water of life. Around the end of the seventeenth century the more prosaic Dutch called the liquid *brandy*, meaning burnt wine.

Between the table wines, which are produced by fermentation, and brandies, the distillate of wine, are the fortified wines. These are fermented wines with enough distillate added to bring the alcohol content up to about 20%. Sherry, port, Madeira, and muscatel are familiar examples.

Originally a liqueur was a distilled wine combined with many herbs and used only for medicinal purposes. These cordials have a high sugar content and are usually taken only in very small quantities. Some of the formulations for these beverages, such as Benedictine, are still secret. Some now are distillates of other products. Drambuie, for example, is a distillate of Scotch whiskey with the addition of heather, honey, and herbs.

All "hard liquors" start from a mash composed of a starchy grain (or other starchy plant, such as potatoes) and malted barley to which yeast is added. Unlike the process of making beer, hops are not added, and the solid material is not strained out before fermentation is started. This mash is then heated and the distillate condensed.

The name "whiskey" comes from the Irish-Gaelic equivalent of aqua vitae and was already commonplace around 1500. The distillation of whiskey in America started on a large scale toward the end of the eighteenth century and was the basis for the first major political-social drug problem in this country. The chief product of the area just west of the Appalachian Mountains—western Pennsylvania, western Virginia, eastern Kentucky—was grain. It was not profitable for the farmers to ship the grain or flour across the mountains to the markets along the eastern seaboard. Since 10 bushels of corn could be converted to 6 barrels of flour, which could then be converted to 1 barrel of whiskey, which could be profitably shipped east, distillation started on a grand scale.

In 1789 one of the early distillers who established a good reputation was Elijah Craig, a Baptist minister living in what was then Bourbon County, Kentucky. He began storing his whiskey in charred new oak barrels, originating a manufacturing step still used with most American whiskeys (but not with Canadian whiskeys, which are stored in uncharred barrels).

Today's Scotch is the distillate of fermented malted barley. The distinctive "smoky" flavor of Scotch comes from two sources. The malted barley is dried in kilns in which burning peat provides the heat, and some of the distinctive characteristics of peat are probably picked up by the barley. After distillation the product is stored for at least 3 years in uncharred barrels that were originally used to transport sherry.

A few other distillates will be mentioned briefly. By the seventeenth century distillation techniques made possible the production of relatively pure alcohol. To soften the raw taste of pure alcohol (and possibly to increase its medicinal value), the distillate was filtered through juniper berries and named "jenever" by the Dutch and "genievre" by the French. The British shortened the name first to "geneva" and finally to gin. In its present form gin is merely flavored alcohol, made primarily from corn to which water is added to give the desired alcohol content. Schnapps is manufactured in the same way but is not as thoroughly distilled, thus still retaining some of the flavor of the potatoes. Pure alcohol diluted with water to the desired alcoholic content is vodka, meaning "little water" in Russian. None of these liquors is aged; instead they are bottled for consumption immediately after distillation.

Rum is the distillate from the fermentation of molasses made from sugar cane. The most profitable and largest industry in New England in colonial days was the manufacture of rum. The same ships were used in a very active trade system that carried rum to Africa to pay for slaves, who were then sold in the continental United States to pay for the West Indian molasses that was traded for New England rum, and so on. This triangle, along with the industry, came to an abrupt halt in 1807

when the importation of slaves was forbidden.

One final note. In the United States the alcoholic content of distilled beverages is indicated by the term *proof*. The percentage of alcohol by volume is one half the proof number, that is, 90-proof whiskey is 45% alcohol. The term *proof* developed from a British Army procedure to gauge the alcohol content of distilled spirits before there were modern techniques. The liquid was poured over gunpowder and ignited. If the alcohol content was high enough, the alcohol would burn and ignite the gunpowder, which would go "pooff" and explode! That was proof that the beverage had an acceptable alcohol content, about 57%.

REGULATION OF ALCOHOL USE

Alcohol is different from most of the recent psychoactive drugs in western civilization in that the problem has never been to prevent its introduction—it has always been everywhere! There have been repeated attempts to control its use and, on occasion, to eliminate its availability. Throughout Europe and America, from the fourteenth through the twentieth century, all attempts to suppress alcohol have failed.

Early attempts at regulation of alcohol consumption in England consisted of edicts handed down by religious authorities. Some of these were recorded as early as the sixth century AD. The first national English legislation to curb intemperance was passed in 1327; it tried to limit the number of establishments that could sell alcoholic beverages. It was rapidly repealed, and a different approach was tried over 150 years later in 1494. This was the first licensing law; it gave justices of the peace the authority to determine where alcoholic drinks could be sold. Nothing succeeded. The consumption of alcohol in one form or another increased regularly. When legal production or sale was prohibited or highly taxed, illegal quantities increased.

In 1688 distillation was opened wide in England; upon paying a small tax, anyone could become a distiller—and almost everyone did! Gin drinking became a national passion, and, although laws changed and home distillation was made illegal, consumption increased. The crowding of urban central-city poverty areas with the workers of the industrial revolution, coupled with low-cost, easily available alcohol, contributed to the increase in alcohol consumption and in public drunkenness.

Parallel to this increased drinking was a negative reaction that resulted in the formation of temperance groups. In 1825 concern was expressed[1,pp.21-24] that "women of the middle and high classes of society entered the small private doors of gin shops to take their drams with the common women." In 1834 one report on drunkenness comments on the "great number of women and sometimes decent women" and of "the young prostitutes from twelve to fourteen years of age who were charged with being drunk and disorderly." One well-enforced act in 1839 started the decline in public drunkenness in England by placing penalties on selling spirits to those under 16 years of age and establishing closing times for Saturday and Sunday, the days of greatest drunkenness.

Meanwhile, across the Atlantic a new nation was developing. Remembering that one of the reasons the Pilgrims settled for Massachusetts was that "our victuals were much spent, especially our beer," it will be worthwhile to trace some of the high spots in this country's concern over the use of alcohol. The very first law was passed in Maryland in 1642, which made drunkenness punishable by a fine of 100 pounds of tobacco. Shortly thereafter, in 1650, Connecticut passed a law forbidding drinking more than a half hour at a time. Connecticut in 1659 followed with a $5 fine for being drunk in one's own home!

Virginia had other problems. In 1664 the colony passed a law prohibiting ministers from drinking to excess. Virginia ministers were a difficult group to change, though, and 100 years later Virginia had to pass another law prohibiting ministers from "drinking to excess and inciting riot." At about the same time, 1755, Georgia indicated what it thought about tavern keepers by forbidding a liquor license "to any tradesman who was capable of making his livelihood by honest labor"!

When the United States of America was a year old, Congress passed the first federal law regarding

TABLE 8-3 Alcoholic beverage consumption (gallons per person 15 years of age and older)

Year	Distilled spirits	Beer*	Wine
1800	7.2	32	0.6
1850	4.2	3	0.5
1900	2.0	24	0.7
1915	2.0	29	0.7

Data from Keller, M., and Gurioli, C.: Statistics on consumption of alcohol and alcoholism (mimeographed booklet), New Brunswick, N.J., 1976, Journal of Studies on Alcohol, Inc.
*In 1800 "beer" is mostly hard cider.

alcohol. This 1790 law authorized giving every soldier a daily ration of a fourth of a pint of rum, brandy, or whiskey. This fringe benefit was lost in the army in 1830, but the navy in its wisdom continued to dole out the ration until 1862. (It was over a hundred years later that the British sailors lost their grog ration!)

At no time did drinking in the United States reach the epidemic levels it had in England. An expanding frontier, fewer overcrowded slum areas, and a pioneer ideology resulted in almost everyone in the colonial period drinking, but moderately. As society changed in the early part of the nineteenth century, heavy drinking increased, and with each new public drunkard, there appeared two or three temperance workers. Temperance movements were everywhere in this period, acquiring national status with the formation of the American Temperance Society in 1827, which, it is important to note, advocated temperance, not abstinence. The changing pattern of alcohol use in this period is indicated in Table 8-3. In 1834 Congress provided the plot for a thousand western movies by passing a law forbidding the sale of liquor to Indians. The evidence is mixed on whether Indians differ in the way they metabolize alcohol. Perhaps Indians are more sensitive to the CNS effects of alcohol. Perhaps, though, they learned to drink from the early fur trappers and explorers, whose drinking pattern was to get "bombed." This is still an open question.

In the second half of the nineteenth century

things changed. Up to this time there had been little commercial nondistilled alcohol consumed in the United States. It was only with the advent of artificial refrigeration and the addition of hops, which helped preserve the beer, that there was an increase in the number of breweries. The waves of immigrants who entered this country in this period provided the necessary beer-drinking consumers.

At first, encouraged by temperance groups who preferred beer consumption to the use of liquor, breweries were constructed everywhere. Surprisingly, it was the great number of breweries that made abstaineers out of temperants and brought about the second wave of state prohibition statutes that evolved into national prohibition in 1920. With too many breweries there was an overproduction of beer. To sell their beer many brewers bought taverns or formed partnerships with tavern owners, offering special inducement to bartenders to push the sale of their beer. The brewers also found that it was necessary to supply distilled spirits to the taverns to satisfy the consumers. This alliance worked well; the consumption of malt beverages increased greatly but did not cause a decrease in the consumption of liquor.

The first state prohibition period began in 1851 when Maine passed its prohibition law. Between 1851 and 1855 thirteen states passed statewide prohibition laws, but by 1868 nine had repealed them. There was a continual battle throughout this period between the "wets" and the "drys." The strength of the feeling is seen in an 1865 Presbyterian church decision declaring that liquor manufacturers and sellers were not eligible to be members of a Presbyterian church. Another indication of the pervasiveness of temperance beliefs is that our sixteenth president, Abraham Lincoln, was a temperance organization member.

The National Prohibition Party, organized in 1874, provided the impetus for the second wave of statewide prohibition that developed in the 1880s. From 1880 to 1889 seven states adopted prohibition laws, but by 1896 four had repealed them. In 1895 the American Anti-Saloon League was organized, but it was 12 years later (1907) that the final state prohibition movement began.

Much of the prohibition activity gathered its energy and justification from changes occurring in a bit of Americana.

> The saloon was for centuries an honorable institution. In colonial times, well-meaning legislators made its presence mandatory in certain townships and defined its purpose as the "refreshment of mankind in a reasonable manner". . . . The saloon of the early nineteenth century was dedicated to the values of fellowship, equality, and euphoria. . . . It was a place where one could lift the burdens of caste, of status, and of the more restrictive social inhibitions, and thus freed, could grasp for the dim image of his own individuality. The saloon was also a glittering release from the drab and gray monotonies of an agrarian reality, a momentary refuge from worry or trouble, humiliation or shame. . . . In a society not yet oppressed by the god of precision—when a man could spell his own name differently every day of the week if he wanted to and when no one measured the trueness of a furrow in millimeters—a reasonably soft cloud of alcoholic haze was a luxury one could hardly afford to be without. Until the agrarian America that produced the saloon no longer existed, the saloon sustained many an honorable man.[2,pp.54-55]

In 1899 a group of educators, lawyers, and clergymen described the saloon as "the workingman's club, in which many of his leisure hours are spent, and in which he finds more of the things that approximate luxury than in his home. . . ." They went on to say: "It is a centre of learning, books, papers, and lecture hall to them. It is the clearinghouse for common intelligence, the place where their philosophy of life is worked out, and their political and social beliefs take their beginnings."[3,pp.215-217]

Truth lay somewhere between those statements and the sentiments expressed in a sermon:

> The liquor traffic is the most fiendish, corrupt and hell-soaked institution that ever crawled out of the slime of the eternal pit. It is the open sore of this land. . . . It takes the kind, loving husband and father, smothers every spark of love in his bosom, and transforms him into a heartless wretch, and makes him steal the shoes from his starving babe's

feet to find the price for a glass of liquor. It takes your sweet innocent daughter, robs her of her virtue and transforms her into a brazen, wanton harlot. . . .

The open saloon as an institution has its origin in hell, and it is manufacturing subjects to be sent back to hell. . . .[2,pp.66-67]

Prohibition was not just a matter of "wets" versus "drys," or a matter of political conviction or health concerns. Intricately interwoven with these factors was a middle-class, rural, Protestant, evangelical concern that the good and true life was being undermined by ethnic groups with a different religion and a lower standard of living and morality. One way to strike back at these groups was through prohibition. As one Anti-Saloon League leader puts it, "There is one thing greater than democracy . . . and that is the will of God."[2,pp.66-67]

If you can serve God's will, protect the virtue of your women, reduce temptation, and decrease your anxiety level by voting prohibition, it is not surprising that between 1907 and 1919 34 states enacted legislation enforcing statewide prohibition, while only two states repealed their prohibition laws. By 1917 64% of the population lived in dry territory, and in the 1908 to 1917 period over 104,400 licensed bars were closed. The effect on alcohol consumption? A 16% increase in per capita consumption of distilled liquors to a level higher than it had been for over 45 years! Beer consumption on a per capita basis over this same period decreased 3%.

It should also be remembered that the fact that there was a state prohibition law did not mean that the residents did not drink. They did, both legally and illegally. They drank illegally in speakeasies and other private clubs. They drank legally from a variety of the many patent medicines that were freely available. A few of the more interesting ones were Whisko, "a nonintoxicating stimulant" at 55 proof; Golden's Liquid Beef Tonic, "recommended for treatment of alcohol habit" with 53 proof; and Kaufman's Sulfur Bitters, which "contains no alcohol" but was in fact 20% alcohol (40 proof) and contained no sulfur!

1917 was the beginning of the end. In January the United States Supreme Court upheld a law passed by Congress in 1913 forbidding interstate shipment of alcoholic beverages into areas where the manufacture and sale of liquor was "illegal."[1] In March Congress passed an antiliquor advertising bill, which prohibited the use of the United States mail to advertise "spirituous, vinous, malted, fermented, or other intoxicating liquors of any kind" in an area that locally restricted their advertising. At this time, although only 64% of the population was dry, 90% of the land area was, so this law effectively stopped all but local advertising.

In August, 1917, the Senate adopted the resolution authored by Andrew Volstead, which submitted the national prohibition amendment to the states. The House of Representatives concurred in December, and 21 days later on January 8, 1918, Mississippi became the first state to ratify the Eighteenth Amendment. A year later, January 16, 1919, Nebraska was the thirty-sixth state to ratify the amendment, and the deed was done!

As stated in the amendment, a year after the thirty-sixth state ratified it, national prohibition came into effect: January 16, 1920. The amendment was simple, with only two operational parts:

Section 1. After one year from the ratification of this article the manufacture, sale or transportation of intoxicating liquors within, the importation thereof into, or the exportation thereof from the United States and all territory subject to the jurisdiction thereof for beverage purposes is hereby prohibited.

Section 2. The Congress and the several States shall have concurrent power to enforce this article by appropriate legislation.

The Eighteenth Amendment was repealed by the Twenty-first Amendment proposed in Congress on February 20, 1933, and ratified by 36 states by the fifth of December of that year. So ended an era. The Twenty-first Amendment was also short and sweet:

Section 1. The eighteenth article of amendment of the Constitution of the United States is hereby repealed.

Section 2. The transportation or importation into any State, Territory, or possession of the United States for delivery or use therein of intoxicating liquors, in violation of the laws thereof, is hereby prohibited.

Thus was the control of alcoholic beverages returned to the states. The last state to repeal its state prohibition law was Mississippi in 1966. How effective was national prohibition? There are many ways of approaching this question. One writer has commented that

> prohibition was in many ways the single most effective political move of this century, for its principal goal was to destroy the Irish Catholic-American political clubs (in which a fair bit of drinking was done). . . . The second goal was to try to reduce alcohol use. . . .[4,p.31]

Did it reduce the consumption of alcoholic beverages? In the early years it certainly did, and authoritative estimates place beer consumption in 1920 at about 2 gallons per adult, while in 1917, the last normal consumption year, it was 32 gallons per adult. Distilled spirits dropped from an average of over 2 gallons per adult in 1917 to 0.5 gallon per adult in 1920. Wine consumption, however, may have even shown a slight increase, reaching 0.8 gallon per adult in 1920.

By 1930 things were different. Wine consumption had increased to 1.4 gallons, beer to 11.5, and distilled spirits to 2.2 gallons per adult! On a strictly wet-dry basis it would seem that prohibition failed, since 10 years after initiation, alcohol consumption was almost as high as it was before enactment.

All other measures of the effectiveness of national prohibition seem to follow the alcohol consumption curve. Deaths resulting from alcoholism in 1920 were only about 20% of the rate in 1917. By 1929, though, the rate was 70% of the 1917 level. Cirrhosis of the liver followed the same steep dip and slow rise.

Prohibition did have some effects that lasted beyond 1933. One obvious effect was the elimination of many of the abstinence and temperance groups. With their goal achieved (they believed), their motivation and their membership dwindled to almost

nothing in the early twenties. It is doubtful whether these groups could have withstood the urbanization, industrialization, and education that had progressed continually. Of more importance, however, prohibition showed clearly that to attempt to eliminate an already existing pleasure is a mighty hard thing to do.

ALCOHOL AS A CONSUMER ITEM

Anyway you look at it, booze is big business and, like Gaul, is easily divided into three parts. Today Americans are spending about $35 billion on alcoholic products and, on a per capita basis, drinking about 23.5 gallons of beer and 2 gallons each of distilled spirits and wine. This section discusses some of the major changes that have occurred and are now occurring in the production and use of our number one drug (and our number one causer-of-drug-problems). Because alcohol is widely available and used, its shifting pattern of use probably reflects our changing society better than any other form of drug use. The patterns are clearer than those of other drugs because alcohol production, distribution, advertising, sale, and use are legal. As you read about and observe the changes—to a greater diversity of products, and a greater convenience of use—remember that these changes are in response to changes in our society, our way of life. Changes in the alcoholic beverage industry can speed or slow these social changes to some extent. However, if they don't keep in fairly close step with social changes that section of the industry gets run over. As we'll see, several sections have already been squashed.

The high level of beer and liquor use in 1800 dwindled as the temperance and abstinence advocates had their way in the mid-nineteenth century, only to lose their grip around 1900 as beer consumption rose again as a result of immigration in a crescendo that climaxed in 1920 with prohibition. The consumption of liquor never did regain the popularity it had in 1800, but it moved west with the nation, since it was portable and potable.

The beer-drinking, free-lunch saloon with nickel beer and bucket-of-suds-to-go disappeared forever

TABLE 8-4 Beer production since prohibition

Year	Barrels (millions)	Packaged (%)	Draft (%)
1934	43.2	25	75
1940	53.9	52	48
1950	88.2	72	28
1960	93.4	81	19
1970	133.1	86	14
1975	160.6	88	12
1981	180.0	90	10

Compiled in part from data in A history of packaged beer and its market in the United States, 1969, American Can Company; Statistical highlights, U.S. Brewers Association.

with prohibition. And so did a couple of thousand breweries. Two years after prohibition ended there were only 750 brewers, and by 1941 that had dwindled to 507. From 1960 to the mid-seventies about ten beer makers vanished each year, until in 1976 there were less than 50. This declined to about 40 in the early 1980s. Mechanization, efficiency of large breweries, advertising, and a leveling off of consumption continues to push the smaller, regional brewers, but not necessarily the brands, out of the market. The trend is clear: the top five brewers accounted for 53% of the market in 1971; by 1976 it was 69%. In 1982 the top seven brewers sold 80% of the beer marketed in the United States.

Table 8-4 points out the very clear shifts in patterns of beer consumption since prohibition. In 1934 75% of the beer sold was draft, and it was usually consumed away from the home. By 1982 home consumption had increased greatly, and packaged beer—nondraft—was 90% of the market. To make it possible to put beer in bottles or cans for shipment, it had to be pasteurized to stop all fermentation so the container wouldn't explode. Draft beer in barrels usually contained some active yeast, and fermentation would continue right to the top. Pasteurization, of course, changed the flavor somewhat, and many purists objected. The canned beer you now see labeled *draft* has not been pasteurized, but instead it has been put through filters to remove all the active yeast. It still tastes differ-

ent, as you would expect, since it *is* different. Table 8-4 shows that convenience is the keynote in beer, as in other forms of drug use. It has been a major factor in the type of beer container selected in the past—about 85% of the packaged containers are one-way bottles and cans—but ecological and other factors may reverse the trend and return us to the returnable bottle.

Most of the beer sold today in America is *lager*, from the German word *lagern*, meaning to store. To brew lager, a type of yeast is used that settles to the bottom of the mash to ferment. After fermentation, and before packaging, the beer is stored to age. *Ale* requires a top-fermentation yeast, higher temperatures, and more malt and hops, and it produces a stronger (more flavorful) beverage. *Malt liquor* is brewed much like lager but is aged longer, has less carbonation, more calories (185 per 12 ounces) and 1% to 3% more alcohol.

When there is very little difference in competing products, as in today's commercial beers, you have to spend a lot to sell the image. In 1981 advertising costs for the industry averaged about $3 a barrel. Brewers spend a lot, and we drink a lot—but not as much as some countries. Everyone should be able to guess who drinks the *most* beer, but who drinks the least? Czechoslovakia, Belgium, and Austria are neck and neck, close behind the world leader in beer drinking, West Germany. On a per capita basis (age 15 and over population) Germany (with over 1400 breweries and where beer costs 25% less than apple juice) consumes 50 gallons a year, almost ten times as much as the lowest beer consumer, Spain. Compared to the rest of the world in per capita consumption, the United States is in the middle with 30 gallons a year, about the same as its neighbor to the north, Canada. It is still big business, though, and in 1979 the brewers paid $3.4 billion in taxes to state and federal governments.

That amount is only a drop in the bucket. The distilled spirits industry paid $6.9 billion in the same year. Liquor is a little different, however, and since 1951 there has been a $10.50 per gallon federal tax. Liquor taxes are the largest source of federal revenue other than corporate and individual

TABLE 8-5 Distilled spirits: U.S. manufactured/imported (millions of gallons)*

Year	Whiskey	Brandy	Rum	Gin	Vodka	Gallons consumed (15 years and older)
1934	107.9/5.6	12.5/0.6	2.2/0.3	4.7/0.2	—	0.6
1940	111.7/9.7	25.6/0.8	2.4/0.4	5.3/0.1	—	1.3
1950	174.8/15.3	10.8/0.8	1.9/0.2	6.1/0.1	0.01	1.6
1960	148.9/32.9	9.1/1.8	1.7/0.2	18.0/1.1	9.20	1.9
1970	146.4/79.9	15.3/2.7	1.1/0.4	27.4/3.9	22.20	2.5
1975	59.0/95.0	20.6/2.8	0.8/0.7	28.3/4.8	34.90	2.6
1979	101.2/95.4	18.5/5.0	2.2/0.7	27.3/6.4	37.40	2.6

Data from Distilled Spirits Industry; 1979 Annual Statistical Review, Washington, D.C., 1980, Distilled Spirits Council.
*U.S. manufactured figures are tax gallons produced.

income taxes. When state taxes are added to federal taxes, the average tax bite totals about 53% of what the consumer pays for a bottle of distilled spirits. If you think that's high, buy a bottle of booze in Great Britain: 86% of the cost is tax. Since I've used the term several times, you should know that distilled spirits did *not* acquire booze as a nickname from the E.C. Booz Company, which sold whiskey in bottles shaped like a log cabin. Booze probably came from the old English *bousen:* to carouse or drink heartily.

The battles in the distilled spirits world are not so much between corporations, although that struggle exists, as they are between the type of distilled spirit. Right now it's a slugfest between bourbon and vodka, with vodka in the winner's circle. Since most of the distilled spirit companies produce *both* types of liquor, the major excitement is over whether the trend to convenience, uniformity, and mixability (that is, vodka) will continue in the liquor industry as it has in the other areas of drug use. Table 8-5 contains a summary of the use of distilled spirits in the United States since prohibition.

The interesting facts about distilled spirits are in the manufacturing processes used for the various types of spirits. Several factors are involved: proof at which distillation is done, the grain used in the fermenting mash, and the type of barrel in which the distillate is aged.

The proof at which distillation is carried out determines two things that are related to the taste of the liquor. At high proof, 190 or above, none of the congeners and none of the flavor of the grains used in the mash remain in the distillate. What you have is 95% pure alcohol with little if any taste. *Grain neutral spirits* is the term for alcohol distilled at this proof; it is used primarily in medicine and research. When this 190-proof distillate is diluted, it is sold as *vodka.* The same distillate is filtered through a "ginhead" containing juniper, and perhaps other plant material, to produce gin. Neither gin nor vodka is aged. You may wonder why vodkas of the same proof are priced differently if they are all identical—and they are. The best answer to that question was provided by an official of Heublein's, a company that produces both the high-priced *Smirnoff* vodka, the second best-selling brand in the country, and a medium-priced vodka. "That's a very embarrassing question. Shall we say it's a difference in pricing policy?"[5] Yes, we shall say that—maybe one label costs more?

Whiskey is usually distilled at a lower proof, not more than 160, and thus the distillate contains congeners as well as some of the flavor of the grain used. If 51% or more of the grain used was rye, then the product is labeled *straight rye* whiskey. When corn constitutes over 51% of the grain in the mash, the liquor is called *bourbon.* (To be called *corn whiskey* requires that the mash be 80% or more corn.) Both rye and bourbon are then diluted to 120 to 125 proof and aged in new, charred oak barrels for at least 2, and usually more, years.

Blended rye whiskey must contain at least 51% of straight rye whiskey, the remainder being bourbon or grain neutral spirits.

Whiskey accumulates congeners during aging, at least for the first 5 years, and it is the congeners and the grain used that provide the variation in taste among whiskeys. Until prohibition almost all whiskey consumed in the United States was manufactured in the United States. Prohibition introduced smuggled Canadian and Scotch whisky (spelled without an *e;* America and Ireland added the letter in the early decades of this century) to American drinkers, and they liked them. World War II sent American men around the world, further exposing them to this different type of liquor. Scotch and Canadian whisky are lighter than American whiskey, which means lighter in color and less heavy in taste. They are lighter because Canadian and Scotch whiskys are distilled at 150 to 180 proof and then aged (perhaps up to 5 years) in seasoned oak barrels, which have been used before for holding liquor. These seasoned barrels add fewer congeners to the whisky.

The less flavorful whiskys were more satisfactory in mixed drinks and fitted well with the loosening of life-styles and the decline in the number of people who took their whiskey "neat" after World War II. The result: whisky imports increased 800% from the late 1940s to the mid-1970s. In 1968 American distillers began to fight back when Congress passed laws permitting a new kind of whiskey to be made in the United States: American light whiskey, distilled at more than 160 proof and aged in seasoned barrels that were originally used for bourbon, is an approach to duplicating the whisky from outside the country. The Japanese are imitating the Scotch *exactly*—well, almost. They are even importing peat from Scotland!

Light whiskey hasn't done very well in the marketplace. It was too little and too late. The trend toward lightness that benefited Scotch and Canadian whisky also increased sales of gin and especially vodka. From less than a half million gallons of vodka in 1950, sales of American-produced vodka increased to 85 million gallons in 1975. In 1977 vodka pushed bourbon aside, clearly taking over

as the number one *type* of distilled spirit in America. Even the Russians and the Chinese have moved vigorously into the American vodka market. Some Russian and Chinese vodkas are different from American vodka, however: they may add buffalo grass for flavor or age the vodka for several years in wine casks. Just so you can settle arguments with your mother, the top five best selling brands of distilled spirits in 1980 were: Bacardi rum, Smirnoff Vodka, Seagrams 7-Crown, Seagrams VO, and Canadian Club. You should know that generic—no brand name—whiskey has sold well in test markets!

The newest beverages are in direct competition with one of the oldest. Wine consumption has been increasing by fits and starts in the United States since about 1960 and in 1980, for the first time ever, Americans drank more wine than distilled spirits. They did it again in 1981 and the trend may continue. Wine courses, wine clubs, and wine books have helped to bring the fruit of the vine onto the table in many American homes. They have also escalated prices. The wine experience may be part of the nostalgia craze—things are so bad today, they *had* to be better in earlier years—but there's no going back. The little old winemaker and the happy peasants jumping up and down in their bare feet to crush the grapes are gone, if they ever existed. The straw covering for Chianti bottles will soon be seen only on the late movies. In their place? The multimillion-dollar, stainless steel–vat, Madison Avenue winery of Julio and Ernest Gallo, the General Motors of wine. They sell about 25% of all American-made wine, and about 80% of what we drink is made in America. The top 10 American wine producers are: Gallo, United Vintners (Inglenook, Italian Swiss Colony, and others), Almaden, Wine Spectrum (Taylor and Great Western), Wine Group (Mogen David and others), Paul Masson, Canandaigua, Guild, Monarch, and Sebastiani.

Table 8-6 gives some feel for the variety, as well as our total consumption, of wine over the years. It will be a long time before we have to think about being the number one wine consumer in the world. Portugal is first and Italy second with a per capita consumption (age 15 and over population) of about

TABLE 8-6 Wine consumption in the United States

Year	Production*	Percent of total consumption—imported and domestic			
		Table	Dessert	Vermouth	Sparkling
1960	159	34	52	4	3
1970	237	50	28	4	8
1975	318	57	18	3	6
1979	352	73	11	2	6

Data from Economic Research Report, ER45, San Francisco, October 1, 1980, Wine Institute.
*In millions of gallons.

44 and 38 gallons, respectively, in 1976. France and Spain round out the top four in annual consumption, although all four countries are drinking less wine and more beer every year. In this country California has the highest consumption rate—not too surprising, since it produces about 88% of our wine. About 20 other states also produce wine, including New York (8% to 9%) and Illinois (1% in 1979). You should remember that many American grapevines came originally from France and Spain, but after a late nineteenth century disease destroyed almost all the European vineyards, they used our plants. Today most of the French, Italian, and Spanish grapes are grown from descendants of transplanted American vines.

Even though wine production has been mechanized and sterilized, there is still a greater variety in the product than in any other alcoholic beverage. This has given rise to "I don't know wine, but I know what I like" and "one man's wine is another man's vinegar" type of thinking. It may be true; like many other things in life, what you believe has much to do with what you experience. There are two types of American wines. Some are called *generics* (!) and usually have names taken from European land areas where the original wines were produced: champagne, Burgundy, Bordeaux, Rhine. These are all blended wines, and there is no guarantee that a domestic and a foreign wine with the same name will have a similar taste. The second type of American wine is called *varietals*, named after the one variety of grape that by law must make up at least 51% of the grapes used in producing the wine. There are many of these wines, and they are usually sold only by the bottle, not in gallon jugs, and are more expensive than the generic wines.

Table wines are the wines most people drink, wines with familiar names: Burgundy, Bordeaux, claret, Rhine, Tokay. Most table wines are dry, that is, not sweet. The wine you select for a meal depends on the food that is served. Heavier wines are used with heavier foods and lighter wines with lighter foods. It's all very patriotic: red wine with meat, white wine with fish, and Blue Nun with fowl. Dessert wines are fortified (that is, brandy will be added to bring their alcohol content to near 20%) and are usually sweet, as are most desserts. Port and Madeira are the best known dessert wines. Most people are familiar with the sparkling wines such as *champagne* and *sparkling Burgundy*. Their carbonation is a natural one, in contrast to the less expensive, and usually sweeter, "pop wines" that have the carbonation added, as do soft drinks. ("Pop wines" had 10% of the market in 1975 but only 7% in 1980.) The only other wines you should note are *sherry* and *vermouth;* these are aperitifs and originally were like appetizers, used at the beginning of a meal.

The wine industry is about to take off in several new directions that will probably expand the user population and increase sales. In 1980 several "soft" and "light" wines were introduced with great success. Soft wines have a lower alcohol content (8% to 9%) than regular wine and are easily made: the grapes are harvested early, when they have less

TABLE 8-7 Wine consumption in the United States

	Red	Rosé	White
1960	73%	10%	17%
1979	30%	21%	49%

sugar, or the fermentation is stopped when the desired alcohol content is reached. Light wines have about 25% fewer calories. Whether the market will support two separate lines or force them to combine into a single type—low calorie, low alcohol—remains to be seen. The prediction is that low-calorie wine will be 10% to 15% of the market in the late eighties. One of the first successful low-calorie wines comes from Taylor, which is owned by Coca-Cola, and is under the supervision of the man who introduced Tab (the world's most successful low-calorie item ever).

There's more. Wine is being sold in 6-ounce cans in some areas and seems to be successful. The use of aluminum cans prevents the wine from taking on the taste of tin. Consumers are asking for, or at least waiting for, all of these innovations. On their own they have shifted their pattern of wine drinking from red wine to white, which is compatible with more foods (Table 8-7). The trend is clear—soon white wine, with low calories and low alcohol, will be available in cans and it will compete for the beer market as a thirst quencher and refresher, rather than a drink with meals or meditation. Decisions, decisions. Shall I pick up a cold six-pack of beer or a cold six-pack of wine to take to the tennis court?

One more thing. The head of a household may register with the U.S. Treasury Department and each year legally produce 200 gallons of wine (not beer or any distillate) for personal use. It is not legal to make any alcoholic beverage for sale without federal and state licenses. That point is a bone of contention with some people: in 1977 U.S. Treasury agents closed down 481 illegal stills, which could produce about 2 million gallons of moonshine

a year. Many people still believe that moonshine is so called because it is made by the light of the silvery moon. Not so—the term originated in the nineteenth century and referred to white brandy smugglers in the British North Sea who would bring their illegal cargoes to shore when the moonlight was bright enough to guide their efforts.

My Uncle Bill has a still on the hill
Where he runs off a gallon or two;
The birds in the sky get so drunk they can't fly
On the good old mountain dew.

They call it that old mountain dew,
And them that refuse it are few.
You may go 'round the bend,
But you'll come back again
For that good old mountain dew.[6]

There aren't as many Uncle Bills working any more. From 1950 to 1980 the number of stills seized each year by federal agents dropped from 10,030 to 106. Maybe the Burt Reynolds movies are right: over 90% of the stills were in the southeastern region of the United States and in Appalachia. The high cost of sugar, which is added to the malt, and a variety of socioeconomic factors have almost driven the small independent businessman out of the field. They have also driven the cost of "white lightning" up over $20 a gallon, which is more expensive than some legal whiskeys.

The procedures used to produce moonshine are the same, only cruder, as those used in legal distilleries, but there are two variations you might like to know about. One is that stills have frequently been placed in pigpens—to conceal the odor of the boiling mash—and, as one moonshiner described the process, "it usually takes seventy-two hours on up to three or four days according to how many hogs fall in it. . . ."[7] Into the mash, that is. No joke. Neither is the other variation. Some of the wild yeasts floating in the air will convert starches in the mash into acetic acid (vinegar). In the still the acid combines with the lead in pipes as well as the lead in the solder of automobile radiators frequently used to condense the distillate. Lead is deadly, as you should know from news reports about children eating leaded paint. A 1961 assay of 221 whiskey samples found 86% with a measurable amount of lead salts—one had over 23,000 μg of lead per liter! There are clinical reports of successful and unsuccessful treatments of whiskey-induced lead poisoning.[8,9] A 1980 report of moonshine assays identified arsenic in every sample.[10]

Some legal comments

Repeal of prohibition returned to the states the right to enact laws regulating the sale and use of alcoholic beverages within each state. The federal government, of course, retained control over interstate commerce and the right to tax the production for sale of alcohol. Since prohibition, most of the federal effort in regulating alcohol has been by the Treasury Department—the Bureau of Alcohol, Tobacco, and Firearms. In 1975 a court decision resolved an administrative problem and said that the Bureau, not the FDA, had the authority to control the labels put on containers of alcoholic beverages. The FDA had argued that alcoholic beverages should be treated as foods and have a full ingredient listing on the label. In 1977 the FDA asked the Bureau to require liquor labels to warn pregnant women that excessive use of alcohol might harm their babies. In 1981 the decision was reached *not* to put a health warning label on alcoholic beverages.

Changes are occurring at the state level as well. All states have always had laws that put a lower limit on the age at which an individual could purchase alcohol for consumption. Until 1970, when the national voting age was lowered to 18, all the states had 21 as the minimum age except New York and Louisiana, which lowered the age years ago (1934 in New York). Thirty states changed their laws to permit individuals under 21 to purchase alcoholic beverages on their own. However, by 1981 10 states had raised the lower age from 18 to 19. As of 1983 New York raised its minimum age to 19.

One interesting sidelight in the equalization of the sexes occurred in December, 1976, when the U.S. Supreme Court ruled that Oklahoma could not permit women 18 to 21 to purchase 3.2% beer while prohibiting it to men of the same age. Oklahoma unsuccessfully tried to justify the difference on the basis that more males than females in this age range were arrested for drunk driving and killed in automobile accidents.

Alcohol as a consumer product—yes, it surely is, produced and consumed by the gallons. Most consumers do engage in responsible drinking—some don't. And it will always be that way, no matter what the laws are.

WHO DRINKS? AND WHY?

There are clear differences even between primitive tribes that use alcohol only sparingly and those which are referred to as drinking tribes. The more sober tribes lived in settled communities with structured social systems that spell out social level and social rights and obligations. The drinking tribes typically have a much looser social structure, with property being held communally and few ties to land. These tribes frequently are nomadic or survive by hunting rather than by growing crops. In brief, in primitive societies if one has to account for his behavior, provide for himself, and receive according to his output, drinking is usually well controlled. If there is no need for self-control, then heavy drinking is not atypical.

Such relationships could be seen in the rural Ireland of the eighteenth and nineteenth centuries. Public drunkenness was widespread and has been related to a very diffuse social organization with little attachment to the land. Also, Ireland at that time suffered from outside rule, which resulted in low respect for authority and little interest in self-control. Some of these general attitudes may be reflected in the finding that the highest alcoholism rate in the United States today is among the Irish-Americans.

Differences between countries in drinking patterns are apparent even today. Although Italians consume the equivalent of 13.5 quarts of pure alcohol per year per adult, public intoxication is much less frequent in most of Italy than one might expect. Except in the industrial north, drinking in Italy is associated with meals and family gatherings.

It will be interesting to see whether public drunkenness moves south along with the industrialization of Italy.

France is probably the country that had the greatest drinking problem in the world, although a concerted effort by the government has reduced consumption in recent years. Best estimates in the mid-1970s were that 15% of French adult males were alcoholics and that at least an additional 15% consumed alcohol in levels dangerous to their health. The government's "responsible" drinking efforts have been countered by a strong wine lobby, which put ads in the subway saying, "Water is for frogs," and the French belief that relates wine drinking to virility. All of that seems to be rapidly going by the board. A 1981 study in France reported[11] that wine consumption had dropped by 25% since 1964 and that neighborhood bars were closing by the hundreds. Why? Watching television has taken the place of visiting the bistros, which were places to congregate, drink, and talk in the evening. Automation is the other factor leading to less routine wine drinking. Doing physical labor you can have a glow on and still get the job done—not so when you're working in an automated, mechanized, skilled factory. Wine drinking in France is moving toward the American pattern—a pleasant reward, not a regular morning-noon-and-night beverage. This will probably improve the health of French males.

The United States is a huge melting pot where everything hasn't yet melted. As a result there are educational, socioeconomic, religious, racial, regional, and a thousand other differences in drinking patterns. As we melt together, the differences will decrease.

In 1958 55% of the American adult population said that they used alcohol. That was the low point. The percentage of users climbed to a high of 71% in 1976 and dropped to 69% in 1979. As of 1981[12] about one third of all adults age 18 years and older label themselves as abstainers (25% of men and 40% of women). That means that of those adults who use alcohol there is enough alcohol consumed for each person to have 1½ ounces (about 3 drinks) of pure alcohol every day. Most of us don't use anything near that amount—in fact, 11% of the alcohol users consume about half of all the alcohol. We Americans consume 49% of our alcohol in beer, 12% in wine, and 39% in distilled spirits. The rate at which alcohol use is increasing slowed from 25% in the 1960s to an 8% increase in the 1970s. Of equal importance is the shifting pattern of use—in the late seventies wine showed a 19% increase in use while distilled spirits dropped 4%. Whites are more likely to drink than blacks, Northerners than Southerners, younger than older, Catholics and Jews than Protestants, nonreligious than religious, urban than rural, large city than small city, and college educated than those with only a high school or grade school education.

Some people don't just drink, they drink in amounts and ways that cause problems—for them, you, me . . . all of us. Twenty percent of the males and 10% of the females who drink report signs and symptoms of alcohol addiction or loss of control as a result of alcohol use, and about half of those report serious adverse social consequences (on job, family, etc). One report[13] showed almost a doubling of the percentage of individuals who said that alcohol use, not necessarily theirs, had had a negative effect on their family—from 13% in 1972 to 24% in 1978. The careless drinker causes problems for everyone. Even though 34 states have decriminalized public drunkenness, there are 1 million arrests a year as a result of it—only now it's called disorderly conduct or disturbing the peace.[14]

California has the highest percentage of alcoholics, followed by New Jersey, New Hampshire, and New York. The highest rate of alcoholism in an identifiable ethnic group is in the Irish-Americans. A better predictor of alcoholism than where people live or what their national origins are is the kind of homes they come from. A broken home is the background for 40% of alcoholics, and 40% (some overlapping) report problem drinking in at least one parent. Late birth position in a family is associated with alcoholism, and this may be caused, at least partially, by the greater likelihood of a broken home or loss of a parent early in the life of a later-born child.

One study of juvenile drinkers who had been

TABLE 8-8 Characteristics of a clinical alcoholic personality

Weak ego	Stimulus augmenter	Field dependent	Neurotic
Weak sexual identity	Greater sensitivity to environment	Passive	Anxiety
Psychopathy	Hypochondriasis	Dependent	Depression
Hostility	Fear of death	Undifferentiated	Hysteria
Immaturity			
Impulsiveness			
Low tolerance for frustration			
Present orientation			

From Barnes, G.E.: The alcoholic personality, a reanalysis of the literature. (Reprinted by permission from Journal of Studies on Alcohol, **40**(7):571-634, 1979. Copyright by Journal of Studies on Alcohol, Inc. New Brunswick, NJ 08903

referred to an alcoholism clinic reported that one or both parents of the subjects were alcoholic. Moreover, these juveniles expressed much anxiety over drinking, but since drinking made them less anxious, they continued. One motivation for their drinking was to prove that they could drink better than their alcoholic parent. Another basis was suggested by the fact that they typically engaged in group, not solitary, drinking and may have been looking for a substitute for the family ties they were unable to form at home.

One report suggests that ". . . conditions predisposing to poor self-esteem and low ego strength are prevalent in the personal and family histories of alcoholics."[15,p.621] Particularly clear was the ambiguity in their lives over what they were expected to do, and that in a context of maternal ambivalence and nonaffection toward them. That would certainly make you wonder about yourself: What do *they* want me to do? Do *they* like me?

Alcoholics have been studied extensively but it wasn't until 1979 that the thousands of studies were put together in a way that seems to help us make some sense of them psychologically. Two really good papers on "The Alcoholic Personality"[15,16] said about the same thing—only in different words. Clinicians have always been impressed with the communality of psychological characteristics of individuals in treatment for alcoholism. "Alcoholics do present a fairly common personality pattern when they present for treatment . . . neuroticism, weak ego, stimulus augmenting, and field depen-

dence."[15,p.622] Table 8-8 gives a summary of the components that make up the alcoholic personality. Many of those characteristics are the result of the effects of a history of excessive drinking on the prealcoholic personality—that is, the characteristics are not predictive of alcoholism, they are in part the result of it. The prealcoholic personality is less well defined but some work suggests that the prealcoholic individual is not grossly maladjusted and is more likely to be nonconforming, gregarious, and impulsive. The one factor that appears repeatedly is poor impulse control: ". . . prealcoholic males . . . have been described as fearless and independent, with uncontrolled impulsivity and an overemphasis on masculinity."[16,p.136]

A brief comment must be made of the data in Table 8-9, which is based on a large 1974 national sample of students in grades 7 through 12.[17] Take note of the higher drinking levels of boys and the increasing percentage of heavy drinkers with increasing age: pretty much what you would expect. Many people would also expect to find high religiosity—belief in God, church attendance, etc.—associated with lower levels of alcohol use and abuse, and it was.[18] You may not have expected the relationship between occupational level and drinking level: there is none. It is no longer only the "the kids on the other side of the tracks" who use alcohol and sometimes use too much. A 1981 partial repeat of this survey found things pretty much unchanged from 1974 except that the difference between boys and girls was not as great.[19] One other

TABLE 8-9 Drinking level in junior and senior high school students by selected characteristics*

	Percentages		
	Light	Moderate	Heavy
Sex			
Boys	37	32	31
Girls	50	32	18
Age			
13-14	54	29	17
15-16	36	34	30
17-18	28	35	37
Religiosity			
Low	23	36	41
High	57	29	14
Parents' occupations			
Semiskilled	45	30	25
Skilled and office	42	34	24
Manager-professional	42	34	24

Drinking level combines both frequency and amount as indicated:

Frequency of drinking episodes	Number of drinks each episode		
	1	2-4	5-12
None, less than 1/year	Light		
1/month at most	Light	Moderate	Moderate
No more than 3-4/ month	Moderate	Moderate	Heavy
At least 1/week	Moderate	Heavy	Heavy

*From Summary of final report: A national study of adolescent drinking behavior, attitudes and correlates, Research Triangle Park, N.C., April, 1975, Center for the Study of Social Behavior, Research Triangle Institute.

point was made—states that allow 18-year-olds to purchase alcohol have heavier drinking. That has been long known, although the data are not complete.[20] The homogenizing process goes on, and we all become more and more alike; every year the melting pot looks more like a puree than a stew. Studies on the characteristics of problem drinkers suggest that they are pretty much the same whether in Iceland[21] or San Francisco.[22]

It is fairly well accepted now that there is a genetic component, a predisposition to alcohol addiction. The exact nature of the contribution from heredity is not known, but researchers are closng in: ". . . variations in the rates of ethanol elimination and total alcohol intake in laboratory animals can be adequately explained by the known kinetic constants of a single enzyme, alcohol dehydrogenase, the only enzyme to metabolize alcohol to any extent in vivo in animals or in man."[23,p.1141] There are studies on both sides of the American Indian–alcohol question. One problem may be that American Indians are not a clear genetic entity and that the idea of "an American Indian" may have no more biological value than the concept of "the white man." Another problem may be that compared to "white men" American Indians absorb alcohol more rapidly and thus have a higher blood alcohol level (BAL). However, they also metabolize the alcohol 15% to 20% faster![24] The more acute responses to alcohol intake by Orientals as compared to Caucasians could be the result of a lower level of aldehyde dehydrogenase, the enzyme that breaks down the aldehyde that accumulates during alcohol metabolism.[25] Most adoption studies show that the probability of a child growing into an alcohol abuser is better predicted by the drinking pattern of his biological parents than that of his foster parents.[26] Debate over whether this was true of females as well as males seems to have been answered in the affirmative.[27]

Do not believe that all the answers are in on the question of why people drink, or drink to excess. It may be that alcohol is no different from other drugs and availability, peer group, and role models are the primary keys to understanding. It may also be that alcohol is different, with a strong biological component.

SOME APERITIFS

The next few sections focus on some of the many behavioral and physiological effects of alcohol. The discussion is limited, unless otherwise noted, to *ethyl* alcohol (that is, *ethanol*, C_2H_5OH), and the term *alcohol* refers specifically and only to ethyl alcohol.

Absorption

Alcohol is unique in that it requires no digestion and can be absorbed unchanged from the stomach and, more rapidly, from the small intestine. In an empty stomach the overall rate of absorption depends on the concentration of alcohol. Even though concentration is the primary factor, the absorption rate can be altered. For example, alcohol taken with or after a meal is absorbed more slowly. This is because the food remains in the stomach for digestive action, and the protein in the food retains the alcohol with it in the stomach.

Plain water, by decreasing the concentration, slows the absorption of alcohol, but carbonated liquids speed it up. The carbon dioxide acts to move everything quite rapidly through the stomach to the small intestines. It is this emptying of the stomach and the more rapid absorption of alcohol in the intestines that give champagne and sparkling Burgundy a faster onset of action than wine. Once absorbed into the bloodstream, alcohol passes almost immediately through the liver.

Peripheral blood effects

One effect of alcohol on the CNS is the dilation of the peripheral blood vessels. This increases the heat loss from the body but makes the drinker feel warm. The heat loss and cooling of the interior of the body is great enough to cause a slowdown in some biochemical processes. It is this dilation of the peripheral vessels that argues against the use of alcohol in individuals in shock or extreme cold. Under these conditions blood is needed in the central parts of the body, and heat loss must be diminished if the person is to survive.

Hangovers

The Germans call it "wailing of cats" (Katzenjammer), the Italians "out of tune" (stonato), the French "woody mouth" (gueule de boise), the Norwegians "workmen in my head" (jeg har tommermenn) and the Swedes "pain in the roots of the hair" (hont i haret).[28]

Hangovers aren't much fun. And they aren't very well understood, either. The symptoms are well known to a high percentage of even moderate drinkers who occasionally overindulge: upset stomach, fatigue, headache, thirst, depression, anxiety, general malaise.

Some authorities believe that the symptoms of a hangover are the symptoms of withdrawal from a short- or long-term addiction to alcohol. The pattern certainly fits. Some alcoholics report continuing to drink just to escape the pain of the hangover. This behavior is not unknown to moderate drinkers, either: many believe that the only "cure" for a hangover is some of "the hair of the dog that bit you"—alcohol. And it may work to minimize symptoms, since it spreads them out over a longer period of time. There is no evidence that any of the "surefire-this'll-fix-you-up" remedies are effective. An analgesic for the headache, rest, and time are the only known "cures." Some of the ways to reduce the probability and the severity of a hangover will be evident from the following.

A 1970 study, "Experimental Induction of Hangover,"[29] provided support for two factors contributing to the hangover syndrome: (1) the higher your BAL, the more likely you are to have a hangover and (2) with the *same* BAL, bourbon drinkers were more likely (2 out of 3) than vodka drinkers (1 out of 3) to have a hangover. This fits in with the belief that some hangover symptoms are reactions to congeners. *Congeners* are natural products of the fermentation and preparation process, some of which are quite toxic. Congeners make the various alcoholic beverages different in smell, taste, color, and, possibly, hangover potential. Beer, with a 4% alcohol content, has only a 0.01% congener level, whereas wine has about 0.04% and distilled spirits between 0.1% and 0.2%. Gin, being almost a mixture of pure alcohol and water, has a congener content about the same as wine, while a truly pure mixture of alcohol and water (vodka) has the same congener level as beer. Aging distilled spirits does not decrease the level of congeners but, in fact, increases their level about threefold.

A personally conducted survey, as well as an experiment with a subject population of one, allows me to state that both the incidence and the severity of hangover increase as a function of age. One study[30] showed that the same amount of alcohol in young and old males resulted in a higher BAL in the older subjects because they had more fat at a given body weight. Still other factors contribute to the trials and tribulations of the "day after the night before." One of the actions of alcohol on the brain is to decrease the output of the antidiuretic hormone responsible for retaining fluid in the body. This action probably means that the body excretes more fluid than is taken in with the alcoholic beverages. However, this does not seem to be the only basis for the thirst experienced the next day. Another cause may be that alcohol causes fluid inside cells to move outside the cells. This cellular dehydration, without a decrease in total body fluid, is known to be related to, and perhaps to be the basis of, an increase in thirst.

The nausea and upset stomach typically experienced can most likely be attributed to the fact that alcohol is a gastric irritant. The consumption of even moderate amounts causes local irritation of the mucosa covering the stomach. It has been suggested that the accumulation of acetaldehyde, which is quite toxic even in small quantities, contributes to the nausea and headache. The headache may also be a reaction to fatigue. Fatigue some times results from a higher than normal level c activity while drinking. Increased activity frequently accompanies a decrease in inhibitions, a readily available source of energy, and a high blood sugar level. One of the effects of alcohol intake is to increase the blood sugar level for about an hour after ingestion. This may be followed several hours later by a low blood sugar level and an increased feeling of fatigue. Although hangover cures may be just around the corner, for now the only sure cure is time.

Suicide and homicide

The relationship between alcohol use and homicides is well known to police and the judicial system. One review of the world literature[31] did not deal with background factors but noted several studies which found that in at least 50% of the homicides the slayer, the victim, or both had measurable blood alcohol levels. Drinking *is* involved with homicide, but alcoholism is not. Most homicides occur between friends or acquaintances—family quarrels, neighborhood disputes—so the relationship to drinking is easy to understand.

Suicide and suicide attempts seem to have a different background, but most agree that alcohol is involved in about one third of all suicides. Alcoholism is second only to depression as the diagnosis in suicide attempters, and there are some who believe that all alcoholics are seriously depressed. A report on "Alcoholism, Alcohol Intoxication, and Suicide Attempts"[32] studied a group of suicide attempters, 75% of whom were drinking at the time of the attempt, and identified two types of alcohol-suicide situations. One type, the most common and most likely to succeed, involves the solitary, chronic heavy use of alcohol accompanied by increasing depression and withdrawal. The second type consists of individuals who become intoxicated quite rapidly in a situation involving interpersonal aggression and activity. It is probable that the superficial explanation has considerable validity in these two types: the use of alcohol increases the chronic drinker's feelings of being no-damn-good, and the disinhibiting effect of alcohol allows the aggressive drinker to turn his anger on himself.

Blackouts

Alcohol-induced blackouts are periods of time during alcohol use in which the individual appears to function normally but later, when the individual is sober, the events cannot be recalled. The drinker may drive home or dance all night interacting in the usual way with others. When the individual cannot remember the activities, the people, or anything—that's a blackout. Most authorities include it as one of the danger signs suggesting excessive use of alcohol. Amazingly, it has not been studied extensively. An 1884 article titled "Alcoholic Trance" refers to the syndrome:

> This trance state is a common condition in inebriety, where . . . a profound suspension of memory and consciousness and literal paralysis of certain brain-functions follow.
>
> This trance state may last from a few moments to several days, during which the person may appear and act rationally, and yet be actually a mere automaton, without consciousness or memory of his actual condition.[33]

Two of the examples used to show how sometimes we do strange things in an alcoholic trance were "a drinking man drank early in the morning, then killed his wife, and went about his work in the vicinity, as if nothing had happened, all unconscious until arrested" and "a college graduate enlisted in the army."

There is no accepted basis for blackouts, but it is unlikely that they only reflect short-term memory deficits, although protein synthesis is inhibited by high alcohol levels. Still unknown is whether experiences during the blackout are recorded in memory, but very inaccessible, or whether nothing is recorded.

Interactions with other drugs

Drug interactions are very "in" because of the increased information available about drugs and very important because everyone seems to be taking more drugs, increasing the number of interactions. Alcohol is a drug of particular concern because it is widely used and is not generally considered to be a drug. There is no way that any of the interactions can be discussed in detail, and only brief comment can be made on the types of drug interactions that occur with alcohol. Of particular concern is the summation of the CNS effects of alcohol with those of the sedatives and hypnotics, especially the barbiturates. Both are CNS depressants, and the combined action is at least additive, and sometimes synergistic.

A partial explanation of this potentiating effect may be that high levels of alcohol in the system, or existing liver damage from previous alcohol use, will depress the microsomal enzymes that metabolize drugs. This results in an increase in the duration and perhaps the peak effect of the drug. Continued use of alcohol generally, and most importantly, causes an increase in the activity of the microsomal enzymes. This usually results in more rapid metabolism and thus a decreased effect of drugs. Two other interactions are only now being explored: alcohol increases the absorption of some drugs, giving higher blood levels of the drug; in some cases alcohol will decrease the sensitivity of a receptor to other drugs, thereby making the drug less effective.

The complexity of the interactions should be apparent. Much work needs to be done, and the wide variety of the drugs that interact with alcohol can be seen in a number of reviews.[34] The moral of the story is make sure you tell your physician honestly about your alcohol-use habits before medication is prescribed.

CENTRAL NERVOUS SYSTEM EFFECTS

> The body of *information* concerning the action of ethanol in the brain is enormous; however, the body of *knowledge* is still disappointingly small.[35]

Alcohol is like any other general anesthetic: it depresses the central nervous system. It was used as an anesthetic until the late nineteenth century, when nitrous oxide, ether, and chloroform became more widely used. However, it was not just new compounds that decreased alcohol's use as an anesthetic; it has some major disadvantages. In contrast to the gaseous anesthetics, alcohol is almost completely metabolized in the body, and the rate of oxidation is slow. This gives alcohol a long duration of action that cannot be controlled. A second disadvantage is that the dose effective in surgical anesthesia is not much lower than the dose that causes respiratory arrest and death. Finally, alcohol slows the blood clotting time.

The exact mechanism for the CNS effect of alcohol is not clear, but the best evidence is that alcohol acts directly on neuronal membranes and not at the synapse.[36] It is known that alcohol acts on the neuron's capability to produce electrical impulses and thus process information properly. Furthermore, the effect of alcohol on the CNS is directly proportional to the level of alcohol in the blood.

At the lowest effective blood level, the reticular system begins to malfunction. This disruption results in the cerebral cortex not being regulated and losing its integrational and inhibitory ability even before the alcohol blood level reaches the point at which the cerebral cortex is directly affected. The general sequence of behaviors affected is the same with alcohol as with all depressant drugs. Complex, abstract, and poorly learned behaviors are disrupted at the lower alcohol levels, and, as the dose increases, better-learned and simpler behaviors are also affected. Certain inhibitions may be reduced with the result that performance improves in some areas. Even though there may be an increase in behavior, alcohol is not a stimulant. "The apparent stimulation results from the unrestrained activity of various parts of the brain that have been freed from inhibition as a result of the depression of inhibitory control mechanisms."[37,p.137] Not everyone agrees with this position. One researcher has shown, after alcohol intake, an increase in EEG activity that suggests an alerting and activation in some individuals. He proposes that this is the result of the catecholamine release known to be caused by alcohol. If these and other similar results obtain wide support in many laboratories, it may be that future discussions of alcohol will talk about both stimulant and depressant effects on the CNS, with the stimulant effects gradually being overridden by the more slowly developing and greater depression of activity.

Perhaps it speaks to the magnificent resiliency of the brain that it was not until the late 1970s that the data were obvious: alcohol use does cause changes in brain structures and morphology, as well as in its functioning. Microscopic work with animals support this but *most importantly:* use of new techniques for visualizing the brain from outside the skull show that *the use of alcohol is associated with enlargement of the empty spaces in the brain—that is, the ventricles and the space between folds in brain tissue.* Computer-assisted tomography (CAT or CT scans) have made it possible to show that this "enlargement of the brain ventricles and widening of the sulci"[12,p.14] is dose dependent, that is, related to the extent of drinking from nondrinkers through light and heavy social drinkers to alcoholics.

It is not clear if this is a result of the loss of neurons. In younger alcohol users there is a return toward normal when alcohol use stops. Something is happening and it isn't good. Along with these brain changes there are cognitive and behavioral changes but it's not possible to show a 1-to-1 relationship. Changes in brain morphology—that's one. Add to that a lower level of blood flow in the brain in alcoholics—that's two—and the problems that can arise from possibly lower levels of oxygen, nutrients, and waste removal are obvious. Number three is the finding that stimulus inputs to young alcoholics have the same effect on brain activity as is found in normal elderly persons.[38]

The fact that alcohol impairs functioning of the reticular system, which disrupts cortical functions, resulting in behavioral changes, makes it impossible to predict specific behavioral effects that follow alcohol intake. Which behaviors are suppressed and which will be released from inhibition depend on the individual's history. Some individuals, after taking a moderately depressant dose of alcohol, turn from passive, nonaggressive comrades into belligerent, hostile combatants. Others become convinced that they are Don Juans, Casanovas, or Lolitas.

If the alcohol intake is "just right," most people experience a "high," a happy feeling. Below a certain BAL there are no mood changes, but at some point we become uninhibited enough to enjoy our own charming selves and uncritical enough to accept the clods around us. This point seems to occur when the alcohol has disrupted social inhibitions and impaired good judgment but has not depressed most behavior. We become witty, clever, true continentals! Fortunately, most of those around us at this time also have impairment of judgment, so they can't say any differently!

Another factor contributing to the feeling of well-being is the reduction in anxieties as a result of the disruption of normal critical thinking. The reduction in concern and judgment may range from not worrying about who'll pay the bar bill (another round, garçon—and be quick about it!) to being sure that you can beat the train to the crossing (watch me scare that engineer!). A final effect of alcohol that may make the older person feel better is the anesthetizing of minor aches and pains.

No blood levels were suggested for the points at which an individual begins to feel good or happy or becomes amorous, or when sensory and motor functions are seriously impaired. BALs are reported as the number of grams of alcohol in each 100 ml of blood and are expressed as a percentage. Since 100 g in 100 ml would be 100%, 100 mg of alcohol in 100 ml of blood is reported as 0.1%.

Before suggesting blood alcohol level/behavioral change relationships, two factors must be mentioned. One is that the rate at which the blood alcohol rises is a factor in determining behavioral effects. The more rapid the increase, the greater the behavioral effects. Second, it is well to note that a classic study using a variety of simple visual, motor, and visual-motor tests showed disruption of performance at an average blood level of 0.05% in abstainers, 0.07% in moderate drinkers, and 0.1% in heavy drinkers.[39]

These results show clearly that behavioral and CNS tolerance to alcohol does develop. They also indicate that the better performance of the heavy drinker compared to the moderate drinker after equal amounts of alcohol is not caused solely (if at all) by the greater rate of alcohol metabolism in heavy drinkers. A higher BAL is necessary to impair the performance of a chronic heavy drinker than to impair a moderate drinker's performance!

A partial explanation might be that the heavy drinker is better motivated to conceal the alcohol-induced impairment and probably has had more practice. Performance differences may only reflect the extent to which the two groups have learned to overcome the disruption of nervous system functioning. There are both animal[40] and human[41] data to support this learning explanation. Another explanation may be that the CNS in the heavy drinker develops a tolerance to alcohol that does not exist in the moderate drinker. It is established that neu-

TABLE 8-10 Blood alcohol level and behavioral effects

Percent blood alcohol level	Behavioral effects
0.05	Lowered alertness, usually good feeling, release of inhibitions, impaired judgment
0.10	Slowed reaction times and impaired motor function, less caution
0.15	Large, consistent increases in reaction time
0.20	Marked depression in sensory and motor capability, decidedly intoxicated
0.25	Severe motor disturbance, staggering, sensory perceptions greatly impaired, smashed!
0.30	Stuporous but conscious—no comprehension of the world around them
0.35	Surgical anesthesia; about LD 1, minimal level causing death
0.40	About LD 50

ral tissue becomes tolerant to alcohol, and tolerance can apparently develop even when the alcohol intake is well spaced in time.

Any dose-response curve contains considerable variability, and Table 8-10 reports some general behavior. These relationships are approximately correct for moderate drinkers. There are some reports that changes in nervous system function have been obtained at blood levels as low as 0.03% to 0.04%.

There is reason to believe that performance impairment in the 0.1% BAL range is the result of a decrement in decision-making capability. The evidence suggests that these BALs do not impair perception of the situation or the capability of responding. In these experiments "one important source of impairment with moderate alcoholic intoxication is a difficulty in selecting and organizing the correct response."[42] The integration of information and behavior seems to be the critical factor. It should be noted, however, that some changes in stimulus processing may occur even at low dose levels. One study presented a mild shock stimulus to the skin. The response elicited in the brain showed an increase in variability and a decrease in magnitude after alcohol ingestion.[43]

The vomiting reflex may be activated by alcohol at a blood level of about 0.12% or even lower, but only if that level is approached rapidly. With slow, steady drinking the 0.12% level is reached gradually, and the vomiting center is depressed. The individual can then continue drinking up to lethal levels if he remains conscious!

The surgical anesthesia level and the minimum lethal level are perhaps the two least precise points in the table. In any case they are quite close, and the safety margin is less than 0.1% blood alcohol. Death resulting from acute alcohol intoxication usually is the result of respiratory failure when the medulla is depressed. With respect to this last point, caffeine is an effective respiratory stimulant in cases of alcohol depression of respiration. There is mixed evidence regarding any antagonistic actions on the behavioral effects that occur at lower BALs. There is no basis for believing that making an intoxicated person move around will help reduce BALs. The standard "on your feet, keep walking, drink this black coffee" does not accelerate the sobering-up process.

The blood alcohol level and behavior relationship is similarly but more enjoyably described in the following, which is modified from Bogen.[44]

At less than 0.03%, the individual is dull and dignified.
At 0.05%, he is dashing and debonair.
At 0.1%, he may become dangerous and devilish.
At 0.2%, he is likely to be dizzy and disturbing.
At 0.25%, he may be disgusting and disheveled.
At 0.3%, he is delirious and disoriented and surely drunk.
At 0.35%, he is dead drunk.
At 0.6%, the chances are that he is dead.

The relationship between BAL and alcohol intake, the oral consumption of an alcoholic beverage, is not simple but is reasonably well understood. Remember, alcohol is not appreciably excreted from, or stored anywhere in, the body prior to metabolism. When taken into the body, alcohol is distributed throughout the body fluids, including the blood. The heavier the person, the more body fluid and the lower the concentration of blood alcohol. Sex is also important, since women have less fluid than men of the same weight because women have more fat. With less fluid the concentration of alcohol will be higher. In individuals of either sex with the same body weight, as the amount of fat increases there is a corresponding decrease in body fluid and thus a higher concentration of alcohol. It cannot be emphasized too often that CNS effects of alcohol are related directly to the blood alcohol concentration.

It is important to appreciate that the relationships and numbers presented here are only typical and cannot be applied directly to a specific individual. Additional points to remember are that distilled spirits are absorbed more rapidly than wine, which is absorbed more rapidly than beer, and that, although eating while drinking will slow the absorption of alcohol and reduce peak blood concentrations, the absorption will continue for a longer period of time.

The relationships among alcohol intake, blood alcohol level, sex, and weight are indicated in Table 8-11. In the 150-pound person, the *average* rate of metabolism of alcohol is about 0.3 ounce per hour of absolute alcohol; this lowers the BAL *approximately* 0.01% per hour. Thus, if a 150-pound man has six drinks over a 4-hour period, his BAL would roughly be 0.11%. Fig. 8-1 is included to give you a better feel for the absorption and metabolism time curve following alcohol intake. Sixty milliliters of 95% ethanol is the same as 2 ounces of absolute alcohol.[45] (See Table 8-10.) Although not completely studied, the rate of metabolism possibly depends on the size of the liver and thus the size of the body. As a result, the rate of alcohol metabolism may be higher in the heavier person than in the lower-weight individual, but this has not yet been shown.

One rule of thumb is often used to approximate how much an individual can (should) drink. It concerns itself with the amount of the alcohol beverage a person can metabolize in an hour and is determined by dividing body weight in pounds by five

TABLE 8-11 Relationships among sex, weight, oral alcohol consumption, and blood alcohol level

Absolute alcohol (ounces)	Beverage intake*	Blood alcohol levels (mg/100 ml)					
		Female (100 lb)	Male (100 lb)	Female (150 lb)	Male (150 lb)	Female (200 lb)	Male (200 lb)
½	1 oz spirits† 1 glass wine 1 can beer	0.045	0.037	0.03	0.025	0.022	0.019
1	2 oz spirits 2 glasses wine 2 cans beer	0.090	0.075	0.06	0.050	0.045	0.037
2	4 oz spirits 4 glasses wine 4 cans beer	0.180	0.150	0.12	0.100	0.090	0.070
3	6 oz spirits 6 glasses wine 6 cans beer	0.270	0.220	0.18	0.150	0.130	0.110
4	8 oz spirits 8 glasses wine 8 cans beer	0.360	0.300	0.24	0.200	0.180	0.150
5	10 oz spirits 10 glasses wine 10 cans beer	0.450	0.370	0.30	0.250	0.220	0.180

*In 1 hour.
†100-proof spirits.

times the percentage of alcohol in the beverage. For the hypothetical 150-pound person, that yields about 7.5 ounces of beer.

BAL gives a good estimate of the alcohol concentration acting on the brain, and the concentration of alcohol in the breath gives a good estimate of the alcohol concentration in the blood. There is a ratio of 1:2100 between the concentration of alcohol in breath (1) and the concentration in blood (2100). These relationships between breath level–blood level–central nervous system effects–behavioral effects are put to practical use by police. By determining alcohol level in the breath, statements can be made about BALs, which form the basis in most states for conviction as a drunken driver.[46]

Everyone should appreciate that some individuals are quite sensitive to alcohol, and their performance is impaired at very low BALs. Don't depend on the average; learn your own limit and stick to it. (See Chapter 4 for a discussion of alcohol use and driving.)

METABOLISM

What is the size of a pumpernickel, has the shape of Diana's helmet, and crouches like a thundercloud above its bellymates, turgid with nourishment? What has the industry of an insect, the regenerative powers of a starfish . . .? It is . . . the liver, doted upon by the French, as-

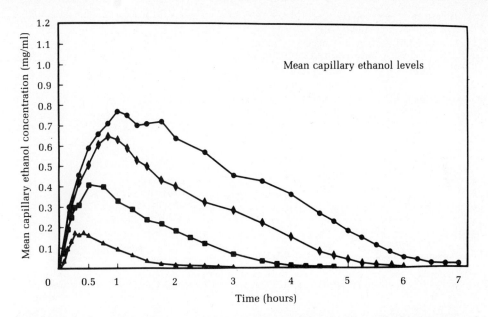

FIG. 8-1 Mean capillary blood ethanol concentrations following the oral administration of four different doses of ethanol to eight male subjects: ▲ 15 ml, ■ 30 ml, ♦ 45 ml, and ● 60 ml 95% ethanol diluted to 150 ml with orange juice. (From Wilkinson, P.K.: Pharmacokinetics of ethanol: a review, Alcoholism: Clinical and Experimental Research 4(1):6-21, 1980. Copyright 1980, American Medical Society on Alcoholism.)

saulted by the Irish, disdained by the Americans, and chopped up with egg, onion, and chicken fat by the Jews.[47]

Yes, the liver is all that and more and it still remains one of the unsung heroes of our innards. Our interest in the liver here is that it contains two enzyme systems (one just identified in 1972) that are responsible for the metabolism of alcohol. Alcohol has two unique characteristics as a calorie container. It requires no digestion and is absorbed unchanged into the bloodstream. Second, it can be neither stored nor bound, nor can its calories be converted into lipids or protein and stored. Once absorbed, alcohol remains in the bloodstream and body fluids until it is metabolized, and over 90% of this occurs in the liver. Very little alcohol is normally excreted unchanged, perhaps 2%, but with a very high alcohol intake, the kidneys, lungs, and skin may eliminate 10% to 15%.

The better-known metabolic system is diagrammed in Fig. 8-2 and involves a simple process

that finally results in energy, carbon dioxide, and water. The critical enzyme here is *alcohol dehydrogenase*, which converts alcohol to *acetaldehyde*. *It is mostly this step, alcohol to acetaldehyde, that limits the rate of disappearance of alcohol from the body.* The rate of oxidation of alcohol is not influenced by its level in the blood. The determining factor is the activity of the enzyme, alcohol dehydrogenase, which is determined by the rate of oxidation of NADH, another enzyme. In moderate drinkers the maximum amount of alcohol that can be metabolized is between 0.25 and 0.33 ounce per hour. If intake is faster than oxidation, blood alcohol concentration increases.

Recent work[48,49] has suggested that acetaldehyde may be more than *just* an intermediate step in the oxidation of alcohol. Acetaldehyde is quite toxic and, even though blood levels are only one one-thousandth of those of alcohol, may in fact be the cause of some of the physiological effects now attributed to alcohol. Although more work needs to

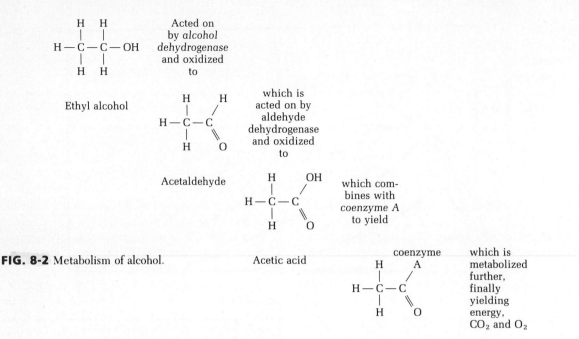

FIG. 8-2 Metabolism of alcohol.

be done in this area, it is an intriguing finding that acetaldehyde blood levels are higher in alcoholic patients than in nonalcoholic.[50] The danger in heavy alcohol use may be in the higher blood levels of acetaldehyde. There may be other indices of alcohol in the blood.[51,52]

The second enzyme system is much more complicated and, at this time, has many more known ramifications. The liver responds to chronic intake of alcohol by increasing production of a certain type of membrane: endoplasmic reticulum. This increase in endoplasmic reticulum is associated with increased levels of the *microsomal drug metabolizing enzymes* (Chapter 7). This gives rise to some interesting situations. In the long-term, heavy-alcohol-intake person there is an increase in the activity of the microsomal enzymes. As long as there is alcohol in the system, alcohol gets preferential treatment and the metabolism of other drugs is slower than normal.[53,55] When heavy alcohol use stops and the alcohol has disappeared from the body, the high activity level of the enzymes continues for 4 to 8 weeks. During this time drugs are metabolized *more* rapidly.[56] To obtain therapeutic levels of the drugs metabolized by this enzyme

system (for example, the benzodiazepines) it is necessary to administer *less* drug to the drinking alcoholic and more drug to the just-nondrinking alcoholic.

One of the enzymes that increases is the *microsomal ethanol oxidizing system*, MEOS. Thus, alcohol increases the activity of one of the two enzyme systems responsible for its own oxidation. The increased activity of this MEOS pathway may be a partial basis for the tolerance to alcohol that is shown by heavy users of alcohol.

Another reason why it is important to know about the MEOS is that it is part of the indirect cause of the *fatty liver* that develops in alcohol consumers. For most of us this is not a serious problem. Fatty acids are the usual fuel for the liver. When alcohol is present, it has higher priority and is used as fuel. As a result, fatty acids (lipids) accumulate in the liver and are stored as small droplets in liver cells. Sometimes the droplets increase in size to the point where they rupture the cell membrane (and pour lipids into the bloodstream, which may have serious effects on the cardiovascular system), causing death of the liver cells. Up to the point where the liver cells die, a fatty liver is completely reversible and usually of minor medical concern. If alcohol input ceases, the liver uses the stored fatty acids for energy.

Sometimes, with prolonged and/or high-level alcohol intake, another phase of liver damage is observed. This is alcoholic hepatitis, which is a serious disease and includes both inflammation and impairment of liver function. Usually this occurs in areas where there are dead and dying liver cells, but it is not known if an increasingly fatty liver leads to alcoholic hepatitis. It is known that you can have alcoholic hepatitis in the absence of a fatty liver.

Cirrhosis is the liver disease everyone knows is related to high and prolonged levels of alcohol consumption. It's not easy to get cirrhosis from drinking alcohol—you have to work at it. Usually it takes about 10 years of steady drinking of the equivalent of a pint or more of whiskey a day. Not all cirrhosis is alcohol related, but a high percentage is, and cirrhosis is the seventh leading cause of death in the United States. In large urban areas it is the fourth or fifth leading cause of death in men ages 25 to 65. In cirrhosis, liver cells are replaced by fibrous tissue, which changes the structure of the liver. These changes decrease blood flow and, along with the loss of cells, result in a decreased ability of the liver to function. When the liver does not function properly, fluid accumulates in the body, jaundice develops, and cancer may develop in the liver. The yellow color of the jaundiced individual is the result of bile pigment distributed through the body, but, most importantly, it is a sign that the liver is not functioning properly, and toxins are beginning to accumulate in the blood. Cirrhosis is not reversible, but stopping the intake of alcohol will retard its development and decrease the serious medical effects. The liver has a large reserve capacity and is able to function adequately with mild cirrhosis. One of the important, unanswered questions is why not all alcoholics develop cirrhosis.

This is a good place to clear up some possible confusion over the role of diet, vitamin deficiency, alcohol intake, and impairment of liver function. For many years it was believed that the negative effects of alcohol consumption on the liver were secondary to vitamin deficiency. The reasoning was that a high alcohol intake meant that the individual received a substantial number of calories (about 200 per ounce) without any accompanying vitamins or proteins. Since some people would take in over half their daily calories through alcohol, they usually ate poor diets—and had vitamin deficiencies. It was thought that protein and perhaps vitamin deficiency caused the liver damage. There was support for this from animal research: animals fed diets severely deficient in vitamins and proteins developed liver disease in the absence of alcohol. The other side of the coin also matched: animals fed alcohol *and* adequate diets did not develop liver disease.

That position was altered considerably, if not reversed, with the use of new behavioral techniques and the finding that baboons[57] would develop liver disease—fatty liver, alcoholic hepatitis, and cirrhosis—if the alcohol intake was high enough, even though they had adequate diets. Both dietary deficiencies and alcohol consumption probably interact in most cases to cause human liver disease.[58] It seems now that severe protein and vitamin deficiencies by themselves are not enough to damage the liver.

It should have been noticed a few paragraphs back that alcohol use per se cannot make you fat, no matter how much you drink! Be careful, though. Since it is the nonstorable calories in alcohol which meet the energy requirements of the body, it is the food you eat in addition to the alcohol that may cause a weight gain—even a beer belly! These other foods can be, and are, converted to fat and stored if their energy is not needed for ongoing body needs. As should be evident by now, alcohol and its calories are not enough; it is only through a good diet that you can obtain protein, vitamins, and other dietary components essential for health and life.

Finally, in 1976, a national organization was formed to herald the liver so it can take its rightful place below the heart and lung associations. You have to admit, it is difficult not to have a fondness for our very own personal antipollution device with all its microsomal enzymes. It may be a bit much but—take care of your liver and it will take care of you!

PHYSIOLOGICAL EFFECTS

When alcohol intake occurs regularly and in large quantities over a period of years, physical dependence on the drug occurs. Abrupt withdrawal from alcohol results in dangerous changes in body physiology. Before the addiction to alcohol reaches this point, physical symptoms sometimes develop, with facial appearance the first to be affected. The capillaries around the conjunctiva of the eyes become enlarged, and the skin of the face, forehead, and under the eyes becomes puffy and filled with fluid.

In an individual with a fair complexion, the skin may appear continually flushed and, after prolonged use, a "whiskey nose" may develop. The frequent hoarseness of the alcoholic results from the accumulation of fluid in the mucous membranes of the nose, pharynx, larynx, and vocal cords. Continual ingestion of alcohol leads to an inflamed stomach associated with nausea and loss of appetite.

The relationship of alcohol use to many diseases has been studied extensively and still continues.[59,60] An excellent summary appeared in 1981 of the "Health Hazards Associated with Alcohol Consumption"[61] and cross-cultural data provide an interesting perspective.[62] One long-term study of white middle-aged males (40 years and over) with good jobs showed that there was an increased mortality from all causes only ". . . at the level of six or more drinks per day."[63,p.78] Keeping all of this in mind, the following are quotes from the NIAAA's 1981 report to Congress.[12] If nothing else, comparing the size of the two lists should tell you something.

Bad news

The actual mortality rate of alcoholics is 2.5 times greater than expected . . . (p.10)

Many investigators have seen association between chronic substantial alcohol use and heart muscle failure . . . (p.11)

. . . regular use of large amounts of alcohol is as-

sociated with a substantially higher prevalence of hypertension . . . (p.12)

A positive correlation between drinking and stroke incidence has been reported . . . (p.13)

. . . testosterone clearance is enhanced in chronic alcoholic humans . . . (p.13)

. . . alcohol administration also depresses testosterone synthesis in the testes. (p.14)

Neuropsychological tests show cognitive and perceptual deficits in alcoholics similar to those in patients with brain damage unrelated to alcohol. (p.14)

The Wernicke-Korsakoff syndrome represents an extreme on the continuum of cognitive impairment resulting from alcohol-induced brain damage. (p.15)

. . . heavy alcohol consumption has been related to an increased risk of cancer at various sites in the human body, particularly the mouth, pharynx, and larynx. (p.16)

Alcohol and tobacco appear to act synergistically in the pathogenesis of cancer in the upper digestive tract. (p.16)

Good news

. . . recent studies have reported an inverse relationship between alcohol use and heart attacks (myocardial infarctions), the largest difference in coronary risk was between current nondrinkers (including past drinkers) and light to moderate drinkers (two or fewer drinks per day) . . . (p.12)

Alcohol raises high-density lipoprotein-cholesterol (HDL-C) levels in blood . . . elevated HDL-C is inversely related to coronary atherosclerotic disease . . . (p.13)

After all is said and done, there is no evidence that moderate alcohol use—one to three drinks a day—has overall negative effects on your physical health. If you are or might be pregnant, then you should drink rarely, if at all. (See Chapter 4.) If you start combining moderate alcohol use with other drug use it may mean problems. If you engage in moderate alcohol use before operating heavy machinery—like an automobile—the combination may kill you. As with any other form of drug use: (1) There is lots we don't know; (2) You may be a particularly sensitive person and not fit into the above generalizations and averages; and (3) Think before you use the drug.

ALCOHOLISM: DIAGNOSIS AND TREATMENT

Defining *alcoholism* gets harder each year, since it has different meanings to different authorities, and there seem to be more and more authorities. Another problem is that the definition of both alcoholism and an alcoholic has been changing. In this last quarter of the twentieth century an acceptable definition of an *alcoholic* is *an individual who uses alcohol to such an extent, and in such a way, that it interferes with his personal, social, or occupational behavior*. This is obviously a psychosocial definition, since it does not talk of blood alcohol levels, medical problems, or quantities of alcohol consumed. It does not say the alcoholic is suffering from an illness. It just says that when alcohol mucks up a person's life in any way, let's call him an alcoholic and see if the problem can't at least be reduced.

There are other definitions that emphasize the medical and physiological signs and symptoms of alcoholism. The National Council on Alcoholism has taken this approach and tentatively identified ten physiological or medical signs and two behavioral signs that are clearly related to alcoholism and critical to the diagnosis of alcohlism.[64] Most of their signs and symptoms appear in different sections of this chapter.

Alcoholism is partially a sociological condition, and there are interesting cross-cultural differences. A recent study compared male French and American alcoholics.[65] Compared to the French, the Americans (1) engaged in more periodic drinking—large amounts consumed at one time and then no alcohol for a while; (2) had more symptoms and signs of alcoholism—drinking in the morning and before going to a party, blackouts, etc; and (3) showed more loss of control—trouble with the law, unable to stop after the first, etc. The Americans exhibited the "Anglo-Saxon" variety of alcoholism with its high use of distilled spirits and spree drinking, with the usual effects after the party. The

French alcoholics mostly drank wine and drank more consistently day in and day out. Even with these two very different drinking patterns, the average daily pure alcohol intake was nearly the same for these alcoholics: the Americans, 8.5 ounces, and the French, 9.2 ounces.

Cultural factors are potent. Comparison of American male and female alcoholics showed only one major difference: females have more guilt and shame over their drinking.[66] This is not too surprising, since alcoholism has not been as common or as acceptable for women as it is for men. That is changing, and the differences will probably soon disappear. Today one out of three alcoholics is a woman, up sharply from the one in six estimate in the mid-1960s.

It should be remembered that this country has come a long way in this century in our attitudes toward alcoholism and the alcoholic. A nice article[67] analyzed the image of the alcoholic in popular opinion, and the analysis shows two important changes. We have become much less moralistic about the alcoholic—we are less likely to blame him for his alcoholism today than in 1900. The second change came in the 1940s, when attitudes shifted from the previous sociological explanation that it was factors outside the individual that made him an alcoholic (it's those saloons—let's close them all down!) to a more inner, psychological explanation. Fortunately the pendulum reversed itself again so that we now appreciate the many factors, both internal and external, that contribute to making a person an alcoholic.

As attitudes change, so also do laws. When you believe that it is a moral defect that makes a person an alcoholic or that "it's his own fault," then you blame him, treat him as a criminal, and arrest him for public drunkenness. After all, "if he wanted to stop drinking, he could. It's his choice; if he doesn't want to obey the laws, he should go to jail!" And so it was. As the police used to say, "Half of the crimes committed involve alcohol." True, as long as you defined public intoxication as a crime. Things are changing.

In 1971 the Commission on Uniform State Laws suggested a law for each state to enact that decriminalized public drunkenness. Section One of that proposed legislation said:

> It is the policy of this State that alcoholics and intoxicated persons may not be subjected to criminal prosecution because of their consumption of alcoholic beverages but rather should be afforded a continuum of treatment in order that they may lead normal lives as productive members of society.[68]

Those treatment programs are needed. There are between 8 and 12 million alcoholics in the United States. You can never be sure who should be counted, but they come in all shapes, sizes, sexes, and colors. They are much like the rest of us. The only thing that is definitely different about an alcoholic is that he drinks too much. The skid-row bum with a week's growth of beard, dirty clothes, bloodshot eyes, and trembling hands is the stereotype of the alcoholic. Nothing could be more wrong—this group probably makes up less than 5% of those who would today be called alcoholics. Probably equally unique is the alcoholic who never caused anyone any trouble except himself. One of the best examples is the TV and movie actor, Dick Van Dyke. These comments are taken from a longer interview,[69] but the important thing is that Van Dyke is an alcoholic because he decided he was an alcoholic.

> *Van Dyke:* I didn't miss work ever because of drinking. And I never drank at work. Never drank during the day—only at home and only in the evenings. . . .
>
> I never craved a drink during the day. I was never a morning drinker—I didn't want one then. The idea made me as sick as it would make anyone else. But evening drinking is a form of alcoholism, just like periodic drinking is a form of alcoholism.
>
> *Question:* Did your drinking problem have a big effect on your home life?
>
> *Van Dyke:* It was a funny thing. My 19-year-old daughter was on the Tom Snyder "Tomorrow Show". . . . Tom asked my daughter about my drinking—my alcoholism—"How did that affect you?" She said, "I never knew it. My father was

so quiet about it, never made any noise. As a matter of fact, some of the best talks we ever had were when my father was drinking." Which is a very strange reaction. When I asked her afterwards, she said, "I never knew a thing about it."

> *Question:* For 5 years you had a drinking problem without really admitting it to yourself. What finally happened to make you realize that you were an alcoholic?
>
> *Van Dyke:* I don't know. . . . I said to myself, "What am I doing?" My wife had long gone to bed. I was sitting alone, drinking, lost in what I took to be deep thought. I realized suddenly, "Why, I am thinking gibberish here—my mind is completely out of it." When I woke up the next morning, I got up and went to a hospital. Went straight into a treatment center.

Near the other end of the alcoholic spectrum and a much more frequent type is the unemployed man described below. Although admitting to being a spree drinker, he repeatedly refused treatment.

> This 45-year-old white male had 8 years of education and 2 years in the army. He started drinking at 18 and, although he was court martialed three times and spent 6 months in the stockade for alcohol-related offenses, he says his drinking has been a problem only for the last 10 years.
>
> His drinking sprees now last 3 to 4 weeks and occur about six times a year. During these sprees he reports consuming at least a quart of whiskey, a gallon of wine, and 1 to 3 six-packs of beer every day. He has had blackouts, extreme shakes, and hallucinations on a "few" occasions. He has had more arrests for public drunkenness than he can remember.
>
> On his first admission to the hospital 5 years ago he said he only drank a few beers a day, but his wife brought him to the hospital because he was talking to the TV, hearing strange music, and seeing bugs and snakes. On his next admission 2 years later, he said he was ready for treatment but managed to miss all of his scheduled appointments. When confronted, he dressed and left the hospital.

There are three phases to a program for an individual who has been drinking heavily. The first phase is *detoxification*. This is aimed at withdrawing the individual from his addiction to alcohol. Phase two is the formal *treatment* program itself: the focus here is on helping the individual find ways and reasons to reduce or stop completely his destructive drinking. The last part of the program is called *aftercare*, or maintenance therapy, and usually involves less frequent, and sometimes, a less structured treatment relationship between the individual and the therapists.

Detoxification

The physical dependence associated with prolonged heavy use of alcohol is best seen when alcohol intake is stopped. *The abstinence syndrome that develops is medically more severe and more likely to cause death than withdrawal from narcotic drugs.* In untreated advanced cases, mortality may be as high as one in seven. Withdrawal symptoms do not appear until the BALs drop below the intoxication level, and these withdrawal symptoms alone may be enough to keep the drinker drinking.

One physician[70] has described the progression of withdrawal, the abstinence syndrome, in the following way:

Stage 1: Tremors, excessively rapid heartbeat, hypertension, heavy sweating, loss of appetite, and insomnia.

Stage 2: Hallucinations—auditory, visual, tactile, or a combination of these; and, rarely, olfactory signs.

Stage 3: Delusions, disorientation, delirium, sometimes intermittent in nature and usually followed by amnesia.

Stage 4: Seizure activity.

The belief was expressed that the term *delirium tremens* should be used only when the syndrome progresses through all four stages. In fact, medical treatment is usually sought in either stage 1 or 2, and rapid intervention will prevent stage 3 or 4 from occurring.

Tremors are one of the most common physical changes associated with alcohol withdrawal and may persist for a long period after alcohol intake has stopped. The classic drunk, bending over to sip from his cup, attests to the frequency of tremors. Anxiety, insomnia, feelings of unreality, nausea, vomiting, and many other symptoms are also common.

The withdrawal symptoms do not develop all at the same time or immediately after abstinence begins. The initial signs may develop within a few hours (tremors, anxiety), but the individual is relatively rational. Over the next day or two, hallucinations appear and gradually become more terrifying and real to the individual. Huckleberry Finn has described these quite vividly in his pap.[71]

Pap took the jug, and said he had enough whisky there for two drunks and one delirium tremens. . . . He drank and drank. . . .

I don't know how long I was asleep, but . . . there was an awful scream and I was up. There was a pap looking wild, and skipping around every which way and yelling about snakes. He said they was crawling up on his legs; and then he would give a jump and scream, and say one had bit him on the cheek—but I couldn't see no snakes. He started and run round . . . hollering "Take him off! he's biting me on the neck!" I never see a man look so wild in the eyes. Pretty soon he was all fagged out, and fell down panting; then he rolled over . . . kicking things every which way, and striking and grabbing at the air with his hands, and screaming . . . there was devils a-hold of him. He wore out by and by. . . . He says . . .

"Tramp-tramp-tramp; that's the dead; tramp-tramp-tramp; they're coming after me; but I won't go. Oh, they're here; don't touch me—don't! hands off—they're cold; let go . . . ."

Then he went down on all fours and crawled off, begging them to let him alone . . .

By and by he . . . jumped up on his feet looking wild . . . and went for me. He chased me round and round the place with a claspknife, calling me the Angel of Death, and saying he would kill me, and then I wouldn't come for him no more. . . . Pretty soon he was all tired out . . . and said he would rest for a minute and then kill me. . . .

• • •

"Git it up! . . ."

I opened my eyes and look around. . . . Pap was

standing over me looking sour—and sick, too. He says:

"What you doin'. . . ?"

I judged he didn't know nothing about what he had been doing. . . .

In one double-blind, multiple hospital study, 7% of the patients given placebos suffered convulsions during withdrawal, while 6% showed delirium tremens.[72] In another study convulsions were reported in 12% of the patients, delirium tremens in 5%, and hallucinations in 18%.[73]

The symptoms that do develop seem to result from the fact that the cells of the body, and particularly the CNS, have been functioning reasonably normally in spite of the depressant action of alcohol. When the alcohol is reduced, the cells become hyperactive. Released from the depression induced by the drug, the cells overreact and become hyperexcitable.

Optimal treatment of the patients seems to be the administration of antianxiety agents such as chlordiazepoxide or diazepam (Chapter 13), although not everyone agrees.[74] In comparing the effectiveness of several compounds in blocking withdrawal symptoms, chlordiazepoxide reduced the incidence of convulsions and delirium tremens to less than 1%.[72] This probably is a result of a high degree of cross-tolerance (cross-dependence) between alcohol and chlordiazepoxide, so one drug can be substituted for the other and withdrawal continued at a safer rate. The use of drugs to decrease alcohol withdrawal signs is clearly only symptomatic treatment. To keep the alcoholic from resuming drinking is a difficult task and will be discussed briefly.

Treatment

There is much discussion among staff members involved in alcohol treatment programs over the ability of a recovered (that is, nondrinking) alcoholic to engage in "controlled drinking." Controlled drinking has several very different, and very specific, definitions, but they all refer to the ability of an alcoholic to control his drinking: to use alcohol normally under some conditions without using it to excess. Much fuel was added to this fire by a NIAAA-sponsored study completed by the Rand Corporation in 1976 on treatment effectiveness in eight large treatment centers.[75] They summarized the alcoholics who went into these treatment programs, as well as the 18-month results:

They drink nine times more alcohol than the average person, and they experience adverse behavioral consequences at a rate nearly twelve times that for nonalcoholic persons. They are also socially impaired, with more than half unemployed and more than half separated or divorced. These alcoholics also tend to be engaged in more blue collar occupations and to have lower income and less education than the average person. . . .

The rate of improvement is on the order of 70 percent for several different outcome indicators. . . .

It is important to stress that the improved clients include only a relatively small number who are long-term abstainers. . . . The majority of improved clients are either drinking moderate amounts of alcohol—but at levels far below what could be described as alcoholic drinking—or engaging in alternating periods of drinking and abstention.[75,p.V]

Four years later[76] 46% were in remission (down from 70%)—28% were abstaining and 18% were drinking socially. Only 28% were free of alcoholism at both the 18- and the 48-month follow-up. More importantly the 4-year data suggested that the only hope of avoiding problems for males over 40 with severe alcohol dependency was complete abstinence. That last statement was satisfying for the people at Alcoholics Anonymous (AA). They had strongly objected to the early report's suggestion that controlled drinking might be a possible way of life for recovered alcoholics.

The AA position has always been clear: they support only total abstinence as a life-style for recovered alcoholics. Their statement, "For an alcoholic, one drink is too many and a thousand not enough," summarizes that belief. They even go one step further and believe that any alcoholic who is able to return to moderate (controlled) drinking was not really an alcoholic to begin with!

Most other treatment programs believe that some alcoholics must always abstain, whereas others can return to moderate alcohol consumption. Many treatment programs put a great emphasis on abstinence, although their results suggest that most people who complete a treatment program do not abstain but do have less destructive drinking patterns.

A 1975 review of "384 studies of psychologically oriented alcoholism treatment showed that differences in treatment methods did not significantly affect long term outcome."[77] The evidence from other sources, such as the Rand study, is also overwhelming: the specific type of treatment used does not change the likelihood of successful treatment, successful treatment being either a reduction in problem drinking or abstinence.

The 1975 review also found that:

> Mean abstinence rates did not differ between treated and untreated alcoholics, but more treated than nontreated alcoholics improved, suggesting that formal treatment at least increases an alcoholic's chances of reducing his drinking problem.[77]

This is an important conclusion. Participation in a formal treatment program resulted in 25% of the members being abstinent 6 months after treatment, compared to 16% of those individuals who were not in a formal program. The difference is not statistically significant but is in the hoped-for direction. Total improvement—abstinence or a reduction in destructive drinking—was found in 65% of the formal treatment participants and in only 42% of those not in a formal program. This is not only significant but meaningful: the efforts put forth in alcohol treatment programs all over this country are helping an additional 23 out of every 100 alcoholics reduce the amount of their problem drinking. Regardless of whether programs want to be, they are controlled drinking programs. No one has yet done a study in which alcoholics are randomly assigned to treatment and no-treatment conditions. It may be, and probably is, that alcoholics who select treatment are more motivated and have better social support systems.

Because it is the oldest, the largest, the best-known, and probably one of the best treatment programs for alcoholism, special note must be made of AA. It was started in Akron, Ohio, in 1935 by two alcoholics, a stockbroker and a surgeon, and has grown to a worldwide organization of over 22,000 local groups and 1 million members. There are 500,000 members in the United States—one third are women.

> Its approach is concerned with the physical, psychological, and spiritual well-being of the individual. Total abstinence is stressed, with each day lived in itself—24 hours of sobriety. AA has a buddy system. If a person feels he's going to go out and drink, he can call up a buddy who will come right to him and help him. It's a sort of ego support. AA provides camaraderie in a group setting.[78]

One obvious question arises: If there are no significant differences among the various treatment approaches, are there any ways of predicting treatment outcome? Probably. Most individuals working in this area would agree "that a vital part of any treatment program is the opportunity offered the alcoholic person to develop trust in someone.[59]

More specific factors are cited in an article titled "Prognostic Factors in the Evaluation of Addicted Individuals,"[79] which contains succinct comments on predicting successful treatment outcome, that is, either a reduction in problem drinking or abstinence. The five variables that are related to successful completion of treatment programs are well supported by much literature and apply equally to programs for other addictions.

1. *Age*. As age increases so does the probability of success.

2. *Drinking style*. Periodic drinkers will have fewer relapses than daily drinkers.

3. *Social stability*. The support of a wife, family, job, etc. increases the likelihood of a permanent reduction in problem drinking.

4. *Diagnostic category*. Obsessive-compulsive types (conscientious, overcontrolling) and neurotics generally do better than individuals with sociopathic or psychotic disorders.

5. *Motivation*. This is the key factor, and the hardest to evaluate, since if the person doesn't want to stop drinking, he won't. Of course, many say

they *do* want to stop, but are unwilling (unable?) to do what is necessary.

Alcoholics are like the rest of us: we all want a better life, better jobs, better grades—until we learn what we have to do to achieve them. Then many of us back off. Treatment programs provide a social support setting and a social motivation to do what we want to do, but have difficulty without help.

One recent, large scale, good study was quite pessimistic about the role of alcoholic treatment programs in dealing with the problem of alcoholism—maybe it was just realistic:

> If we consider the large number of alcoholics in this country, the relatively small fraction of them who come for treatment, and the small fraction of those who come for treatment who benefit from it, it is clear that no extension of current treatment methods can possibly catch up with the alcoholism problem.[80,p.521]

In attempting to locate factors that would be predictive of a positive outcome from treatment, the authors state, "Having a paying job at admission was the only one of the many social variables examined which was significant enough for inclusion in the predictor model."[80,p.520] That's particularly interesting because of the next section.

Occupational alcoholism programs. A new trend that has developed since the late 1960s may solve some of the problems found in most treatment programs: motivation of the individual and maintenance of the family and work support systems.[81,82] It has been estimated that 6%[83] of the work force in this country engages in destructive drinking, and losses to productivity in illness, accidents, and personal problems amount to billions of dollars each year. With the encouragement of the federal government, many large corporations have organized treatment programs for their alcoholic and potentially alcoholic employees. As of 1980 there were 4400 occupational alcoholism programs. The federal government has done the same thing for civilian employees. In March, 1972, the Pentagon announced that treatment programs would be available for members of the military. Most of the programs—military, government, and industry—

are based on the same principles as those listed here[84]:

1. The company makes it plain that it considers alcoholism a disease and will treat alcoholics just as it does employes with any other illness.
2. Supervisors are told to report poor job performance, often the first indicator of alcoholism, to trained counselors in medical or personnel units.
3. If the problem is diagnosed as alcoholism, the employe is given the choice of entering a treatment program or losing his job for poor performance.
4. A worker who enters treatment gets sick leave and medical benefits.
5. Medical records on alcoholism are kept confidential.

The programs seem to be no more effective than voluntary programs outside the vocational setting. But they are a boon for industry: a program in the Oldsmobile Division of General Motors found that among the participants there was an 82% drop in job-related accidents, a 56% drop in leaves of absence, and a 30% decrease in sickness and accident benefits paid. GM expects to save $3 to $10 for every dollar they invest in the program. Even a city can make money by providing alcoholism treatment. A cost-benefit analysis showed that one state would recover $1.98 for every dollar invested in alcoholism treatment.[85]

For both alcohol and drug treatment this approach seems to be the rising star—great hopes exist, but there is no evidence that the big problem of motivation is solved, in spite of how logical it seems.

> The biggest difficulty in the treatment of an alcoholic is motivating him to seek help. For this purpose . . . no one is in a better position than his employer, who has the power—through the threat of firing or demotion—to intervene in a worker's life, as well as the right to do so once the problem begins to interfere with his work. Neither logic nor tears has the same effect on a problem drinker as the fear of losing what may be his last link to respectability—his job.[86]

Use of disulfiram. It may be that the constructive coercion of the occupational programs will work. In closing this section on treatment one more treatment technique needs to be mentioned: the use of disulfiram (Antabuse). Disulfiram inhibits the enzyme aldehyde dehydrogenase (Fig. 8-2) so that alcohol is still metabolized to acetaldehyde, but the acetaldehyde is not metabolized, and it accumulates. High levels of acetaldehyde usually produce a severe reaction: headache, nausea, vomiting, throbbing in head and neck, breathing difficulties, and a host of other unpleasant symptoms.[87] Even the alcohol in a wine sauce used in cooking may be enough to cause a severe reaction, so much care is needed in the use of disulfiram.

Many treatment programs urge or require their alcoholics to take disulfiram daily in the belief that it reduces the chance of someone impulsively taking a drink.[88] If you plan to drink, it is necessary to stop taking disulfiram 2 or 3 days before using alcohol, or all the bad things just mentioned will happen to you. It's a good theory, but there are no good data to support it. The alcoholics who continue to take their disulfiram daily after they finish the treatment program—and thus can't drink without a reaction—are those who don't usually drink anyway. They are treatment successes with or without disulfiram.[89,90]

Aftercare

The final step in the rehabilitation, or habilitation, of the alcoholic is the aftercare program. This usually involves follow-up meetings or therapy sessions every week or month to help maintain motivation levels, solve personal and family problems, or whatever continuing assistance the individual needs. The duration of the aftercare phase may be 6 to 12 months or a lifetime. AA encourages its members to continue participation in its meetings forever.

This section has covered a lot of ground. To put it in a capsule form: existing treatment programs do not differ in effectiveness, but most are more effective than no formal treatment. Many alcoholics do not abstain from the use of alcohol after treatment but do drink less, and less often, and with fewer negative consequences. Some of them have learned a few of the techniques for decreasing the physiological impact of alcohol. You may have

gleaned most of them from this chapter: eat before you drink, preferably foods high in fat or protein; dilute your drink with water (ice cubes), not a carbonated beverage; always take into account other legal and illegal drugs you might be using—they'll probably increase the effect of the alcohol; pace yourself; don't try to match drinks with the lush in the group; remember your size and sex: women are more affected than men and small people more than large.

The newest approach to treatment and aftercare is to tie it in with the individual's occupational setting. It is important to realize that neither the off-the-job use of alcohol nor alcohol addiction is sufficient reason to terminate an individual's employment. (As of September, 1977, this is also true of the use of any drug.) Poor performance *is* justification for termination. If the poor performance is based on alcohol or drug use, then the individual may be offered treatment rather than termination. This procedure is not as successful as was hoped for, but anything that increases the number of problem drinkers who are rehabilitated is better than nothing.

A SHORT CHASER

Alcohol. Our best-selling tranquilizer. Our most used, most abused, and most deadly recreational drug. There is no way to separate use from abuse—any time any drug is used, there will be those who abuse it. The pattern of use and abuse that has been developing has reduced the generation gap from kilometers to micrometers. Those who are having trouble with alcohol are getting younger every year according to NIAAA, which estimates that about 1.3 million preteens and teenagers have serious drinking problems.[91]

Can anything be done? Is there any hope of reducing the personal and social cost of alcohol misuse and abuse? Yes. And it's simple to do. But probably impossible. Some work[92] suggests that making alcohol a little more difficult to buy would decrease use of the alcoholic beverage. Translated that means if you don't sell it in fast food markets and grocery stores, less will be sold. An excellent book[93] that looked at patterns around the world of alcohol use, levels of use, attitudes about use, and damage resulting from use had two important rules that are applicable here: the more moderate alcohol use is integrated into society, the greater will be the incidence of alcohol-related damage and the best way to reduce alcohol-related damage is to decrease availability, and thus per capita use, of alcohol.

REFERENCES

1. Gordon, L.: The new crusade, Cleveland, 1932, The Crusaders, Inc.
2. Clark, N.H.: The dry years: prohibition and social change in Washington, Seattle, 1965, University of Washington Press.
3. Koren, J.: Economic aspects of the liquor problem, New York, 1899, Houghton Mifflin & Co.
4. Milner, G.: An overview of the drug/driving problem. In Report of an International Symposium on Drugs and Driving, Bloomington, Ind., 1975, Indiana University.
5. Nagle, J.J.: Vodka gains on bourbon: New York Times, January 13, 1975.
6. *Old mountain dew* (country song).
7. Gordon, J.: Slingings and high shots: moonshining in the Georgia mountains. In Morland, J.K.: The not so solid south, Athens, Ga., 1971, University of Georgia Press.
8. Escew, A.E., and others: Lead poisoning resulting from illicit alcohol consumption, Journal of Forensic Sciences 6(3):337-350, 1961.
9. Crutcher, J.C.: Clinical manifestations and therapy of acute lead intoxication due to the ingestion of illicitly distilled alcohol, Annals of Internal Medicine 59(5):707-715, 1963.
10. Gerhardt, R.E., and others: Moonshine-related arsenic poisoning, Archives of Internal Medicine 140:211-213, February 1980.
11. Prial, F.J.: Wide study finds the French drink less wine than before, New York Times, November 18, 1981, p. C21.
12. Focus on the Fourth Special Report to the U.S. Congress on Alcohol and Health, DHHS Pub. No. (ADM) 81-151, Alcohol Health and Research World, vol. 5, no. 3, Spring 1981.
13. More Americans found with alcohol problem, New York Times, July 2, 1978, p. 19.
14. One million are reported held for public drunkenness yearly, New York Times, July 20, 1980, p. 31.
15. Barnes, G.E.: The alcoholic personality, a reanalysis of the literature, Journal of Studies on Alcohol 40(7):571-634, 1979.
16. Cox, W.M.: The alcoholic personality: a review of the evidence. In Maher, B., editor: Progress in experimental personality research, vol. 9, New York, 1979, Academic Press, Inc.
17. Summary of final report: A national study of adolescent drinking behavior, attitudes and correlates, Research Triangle Park, N.C., 1975, Center for the Study of Social Behavior, Research Triangle Institute.
18. Donovan, J.E., and Jessor, R.: Adolescent problem drinking: psychosocial correlates in a national sample study, Journal of Studies on Alcohol 39(9):1506-1524, 1978.
19. Rise in teen-age drinking found, New York Times, March 20, 1981, p. A16.
20. Smart, R.G., and Goodstadt, M.S.: Effects of reducing the legal alcohol-purchasing age on drinking and drinking problems, Journal of Studies on Alcohol 38(7):1313-1323, 1977.
21. Helgason, T., and Asmundsson, G.: Behavior and social characteristics of young asocial alcohol abusers, Neuropsychobiology 1:109-120, 1975.
22. Cahalan, D., and Room, R.: Problem drinking among American men, New Brunswick, N.J., 1974, Rutgers Center of Alcohol Studies.
23. Rutstein, D.D., and Veech, R.L.: Genetics and addiction to alcohol, New England Journal of Medicine 298(20):1140-1141, 1978.
24. Farris, J.J., and Jones, B.M.: Ethanol metabolism in male American Indians and whites, Alcoholism: Clinical and Experimental Research 2(1):77-81, 1978.
25. Agarwal, D.P., and others: Racial differences in biological sensitivity to ethanol: the role of alcohol dehydrogenase and aldehyde dehydrogenase isozymes, Alcoholism: Clinical and Experimental Research 5(1):12-16, 1981.
26. Goodwin, D.W.: Genetics of alcoholism. In Pickens, R.W., and Heston, L.L., editors: Psychiatric factors in drug abuse, New York, 1979, Grune & Stratton.
27. Gallant, D.M.: Current literature reviewed and critiqued, Alcoholism: Clinical and Experimental Research 6(1):130-131, 1982.
28. Brody, J.: Personal health, New York Times, December 27, 1976, p. C13.
29. Chapman, L.F.: Experimental induction of hangover, Quarterly Journal of Studies on Alcohol, Suppl. 5, pp. 67-86, March 10, 1970.
30. Vestal, R.E., and others: Aging and ethanol metabolism, Clinical Pharmacology and Therapeutics 21(3):343-354, 1977.
31. Goodwin, D.W.: Alcohol in suicide and homicide, Quarterly Journal of Studies on Alcohol 34:144-156, 1973.
32. Mayfield, D.G., and Montgomery, D.: Alcoholism, alcohol intoxication, and suicide attempts, Archives of General Psychiatry 27(3):349-353, 1972.
33. Crothers, T.D.: Alcoholic trance, Popular Science Monthly 26:189, 191, 1884.
34. Interactions of drugs with alcohol, The Medical Letter 23(7):33-34, 1981.
35. Deitrich, R.A.: Neurochemistry of ethanol, Federation Proceedings 34:1929, 1975.
36. Goldstein, D.B., and Chin, J.H.: Interaction of ethanol with biological membranes, Federation Proceedings 40(7):2073, 1981.

37. Ritchie, J.M.: The aliphatic alcohols. In Goodman, L.S., and Gilman, A., editors: The pharmacological basis of therapeutics, ed. 5, New York, 1975, Macmillan Publishing Co.

38. Begleiter, H.: Brain dysfunction and alcoholism: problems and prospects: Alcohol Symposium, Alcoholism: Clinical and Experimental Research 5(2):264-266, 1981.

39. Goldberg, L.: Quantitative studies on alcohol tolerance in man, Acta Physiologica Scandinavica 5(suppl. 16):1-128, 1943.

40. Wenger, J.R., and others: Ethanol tolerance in the rat is learned, Science 213:575-577, July 1981.

41. Mann, R.E., and Vogel-Sprott, M.: Alcohol tolerance development in humans: tests of the learning hypothesis. In Problems of Drug Dependence 1980, NIDA Research Monograph 34, Washington, D.C., February 1981, U.S. Government Printing Office.

42. Tharp, V.K., and others: Alcohol and information processing, Psychopharmacologia 40:33-52, 1974.

43. Salamy, A.: The effects of alcohol on the variability of the human evoked potential, Neuropharmacology 12:1103-1107, 1973.

44. Bogen, E.: The human toxicology of alcohol. In Emerson, H., editor: Alcohol and man, New York, 1932, The Macmillan Co.

45. Wilkinson, P.K.: Pharmacokinetics of ethanol: a review. Alcoholism: Clinical and Experimental Research 4(1):6-21, 1980.

46. Lovell, W.S.: Breath tests for determining alcohol in the blood, Science 178:264-273, 1972.

47. Selzer, R.: The drinking man's liver, Esquire, p. 126, April 1976.

48. Korsten, M.A., and others: High blood acetaldehyde levels after ethanol administration, New England Journal of Medicine 292(8):385-389, 1975.

49. Raskin, N.H.: Alcoholism or acetaldehydism, New England Journal of Medicine 292(8):422-423, 1975.

50. Screening tests for alcoholism? Lancet, p. 1117-1118, November 22, 1980.

51. Papoz, L., and others: Alcohol consumption in a healthy population, Journal of the American Medical Association 245(17):1748-1751, 1981.

52. Eckardt, M.J.: Biochemical diagnosis of alcoholism, Journal of the American Medical Association 246(23):2707-2710, 1981.

53. Hoyumpa, A., and others: Effect of ethanol on benzodiazepine disposition in dogs, Journal of Laboratory and Clinical Medicine 95:310-322, 1980.

54. Desmond, P., and others: Short-term ethanol administration impairs the elimination of chlordiazepoxide (Librium) in man, European Journal of Clinical Pharmacology 18:275-278, 1980.

55. Hoyumpa, A., and others: Effect of short term ethanol administration on lorazepam clearance, Hepatology 1:47-53, 1981.

56. Iber, F.L.: Drug metabolism in heavy consumers of ethyl alcohol, Clinical Pharmacology and Therapeutics 22(5, part 2):735-742, 1977.

57. Rubin, E., and Lieber, C.S.: Fatty liver, alcoholic hepatitis and cirrhosis produced by alcohol in primates, New England Journal of Medicine 290:128-135, 1974.

58. Patek, A.M., and others: Alcohol and dietary factors in cirrhosis, Archives of Internal Medicine 135:1053-1057, 1975.

59. First special report to the U.S. Congress on Alcohol and Health from the Secretary of H.E.W., Publication No. (ADM) 74-68, Department of Health, Education, and Welfare, Washington, D.C., 1971, U.S. Government Printing Office.

60. Alcohol and health: new knowledge, National Institute on Alcohol Abuse and Alcoholism, Publication No. (ADM) 75-212, Department of Health, Education, and Welfare, Washington, D.C., 1975, U.S. Government Printing Office.

61. Eckardt, M.J.: Health hazards associated with alcohol consumption, Journal of the American Medical Association 246(6):648-666, 1981.

62. LaPorte, R.E., and others: The relationship of alcohol consumption to atherosclerotic heart disease, Preventive Medicine 9:22-40, 1980.

63. Dyer, A.R., and others: Alcohol consumption and 17-year mortality in the Chicago Western Electric Company Study, Preventive Medicine 9:78-90, 1980.

64. Filstead, W.J., Goby, M.J., and Bradley, N.J.: Critical elements in the diagnosis of alcoholism, Journal of the American Medical Association 236:2767-2769, 1976.

65. Babor, T.F., and others: Patterns of alcoholism in France and America: a comparative study. In Chafetz, M., editor: Proceedings of the Third Annual Alcohol Conference of the National Institute on Alcohol Abuse and Alcoholism, Washington, D.C., 1974, U.S. Government Printing Office.

66. Horn, J.L., and Vanberg, K.W.: Females are different: on the diagnosis of alcoholism in women, Proceedings of the First Annual Alcoholism Conference of the National Institute on Alcohol Abuse and Alcoholism, Washington, D.C., 1971, U.S. Government Printing Office.

67. Linsky, A.S.: Theories of behavior and the image of the alcoholic in popular magazines, 1900-1966, The Public Opinion Quarterly 34(4):573-581, 1970-1971.

68. Uniform act or similar laws passed by 16 states and D.C., Alcohol and Health Notes, p. 1, November 1973.

69. Even my kids didn't know I was an alcoholic: an interview with Dick Van Dyke, The Drinking American, Publication No. (ADM) 76-348, Department of Health, Education, and Welfare, Washington, D.C., 1976, U.S. Government Printing Office.

70. High degree of morbidity, mortality found in acute alcohol withdrawal, Alcohol and Health Notes, p. 2, October 1973.

71. Twain, M.: The adventures of Huckleberry Finn, 1885.

72. Kaim, S.C., Klett, C.J., and Rothfeld, B.: Treatment of the acute alcohol withdrawal state: a comparison of four drugs, American Journal of Psychiatry 125:1640-1646, 1969.

73. Victor, M., and Adams, R.D. Cited by Fraser, H.F.: Tolerance to and physical dependence on opiates, barbiturates and alcohol, Annual Review of Medicine 8:427-440, 1957.

74. Coleman, J.H., and Evans, W.E.: Pharmacotherapy of the acute alcohol withdrawal syndrome, Diseases of the Nervous System 36(4):151-154, 1975.

75. Armor, D.J., Polich, J.M., and Stambul, H.B.: Alcoholism and treatment, R-1739-National Institute on Alcohol Abuse and Alcoholism, Washington, D.C., June, 1976, U.S. Government Printing Office.

76. Brody, J.E.: Alcoholic study supports finding that some can resume drinking, New York Times, January 25, 1980, p. A14.

77. Emrick, C.D.: A review of psychologically oriented treatment of alcoholism. II. The relative effectiveness of different treatment approaches and the effectiveness of treatment versus no treatment, Quarterly Journal of Studies on Alcohol 36(1):88-108, 1975.

78. Noble, E.P.: Your role in alcoholism detection and treatment, Practical Psychology for Physicians, p. 16, July 1976.

79. Neumann, C.P., and Tamerin, J.S.: Prognostic factors in the evaluation of addicted individuals, International Pharmacopsychiatry 6:59-76, 1971.

80. Gordis, E., and others: Outcome of alcoholism treatment among 5578 patients in an urban comprehensive hospital-based program: application of a computerized data system, Alcoholism: Clinical and Experimental Research 5(4):509-522, 1981.

81. Rachin, R.L., editor: Job-based programs for alcohol and drug problems, Part I, Journal of Drug Issues 2(2):1, 1981.

82. Rachin, R.L., editor: Job-based programs for alcohol and drug problems, Part II, Journal of Drug Issues 2(2):1, 1981.

83. Hearings on Occupational Alcoholism Programs, House of Representatives, April 24-25, 1974.

84. How business grapples with problem of the drinking worker, U.S. News and World Report, p. 76, June 15, 1974.

85. Rundell, O.H., and Paredes, A.: Benefit—cost methodology in the evaluation of therapeutic services for alcoholism, Alcoholism: Clinical and Experimental Research 3(4):324-333, 1979.

86. Holden, C.: Alcoholism: on-the-job referrals mean early detection, treatment, Science 179:363, 1973.

87. Kitson, T.M.: The disulfiram—ethanol reaction, a review, Journal of Studies on Alcohol 38(1):96-113, 1977.

88. Kwentus, J., and Major, L.F.: Disulfiram in the treatment of alcoholism, a review, Journal of Studies on Alcohol 40(5):428-446, 1979.

89. Gallant, D.M.: Disulfiram: a valuable study and a thoughtful statistical approach, Alcoholism: Clinical and Experimental Research 5(2):344-345, 1981.

90. Baekeland, F., and others: Correlates of outcome in disulfiram treatment of alcoholism, Journal of Nervous and Mental Disease 153(1):1-9, 1971.

91. Study finds drinking—often to excess—now starts at earlier age, New York Times, March 27, 1977, p. 38.

92. Europeans imbibe more than ever, Medical World News, p. 42-43, September 17, 1979.

93. Frankel, B.G., and Whitehead, P.C.: Drinking and damage: theoretical advances and implications for prevention, Monograph of the Rutgers center of alcohol studies, vol. 14, New Brunswick, N.J., 1981, Rutgers Center of Alcohol Studies.

CHAPTER 9

NICOTINE

TOBACCO WAS A PLANT JUST WAITING for civilization to discover it—so it could conquer civilization. Long before Columbus stumbled on the Western Hemisphere, the Indians here were using tobacco. It was one of the many contributions of the New World to Europe: corn, sweet potatoes, white potatoes, chocolate, and—so you could lie back and enjoy it all—the hammock. Christopher Columbus recorded that the natives of San Salvador presented him with tobacco leaves on October 12, 1492. A fitting birthday present.

In 1497 a monk who had accompanied Columbus on his second trip wrote a book on native customs that contained the first printed report of tobacco smoking. Only it wasn't called tobacco, and it wasn't called smoking. Inhaling smoke was called drinking. In that period you either "took" (used snuff) or "drank" (smoked) tobacco.

The word tobacco came from one of two sources. "Tobaco" referred to a two-pronged tube used by natives to take snuff. Some early reports confused the issue by applying the name to the plant they incorrectly thought was being used. Another idea is that the word developed its current usage from the province of Tobacos in Mexico where everyone used the herb. Be that as it may, in 1598 an Italian-English dictionary published in London translated the Italian "Nicosiana" as the herb "Tobacco," and that spelling and usage gradually became dominant.

History has taken little note of Rodrigo de Jerez, but students frequently see parallels between him and current users of marijuana. Rodrigo was the poor fellow who introduced tobacco drinking to Europe. He was also the first European to touch Cuba and possibly the first to smoke tobacco. When he continued his habit in Portugal, his friends were convinced the devil had possessed him as they saw the smoke coming out his mouth and nose. The priest agreed, and Rodrigo spent the next several years in jail, only to find on his release that people were doing the same thing for which he had been jailed!

The major interest in tobacco during this period was medical, not recreational. A 1529 report[1] indicated that tobacco was used for "persistant headaches," "cold or catarrh," "abscesses and sores on the head." Everyone wanted to have a say: between 1537 and 1559 14 books mentioned the medicinal value of tobacco. With the medical use of tobacco already well publicized, and importation of the plant from Brazil to Portugal before 1550, everything was set for a French ambassador to Portugal to make a name for himself. And that's just what Jean Nicot did.

Nicot was sent to Lisbon in 1559 to arrange a royal marriage that never took place, but he became enamored with the medical uses of tobacco. He tried it on enough people to convince himself of its value and sent glowing reports of the herb's effectiveness to the French court. He was successful in "curing" the migraine headaches of Catherine de Medicis, Queen of Henry II of France, which made tobacco use very much "in." It was called the *herbe sainte*, the holy plant, and the *herbe a tous les maux*, the plant against all evils, pains, and other bad things. The French loved it, and, although tobacco had been introduced earlier to Paris, Nicot received the credit. By 1565 the plant had been called nicotiane, and Linnaeus sanctified it in 1753 by naming the genus *Nicotiana*. When a pair of French chemists isolated the active ingredient in 1828, they acted like true nationalists and called it nicotine.

To fully appreciate the history of tobacco you must know that there are over 60 species of *Nicotiana*, but only two major ones. *Nicotiana tobacum*, the major species grown today in over 100 countries, is large leafed. Most importantly, *tobacum* was indigenous only to South America, so the Spanish had a monopoly on its production for over a hundred years. *Nicotiana rustica* is a small-leaf species and was the plant existing in the West Indies and eastern North America when Columbus arrived.

MEDICAL HISTORY—ABBREVIATED

Tobacco was formally introduced to Europe as an herb useful for treating almost anything. In the late sixteenth century

> it was more likely than not that . . . the doctor would prescribe tobacco. . . . Did the patient suffer from flatulence? The remedy was a tobacco emetic. . . . A heavy cough? Smoke of tobacco, deeply inhaled. Pains accompanying gestation or labor? Place a leaf of tobacco, very hot, on the navel. If a form of delirium ensued, blow smoke up the nostrils[2,pp.38-39]

In this period Sir Anthony Chute[1,p.238] summarized much of the earlier material and said, "Anything that harms a man inwardly from his girdle upward might be removed by a moderate use of the herb." Others, however, felt differently: "If taken after meals the herb would infect the brain and liver," and, "Tobacco should be avoided by (among others) women with child and husbands who desired to have children."[1,p.238]

A few years later in 1617 Dr. William Vaughn phrased the last thought a little more poetically:

> Tobacco that outlandish weede
> It spends the braine and spoiles the seede
> It dulls the spirite, it dims the sight
> It robs a woman of her right.[3]

There was much discussion over the medical value of tobacco, but even more over the increasing social use. The opening speech in Molière's famous play. *Don Juan*, was quite topical, and debatable, for 1665:

> No matter what Aristotle and the "Philosophers" say, there is nothing like tobacco. It's the passion of the virtuous man and whoever lives without tobacco isn't worthy of living. . . . Haven't you noticed how well one treats another after taking it . . . so true it is that tobacco inspires feelings, honor and virtue in all those who take it.[4,pp.33-34]

The argument over the value of the recreational use of tobacco has waxed and waned throughout the years, even to the present. The slow advance of medical science through the eighteenth and nineteenth centuries gradually removed tobacco from the doctor's black bag, and nicotine was dropped from *The United States Pharmacopeia* in the 1890s. Special note must be made of a series of experiments reported in 1805 by Dr. D. Legare, since his work pushed back the boundaries of ignorance and clearly disproved an old folk remedy. Beyond the shadow of a doubt, Dr. Legare personally proved that, contrary to general opinion, blowing tobacco smoke into the intestinal canal did *not* resuscitate drowned animals or people! Another unsung hero of the men in white coats.

EARLY HISTORY

In the sixteenth century the English had real heroes to love and to emulate, men like Sir Walter Raleigh (who wasn't always a pipe tobacco) and Sir Francis Drake (who never was). They sailed the seven seas and, unlike most sailors of the day, took up pipe smoking. During the Elizabethan era, smoking became a national pleasure for the English, even though few people smoked on the continent.

One thorn in the British side was the Spanish monopoly on tobacco. When the settlers returned to England in 1586 after failing to colonize Virginia, they brought with them seeds of the *rustica* species and planted them in England, but this species never grew well. The English crown again attempted to establish a tobacco colony in 1610 when they sent John Rolfe as leader of a group to Virginia. From 1610 to 1612 Rolfe tried to cultivate *rustica* for sale in London, but it wouldn't sell. The small-leafed plant was weak, poor in flavor, and had a sharp taste.

In 1612 Rolfe's wife died, but, more important, he somehow got hold of some seeds of the Spanish *tobacum* species. This species grew beautifully and sold well in 1613. The colony was saved, and every available plot of land was planted with *tobacum*. By 1619, as much Virginia tobacco was sold in London as Spanish tobacco. That was also the year that King James prohibited the cultivation of any tobacco in England and declared the tobacco trade a royal monopoly.

Tobacco became one of the major exports of the American colonies to England. The Thirty Years' War spread smoking throughout central Europe, and nothing stopped its use. Measures such as one in Bavaria in 1652 probably slowed tobacco use, but only momentarily. This law said that "tobacco-drinking was strictly forbidden to the peasants and other common people . . . " and made tobacco available to others only on a doctor's prescription from a druggist.[5,pp.112-114]

In 1660 England raised the duty on tobacco, and for the first time tobacco appeared on the tax books.

Rising costs made adulteration a worthwhile occupation, causing Parliament to pass the "Pure Tobacco Act" in 1716 to control adulteration. That this is a never-ending problem is suggested by a 1918 decision of the Mississippi Supreme Court, which said:

> We can imagine no reason why, with ordinary care, human toes could not be left out of chewing tobacco, and if toes are found in chewing tobacco, it seems to us that somebody has been very careless.[2,p.303]

During the eighteenth century smoking gradually diminished, but the use of tobacco did not. Snuff replaced the pipe in England. At the beginning of that century the upper class was already committed to snuff. The middle and lower classes only gradually changed over, but by 1770 very few people smoked. The reign of King George III (1760 to 1820) was the time of the big snuff. His wife Charlotte was so addicted to the powder that she was called "Snuffy Charlotte," although for obvious reasons not to her face. On the continent Napoleon had tried smoking once, gagged horribly, and returned to his 7 pounds of snuff a month.

A 1980 article titled "A New Age for Snuff" took note of the increase in snuff use by athletes and male teenagers and concluded that "Snuff could be an acceptable and less harmful substitute for cigarette smoking."[6,p.474] There are two forms and uses of snuff. One type (a la King George) involves "inserting powdered tobacco in to the nose" and yields blood nicotine levels in 5 minutes that are comparable to those obtained with cigarette smoking. And that's without the products of combustion: carbon monoxide, tars, etc. Reduction of lung cancer would certainly follow—although what illnesses would increase with the snuffing is at present unknown. Snuff dipping involves putting a small wad of tobacco between the gum and the cheek—not chewing—and absorbing nicotine through the mouth tissues. This results in an increase in mouth and pharnyx cancer that is related to the amount and years of use.[7]

MIDDLE HISTORY

Trouble developed in the colonies, which, being democratic, made the richest man in Virginia (perhaps the richest in the colonies) commander in chief of the Revolutionary Army. In 1776 George Washington said in one of his appeals, "if you can't send money, send tobacco."[8,p.73] Another American commander in chief was to echo those words 141 years later when Pershing said, "You ask me what we need to win this war. I answer tobacco as much as bullets."[8,p.226] These sentiments were reaffirmed by Pershing's protégé, General Douglas MacArthur, in World War II.[8,p.242] Tobacco played an important role in the Revolutionary War, since it was one of the major products for which France would lend the colonies money. Knowing the importance of tobacco to the colonies, one of Cornwallis' major campaign goals in 1780 and 1781 was the destruction of the Virginia tobacco plantations.

After the war, the American man in the street rejoiced and rejected snuff as well as tea and all other things British. The aristocrats who organized the republic were not as emotional, though, and installed a communal snuff box for members of Congress. Only in the mid-1930s did this remembrance of things past disappear. However, to emphasize the fact that snuff was a nonessential, the new Congress put a luxury tax on it in 1794.

If you don't smoke and you don't snuff
How can you possibly get enough?

By chewing, which gradually increased in the United States. Chewing was a suitable activity for a country on the go; it freed the hands, and the wide open spaces made an adequate spittoon. There were also other considerations: Boston, for example, has passed an ordinance in 1798 forbidding anyone from being in possession of a lighted pipe or "segar" in public streets. The original impetus was a concern for the fire hazard involved in smoking, not the individual's health, and the ordinance was finally repealed in 1880. Today it is difficult to appreciate how much of a chewing country we were in the nineteenth century. In 1860

only 7 of 348 tobacco factories in Virginia and North Carolina manufactured smoking tobacco. The amount of tobacco for smoking did not equal the amount for chewing until 1911 and did not surpass it until the 1920s. Even as cigarettes began developing in Europe, American chewing tobacco was expanding.

The Civil War shut southern *bright* (that is, light colored when cured) tobacco out of northern markets, but Ohio and Kentucky had a different variety of tobacco, *burley*, that was darker and better suited for chewing. Burley had a low sugar content and thus could absorb up to 25% of its weight in licorice, rum, and molasses, whereas the bright tobacco from Virginia and North Carolina could only absorb about 4% of its weight. The tobaccos from west of the Appalachian Mountains reached their peak in the 1890 to 1910 period. The 1890s particularly were times of price wars and intense competition. By selling at less than cost, consumption of chewing tobacco increased so that by 1897 one half of all tobacco in the United States was prepared for chewing. The names of some of the brands suggest the savageness of the competition: "Battle Ax," "Scalping Knife," "Crossbow."

Although the writing was on the wall before the turn of the century, it was not until 1945 that the last bow was made to the chewer when cuspidors were removed from all federal buildings. In that same year, however, at the National Tobacco Spitting Contest the winner spat 21 feet 2 inches. That wasn't as good as Mark Twain, but they're slowly getting there. The 1975 competition established a world's record that still stands: 31 feet 1 inch.[9]

Smokeless tobacco (snuff and chewing tobacco) began its return in the early 1970s in response to health concerns over cigarette smoking. In 1980 there were about 22 million users of smokeless tobacco.[10] Red Man is the best selling chewing tobacco. Levi Garrett is number two and Beech Nut is third. However, Mail Pouch will be remembered in history as *the* chewing tobacco of the twentieth century—the Mail Pouch signs painted on the sides of barns all over America were designated as national landmarks by the U.S. Congress in 1966![11]

RECENT HISTORY

The transition from chewing to cigarettes had a middle point, a combination of both smoking and chewing: cigars. Cigarette smoking was coming, and the cigar manufacturers did their best to keep cigarettes under control. They suggested that cigarettes were drugged with opium so you could not stop using them and that the paper was bleached with arsenic and thus was harmful to you. They had some help from Thomas Edison in 1914:

> The injurious agent in Cigarettes comes principally from the burning paper wrapper. . . . It has a violent action in the nerve centers. producing degeneration of the cells of the brain, which is quite rapid among boys. Unlike most narcotics, this degeneration is permanent and uncontrollable. I employ no person who smokes cigarettes.[12,p.274]

They made cigarette smokers so nervous they had to smoke more to stay calm!

Most cigars had been hand rolled or at least made by hand shaping in a mold, but as sales increased, machines had to be used. Today, a good worker hand rolls about 200 cigars in an 8- to 9-hour day. There was an aversion to machine-made cigars, so some advertising was educational in nature. As an example of the high level of advertising before television and Madison Avenue:

> Spit is a horrid word, but it's worse on the end of your cigar. Why run the risk of cigars made by dirty yellowed fingers and tipped in spit?[22,p.273]

Buy a machine-made cigar with clean toes in it!

The efforts of the cigar manufacturers worked for a while, and cigar sales reached their highest level in 1920, when 8 billion were sold. As sales increased, though, so did the cost of the product. The whole world knows that "what this country *needs* is a really good five-cent cigar," but how many know that this statement was made by a vice president of the United States as an aside in the Senate when one of the members was going on at great length about the needs of the country. If the country got one, it was not enough. The dudes, the effete, were beginning to have their day.

Not even the great John L. Sullivan could stem the tide. He wasn't exactly a diplomat, but in 1905 you didn't have to be!

> Smoke cigarettes? Not on your tut-tut. . . . You can't suck coffin-nails and be a ring-champion. . . . You never heard of . . . a bank burglar using a cigarette, did you? They couldn't do it and attend to biz. Why, even drunkards don't use the things. . . . Who smokes 'em? Dudes and college stiffs—fellows who'd be wiped out by a single jab or a quick undercut. It isn't natural to smoke cigarettes. An American ought to smoke cigars, an Englishman a briar, a Harp a clay pipe and a Dutchy a Meerschaum. It's the Dutchmen, Italians, Russians, Turks and Egyptians who smoke cigarettes and they're no good anyhow.[13,p.259]

Thin reeds filled with tobacco had been seen by the Spanish in Yucatan in 1518. In 1844 the French were using them, and the Crimean War circulated the cigarette habit throughout Europe. The first British cigarette factory was started in 1856 by a returning veteran of the Crimean War, and in the late 1850s an English tobacco merchant, Phillip Morris, began producing handmade cigarettes. On the continent the use of this new dose form must have developed fairly rapidly. One company in Austria began making double cigarettes in 1865—both ends had a mouthpiece, and the consumer cut them in two—and sold 16 million in 1866.

In the United States cigarettes were being produced during this same period (14 million in 1870), but it was in the 1880s that their popularity increased rapidly. The date of the first patent on a cigarette-making machine was 1881, and by 1885 over a billion cigarettes a year were being sold. By the turn of the century there was a preference for cigarettes with an aromatic component, that is, Turkish tobacco. A new cigarette in 1913 capitalized on the lure of the Near East while rejecting it in actuality. Three hundred years after John Rolfe saved the Virginia colony with American-grown Spanish tobacco, a truly American cigarette was created, Camels. Camels were a blend of burley

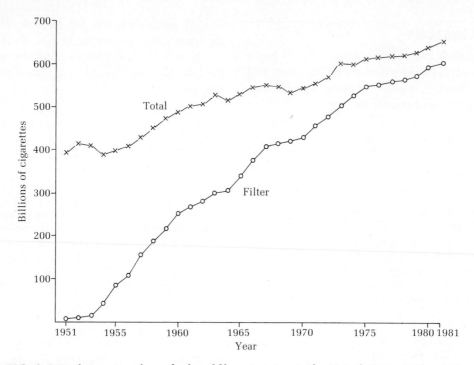

FIG. 9-1 Total cigarette sales and sales of filter cigarettes in the United states, 1951 to 1981. (From Robert Miller, Economics, Statistics and Cooperatives Service, USDA.)

and bright with just a hint of Turkish tobacco—you had the camel and pyramid on the package, what more could you want? Besides, eliminating most of the imported tobacco made the price lower. Low price was combined with a big advertising campaign: "The Camels are coming. Tomorrow there'll be more CAMELS in town than in all of Asia and Africa combined." By 1918 Camels had 40% of the market and stayed in front until after World War II. In the early 1980s Camels were holding steady with about 4% to 5% of the market.

Chesterfield had been started in 1912, and the name Lucky Strike, which started as a smoking plug after the Civil War, was revived in 1916 as a cigarette. The name didn't have the relevance it had had in the 1860s and 1870s during the gold rushes, but neither did Old Gold, which appeared first in 1885 and then in 1926 as a cigarette. The year 1919 was marked by the first ad showing a woman smoking. To make the ad easier to accept, the woman was oriental looking and the ad was for Turkish-

type cigarettes. King-size cigarettes appeared in 1939 in the form of Pall Mall, which became the number one seller. Filter cigarettes as filter cigarettes, not cigarettes that happen to have filters along with a mouthpiece, appeared in 1954 with Winston, which rapidly took over the market and continued to be number one until the mid-1970s.

Increasing cigarette sales, decreasing per capita cigarette use, people starting, people quitting, and our aging population make it difficult to give a simple answer to the question: What are the trends in cigarette smoking? Fig. 9-1 shows the total number of cigarettes, as well as the number of filter cigarettes, sold in the United States since 1951. The general trend is up: more cigarettes are being sold today than ever before, and over 90% are filter cigarettes. Worldwide, almost 4½ trillion cigarettes were sold in 1981. Sales figures, starting in the 1950s, for the current top four brand names are shown in Fig. 9-2.

Even though more cigarettes are being sold, the

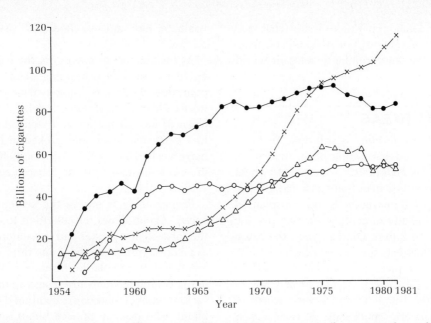

FIG. 9-2 Sales of cigarettes (filter and nonfilter); ● Winston, ✕ Marlboro, Δ Kool, ○ Salem.

TABLE 9-1 Cigarette smokers at selected ages (percent who are smokers)

A Year	12-14 Male	12-14 Female	15-16 Male	15-16 Female	17-18 Male	17-18 Female	B Year	19 and older Male	19 and older Female
1968	3	1	17	10	30	19	1955	53	25
1974	4	5	18	20	31	26	1970	44	31
1979	3	4	14	12	19	26	1975	39	29
							1980	37	29

Compiled from 1982 Cancer facts and figures; New York, 1981; American Cancer Society; and Dangers of Smoking benefits of quitting; rev. ed., New York, 1980, American Cancer Society.

percentage of people who smoke cigarettes is declining. The explanation is that our population is still expanding.

Table 9-1 shows the percentage of smokers by age and sex for several time periods. Part A shows that the percentage of teenage male smokers was level from 1968 to 1974 and then declined from 1974 to 1979. The percentage of teenage female smokers may now be leveling off, 1974 to 1979, and may begin to decline. Check back in 1984. Part B shows a continual decline in the percentage of

adult male smokers since 1955. The percentage of adult female smokers increased from 1955 to 1970 and has leveled off since that time. Perhaps the decline will come soon.

A significant number of young and middle-aged adults have quit smoking, and surveys identify them as having better educations and higher incomes.

The reduction in the percentage of smokers combined with the increasing concern that nonusers may be negatively affected when exposed to smoke has resulted in a major civil rights issue. That story is told in another section, but it should be made clear here that the same trend is developing world-wide.

FROM FARM TO FAG

Much of tobacco farming is still done by hand. The cultivation and harvesting of an acre of tobacco require 300 man-hours, in contrast to wheat, which requires only 3 man-hours per acre. Tobacco seeds are started in seed beds and transplanted, 5000 to 10,000 plants an acre, when they are 6 to 8 inches high. In 2 to 3 months, when the tobacco is ready to harvest, the leaves will be 1 to 2½ feet long, and a typical burley tobacco plant will have 10 leaves. The nicotine content of a raw tobacco leaf ranges from 0.3% to 7% and varies with the variety, climatic conditions, fertilizer used, and many other factors. Nicotine levels can be manipulated during processing to any desired level.

Burley is one of the major tobaccos used in cigarettes. It is harvested by cutting the stalk close to the ground, then hanging the entire stalk in a curing barn for 4 to 6 weeks. The plant uses its stored food, dies, and loses about 80% of its weight through moisture loss. This is "air-curing," the method used for most cigarette tobacco grown west of the Appalachians. East of the mountains "flue-curing" is used to produce bright tobacco. Tobacco that is to be flue-cured has the leaves separated from the stalks during harvesting, and heat is added to the curing barn so that the process is complete in less than a week.

After curing, the burley leaves are removed from the stalk and sorted on the basis of color, size, and stalk position. Almost all tobacco is still sold at one of the 176 auction houses in this country. Each farmer puts his sorted leaves in different stacks called baskets, up to 600 pounds a basket, and a Department of Agriculture employee grades the quality of each basket from choice to poor. The auction itself is bedlam, it seems, but spirited bidding, fast action, and a very efficient system let the auctioneer, his assistants, and the buyers walk by,

evaluate, bid, and sell about 360 baskets of burley an hour.

As the auctioneer moves on, the baskets are taken to the buyer's processing plant. Only at this point does modern technology take over. Here the tobacco leaves are shredded, dried, picked, blown clean of foreign matter and stems, remoisturized to a particular level, and packed in huge wooden barrels called *hogsheads*. The hogsheads are placed in storehouses, where the tobacco ages for 2 to 3 years.

Proper aging is one of the secrets to good tobacco. Aging allows fermentation to occur so that the tobacco gets darker and loses moisture, as well as nicotine (probably about one third of its original level) and other volatile substances. When the aging is complete, moisture is again added, and the various types of tobacco are combined to the correct blend. The makeup of each blend is a deep, dark trade secret, but the typical cigarette today contains about 47% flue-cured bright, 35% burley, 1% Maryland, and 17% imported tobacco. The percentage of imported tobacco has tripled since the late 1950s. Most of it comes from Turkey, although Greece also exports a substantial amount to the United States. In 1981 the United States imported 450 million pounds of tobacco and exported 599 million pounds.

During the blending process the tobacco receives any additives that are necessary. Glycerine is one chemical that is almost universally added to help stabilize the moisture content. The blended material is compressed and then cut into hangnail-size strips to prepare it for the cigarette machine.

A century ago James Buchanan Duke thought his cigarette girls were doing very well if they could consistently roll four cigarettes a minute. In 1881 he started the cigarette revolution by using a machine that had just been patented. It produced 200 cigarettes a minute! He would love today's machine. It starts with a roll of cigarette paper 3½ miles long, makes a continuous clothesline-like tube filled with tobacco, cuts it to length, weighs the cigarette, rejecting those over or under the correct weight, and checks it for uniformity. It does everything but salute, and still turns out 3,600 cigarettes a minute. Filter cigarettes are made by adding a machine that attaches a double-size filter between two cigarettes and then cuts them apart at the same rapid rate.

Packaging is just as neat and efficient, although only one twentieth as fast. The packs go into cartons, the cartons into boxes, the boxes into trucks, and the trucks into traffic jams as they speed their load to the consumer. Amazingly, the cost of producing a pack of cigarettes, exclusive of tobacco, is only 2 to 3 cents.[14]

Someone, somewhere, must have made the observation that a plant that is America's fifth largest money crop can't be all bad. The industry is enormous. Consumers now spend about $24 billion a year for tobacco products, and the amount goes up by about a billion dollars a year. Over 90% of this is for cigarette purchases.

Uncle Sam gets his share of that money about $3 billion in 1981. That will increase in the future since the tax on cigarettes will probably increase from the 1981 level of 8 cents a pack. Each of the states, and even some cities, also adds taxes, and together their bill was over $4 billion in 1981. In some states the tax is more than a penny a cigarette. In others the tax is much less, and, not too surprisingly, the tax in North Carolina, where the largest industry is tobacco growing and manufacturing, is 2 cents a pack.

There is a problem when a product can be bought for much less money in one state than in another. The problem is called bootlegging and in 1977 states in the Northeast claimed that bootleg cigarettes were costing them millions in lost tax revenues.[15] Cigarettes bought legally in North Carolina were illegally transported to the Northeast and sole there without the high state and city taxes being paid. The U.S. Treasury Department investigated but in 1981 the Bureau of Alcohol, Tobacco and Firearms bowed out saying they "had found little evidence of large scale cigarette smuggling."[16]

There are regular proposals made to increase the federal tax on cigarettes, which has remained unchanged since 1951, and one suggestion is: the higher the tar and nicotine content, the higher the tax. Smuggling and talk of higher taxes make many people very nervous, and not just the tobacco companies. Many groups get substantial pieces of the $24 billion pie. Tobacco products are sold in over 1.4 million retail outlets, and tobacco is grown on over 200,000 farms and provides 69,000 jobs in the manufacturing process. To counter some of the anxiety and provide job security cigarette companies spent $1 billion on advertising in 1981—three times the amount spent in 1970 when ads were still allowed on radio and television. To buffer declining profits the tobacco companies diversified into many products throughout the 1970s. They really didn't need to—profits from cigarette manufacturing and sales have remained high.

There must be a moral somewhere in the fact that as cigarette consumption is increasing, tobacco use is declining. In the 20-year period between 1956 and 1976, the amount of leaf tobacco used per cigarette decreased 25%! Filter tips cause even more problems, since they use about one-third less tobacco than plain-tip cigarettes of the same length.

Two technological changes have decreased the need for leaf tobacco. One is the use of reconstituted sheets of tobacco. Parts of the tobacco leaf and stems that had been discarded in earlier years are now ground up, combined with many added ingredients to control such factors as moisture, flavor, and color, and then rolled out as a flat, homogenized sheet of tobacco. After shredding, this material is combined with normally processed leaf tobacco. Today about 20% of all cigarette tobacco is reconstituted sheet.

The second development that reduced the need for tobacco in cigarettes is "fluffing." Tobacco is freeze dried, and an inert gas such as Freon is used to expand the tobacco cells so that they take up more space and can absorb more additives. One low-tar cigarette introduced in the early 1970s was able to reduce by 35% the tobacco in each cigarette because of its process to "fluff" the tobacco. Fluffing, of course, reduces the tar, nicotine, and carbon monoxide content of a cigarette, but it also reduces smoking time, perhaps by 15%. In the early 1950s,

2¾ pounds of tobacco were needed for 1000 cigarettes. Now only about 1¾ pounds are required to produce the same number.

The additives that are used in cigarettes are, for the most part, unknown secrets. A 1972 publication by the Reynolds Tobacco Company listed 1290 "flavorants" that could be added to cigarettes. Someone should be worrying about them but they are neither analyzed nor regulated by the FDA. European companies must, by law, use pure tobacco. As someone said, "'Pure' may not translate into 'healthy' but it does sound better than shellac"[17]—one additive found in some cigarettes.

Perhaps the end is not yet in sight. Increased health concerns, government regulations, restrictions on advertising, and the onward march of science and technology have resulted in the development and sale of "false fags," as the British call them. These cigarettes have either no, or very little, tobacco and a less expensive, and maybe less toxic, vegetable product, such as wood pulp. It is unlikely that these false fags will engulf the market.

It is quite probable, however, that tobacco cultivation and processing will continue to respond to health and economic pressures. If the consumer cannot tell that his cigarette is made from reconstituted tobacco—and the evidence is that he cannot—why not deal only with sheet tobacco? Why not harvest the entire tobacco plant, chop it up, and process it? The savings in labor costs would be great, better control would be possible over the product, and additives could be used to "improve" the quality of low-grade tobacco. Of course, some might not consider these cigarettes real.

TOWARD A LESS HAZARDOUS CIGARETTE

Research on tar/nicotine (T/N) yields suggest that the lower they are in a cigarette, the lower the health hazard.[18] Even before that evidence was available, T/N levels had been declining regularly. The average cigarette smoker today would probably gag, cough, and become nauseous if forced to smoke a 1955 cigarette.

Fig. 9-3 shows the average tar and nicotine yields—weighted for sales of all domestic brands—from 1954 to 1981. Most of you will see a trend. Beginning in 1981 the Federal Trade Commission, which determines the tar and nicotine amounts that are printed on some cigarette packages and contained in all advertisements, analyzed for carbon monoxide.[19] Correlations between the three measures, tar–nicotine–carbon monoxide, for 200 brands analyzed were: T/N, +.97; N/CM, +.90; T/CM, +.91. Overall, the addition of carbon monoxide levels does not add much new information. The average T/N/CM level of the four best-selling filter brands was 15.5/1.05/15.1 (see Fig. 9-2). Note that if *you* smoke, you may receive much more, or much less, tar and nicotine from the cigarette than the average indicated on the pack.[20] It all depends on your smoking behavior.[21] The levels on different brands can, however, serve as a relative guide.

No one is saying where the race to low T/N levels will end, but it is a race. In 1967 only 2% of the market was made up of "low-tar" cigarettes, those with 15 mg of tar or less. Their share of the market reached was 65% in 1981. The cigarette brands showing greatest gains are the ultralows—less than 4 mg of tar. Cigarette producers may not go too far, since one review of the literature suggests "that the possible acceptance limit of a cigarette lies around 8 mg 'tar' and 0.3 mg of smoke nicotine."[22,p.463] That statement has merit.

There may be other ways to make a cigarette acceptable to the consumer than with tar and nicotine. In 1976 a cigarette was introduced that boldly proclaimed that its "taste" was added. The addition of additives may subtract from the purity of the cigarette but seems sure to multiply profits as well as creating a division of the consumer market. Oh, well, Camels started it all in 1913 with licorice, chocolate, and sugar.

There are probably more breakthroughs coming. Nicotine, which is the chemical basis for the physiological and pharmacological reward in tobacco, exists in two forms in smoke: neutral or positively charged, because of the addition of one proton. Neutral nicotine is absorbed more readily than is

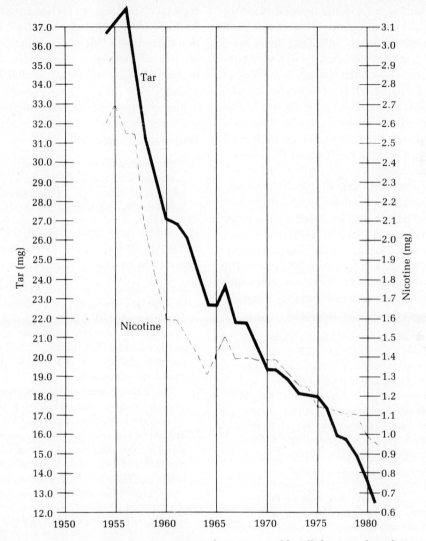

FIG. 9-3 U.S. sales-weighted average tar and nicotine yields (all domestic brands on U.S. market). (From The Tobacco Observer, **7**(1):1,1982.)

the charged nicotine. As the amount of neutral (un-protonated) nicotine increases, so does the pleasure the user obtains from the smoke. More pleasure per puff may mean fewer puffs, less smoke, and less tar and nicotine intake, thus less of a health hazard.[23] Of course, if smoking does not decrease, the increase in nicotine absorption could increase the health risk.

TOBACCO: PRO AND CON

Throughout the history of tobacco use there have been those who praise and those who condemn the vice. Some of these beliefs have already been indicated, but others, particularly the more recent ones, are mentioned here.

In 1600 pipe smoking was *the* thing to do in

England, even though the king opposed it for social, medical, and moral reasons. It was more than a passive opposition, and in 1604 King James (yes, it's *that* King James) wrote and published a very strong antitobacco pamphlet stating that tobacco was "harmefull to the braine, dangerous to the lungs."[8,p.250] Never one to let morality or health concerns interfere with business, he also supported the growing of tobacco in Virginia in 1610, and when the crop prospered, he declared the tobacco trade a royal monopoly.

Even that merry soul, "Ole King Cole," was taken to task 300 years later; there were calls to ban the nursery rhyme because he called for his pipe. New York City made it illegal in 1908 for a woman to use tobacco in public, and in the Roaring Twenties women were expelled from schools and dismissed from jobs for smoking. You must appreciate that these concerns were partly for society and partly to protect women from themselves!

> Smoking by women and even young girls must be considered from a far different stand point than smoking by men, for not only is the female organism by virtue of its much more frail structure and its more delicate tissues much less able to resist the poisonous action of tobacco than that of men, and thus, like many a delicate flower, apt to fade and wither more quickly in consequence, but the fecundity of woman is greatly impaired by it. . . . authorities cannot be expected to look on unmoved while a generation of sterile women, rendered incapable of fulfilling their sublime function of motherhood, is being produced on account of the immoderate smoking of foolish young girls.[24,pp.39-40]

There was some debate in this period about the causes of the lack of fecundity! According to Dr. Tidswell: "The most common cause of female sterility is the abuse of tobacco by males." Old ideas neither die nor fade away, they just lie low for a while. First, Dr. Vaughn, then Dr. Tidswell, and in 1971, Dr. Alton Ochsner.[25] An article was popularized in the January 1975 issue of the *Reader's Digest*[26] which contained a condensation of an American Medical Association magazine article.[27]

Its topic? Smoking can be hazardous to your sexual health. No way. An August 1975 article[28] concluded that there is no evidence that smoking has an effect on sexual activity. Of course, there is that poster: "Kissing a smoker is like licking a dirty ashtray."

The effect of cigarette smoking on fertility could not have been too great since in the 1930s the antitobacco people said:

> Fifty percent of our insanity is inherited from parents who were users of tobacco. . . . Thirty-three percent of insanity cases are caused direct from cigarette smoking and the use of tobacco. . . .[29,p.97]

Those who have lived through the marijuana era of the late 1960s and the 1970s have heard similar statements. In 1931:

> Judge Gimmill, of the court of Domestic Relations of Chicago, declared that, without exception, every boy appearing before him that had lost the faculty of blushing was a cigarette fiend. The poison in cigarettes has the same effect upon girls: it perverts the morals and deadens the sense of shame and refinement. . . .
>
> The bathing beaches have become resorts for women smokers, where they go to show off with a cigarette in their mouths. The bathing apparel in the last ten years has been reduced from knee skirts to a thin tight-fitting veil that scarcely covers two-thirds of their hips. Many of the girl bathers never put their feet in the water, but sit on the shore, show their legs and smoke cigarettes.[29,p.187]

During this period the cigarette industry remained quiet, and sales increased. These were the days of "not a cough in a carload" ads. As early as 1939 a major authority on cancer stated that "the increase in the incidence of pulmonary carcinoma is due largely to the increase in cigarette smoking."[30] The pattern of ever-increasing sales was only slightly disrupted in the early 1950s when scientific reports first linked smoking and lung cancer (Fig. 9-1). There was, however, an increase in cigar smoking and a shift from nonfilter to filter cigarettes that seemed primarily to be linked to health concerns.

Adverse health effects

Each year the Public Health Service of the United States reviews the world scientific literature and reports to Congress on the effects of smoking on health. No concern with bathing suits, insanity, or morality—just sobering facts. The 1979 report[31] marked the fifteenth anniversary of the first report and was bigger and better than usual. Based on over 30,000 articles its 1100 pages were exhaustive and specific and the conclusion very clear, "Cigarette smoking is the single most important environmental factor contributing to premature mortality in the United States."[31] The following are some of the most important findings:

One of every seven deaths in the United States is smoking related.

Overall, a smoker is 70% more likely to die at a given age than a nonsmoker.

Smoking accounts for 80% of all lung cancer deaths (and 70% of lung cancer patients die within the first year).

Smoking is related to 40% of most other cancer deaths.

Smoking doubles the risk of heart attack and accounts for one third of all heart disease deaths (and heart disease accounts for about half of all deaths in the United States).

Smoking accounts for about 75% of emphysema deaths.

Smoking a pack of cigarettes a day decreases life expectancy by 6 years, two packs a day decreases life expectancy by more than 8 years.

There are always doubting Thomases. Who can you trust? There is one source of information that is fairly independent, has its own set of statistics, and is made up of a group that is willing to put its money where its mouth is: life insurance companies. In the early 1900s Phoenix Mutual classed their policy holders as: nonsmokers, light smokers (1 to 5 cigarettes a day), and regular smokers (6 or more a day). No premium reductions were offered but the mortality of light smokers was 107% of nonsmokers, and the regular smokers mortality was 126% of nonsmokers. Since the mid-1960s companies have increasingly offered lower life insurance premiums to nonsmokers. At last count more than 30 companies did so.

The best set of data comes from State Mutual Life Assurance Company.[32] They show that a 32-year-old male smoking 30 cigarettes a day increases his likelihood of death 340% over a nonsmoker. On the average he decreases his life expectancy by 7.3 years (from 46.9 more years to live to 39.6 more years). This difference in life expectancy between male smokers and nonsmokers is greater than the difference in life expectancy between males and females: 5 years! That's the mouth. The money? A 23% reduction in term life insurance premiums for the nonsmoker compared to the smoker![32,p.261]

It is important not to engage in overkill (a bad phrase in this context). Too much doomsaying may result in people just avoiding the facts. One final comment: think of anything related to good physical health; what the research says is that cigarette smoking will impair it! The earlier the age at which you start smoking, the more smoking you do, the longer you do it—the greater the impairment (see Fig. 9-4) .[31] Smoking doesn't do any part of the body any good, at any time, under any conditions.

There is no bright side, but there is a less dark side. The 1981 report of the Surgeon General[18] focused on the low tar/nicotine cigarettes. The conclusions:

1. There is no such thing as safe smoking or a safe cigarette.
2. Smoking low T/N cigarettes reduces the risk of lung cancer and improves life expectancy—if you don't smoke more of the lower T/N cigarettes than you did of the higher T/N cigarettes.
3. No evidence yet exists about the effects of low T/N cigarettes on other diseases.
4. Additives may be a big health problem, particularly in the low T/N cigarettes.

Your best bet? Don't smoke. Save your money, save your health, and give yourself the gift of 7 years of life! Second best bet? If you must smoke, smoke low T/N cigarettes.

Much concern has been expressed over the

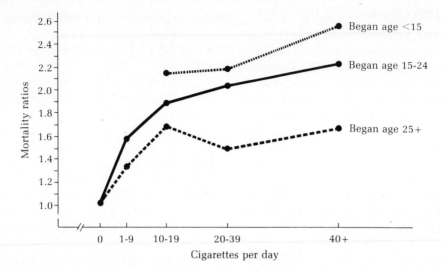

FIG. 9-4 Mortality ratios (total deaths, mean ages 55 to 64) as a function of the age at which smoking started and the number of cigarettes smoked per day.

health effects of "involuntary smoking" or "passive smoking" that is, nonsmokers who inhale cigarette smoke from their environment.[33] It is clear that some individuals are allergic to the components in cigarette smoke and that many more object to smoking because they don't like the smell, etc.[34] That issue is discussed later. The question here is: What is known about the physiological effects of passive smoking? The only hard data (discounting a widely publicized study, later shown to be incorrect)[35,36] are that ". . . chronic exposure to tobacco smoke in the work environment is deleterious to the nonsmoker and significantly reduces small-airways function" in the lungs[37,p.720]; an article in the *Journal of the National Cancer Institute* which concluded, "Compared to nonsmoking women married to nonsmoking husbands, nonsmokers married to smoking husbands showed very little, if any, increased risk of lung cancer."[38,p.1061] More data are needed to make definite statements about passive smoking effects.

The mechanisms whereby cigarette smoking cause all the adverse medical effects are not completely known.[39] There are some good bets, however. Nicotine causes the release of noradrenaline in the cardiovascular system. This increases heart rate and blood pressure causing an increase in the heart's need for oxygen. If there is already poor coronary blood flow, the risk of a heart attack increases. Impairment of coronary heart flow by increased atherosclerosis is made more likely with the finding that cigarette smoking is linked to low levels of HDL (high density lipoproteins).[40] High levels of HDL protect the circulatory system to some degree from the effects of high cholesterol levels (which cause atherosclerosis). Perhaps the most important factor, however, is the blood's decreased oxygen-carrying capacity as a result of the carbon monoxide in the cigarette smoke.[41] Each of these effects reverses fairly rapidly when a cigarette smoker stops smoking. That fits with the finding that 1 to 2 months after a smoker stops, his risk for coronary heart disease is almost equal to a nonsmoker.[42]

The rapid decrease in the risk of coronary heart disease when smoking stops does not hold for lung cancer. If you smoke a pack or more a day for about 10 years and then stop, it may take 15 years for your lungs to return to normal. The tars—a number of various carcinogens (cancer-causing substances)—act on the tissues of the lung and cause damage to cell nuclei.[43] Phlegm production increases (in proportion to the tar level and number of cigarettes smoked) but it does not provide complete protection. Irritants in the smoke, other than tar, also elicit protective responses and these cause lung airways to decrease in size.[44] The importance of this last statement is that low tar cigarettes may not reduce the risk for emphysema.

The 1982 report by the Surgeon General concluded: "Cigarette smoking is clearly identified as the chief preventable cause of death in our society and the most important public health issue of our time." In 1982, 111,000 will die from lung cancer. The report states, "It is estimated that 85% of lung cancer mortality could have been avoided if individuals never took up smoking."

To smoke or not to smoke. That choice may not always be around. The winds keep shifting and the action against cigarette smoking in this and other countries is taking on a different flavor. Until the mid-1970s the emphasis was solely on health considerations: smoking increases the chances that you will become sick, stay sick, die earlier. Only a certain percentage of people will respond to this rational-scare approach, although it will certainly continue as long as there are tobacco users.

Adverse social effects

The new trend is to decrease the social acceptability of smoking and the ease with which a person can smoke. Every year social stigma increases against the smoker. This has been supported by health facts, social action, legislative action, and judicial rulings. The United States has traveled this road before. In the last two decades of the nineteenth century, pure food and pure body zealots began to prowl the American landscape and were successful in setting the stage for the 1906 Pure Food and Drugs Act. As cigarette use increased, so did the antitobacco crusaders. From 1895 to 1907, 12 states banned cigarettes. In 1921 14 states had cigarette prohibition laws, and over 90 anticigarette bills were being considered by the legislative bodies of 28 states. By 1928, however, all the cigarette prohibition laws had been repealed.

The antismoking groups received a major boost in 1972 when the HEW report on smoking and health[45] discussed at length the dangers that the nonsmoker might be exposed to when in areas where other individuals are smoking. There were lots of qualifiers in the original scientific report, but they were lost in most of the translations to the public. Another point also hit home with the man in the street: a pregnant woman smoking beyond the fourth month of gestation endangers the life and health of the fetus.

The strategy of today's antismokers was nicely stated in 1975:

> Our campaign for the right of the non-smoker to breathe pure air has upset the tobacco companies more than anything we have done medically, educationally, scientifically, by legislation or by governmental regulation. The reason for the tobacco merchant's concern is as simple as it is important. If smoking is unacceptable social behavior—relegated to bathrooms, poolrooms, and bar-rooms, then the cigarette will follow the spittoon to oblivion. So long as smoking is regarded as a private form of slow suicide or self pollution, it will be difficult to generate the societal forces needed to combat, what is afterall, a societal problem; our goal is not to reform sinners, but to combat society's number one public health problem. To do that, we must marshall all possible social forces to achieve that goal.[46]

It is an interesting sociocultural, philosophical, medical, and legal question: to what extent and to what degree can cigarette and other tobacco users pollute the air, and then the people around them? The other side of the coin is how much can noncigarette users restrict the personal freedom of a cigarette or tobacco user?

The answer is not yet final, but the trend seems clear. A 1981 guideline in Great Britain would prohibit those who smoke more than 10 cigarettes a day from adopting healthy newborns. They could still adopt "imperfect" babies! Table 9-2 is a chronology of the significant governmental actions in the area of cigarette, and other, smoking. In 1973 the Chairman of the Consumer Product Safety Commission said that "cigarettes would rank at or near the top of our consumer product hazard act

TABLE 9-2 Governmental actions on smoking

1964	Surgeon General's report on smoking and health determines that cigarette smoking is a health hazard.
1966	Federal Cigarette Labeling and Advertising Act requires, as of January 1, cigarette packs to carry statement: CAUTION: CIGARETTE SMOKING MAY BE HAZARDOUS TO YOUR HEALTH.
1967	Federal Communications Commission rules that the "Fairness Doctrine" applies to cigarette advertising, and TV and radio must carry antismoking messages.
1970	Cigarette pack statement changed to WARNING: THE SURGEON GENERAL HAS DETERMINED THAT CIGARETTE SMOKING IS DANGEROUS TO YOUR HEALTH.
1971	Radio and TV ads banned as of January 2. Interstate Commerce Commission restricts smoking to rear five rows of interstate buses.
1972	All cigarette advertising must carry the same health warning as on packs, as well as the tar and nicotine content of a cigarette. The Consumer Product Safety Act specifically excludes cigarettes from being considered under the act.
1973	Arizona becomes first state to prohibit smoking in all elevators, indoor theaters, libraries, art galleries, museums, concert halls, and buses; all airlines required to designate smoking and no smoking areas in planes.
1975	Minnesota passes Indoor Clean Air Act, which makes smoking illegal in all public places and public meetings except where designated.
1978	Civil Aeronautics Board bans cigar and pipe smoking on all American commercial airlines.

. . . " but was unable to act officially. The Secretary of HEW asked Congress in 1975 for legislation that would limit the maximum level of T/N and carbon monoxide in cigarettes.

One of the most significant parts of the no-smoking movement is the passage of state and city laws to control smoking in public places. Arizona started it in 1973; by 1978 33 states plus the District of Columbia had passed laws restricting public smoking. Most of the laws made violation a misdemeanor, and people are getting fined.[47] Of particular importance is the way the laws are written: smoking is prohibited unless there are signs that specifically permit it. NO SMOKING signs are on their way out. In their place will be a much smaller number of SMOKING PERMITTED signs. (It has not gone unnoticed that as marijuana decriminalization laws increase, there is a decrease in the number of public places where smoking anything is permitted.)

Every year sees more restrictions placed on the cigarette user and on advertising. Over 20 countries have banned cigarette advertising on radio and TV, and several are considering a total ban on advertising any tobacco product anywhere. The Federal Trade Commission has recommended to Congress that the warning on cigarette packs be changed every 3 months and be much more explicit, for example: Smoking causes death from cancer, heart attack and lung disease.[48] It is hard to believe but a 1980 survey found that 41% of American smokers said they did not know that a typical 30 year old male shortened his life expectancy *at all* by smoking!

Cigarette smoking is a social and medical problem worldwide. The mid-1970s showed the start of many government programs to reduce smoking.[49-51] This leads to interesting situations since in many countries cigarettes are a state monopoly (for example, France and Japan) and a source of great amounts of revenue. (The United States has also been known to send mixed messages on cigarette smoking and other forms of drug use!)[52] As sales level and decline in developed countries, advertising and promotions in Third World countries ("the great taste of America") resulted in a 33% increase in American cigarette sales from 1970 to 1980.[53] There are *no* warnings printed on the packs we sell to them! (Shades of patent medicines in the late nineteenth century.) Realize that these are mostly underdeveloped countries with lots of preventable disease and high infant mortality, and then listen to the World Health Organization: ". . . the control of cigarette smoking could do more to improve health and prolong life in these countries than any single action in the whole field of preventive medicine."[54]

In the United States Congress is reluctant to pass overly restrictive laws, since the tobacco interests and states repeatedly point to the economic tax aspect of the situation. The judicial branch may end up carrying the ball for the antismokers. The date that may go down in history as the beginning of the end of smoking as a simple recreation is December 22, 1976. On that date the Superior Court of New Jersey handed down its decision in the case of *Shimp v. New Jersey Bell Telephone Company.* Mrs. Shimp is allergic to cigarette smoke and worked in a small office of the telephone company along with several other employees, some of whom smoked cigarettes. Several remedies were tried, none of which was successful, so Mrs. Shimp sued for a nonpolluted working environment. The judge's opinion is both interesting and important, since it is the first to establish several principles.

> The evidence is clear and overwhelming. Cigarette smoke contaminates and pollutes the air creating a health hazard not merely to the smoker but to all those around her who must rely upon the same air supply. The right of an individual to risk his or her own health does not include the right to jeopardize the health of those who must remain around him or her in order to properly perform the duties of their jobs. The portion of the population which is especially sensitive to cigarette smoke is so significant that it is reasonable to expect an employer to foresee health consequences and to impose upon him a duty to abate the hazard which causes the discomfort.
>
> In determining the extent to which smoking must be restricted the rights and interests of smoking and non smoking employees alike must be considered. The employees' rights to a safe working environment makes it clear that smoking must be forbidden in the work area. The employee who desires to smoke on his own time, during coffee breaks and lunch hours should have a reasonably accessible area in which to smoke.[55]

What the judge said is that people have a legal right to work and exist in a smokeless environment and that smoking is a privilege granted under certain conditions.

Medical facts, social pressures, and—the coup de grace—psychiatric opinion. The 1981 diagnostic manual of the American Psychiatric Association, which lists disorders considered to be psychiatric problems, contains for the first time several classifications associated with tobacco use. Maybe Szasz is right.[56] Jaffe, a psychiatrist and authority on drug abuse, believes that the person with a "compulsive smoking disorder"—more than a pack of cigarettes a day—has many similarities to alcoholics and opiate abusers.[57] And he is not alone.

NICOTINE

Nicotine is a naturally occurring liquid alkaloid that is colorless and volatile. On oxidation it turns brown and smells much like burning tobacco. Tolerance to its effects develops, along with the dependency that led Mark Twain to remark how easy it was to stop smoking—he'd done it several times!

Nicotine was isolated in 1828 and has been studied irregularly since then. It has no therapeutic actions, so no drug company has exhaustively looked at its effects. Since it has proved to be a valuable pharmacological tool for studying synaptic functions, as well as being the active ingredient in tobacco, there is some relevant information. The structure of nicotine is shown in Fig. 9-5; it should be noted that there are both d and l forms, but they are equipotent. It is of some importance that nicotine in smoke has two forms, one with a positive charge and one that is electrically neutral. The neutral form is more easily absorbed through the mucous membranes of the mouth, nose, and lungs.

Inhalation is a very effective drug-delivery system, with 90% of inhaled nicotine being absorbed. The physiological effects of smoking one cigarette have been mimicked by injecting about 1 mg of nicotine intravenously.

Acting with almost as much speed as cyanide, nicotine is well established as one of the most toxic drugs known. In humans, 60 mg is a lethal dose, and death follows intake within a few minutes. A cigar contains enough nicotine for two lethal doses (who needs to take a second one?), but not all of the nicotine is delivered to the smoker or absorbed in a short enough period of time to kill a person.[58]

Nicotine is primarily deactivated in the liver,

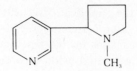

FIG. 9-5 Nicotine (1-methyl-2-[3-pyridly]pyrrolidine).

with between 80% and 90% being modified prior to excretion through the kidneys. Part of the tolerance that develops to nicotine may result from the fact that either nicotine or the "tars" increase the activity of the liver microsomal enzymes which are responsible for the deactivation of drugs. These enzymes increase the rate of deactivation and thus decrease the clinical effects of the benzodiazepines and some antidepressants and analgesics.[59] The final step in eliminating deactivated nicotine from the body may be somewhat slowed by nicotine itself, since it acts on the hypothalamus to cause a release of the hormone that acts to reduce the loss of body fluids.

Physiological effects

Nicotine. The effect of nicotine on areas outside the CNS has been studied extensively. One finding is that it has very clear effects on most cholinergic synapses. Nicotine mimics acetylcholine by acting at the cholinergic receptor site and stimulating the dendrite. Nicotine is not rapidly deactivated, and continued occupation of the receptor prevents incoming impulses from having an effect, thereby blocking transmission of information at the synapse. Thus nicotine first stimulates and then blocks the synapse. This blockage of cholinergic synapses is responsible for some of its effects, but others seem to be the result of a second action.

Nicotine also causes a release of adrenaline from the adrenal glands as well as from other sympathetic sites and thus has in part a sympathomimetic action. An additional action that should be identified is that it stimulates and then blocks some sensory receptors, including the chemical receptors found in some large arteries and the thermal pain receptors found in the skin and tongue.

The symptoms of a low-level nicotine poisoning are well known to beginning smokers and small children behind barns and in alleys: nausea, dizziness, and a general weakness. In acute poisoning, nicotine causes tremors that develop into convulsions, terminated frequently by death. The cause of death is suffocation resulting from paralysis of the muscles used in respiration. This paralysis stems from the blocking effect of nicotine on the cholinergic system that normally activates the muscles. With lower doses there is actually an increase in respiration rate because the nicotine stimulates oxygen-need receptors in the carotid artery. At these lower doses of 6 to 8 mg there is also a considerable effect on the cardiovascular system as a result of the release of adrenaline.[60] Such release leads to an increase in coronary blood flow, along with vasoconstriction in the skin and increased heart rate and blood pressure. The increased heart rate and blood pressure increase the oxygen need of the heart but not the oxygen supply. Another action of nicotine with negative health effects is that it increases platelet adhesiveness, which increases the tendency to clotting.

Within the CNS nicotine seems to act at the level of the cortex to increase somewhat the frequency of the electrical activity, that is, to shift the EEG toward an arousal pattern. In animal studies this alerting pattern after nicotine administration could be increased further by stimulation of the reticular formation so that if the observed cortical arousal is a real effect, it is only a partial basis for the behavioral effect.

Smoking. Many effects of nicotine are easily discernible in the smoking individual. The heat releases the nicotine from the tobacco into the smoke. Inhaling while smoking one cigarette has been shown to inhibit hunger contractions of the stomach for up to 1 hour. That finding, along with a very slight increase in blood sugar level and a deadening of the taste buds, may be the basis for a decrease in hunger after smoking.

In line with the last possibility, it has long been an old wives' tale that when a person stops smoking, he begins to nibble food and thus gains weight. Some reports suggest that this is not the only reason: weight gain is also the result of a lower metabolic rate in the nonsmoking individual. One report showed that when over-a-pack-a-day smokers stopped smoking, there was a three beat per minute decrease in heart rate and a 10% decrease in oxygen consumption. Slowing of the heart rate decreases, to some extent, the energy needs of the body. It seems more probable that the decrease in oxygen consumption results from a general decrease in the rate at which food is used for energy, so that with the same food intake, more will be shifted into fat storage depots.[61]

In a regular smoker, smoking results in a constriciton of the blood vessels in the skin along with a decrease in skin temperature and an increase in blood pressure. The blood supply to the skeletal muscles does not change with smoking, but a routine finding in a regular smoker is a higher than normal amount of carboxyhemoglobin (up to 10% of all hemoglobin) in the blood. All smoke contains carbon monoxide, with cigarette smoke being about 1% carbon monoxide, pipe smoke, 2%, and cigar smoke, 6%. The carbon monoxide combines with the hemoglobin in the blood so that it can no longer carry oxygen. It is this effect of smoking, a decrease in oxygen-carrying ability of the blood that probably explains the "shortness" of breath smokers experience when they exert themselves.

It is probable that the decrease in oxygen-carrying ability of the blood and the decrease in placental blood flow is related to the many results showing that pregnant women who smoke greatly endanger their unborn children. (See Chapter 4 for a discussion of smoking and pregnancy.)

Carbon monoxide (CO) may turn out to be a more toxic component in cigarette smoke than nicotine. Hemoglobin has over 200 times the affinity for CO than it does for oxygen, with the half-life in blood being 3 to 4 hours. Smoking one pack of regular cigarettes delivers 260 mg of CO to the user, an amount that the person would get otherwise only by breathing polluted air with CO levels near the warning level set by the government. The smoker in urban areas is in double jeopardy: blood samples were analyzed in Chicago, Los Angeles, Milwaukee, and New York City, and smokers had

3 to 5 times the amount of CO in their blood than did nonsmokers.[62] The risk for major atherosclerotic diseases, such as angina pectoris or myocardial infarction, is about 21 times as great for individuals with carboxyhemoglobin levels of 5% or more, compared to normal levels of 1% to 2%.

Behavioral effects

In spite of all the protests and the cautionary statements you may read or hear, the evidence is overwhelming that nicotine is the primary, if not the only, reinforcing substance in tobacco. Monkeys will work very hard when their only reward consists of regular intravenous injections of nicotine.[63] A superb review of the work up to 1978 shows that the more nicotine in a cigarette, the lower the level of smoking.[64] Intravenous injections and oral administration of nicotine will decrease smoking under some conditions—but not all.

An ongoing debate—in smokers as well as researchers—is whether nicotine acts to arouse and activate the smoker or whether it calms and tranquilizes the drug user. One review of the literature pointed very nicely to the paradoxical effects of nicotine, ". . . a substantial number of studies have shown that nicotine increases heart rate, blood pressure, and numerous other indices of autonomic arousal; yet rather than producing expected increases of emotional behavior and feelings, it usually decreases emotions."[65, p.657]

Most people smoke in a fairly consistent way, averaging one to two puffs per minute, with each puff lasting about 2 seconds with a volume of 25 cc. This rate delivers to the individual about 1 to 2 μg/kg of nicotine with each puff. There must be something optimal or unique about this dose, since smokers could increase the dose by increasing the volume of smoke with each puff or puffing more often.

A study using cats suggested that this dose rate is optimal in causing a release of acetylcholine from the cortex and an increase in EEG activation. When cats were given 2 μg/kg of nicotine intravenously every 30 seconds, 70% of the animals showed EEG activation, more than with other tested doses or delivery times. The similarity of this nicotine dose and administration interval to the human self-selected dose and interval was intentional. Thus it may be that one of the rewards a smoker receives that keeps him smoking is cortical arousal and an alerting of functions.[66] Some studies with humans point in this direction, but gross EEGs do not permit clear separation of the cortical arousal resulting from the pharmacological effect of nicotine and the arousal that is a result of the smoking behavior.

Other work points in another direction as an explanation for smoking behavior.[67] Heavy smokers compared to nonsmokers show a higher level of cortical activation even in the absence of smoking. On the basis of the frequent finding that nicotine causes an initial stimulation and then a transient depression of synaptic activity, it has been suggested that smokers may be inducing brief periods of tranquilization, that is, a decrease in cortical arousal. This would agree with reports that cigarette smoking increases during periods of stress and tension.

One very important point must be made in connection with that last statement. In times of stress the acidity of the urine increases. Nicotine is filtered from the body and excreted more rapidly in acidic urine.[68] Smoking increases under stress to maintain the nicotine level of the body. Since that may be an important part of the control of smoking someone has suggested that the mind of a smoker is in his bladder.

SMOKING—HOW NOT TO

A lot of people want to stop smoking. A lot of people have already stopped. Are there ways to efficiently and effectively help those individuals who want to stop smoking to stop? With any form of pleasurable drug use it is easier to keep people from starting to use the drug than it is to have them stop once they have started. All the educational programs have had an effect on our society and on our behavior. One analysis of the impact of this nation's antismoking campaign concluded that ". . . in the absence of the antismoking campaign

consumption (of cigarettes) would have exceeded its 1978 level by more than a third."[69,p.729] That's not bad for starters. Those individuals who stop smoking on their own seem to stay stopped longer than those who enter stop-smoking programs.[64] One review of 89 studies showed that only 20% to 30% of smokers who completed a program were still abstinent 6 months later.[70] The data are less promising for some of the bad programs—such as acupuncture.[71,72] The data are *even less* promising if you monitor urine nicotine levels, rather than just ask people about their smoking habits. I know it will shock most of the readers of this book but: people lie. At least people say they aren't smoking but there is still nicotine in their urine.[73]

What to do? Why is it so hard? One reason is that the pack-a-day smoker puffs at least 50,000 times a year. That's a lot of rewarded (pleasurable) behavior. How about cutting down? Many smokers who switch to lower T/N cigarettes increase the number of cigarettes they smoke each day. It's possible to keep the same brand, and thus same T/N, and use shorter cigarettes (by cutting off their ends). When that's done smokers puff harder and smoke more cigarettes.[74] The critical thing is keeping that body nicotine level up! As mentioned earlier, snuff will do that but it has some disadvantages.

Someone is going to make a lot of money by providing a rewarding level of nicotine without the negative side effects that are the result of the tars and carbon monoxide. Reduction in tar is easy; carbon monoxide reduction is a bit harder if you're burning something. Some individuals are now trying a smokeless smoking device that delivers vaporized nicotine.[75] The other approach, and much farther along, is nicotine-containing chewing gum.[76] Nicotine-containing gum is available on prescription in Britain and Canada. It has been approved only for experimental use in the United States and comes in sticks containing 1, 2, or 4 mg of nicotine. Early use suggests that the chewing gum may be particularly helpful with individuals who have high intakes of nicotine from their cigarettes. One study[77] monitored carboxyhemoglobin levels to ensure truthfulness and found that 1 year after treatment 38% of nicotine gum users were still not smoking while 14% of those who received only "psychological" treatment were still abstinent.

Is there a nondrug program that can be recommended to others, or used on one's self? Yes and no. A review of programs and techniques, "Behavioral Treatment of Smoking Behavior",[78] makes two points that are relevant here: There is a lot of variability in the effect of a given program—some people do very well, some very poorly and if one program won't work for an individual, maybe another one will. Fact is, we don't know enough yet to place a smoker in a program that is best for him. If you want—that is, are *really* motivated—to stop smoking, keep trying programs; odds are you'll find one that works . . . eventually.

It *is* possible to stop and it's well worth the effort.[79,80] After everything has been said, stopping smoking—or any other habit—depends on the motivation to stop, the conviction that it's possible to stop, and the availability of a substitute or an adequate reward for stopping. All the rehabilitation, therapy, behavior modification, and other procedures are just devices to make the process easier. But remember, if one technique doesn't work, try another, and another, and. . . .

ONE LAST PUFF

When you're young and healthy it's difficult, if not impossible, to think about death, being chronically ill, or having emphysema so bad you can't get enough oxygen to walk across the room without having to stop to catch your breath. By the time you start to think and worry about those things it's difficult to change your health habits.

Think about these things. If you smoke about a pack a day you probably increase the probability of dying of lung cancer 1100%, of any other cancer 200%, of respiratory disease 400%, and of other causes 200%.[81] Looked at another way, smoking 2 packs of cigarettes a day you decrease the remaining years of your life by 20% if you're 35, by 24% if you're 45, 29% at 55, and 34% at 65.[82] At the least, tell your parents how much of their lives they are throwing away by smoking. Tell them one more

thing. A study in the early 1980s showed that the level of intake of "dietary provitamin A (carotene) was inversely related to the 19-year incidence of lung cancer."[83] Not true for other cancers, other nutrients. Only lung cancer was down when the carotene intake was up. That is not a solitary finding and there is considerable other evidence to support the relationship. Researchers are not sure of the mechanisms that may be operating but, if you smoke, smoke low tar/nicotine cigarettes and eat lots of dark-green leafy vegetables and carrots.

You will have to make your own decision about smoking, since we still have the choice. The mixed messages that descend from the highest pinnacles of government don't make decisions any easier for the consumer and potential consumer. Remember, though, that *all* the messages are true: cigarette smoking *is* bad for your health; cigarette smoking may not have *any* negative effects on your performance in the absence of a health problem; cigarette smokers and nonsmokers *do* have rights, and those rights should not be denied or reduced without good justification.

REFERENCES

1. Stewart, G.G.: A history of the medicinal use of tobacco, 1492-1860, Medical History **11**:228-268, 1967.
2. Brooks, J.E.: The mighty leaf, Boston, 1952, Little, Brown & Co.
3. Vaughn, W.: Quoted in Dunphy, E.B.: Alcohol and tobacco amblyopia: a historical survey, American Journal of Ophthalmology **68**:573, 1969.
4. Molière: Don Juan ou le festin de Pierre, Paris, 1969, Éditions Bordas (free translation from the French).
5. Corti: A history of smoking, London, 1931, George G. Harrap & Co. Ltd.
6. Russell, M.A.H., and others: A new age for snuff? Lancet **1**:474-475, March 1, 1980.
7. Winn, D.M., and others: Snuff dipping and oral cancer among women in the southern United States, New England Journal of Medicine **304**(13):745-749, 1981.
8. Heimann, R.K.: Tobacco and Americans, New York, 1960, McGraw-Hill Book Co.
9. Guinness book of records, New York, 1981, Bantam Books, Inc.
10. Moore, M.: Smokeless tobacco is "burning" young athletes, Physician and Sports Medicine **9**(3):21, 1981.
11. Shaw, B.: Enduring American symbol, 1,000 barn walls of art, Tobacco Observer, **6**:5, October 1981.

12. Edison, T.A. Quoted in Brooks, J.E.: The mighty leaf, Boston, 1952, Little, Brown & Co.
13. Sullivan, J.L. Quoted in Brooks, J.E.: The mighty leaf, Boston, 1952, Little, Brown & Co.
14. Hoffman, P.: Tobacco: leaf to cigarette, New York Times, September 26, 1976, pp. 11, 19.
15. King, W.: Millions in sales taxes lost to cigarette smugglers, New York Times, September 4, 1977, p. 1.
16. Raab, S.: Tax loss in north feared, New York Times, October 13, 1981, p. B17.
17. Foreign cigarettes ride an easy road to sales, New York Times, August 9, 1981, p. F21.
18. The health consequences of smoking: the changing cigarette, a report of the Surgeon General, U.S. Department of Health and Human Services, Washington, D.C., 1981, U.S. Government Printing Office.
19. Report of "tar", nicotine and carbon monoxide of the smoke of 200 varieties of cigarettes, Federal Trade Commission, December 1981.
20. Brecher, E.M.: Smoking for most, a sentence to nicotine addiction, Medical World News, p. 61, March 5, 1979.
21. Kozlowski, L.T.: Tar and nicotine delivery of cigarettes, Journal of the American Medical Association 245(2):158-159, 1981.
22. Kuhn, H., and Klus, H.: Possibilities for the reduction of nicotine in cigarette smoke, Proceedings of the Third World Conference on Smoking and Health, vol. 1, Publication No. (NIH) 76-1221, U.S. Department of Health, Education, and Welfare, Washington, D.C., 1976, U.S. Government Printing Office.
23. Gori, G.B.:Low-risk cigarettes: a prescription, Science 194:1243-1245, 1976.
24. Lorand, A.: Life shortening habits and rejuvenation, Philadelphia, 1927, F.A. Davis Co.
25. Ochsner, A.: Influence of smoking on sexuality and pregnancy, Medical Aspects of Human Sexuality 5:81-92, November 1971.
26. Subak-Sharpe, G.J.: Is your sex life going up in smoke? Readers Digest, pp. 104-107, January 1975.
27. Subak-Sharpe, G.J.: Is your sex life going up in smoke? Today's Health, pp. 50-53, 70, August 1974.
28. Sterling, T.D., and Lobayashi, D.: A critical review of reports on the effect of smoking on sex and fertility, Journal of Sex Research 11(3):201-217, 1975.
29. Eaglin, J.: The CC cough-fin brand cigarettes, Cincinnati, 1931, Raisbeck & Co., Printers.
30. Ochsner, A.: Comment at the International Cancer Congress of 1939, cited in new release of the American Cancer Society, December 1970.
31. Smoking and health: a report of the Surgeon General, U.S. Department of Health, Education, and Welfare, Washington, D.C. 1979, U.S. Government Printing Office.
32. Cowell, M.J., and Hirst, B.L.: Mortality differences between smokers and nonsmokers, State Mutual Life assurance Company of America, 1979.
33. Aronow, W.S.: The effect of smoke on the nonsmoker, Family Practice 1(7):47, 1979.
34. Repace, J.L., and Lowrey, A.H.: Indoor air pollution, tobacco smoke, and public health, Science 203:464-472, May 2, 1980.
35. Hirayama, T.: Non-smoking wives of heavy smokers have a higher risk of lung cancer: a study from Japan, British Medical Journal 282:183-185, January 17, 1981.
36. Miscalculation reported in study on cancer in wives of smokers, New York Times, June 15, 1981, p. B7.
37. White, J.R., and Froeb, H.F.: Small-airways dysfunction in nonsmokers chronically exposed to tobacco smoke, New England Journal of Medicine 302(13):720-723, 1980.
38. Garfinkel, L.: Time trends in lung cancer mortality among nonsmokers and a note on passive smoking, Journal of the National Cancer Institute 66(6):1061-1066, 1981.
39. Aronow, W.S.: Cigarette smoking and heart disease: an update, Consultant, p. 47, July 1980.
40. Criqui, M.H., and others: Cigarette smoking appears to decrease HDL levels, American Family Physician, 21(3):165-166, 1980.
41. Laties, V.G., and Merigan, W.H.: Behavioral effects of carbon monoxide on animals and man, Annual Review Pharmacologic Toxicology 19:357-392, 1979.
42. Gordon, T., Kannel, W.B., McGee, D., and Dawber, T.R.: Death and coronary attacks in men after giving up cigarette smoking. A report from the Framingham study, Lancet 2:1345-1348, 1974.
43. Averbach, O., and others: Changes in bronchial epithelium in relation to cigarette smoking, 1955-1960 vs 1970-1977, New England Journal of Medicine 300(8):381-386, 1979.
44. Higenbottom, T., and others: Lung function and symptoms of cigarette smokers related to tar yield and number of cigarettes smoked, Lancet 1:409-412, February 23, 1980.
45. The health consequences of smoking, U.S. Department of Health, Education and Welfare; Public Health Service, Washington, D.C., 1972, U.S. Government Printing Office.
46. Steinfeld, J.: The health consequences of smoking, Proceedings of the Third World Conference on Smoking and Health, vol. 1, Publication No. (NIH) 76-1221, U.S. Department of Health, Education, and Welfare, Washington, D.C., 1976, U.S. Government Printing Office.
47. Kneeland, D.E.: Antismoking drive keeps gaining, but impetus seems to have slowed, New York Times, January 26, 1979, p. A8.
48. Myers, M.L., and others: Staff report on the cigarette advertising investigation, Federal Trade Commission, May 1981.
49. French agencies clash on antismoking campaign, New York Times, March 12, 1978, p. L7.
50. Yoshizaki, H.: Antismoking drive is penetrating a thick haze in Japan, New York Times, May 13, 1978, p. M25.
51. Swedish anti-smoking campaign success, Tennessean, 73(76):11, June 23, 1978.

52. HEW Secretary Califano's anti-smoking campaign puts to-bacco addiction studies on "hold," Washington Drug Review 3(1):5, 1978.

53. Broad, W.J.: Use of killer weed grows in third world, Science **208**:474, May 1980.

54. Broady, J.E.: Personal health, New York Times, July 8, 1981, p. C18.

55. *Shimp* v. *New Jersey Bell Telephone Company*, Superior Court of New Jersey, Chancery Division, Salem County, Docket No. C-2904-75, filed December 22, 1976.

56. Szasz, T.S.: The myth of mental illness, rev. ed., New York, 1974, Harper & Row, Publishers, Inc.

57. Jaffe, J. Quoted by Bordy, J.E., in New York Times, June 5, 1975.

58. Armitage, A., and others: Absorption of nicotine from small cigars, Clinical Pharmacology and Therapeutics 23(2):143-151, February 1978.

59. Decreased clinical efficacy of propoxyphene in cigarette smokers, Clinical Pharmacology and Therapeutics **14**:259-263, 1973.

60. Jarvik, M.E.: Biological influences on cigarette smoking. In Krasnegor, N.A., editor: The behavioral aspects of smoking, NIDA Research Monograph 26, Washington, D.C., August 1979, U.S. Government Printing Office.

61. Glauser, S.C., and others: Metabolic changes associated with the cessation of cigarette smoking, Archives of Environmental Health **20**:377-381, 1970.

62. Carboxyhemoglobin concentrations in blood from donors in Chicago, Milwaukee, New York, and Los Angeles, Science **182**:789-796, 1973.

63. Goldberg, S.R., and others: Persistent behavior at high rates maintained by intravenous self-administration of nicotine, Science **214**:573-575, October 30, 1981.

64. Jarvik, M.E.: Biological factors underlying the smoking habit. In Jarvik, M.E., and others, editors: Research on smoking behavior, NIDA Research Monograph 17, Washington, D.C., December 1977, U.S. Government Printing Office.

65. Gilbert, O.G.: Paradoxical tranquilizing and emotion-reducing effects of nicotine, Psychological Bulletin 86(4):643-662.

66. Armitage, A.K., Hall, G.H., and Morrison, C.F.: Pharmacological basis for the tobacco smoking habit, Nature **217**:331-334, 1968, Hall, G.H.: Effects of nicotine and tobacco smoke on the electrical activity of the cerebral cortex and olfactory bulb, British Journal of Pharmacology **38**:271-286, 1970.

67. Brown, B.B.: Some characteristic EEG differences between heavy smoker and non-smoker subjects, Neuropsychologia **6**:381-388, 1968.

68. Schachter, S., and others: Effects of urinary pH on cigarette smoking, Journal of Experimental Psychology, General **90**1(1):13, 1977.

69. Warner, K.E.: Cigarette smoking in the 1970's: the impact of the antismoking campaign on consumption, Science **211**:729-731, February 13, 1981.

70. Hallam, K.: How to become a nonsmoker: the behavioral approach, Current Prescribing, p. 99, February, 1979.

71. Lamontagne, Y., and others: Acupuncture for smokers: lack of long-term therapeutic effect in a controlled study, Canadian Medical Association Journal, **122**:787, April 5, 1980.

72. Tichenor, W.S., and Solomon, N.: Cessation of smoking, Journal of the American Medical Association 245(4):341, 1981.

73. Kozlowski, L.T., and others: What researchers make of what cigarette smokers say: filtering smokers' hot air, Lancet, 1(8170):699, March 29, 1980.

74. Russell, M.A.H., and others: Smokers' response to shortened cigarettes: dose reduction without dilution of tobacco smoke, Clinical Pharmacology and Therapeutics 27(2):210, 218, February 1980.

75. Gonzalez, E.F.: Snuffing out the cigarette habit: how about another source of nicotine? Journal of the American Medical Association 244(2):112, 1980.

76. Schneider, N.G., and others: The use of nicotine gum during cessation of smoking, American Journal of Psychiatry **134**(4):439, 1977.

77. Raw, M., and others: Comparison of nicotine chewing-gum and psychological treatments for dependent smokers, British Medical Journal, 281(6238):481, August 16, 1980.

78. Glasgow, R.E., and Bernstein, D.A.: Behavioral treatment of smoking behavior. In Prokop, C.K., and Bradley, L.A., editors: Medical psychology, New York, 1981, Academic Press, Inc.

79. Ockene, J.K., and Ockene, I.S.: 9 ways to help your patients stop smoking, Your Patient and Cancer, p. 47, January 1982.

80. Wynder, E.L.: Tobacco as a carcinogen, Your Patient and Cancer, p. 40, August 1981.

81. Doll, R., and Peto, R.: The causes of cancer: quantitative estimates of avoidable risks of cancer in the United States today, Journal of National Cancer Institute 66(6):1221, 1981.

82. Rogot, E.: Smoking and life expectancy among U.S. veterans, Public Health Briefs, American Journal of Public Health 68(10):1023-1025, 1978.

83. Shekelle, R.B., and others: American Journal of Public Health: Dietary vitamin A and risk of cancer in the Western Electric study, Lancet, 2(8257):1185-1189, November 28, 1981.

CHAPTER 10

CAFFEINE

HOW MANY DRUGS CAN LAY CLAIM to divine intervention in their introduction to mankind? The xanthines, of which caffeine is the best known, have three such legends, and that fact alone tells you that this has been an important class of drugs throughout the ages. Caffeine is the psychoactive agent in coffee.

COFFEE

The legends surrounding the origin of coffee are at least geographically correct. The best concerns an Arabian goatherd named Kaldi who couldn't understand why his goats were bouncing around the hillside like a bunch of kids. One day he followed them up the mountain and ate some of the red berries the goats were munching. "The results were amazing. Kaldi became a happy goatherd. Whenever his goats danced he danced and whirled and leaped and rolled about on the ground." Kaldi took the first coffee trip! A holy man took in the scene, and "that night he danced with Kaldi and the goats." A veritable orgy. The legend continues with Mohammed telling the holy man to boil the berries in water and have the brothers in the monastery drink the liquid so they could keep awake and continue their prayers.[1]

Around 900 AD an Arabian medical book sug-

gested that coffee was good for just about everything, including measles and reducing lust. Once something gets into the literature, it's very difficult to change people's minds; women in England argued against the use of coffee over 700 years later. They published a 1674 pamphlet titled "The Women's Petition Against Coffee, representing to public consideration the grand inconveniences accruing to their sex from the excessive use of the drying and enfeebling liquor." The women claimed men used too much coffee, and as a result the men were as "unfruitful as those *Desarts* whence that unhappy *Berry* is said to be brought." The women were *really* unhappy, and the pamphlet continued:

> Our Countrymens pallates are become as *Fanatical* as their Brains; how else is't possible they should *Apostatize* from the good old primitive way of Ale-drinking, to run a *Whoreing* after such variety of distructive Foreign Liquors, to trifle away their time, scald their *Chops*, and spend their *Money*, all for a little *base, black, thick, nasty bitter stinking, nauseous* Puddle water. . . .[2]

Some men probably sat long hours in one of the many coffee houses composing "The Men's Answer to the Women's Petition Against Coffee," which said in part:

Why must innocent COFFEE be the object of your Spleen? That harmless and healing Liquor, which Indulgent Providence first sent amongst us. . . . Tis not this incomparable fettle Brain that shortens Natures standard, or makes us less Active in the Sports of Venus, and we wonder you should take these Exceptions. . . .[2]

We can all rest easier today and discuss over a cup of coffee the fact that gradually became clear: there is no truth to the idea that coffee diminishes sexual excitability or reduces lust. It is doubtful that the Arabians beleved it either, since the use of coffee spread throughout the Muslim world. However, some animal studies do show a decrease in fertility from caffeine.[3] In Mecca people spent so much time in coffeehouses that the use of coffee was outlawed, and all supplies of the coffee bean were burned. Prohibition rarely works, and coffee speakeasies began to open. Wiser heads prevailed, and the prohibition was lifted.

The middle of the seventeenth century saw the same play enacted but with a new cast of characters and a different locale. Coffeehouses began appearing in England (1650) and France (1671), and a new era began. Coffeehouses were all things to all people: a place to relax, to learn the news of the day, to seal bargains, to plot! This last possibility made Charles II of England so nervous that he outlawed coffeehouses, labeling them "hot-beds of seditious talk and slanderous attacks upon persons in high stations." King Charles was no more successful than the women. In only 11 days the ruling was withdrawn, and the coffee houses developed into the "penny universities" of the early eighteenth century. For a penny a cup you could listen to and learn from most of the great literary and political figures of the period. Lloyds of London, the insurance house, started in Edward Lloyd's coffeehouse around 1700.

Across the channel, cheap wine made the need for another social drink less essential in France than in England. French coffeehouses made at least one contribution to Western culture, the cancan! French cabaret owners were not ready to turn the other cheek, and they fought back: one owner was able to persuade his cancan girls to perform without bloomers! In spite of this, coffeehouses survived, and coffee consumption increased. In 1974 France was consuming almost 12 pounds of coffee per person per year.

Across the Atlantic, coffee drinking increased in the English colonies, although tea was still their thing. Cheaper and more available than coffee, tea had everything, including, beginning in 1765, a 3-pence-a-pound tax on its importation!

The British Act that taxed tea helped fan the fire that lit the musket that fired the shot heard around the world. That story is better told in connection with tea, but the final outcome was that to be a tea drinker was to be a Tory. Coffee became the new country's national drink.

Coffee use expanded as the West was won, and the amount consumed by each person showed steady increases. Some experts became worried about the tendency to "have another cup of coffee," although they believed they could explain it. One wrote:

> The absolute coercion which is imposed on the Americans of the United States by the Prohibition Act with respect to alcohol has necessarily had the result of greatly increasing the use of other excitants and also narcotics. . . . The consumption of coffee has also developed in an undreamt-of manner. In 1919 929.2 million pounds were consumed and in 1920 as many as 1,360 million pounds. The consumption therefore increased from 9 to 12.9 pounds per head per year, and is approaching the threshold of abuse.[4,p.253]

Funny thing: prohibition went away, and coffee consumption continued to rise. We must have been well over the "threshold of abuse" in 1946 when coffee consumption reached an all-time high of 20 pounds per person. The trend has been downhill since then (although the population growth has blunted the impact of decreased use): the United States consumed 11 pounds of coffee per person in 1981.

Some of the decrease can be attributed to changing life-styles—sun and fun and convenient cold canned drinks seem to fit together better. It probably isn't true that people are using fewer bever-

TABLE 10-1 Consumption of beverages (percent of persons)

	1950	1962	1976	1981
Coffee	75	75	59	56
Milk, milk drinks	51	53	50	50
Juices	33	41	44	48
Soft drinks	29	33	49	52
Tea	24	25	26	33
Cocoa, hot chocolate	5	5	4	4

ages, they are just shifting what they drink. Table 10-1 shows the percentage of Americans over the age of 10 who drank different beverages on typical winter days in 1950, 1962, 1976, and 1981.[5]

If the national drink is not as national as it once was, neither is it as simple. Kaldi and his friends could just munch on the coffee beans or put them in hot water and be content. Somewhere in the dark past, probably when the warehouses were burned down, the Middle East discovered that roasting the green coffee bean did not ruin it but, in fact, improved the flavor, aroma, and color of the drink made from the bean. For years housewives, storekeepers, and coffeehouse owners bought the green bean, then roasted and ground it just before use. Everyone made coffee in the hobo way, which many experts still believe is the best method: put freshly ground coffee in cold water in a nonmetallic container, bring to nearly a boil, let cool 3 to 5 minutes, use salt or egg shells to settle the grounds, and drink.

What could be simpler? Well, it really is quite a chore to roast your own coffee beans. In addition to turning them regularly, it is difficult to achieve the 400° F temperature for just the right amount of time and then rapidly cool the beans. Commercial roasting started in 1790 in New York City, and the process gradually spread through the country. One problem is that, while the green bean can be stored indefinitely, the roasted bean deteriorates seriously within a month. Ground coffee can be maintained at its peak level in the home only for a week or two, and then only if it is in a closed

container and refrigerated. Vacuum packing of ground coffee was introduced in 1900, a process that maintains the quality until the seal is broken.

Coffee growing spread worldwide when the Dutch began cultivation in the East Indies in 1696. Latin America had an ideal climate for coffee growing, and with the world's greatest coffee-drinking nation just up the road several thousand miles, it became the world's largest producer. Different varieties of the coffee tree and different growing and processing conditions provide many opportunities for varying the characteristics of coffee.

No one really went commercial with a combination of different coffee beans until J.O. Cheek developed a blend in 1892 and introduced it through a famous Nashville hotel: Maxwell House. The coffee was so well received that the hotel owners let the coffee be named after the hotel. Today Maxwell House sells about 22% of all coffee consumed in the United States, second to Folgers (as of 1978), which sells about 27% of the total.

In the early 1950s about 94% of American coffee was from Latin America, but that percentage has steadily declined; today less than half is grown in this hemisphere. Brazil is the principal exporter to the United States, with Colombia second. Both countries grow *arabica,* which has a caffeine content of about 1%. *Robusta,* with a caffeine level at 2%, is the variety grown in Africa and is usually of a lower grade and price.

The economics of coffee (it is number two in international trade, far behind oil) have as much to do with coffee consumption as does our changing life-style. A price increase in the early fifties—to a dollar a pound!—shifted us from a 40-cups-per-pound to a 60-cups-per-pound nation. This dilution reduced the cost but also the quality of the beverage. Two things happen when prices go up: the quality of the coffee decreases and people drink less coffee. Instant coffee has been around since before the turn of the century, but sales began their marked increase in the hustle and bustle following World War II: another decrease in the quality of the beverage, but an increase in the convenience. Interestingly, Brazil imports many inexpensive African coffee beans to use in manufacturing instant coffee, since they believe that their coffee is too good to be used in that way.

Sales of instant coffee have remained constant for many years and constitute between 40% and 45% of consumer purchases. Expanding rapidly but still a small part of the total market is decaffeinated coffee. About 18% of home-used coffee is now decaffeinated. Caffeine is removed from the green bean by using alcohol as the solvent; decaffeinated coffee has a slightly different taste, since some oils and waxes are also removed. The alcohol is then distilled away and the caffeine collected. Like the squeal in a slaughterhouse, nothing is wasted: the caffeine is used in soft drinks. One of the largest decaffeinating companies is owned by Coca-Cola.

Where can we go from here? Coffee without roasting, then coffee without grinding, then coffee without grounds, then coffee without caffeine. There have been several coffee substitutes without coffee patented. Man triumphs over nature again— or does he?

TEA

Tea and coffee are not like day and night, but their differences are reflected in the legends surrounding their origins. The bouncing goatherd of Arabia suggests that coffee is a boisterous, blue-collar drink. Tea is a different story: much softer, quieter, more delicate. According to one legend, Daruma, the founder of Zen Buddhism, fell asleep one day while meditating. Resolving that it would never happen again, he cut off both eyelids. From the spot where his eyelids touched the earth grew a new plant. From its leaves a brew could be made that would keep a person awake. Appropriately the tea tree, *Thea sinensis* (now classed as *Camellia sinensis*) is an evergreen, and *sinensis* is the Latin word for Chinese.

The first report of tea that seems reliable is in a Chinese manuscript around 350 AD when it was primarily seen as a medicinal plant. The nonmedical use of tea is suggested by a 780 AD book on the cultivation of tea, but the real proof that it was in wide use in China is that a tax was levied on it in the same year. Before this time Buddhist monks had carried the cultivation and use of tea to Japan.

Europe had to wait eight centuries to savor the herb that was "good for tumors or abscesses that come from the head, or for ailments of the bladder . . . it quenches thirst. It lessens the desire for sleep. It gladdens and cheers the heart." The first European record of tea, in 1559, says, "One or two cups of this decoction taken on an empty stomach removes fever, headache, stomach-ache, pain in the side or in the joints. . . ." It was 50 years later in 1610 that the Dutch delivered the first tea to the continent of Europe.

An event occurred 10 years before that which had tremendous impact on the history of the world and on present patterns of drug use. In 1600 the English East India Company was formed, and Queen Elizabeth gave the company a monopoly on everything from the east coast of Africa across the Pacific to the west coast of South America! In this period the primary imports from the Far East were spices, and the company prospered. A major conflict developed between the Dutch and English trade interests over who belonged where in the East. In 1623 a resolution "gave" the Dutch East India Company the islands (the Dutch East Indies), while the English East Indian Company had to be content with India and other countries on the continent!

The English East India Company concentrated on importing spices, so the first tea was brought to England by the Dutch. As the market for tea increased, the English East India Company expanded its imports of tea from China. Coffee had arrived first, so most tea was sold in coffeehouses. Even as tea's use as a popular social drink expanded in Europe, there were some prophets of doom. A 1635 publication by a physician claimed that, at the very least, using tea would speed the death of those over 40 years old. The use of tea was not slowed, though, and by 1657 tea was being sold to the public in England. This was no more than 10 years after the English had developed the present word for it: tea. Although spelled *tea*, it was pronounced *tāy* until the nineteenth century. Prior to this period the Chinese name *ch'a* had been used, anglicized to either *chia* or *chaw*.

With the patrons of taverns off at coffeehouses living it up with tea, coffee, and chocolate, tax revenues from alcoholic beverages declined. To offset this loss, coffeehouses were licensed, and a tax of 8 cents was levied on each gallon of tea and chocolate sold. To keep the profits from the expanding tea trade at home, Britain banned Dutch imports of tea in 1669, which gave the English East India Company a monopoly. Profit from the China tea trade colonized India, brought about the Opium Wars between China and Britain, and induced the English to switch from coffee to tea. In the last half of the eighteenth century, the East India Company carried out a "Drink Tea" campaign unlike anything ever seen before that time. Advertising, patriotism, low cost on tea, and high taxes on alcohol made Britain a nation of tea drinkers.

It was the same profit motive that led to the American Revolution. Because the English East India Company had a monopoly on importing tea to England and thence to the American colonies, the British government imposed high duties on tea when it was taken from warehouses and offered for sale. But, as frequently happens, when taxes went up, consumption did not go down, but smuggling increased. It reached the point in Britain where more smuggled tea than legal tea was being consumed. The American colonies, though, ever loyal to the king, were becoming big tea drinkers, which helped the king and the East India Company stay solvent. The Stamp Act in 1765, which included a tax on tea, changed everything. Even though the Stamp Act was repealed in 1766, it was replaced by the Trade and Revenue Act of 1767, which did the same thing.

These measures made the colonists unhappy over paying taxes they had not helped formulate (taxation without representation), and in 1767 this resulted in a general boycott on the consumption of English tea. Coffee use increased, but the primary increase was in the smuggling of tea. The drop in legal tea sales filled the tea warehouses and put the East India Company in financial trouble. To save the company, in 1773 Parliament gave the East India Company the right to sell tea in the American Colonies without paying the tea taxes.

The company was also allowed to sell the tea through its own agents, and this would eliminate the profits of the merchants in the colonies.

Several boatloads of this tea, which would be sold cheaper than any before, sailed toward different ports in the colonies. The American merchants would not have made any profit on this tea, and they were the primary ones who rebelled at the cheap tea. Some ships were just turned away from port, but the beginning of the end came with the 342 chests of tea that turned the Boston harbor into a teapot on the night of December 16, 1773.

The revolution in America and the colonists' rejection of tea helped tea sales in Great Britain, since to be a tea drinker was to be loyal to the Crown. Many factors contributed to change the English from coffee to tea drinkers, and the preference for tea persists today. Although their use of coffee increases yearly and that of tea declines, the English are still tea drinkers. In 1981 the per capita consumption in the United Kingdom was 8 pounds of tea, second in the world only to Ireland. Oddly enough, over 80% of the coffee sold in the United Kingdom is instant coffee. In 1981 Americans averaged about 8/10 of a pound of tea (enough for 160 cups), this has remained fairly constant for several years.

From plant to pot

Most of the tea (about 70%) that comes to America starts life on a 4- to 5-foot bush high in the mountains of Sri Lanka (Ceylon), India, or Indonesia. Unpruned, the bush would grow into a 15- to 30-foot tree, which would be difficult to pluck, as picking tea leaves is called. The pluckers select only the bud-leaf and the first two leaves at each new growth; these are the "tiny little tea leaves." The bud-leaf is called flowering orange pekoe, the second leaf is larger and called orange pekoe, and the third and largest is pekoe (pekoe is pronounced "peck-ho," *not* "peak-o"). Orange pekoe is not a variety of tea but rather a size and quality of tea leaf, since generally the bud-leaf is of highest quality and the third leaf of lowest quality.

In one day a plucker will pluck enough leaves to

make 10 pounds of tea in the grocery store. Plucking is done every 6 to 10 days in warm weather as new growth develops on the many branches. The leaves are dried, rolled to crush the cells in the leaf, and placed in a cool, damp place for fermentation (oxidation) to occur. This oxidation turns the green leaves to a bright copper color. Nonoxidized leaves are packaged and sold as green tea, the type used in Chinese restaurants in this country. Oxidized tea is called black tea and accounts for about 98% of the tea Americans consume. Oolong tea is greenish-brown, since it consists of partially oxidized, fermented leaves.

After sorting and packing, the tea is shipped in airtight boxes to the U.S. This is when some of the unique rules about tea become evident. It all started in 1869 when the Suez Canal opened, and large, fast steamships began to replace the smaller, famous and beautiful wind-powered clipper ships on the tea run to this country. In the effort to maximize profits and keep the new ships full and busy, low-quality tea was being shipped over the new supply lines.

An 1883 law, but especially the Tea Importation Act of 1897, was designed to set minimum standards of quality in the tea that could be sold in the United States. This may have been the earliest of the consumer protection laws. The 1897 Act required that samples be taken of each tea shipment, and only those which exceeded a certain minimum quality could be released for sale.

How do you determine the quality of a tea? Right, you taste it. The FDA has three official tasters, one each in New York, San Francisco, and Boston, and they brew many cups of tea a day from samples taken from arriving shipments. The mixture is composed of 5 ounces of boiling water and ¼ ounce of tea, which they slurp from (you guessed it) a teaspoon. After swirling it in the mouth, they spit it out and go on to the next cup. The taste test tells the taster if the tea meets minimum taste standards that are established each year in February. Separate standards for each of the seven types of tea are now recognized by the FDA. Tastes in tea change, as does the way in which people like to take their tea.[6]

Until 1904 the only choices available were sugar, cream, and lemon with your hot tea. At the Louisiana Purchase Exposition in St. Louis in 1904, iced tea was sold for the first time. It now accounts for 75% of all tea consumed in America. 1904 was a very good year for tea lovers. Fifteen hundred miles east of the fair, a New York City tea merchant decided to send out his samples in hand-sewn silk bags rather than tin containers. Back came the orders—send us tea, and send it in the same little bags you used to send the samples. From that inauspicious beginning evolved the modern tea bag machinery that cuts the filter paper, weighs the tea, and attaches the tag: all this at a rate of 150 to 180 tea bags a minute.

Convenience continues to be the name of the game in tea sales.[7] In the 1950s instant tea was introduced, and by 1976 instant tea production required over 45 million pounds of leaf tea. Iced tea mix, instant tea with sweeteners and lemon or mint added, was first marketed in the mid-1960s. The tea bag continues to be the most popular way to purchase tea; 83 million pounds of tea leaves were used in this way in 1980 compared to 27 million pounds for iced tea mix, and 38 million pounds for instant tea.[8] The steady loser in all this is the sale of loose tea to the consumer. In 1980 sales of loose tea totaled 8 million pounds, compared to 41 million in 1950 when tea bags used only 28 million pounds of leaf tea.

An interesting study[9] used new assay techniques to look at the caffeine content of tea, as used by the consumer. Since most people judge the strength of the tea by its color the researchers brewed tea to match the color people called: weak, medium, and strong. When package directions are followed the color of the tea was between weak and medium. Instant teas were in the 50- to 60-mg range. Table 10-2 gives some of their results for tea bag tea.

It can only gladden and cheer the hearts of tea drinkers to know that the largest seller of tea in America, with 38% of the market, is a company named after a man, born in Scotland of Irish parents, who emigrated to America, became rich and famous in England, and believed in ships with sails

TABLE 10-2 Caffeine content (mg) in tea (strength established by color comparison)

Brand	Weak	Medium	Strong
Red Rose	45	62	90
Salada	25	60	78
Lipton	25	53	70
Tetley	18	48	70
Twining's English Breakfast	26	78	107

right up to the end: Sir Thomas Lipton (1850-1931).

CHOCOLATE

Long before Columbus landed on San Salvador, Quetzalcoatl, Aztec god of the air, gave man a gift from paradise: the chocolate tree. Linnaeus was to remember this legend when he named the cocoa tree *Theobroma*, food of the gods. The Aztecs treated it as such, and the cacao bean was an important part of their economy, with the cacao bush being cultivated widely. Montezuma, emperor of Mexico in the early sixteenth century, is said to have consumed nothing other than fifty goblets of chocolatl every day. The chocolatl (from the Mayan words *choco* [warm] and *latl* [beverage]) was flavored with vanilla but was far from the chocolate of today. It was a thick liquid like honey that was sometimes frothy and had to be eaten with a spoon. The major difference was that it was bitter; the Aztecs didn't know about sugarcane and had no sweetening material.

Cortez introduced sugarcane plantations to Mexico in the early 1520s and supported the continued cultivation of the *Theobroma cacao* bush. When he returned to Spain in 1528, Cortez carried with him cakes of processed cocoa. The cakes were eaten, as well as being ground up and mixed with water for a drink. Although chocolate was introduced to Europe almost a century before coffee and tea, its use spread very slowly. Primarily this was because the Spanish kept the method of preparing chocolate from the cacao bean a secret until

the early seventeenth century. When knowledge of the technique spread, so did the use of chocolate.

During the seventeenth century chocolate drinking reached all parts of Europe, primarily among the wealthy. Maria Theresa, wife of France's Louis XIV, had a thing about chocolate, and this furthered its use among the wealthy and fashionable. Gradually it became more of a social drink, and by the 1650s chocolate houses were open in England, although usually the sale of chocolate was added to that of coffee and tea in the established coffeehouses.

In the early eighteenth century there were health warnings against the use of chocolate in England, but use expanded. Its use and importance is well reflected in a 1783 proposal in Congress that the United States raise revenue by taxing chocolate as well as coffee, tea, liquor, sugar, molasses, and pepper.

Although the cultivation of chocolate never became a matter to fight over, it too has spread around the world. The New World plantations were almost destroyed by disease at the beginning of the eighteenth century, but cultivation had already begun in Asia, and today a large part of the crop comes from Africa.

Until 1828 all chocolate sold was a relatively undigestible substance obtained by grinding the cacao kernels after processing. The preparation had become more refined over the years, but it still followed the Aztec procedure of letting the pods dry in the sun, then roasting them before removing the husks to get to the kernel of the plant. The result of grinding the kernels is a thick liquid called chocolate liquor. This is baking chocolate. In 1828 a Dutch patent was issued for the manufacture of "chocolate powder" by removing about two thirds of the fat from the chocolate liquor. The chocolate powder was the forerunner of today's breakfast cocoa.

The fat that was removed, cocoa butter, became important when someone found that if it was mixed with sugar and some of the chocolate powder, it could easily be formed into slabs or bars. In 1847 the first chocolate bars appeared, but it was not until 1876 that the Swiss made their contribution to the chocolate industry by inventing milk chocolate, which was first sold under the Nestlé label. By FDA standards, milk chocolate today must contain at least 12% milk solids, although better grades contain almost twice that amount.

If we are to have cigarettes without tobacco and coffee without caffeine, does it surprise you that you may be eating chocolate without chocolate? The "true taste of chocolate made entirely without chocolate" is only the beginning. Check your next Valentine's Day box of chocolates, and you may find you have also bought a variety of artificial flavors, antioxidants (to increase shelf life), and stabilizers.

When chocolate "turns white," it may still be all right to eat, but it is probably old, since the white color comes from the separation of the cocoa butter. Someday when you have the time, you can check on whether your piece of chocolate is all chocolate and properly manufactured. Put it on your tongue: it should melt at body temperature. But be careful! One chocolate lover has said, "Each of us has known such moments of orgastic anticipation, our senses focused at their finest, when control is irrevocably abandoned. Then the tongue possesses, is possessed by, what it most desires; the warm, liquid melting of thick, dark chocolate."[10] Buy a chocolate bar!

The active ingredient in chocolate is theobromine. It has physiological actions that closely parallel those of caffeine but is much less potent in its effects on the central nervous system. The average cup of cocoa contains about 10 mg of caffeine but over 200 mg of theobromine.

COLA DRINKS

Since the beginning and early history of cola drinks is not shrouded in the mists that veil the origins of the other xanthine drinks, there is no problem in selecting the correct legend. And that's what the story of Coca-Cola is: a true legend in our time. From a green nerve tonic in 1886 in Atlanta, Georgia, that did not sell well at all, Coca-Cola has grown into . . . but you *know* what it is—everyone does everywhere! Unbelievable, it must be "the real thing" and provide "the pause that refreshes,"

or else it couldn't sell over 1.5 billion cases a year worldwide. And that includes mainland China where it's called "Ke Koy Ke Le"—which translated means "tasty happiness."[11] Yes, Coke is it!

Dr. J.C. Pemberton's tonic contained caramel, fruit flavoring, phosphoric acid, caffeine, and a secret mixture called Merchandise No. 5. A friend, F.M. Robinson, suggested the name by which it is still known: Coca-Cola. The unique character of Coca-Cola and its later imitators is a blend of fruit flavors that makes it impossible to identify any of its parts.

An early ad for Coca-Cola suggested its varied uses:

> This "INTELLECTUAL BEVERAGE" and TEMPERANCE DRINK contains the valuable TONIC and NERVE STIMULANT properties of the Coca plant and Cola (or Kola) nuts, and makes not only a delicious, exhilarating, refreshing and invigorating Beverage, (dispensed from the soda water fountain or in other carbonated beverages), but a valuable Brain Tonic, and a cure for all nervous affections—SICK HEADACHE, NEURALGIA, HYSTERIA, MELANCHOLY, &c.[12, p. 138]

Coca-Cola was touted as "the new and popular fountain drink, containing the tonic properties of the wonderful coca plant and the famous cola nut." You must remember that this was the period of Sherlock Holmes, Sigmund Freud, and patent medicine—all saying very good things about the product of the coca plant: cocaine. The company admitted to small amounts of cocaine in its beverage in 1903, but a government analysis of Coca-Cola in 1906 did not find any.

The name Coca-Cola was originally conceived to indicate the nature of its two ingredients with tonic properties. This suggestion of the presence of extracts of coca leaves and cola (kola) nuts in the beverage was supposed to be furthered by the use of each bottle of a pictorial representation of the leaves and nuts. Unfortunately the artist-glass blower didn't know that the coca and cocao plants were different, so the bottle had kola leaves and cacao pods! In 1909 the FDA seized a supply of Coca-Cola syrup and made two charges against the company. One was that it was misbranded because it contained "no coca and little if any cola" and, second that it contained an added poisonous ingredient, caffeine.

Prior to the 1911 trial in Chattanooga, Tennessee, the company paid for some research into the physiological effect of caffeine, and when all the information was in, the company won, and the government appealed the decision. In 1916 the Supreme Court of the United States upheld the lower court by rejecting the charge of misbranding, stating that the company has repeatedly said that "certain extracts from the leaves of the coca shrub and the nut kernels of the cola tree were used for the purpose of obtaining a flavor" and that "the ingredients containing these extracts" with the cocaine eliminated is called Merchandise No. 5. The way this is done today is that coca leaves are imported by a pharmaceutical company in New Jersey. The cocaine is extracted for medical use and the decocoainized leaves are shipped to the Coca-Cola plant in Atlanta, Georgia, where Merchandise No. 5 is produced. A 1931 report indicated that Merchandise No. 5 contained an extract of three parts coca leaves and one part cola nuts, but to this day it remains a secret formula.

Then there was the problem of the caffeine:

it is clear that the only question arising under section 7 is whether the caffeine in the Coca Cola is an "added poisonous or other added deleterious ingredient which may render such article injurious to health.". . .[13]

The question of whether caffeine was an "added poisonous ingredient" was not so readily resolved. Caffeine was added, but it was an essential part of the Coca-Cola formula. In that respect it was not added above and beyond the essential ingredients; it was one of them. The Supreme Court said that the lower courts should decide if the caffeine made the drink injurious to health.[13] At that time the company substantially reduced the amount of caffeine in its syrup, and the government never felt it had a case worth pursuing beyond that point.

Caffeine is under attack as a general-purpose food additive. In 1981 the FDA changed its rules so that a "cola" no longer has to contain caffeine.

TABLE 10-3 Top ten soft drinks

Brand	Market share (%)	Caffeine (mg)
Coca-Cola	24.3	34
Pepsi-Cola	18.0	37
Dr. Pepper	5.5	38
7-Up	5.4	0
Tab	3.2	44
Sprite	2.9	0
Mountain Dew	2.9	52
Royal Crown Cola	2.8	36
Diet Pepsi	2.6	34
Sugar Free Dr. Pepper	1.2	37

If it does contain caffeine it may not be more than 0.02%, which is 0.2 mg/ml, or a little less than 6 mg per ounce. There are some consumer and scientist groups that believe that all cola manufacturers should indicate on the label the amount of caffeine the beverage contains. This is in keeping with the trend toward providing more information to the consumer and seems highly probable. The same labeling would probably also be required of coffee, tea, and chocolate, although in these beverages the caffeine is not an added ingredient.

Table 10-3 lists the top 10 soft drinks of 1981, their market share, and the caffeine content in a 12-ounce can.[14,15]

You may not be a cola lover, but colas accounted for 55% of the nondiet soft drink sales in 1980. Lemon-lime drinks (such as 7-Up) had 11% of the market in that year, while pepper-type had 6%, gingerale and orange had 5% each, rootbeer 4%, and grape 1%. Diet soft drinks were only 14% of sales, and colas accounted for 55% of these sales. Whatever you drink, you are part of an expanding group: in 1980 the average per capita soft drink consumption per year was 4915 ounces, up from 2078 ounces in 1965, and 1244 in 1955.[16]

CAFFEINE

Xanthines are the oldest stimulants known to man. Xanthine is a Greek word meaning yellow,

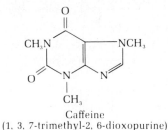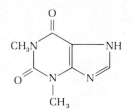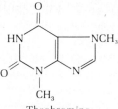

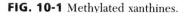

Caffeine
(1, 3, 7-trimethyl-2, 6-dioxopurine)

Theophylline
(1, 3-dimethyl-2, 6-dioxopurine)

Theobromine
(3, 7-dimethyl-2, 6-dioxopurine)

FIG. 10-1 Methylated xanthines.

the color of the residue if the xanthines are heated with nitric acid until dry. The three xanthines of primary importance are caffeine, theophylline, and theobromine.

These three chemicals are methylated xanthines and are closely related alkaloids, as can be seen in Fig. 10-1. Most alkaloids are insoluble in water, but these are unique, since they are slightly water soluble.

These xanthines have similar effects on the body, with caffeine having the greatest and theobromine almost no stimulant effect on the central nervous system and the skeletal muscles. Theophylline is the most potent, and caffeine the least potent, agent on the cardiovascular system. Caffeine, so named because it was isolated from coffee in 1820, has been the most extensively studied and, unless otherwise indicated, is the drug under discussion here.

Few people realize that caffeine is a very common agent in many of our beverages and drugs we use for other purposes, such as relief from pain or an upset stomach. Table 10-4 lists the caffeine content of some of these beverages and drugs. It is relatively easy to consume a gram of caffeine in a day and not be aware of the total consumption. You may want to calculate your approximate caffeine intake for the past several days.

In humans absorption of caffeine is rapid after oral intake; peak blood levels are reached 30 minutes after ingestion. Although maximal CNS effects are not reached for about 2 hours, the onset of effects may begin within half an hour after intake. The half-life of caffeine in humans is about 3 hours,

TABLE 10-4 Caffeine content of certain beverages and drugs

Source	Approximate amount of caffeine per unit (5 oz cup or tablet)
Beverages	
Brewed coffee	80-150 mg
Instant coffee	85-100 mg
Decaffeinated coffee	2-4 mg
Tea (bag or leaf)	30-75 mg
Cocoa	5-15 mg
Nonprescription (OTC) drugs	
Analgesics	
Anacin, Bromo Seltzer, Cope, Empirin Compound	32 mg
Excedrin	60 mg
Stimulants	
No-Doz	100 mg
Vivarin	200 mg
Caffedrine	250 mg
Many cold preparations	32 mg

and no more than 10% is excreted unchanged.

Cross-tolerance exists among the methylated xanthines; loss of tolerance may take more than 2 months of abstinence. The tolerance, however, is low grade, and, by increasing the dose two to four times, an effect can be obtained even in the tolerant individual. There is less tolerance to the CNS stimulation effect of caffeine than to most of its other effects. The direct action on the kidneys, to increase urine output, and the increase of salivary flow do show tolerance.

Dependence on caffeine is real. One withdrawal symptom that has been well substantiated is the headache, which generally develops in habitual users (five cups or more of coffee a day) after about 18 hours of abstinence. Some reports suggest that nausea, lethargy, anxiety, and muscle tension, may precede the actual headache, but the clearest symptom is the headache.[17,18] It has been produced experimentally by giving caffeine chronically to noncaffeine users and then substituting a placebo, as well as by withholding coffee from habitual users.[19,20]

Adverse effects

Caffeine is one of those drugs that seems to always be in trouble. It's always suspected of doing bad things. Since it is probably the most widely used psychoactive drug in the world (it's acceptable to those in the Judaic-Christian as well as Islamic traditions), it is understandable that it would have both good and bad reports. In the early 1970s caffeine was linked with coronary heart disease (CHD) and heart attacks. In 1975 the Public Health Service said, "No association between coffee drinking and the development of CHD, stroke . . . was demonstrated."[21,p.20]

In 1974 the world was introduced to a new term: Caffeinism.[22] As that publication said:

> High intake of caffeine ("caffeinism") can produce symptoms that are indistinguishable from those of anxiety neurosis, such as nervousness, irritability, tremulousness, occasional muscle twitchings, insomnia, sensory disturbances, tachypnea, palpitations, flushing, arrhythmias, diuresis, and gastrointestinal disturbances. The caffeine withdrawal syndrome and the headache associated with it may also mimic anxiety.[22]

There are many studies that show that individuals with psychiatric or emotional problems have those problems intensified by high caffeine intake. Similarly, some of the problems may be the result of high caffeine intake.[23,24] One report showed the same caffeinism effects in college students. This report also found that the students who consumed higher levels of caffeine were those with lower academic performance![25]

In 1977 the FDA appointed a high-level committee of scientists to determine whether caffeine was a health hazard. The scientific evidence was so mixed that two final reports were written. They both agreed that it was impossible to tell for sure whether caffeine was or was not a potential health hazard.[26]

A 1980 statement[27] by the Commissioner of the FDA made many people nervous:

> An experiment recently concluded by the Food and Drug Administration has found that caffeine, when fed to pregnant rats, causes birth defects and delayed skeletal development in their offspring.
>
> The study's implications for people are not known. But the findings have caused enough concern among FDA scientists that today I am advising pregnant women to avoid caffeine-containin foods and drugs, or to use them sparingly.
>
> I want to make clear that we have no conclusive evidence at this time that caffeine has ever caused a birth defect in a human being.

A lot of scientists and clinicians thought the statement was too strong, considering the incomplete evidence.[28]

In 1981 an unexpected finding occurred: "A strong association between coffee consumption and pancreatic cancer was evident in both sexes . . . after adjustment for cigarette smoking, the relative risk associated with drinking up to two cups of coffee per day was 1.8 . . . that with three or more cups per day was 2.7. . . ."[29,p.630] Since tea, colas, etc. don't seem to have an effect, maybe it's not the caffeine. Or maybe it's just not true—there's still debate and more research is needed![30]

Toxic effects

Caffeine is not very toxic, but high doses result in convulsions, whereas still higher doses cause death from respiratory failure. Six deaths in humans have been reported in the literature: one

TABLE 10-5 Comparison of pharmacological activity of the xanthines

	CNS and respiratory stimulation	Cardiac stimulation and coronary dilation	Smooth muscle relaxation	Skeletal muscle stimulation	Diuresis
Caffeine	1*	3	3	1	3
Theophylline	2	1	1	2	1
Theobromine	3	2	2	3	2

*1 means most active.

following an intravenous injection of 3.2 g (the oral dose that would generally be fatal has been estimated at over 10 g).[31] Toxic effects of caffeine can result from taking 1 g in a single dose.[32] The central stimulation and toxic effects can be blocked by CNS suppressants.[33]

Physiological effects

A comparison of the actions of the xanthines is given in Table 10-5. The pharmacological effects on the CNS and the skeletal muscles are probably the basis for the wide use of caffeine-containing beverages.

With two cups of coffee taken close together (about 200 mg of caffeine), the cortex is activated, the EEG shows an arousal pattern, and drowsiness and fatigue decrease. Some research suggests that this effect is the result of a direct action of caffeine on the cortex. Other results attribute the activation to the release of noradrenaline from the adrenal medulla and the brain. This CNS stimulation is also the basis for "coffee nerves," which can occur at low doses in sensitive individuals and in others when they have consumed large amounts of caffeine.

In the absence of tolerance, even 200 mg will increase the time it takes to fall asleep and will cause disturbances in the sleep. There is a good relationship between the mood-elevating effect of caffeine and the extent to which it will keep the individual awake.

For years no one really knew the mechanism whereby the methylxanthines had their effects on the central nervous system. It was known that they blocked the conversion, and thus the inactivation, of cyclic-AMP to AMP (adenosine monophosphate). Since cyclic-AMP is involved in the regulation and modulation of many cellular and metabolic activities this was a plausible primary mechanism of action.[34] It still is, but it's not very specific. It now seems clear that "caffeine affects behavior by countering the effects in the brain of a naturally occurring chemical called adenosine."[35,p.1408] Adenosine acts normally in several areas of the brain to depress neural activity by inhibiting the release of neurotransmitters. Caffeine, by blocking the action of an inhibitor, will therefore cause an increase in neuronal firing at the synapse. It's only a matter of time before new, synthetic, adenosine blockers are developed and tested—and perhaps marketed!

Higher dose levels (about 500 mg) are needed to affect the autonomic centers of the brain, and heart rate and respiration may be increased at this dose. The direct effect on the cardiovascular system is in opposition to the effects mediated by the autonomic centers. Caffeine acts directly on the vascular muscles to cause a dilation, while stimulation of the autonomic centers results in a constriction of blood vessels. Usually dilation occurs, but in the brain the blood vessels are constricted, and this constriction may be the basis for caffeine's ability to reduce hypertensive headaches.[36]

The opposing effects of caffeine, directly on the heart and directly through effects on the medulla, make it very difficult to predict the results of normal (that is, less than 500 mg) caffeine intake. At higher levels there is an increase in heart rate, and continued use of large amounts of caffeine may produce an irregular heartbeat in some individuals.

The basal metabolic rate may be increased slightly (10%) in chronic caffeine users, since 500 mg has frequently been shown to have this effect. This action probably combines with the stimulant effects on skeletal muscles to increase physical work output and decrease fatigue after use of caffeine.

It must be noted in passing that theophylline is a very effective bronchodilator and has definite therapeutic use in humans. Grandma was right—a couple of cups of tea will help the asthmatic breathe easier.[37]

Behavioral effects

A hundred years ago the French essayist Balzac spoke with feeling and described the effects of coffee:

> [It] causes an admirable fever. It enters the brain like a bacchante. Upon its attack, imagination runs wild, bares itself, twists like a pythoness and in this paroxysm a poet enjoys the supreme possession of his faculties; but this is a drunkenness of though as wine brings about a drunkenness of the body.[38,p.65]

In the original French the description is even more stimulating and erotic. Unfortunately it does not refer to the effect most people have with their morning cup of coffee.

Even today essayists sometimes take wing and soar away from the hard research data. One authoritative source[36,p.368] records that caffeine-produces "a more rapid and clearer flow of thought . . . a greater sustained intellectual effort and a more perfect association of ideas." As I write this while drinking a cup of coffee, I'd like to believe that this is true. The data are really not that convincing with respect to cognitive tasks. There are, however, reports that after 200 to 300 mg of caffeine there are increases in the ability to produce associations to words and also in the ability to process sensory information.

There is considerable evidence that 200 to 300 mg of caffeine will partially offset fatigue-induced

decrement in the performance of motor tasks. Like the amphetamines, but to a much smaller degree, caffeine prolongs the amount of time an individual can perform physically exhausting work. In addition to effects on physical work, caffeine seems to slow the onset of boredom and to increase attention. The cortical stimulation and increased alertness and reactivity were very well demonstrated in a 1974 study[39] on simulated automobile driving.

A 1976 report[40] used a personality test to separate undergraduate students into three groups: introverts, ambiverts, and extroverts. On a timed verbal ability test, 200 mg of caffeine improved the performance of extroverts but decreased the performance of introverts. It should not be surprising that a drug with CNS actions will have different behavioral effects depending on the personality of the user, but it is nice to have the effect demonstrated.

Many studies have looked at the effect of caffeine on the behavior of hyperkinetic children (see Chapter 14) and most have not shown any therapeutic effect. One report[41] of the effects of 3 and 10 mg/kg of caffeine on normal 8- to 13-year-old boys showed decreased reaction times and increased vigilance along with increased motor activity. That's pretty much what might be expected from a mild stimulant. It's unfortunate that no one has done comparable studies with adults.

Even the television ads tell you—make that "one last drink for the road," *coffee*. There is not a lot of evidence to support the value of this. Caffeine will not lower blood alcohol level—but it may arouse the drinker. As they say—put coffee in a sleepy drunk, you get a wide-awake drunk. That's probably of some real value. One study[42] showed that in young males with a blood alcohol level of 0.065%, 325 mg of caffeine improved performance on a number of visual-motor tasks important in driving. Performance in the alcohol plus caffeine group was not the same in all tasks as the no-alcohol group so some impairment still existed. This work is being followed up vigorously.

The best simple summary is that 150 to 300 mg of caffeine offsets fatigue-induced performance decrements in both physical and mental tasks, slows the development of boredom, and *may,* in a rested, interested individual, increase motor and mental efficiency above control levels. It may be that the effects of caffeine on cognitive tasks done under stress (as in exams?) varies with personality type. The interesting possibility that performance improves in extroverts and is impaired in introverts needs further confirmation.

CONCLUDING COMMENT

The xanthines have a full-bodied heritage; it is difficult to name a drug that has had more impact on the world than caffeine. Caffeine has remained a popular drug, whether in coffee or cola, because it is easy to adjust the dose level, and there are few adverse side effects. As a mild stimulant it has few peers.

The story is not yet over. As techniques and experimental designs get more sophisticated and users live longer, it may be possible to show that caffeine does in fact have some adverse medical effects. Every year increases our ability to recognize smaller and smaller effects of a drug. With many people now living to 70 and 80 years of age, long-term mild adverse effects may show up as a result of many years of caffeine use. By now you know there are no completely safe drugs. Every drug use is a matter of balancing the advantages against the disadvantages. To this point there are no clear reasons not to use caffeine in moderation. That may change at any time. And the bottom line, as is true with all drugs, is that caffeine is a foreign substance, not a chemical that is necessary for normal body functioning.

REFERENCES

1. Uribe Compuzano, A.: Brown gold, New York, 1954, Random House, Inc.
2. Meyer, H.: Old English coffee houses, Emmaus, Pa., 1954, The Rodale Press.
3. Weatherskee, M.S., and Lodge, J.R.: Caffeine: its direct and indirect influence on reproduction, The Journal of Reproductive Medicine 19(2):55-63, 1977.
4. Lewin, L.: Phantastica narcotic and stimulating drugs, New York, 1931, E.P. Dutton & Co., Inc.
5. Summary of national coffee drinking study, United States of America, 1981, New York, 1981, International Coffee Organization.
6. Dick, R.H., and Hopkins, H.: Putting tea to the taste, FDA Consumer, pp. 18-27, September 1974.
7. Brown, H.L.: Tea workshops, Nielsen Market Research Service, September 1981.
8. Tea Council on the United States of America, Inc.: 1950-1980 statistical history of tea in the U.S.A., February 1981.
9. Groisser, D.S.: A study of caffeine in tea, The American Journal of Clinical Nutrition 31(10):1727-1731, October 1978.
10. Prial, F.J.: Secrets of a chocoholic, New York Times, May 16, 1979, p. C1.
11. Sterba, J.P.: Coke brings "tasty happiness" to China, New York Times, April 16, 1981, p. A3.
12. Huisking, C.L.: Herbs to hormones, Essex, Conn., 1968, Pequot Press, Inc.
13. Sixth Circuit Court of Appeals, 1914: 215 Federal Reporter 539, June 13, 1914.
14. Salmans, S.: Soft-drink wars heating up, New York Times, May 30, 1981, p. 29.
15. Caffeine: how to consume less, Consumer Reports, p. 597, October 1981.
16. Sales survey of the soft drink industry, National Soft Drink Association, 1980.
17. Greden, J.F., and others: Caffeine-withdrawal headache: a clinical profile, Psychosomatics 21(5):411, 1980.
18. White, B.C., and others: Anxiety and muscle tension as consequences of caffeine withdrawal, Science 209(6):1547, 1980.
19. Goldstein, A., and Kaizer, S.: Psychotropic effects of caffeine in man. III. A questionnaire survey of coffee drinking and its effects in a group of housewives, Clinical Pharmacology and Therapeutics 10:477-488, 1969.
20. Goldstein, A.: Wakefulness caused by caffeine, Naunyn-Schmeidebergs Archiv fur Experimentelle Pathologie und Pharmakologie 248:269-278, 1964.
21. Health consequences of smoking, 1975, Public Health Service Publication No. (CEC)76-8704, U.S. Department of Health, Education, and Welfare, Washington, D.C., 1976, U.S. Government Printing Office.
22. Greden, J.F.: Anxiety of caffeinism: a diagnostic dilemma, American Journal of Psychiatry 131:1089-1092, 1974.
23. Mikkelsen, E.J.: Caffeine and schizophrenia, Journal of Clinical Psychiatry, 39(9):83, September 1978.
24. Bezchlibnyk, K.Z., and others: Should psychiatric patients drink coffee?, Canadian Medical Association Journal 124: 357, February 15, 1981.
25. Gilliland, K., and Andress, D.: Ad lib caffeine consumption, symptoms of caffeinism, and academic performance, American Journal of Psychiatry 138(4):512-514, 1981.
26. Select committee report to the FDA: tentative evaluation of the health aspects of caffeine as a food ingredient, Bethesda, Md., 1976, Life Sciences Research Office, Federation of American Societies for Experimental Biology.

27. Goyan, J.E.: Statement FDA release, September 5, 1980.

28. Sun, M.: FDA caffeine decision too early, some say, Science **209**:1500, September 26, 1980.

29. MacMahon, B., and others: Coffee and cancer of the pancreas, New England Journal of Medicine, **304**(11):630-633, March 12, 1981.

30. Storm brews over study tying coffee to pancreatic cancer, Medical World News, p. 10, April 13, 1981.

31. Syed, I.B.: The effects of caffeine, Journal of the American Pharmaceutical Association **NS16**:568-572, 1976.

32. Stillner, V., and others: Caffeine induced delirium during prolonged competitive stress, American Journal of Psychiatry **135**(7):855-856, 1978.

33. Peters, J.M.: Factors affecting caffeine toxicity, Journal of Clinical Pharmacology **7**:131-141, 1967.

34. Levenson, H.S., and Beck, E.C.: Psychopharmacology of caffeine. In Jarvik, M., editor: Psychopharmacology in the practice of medicine, New York, 1977, Appleton-Century-Crofts.

35. Marx, J.L.: Caffeine's sumulatory effects explained, Science **211**:1408, March 27, 1981.

36. Goodman, L.S., and Gilman, A.: The pharmacological basis of therapeutics, ed. 5, New York, 1975, Macmillan Publishing Co., Inc.

37. Nassif, E.G., and others: The value of maintenance theophylline in steroid-dependent asthma, New England Journal of Medicine **304**(2):71-75, 1981.

38. Mickel, E.J.: The artificial paradises in French literature, Chapel Hill, N.C., 1969, University of North Carolina Press. (Free translation from French.)

39. Regina, E.G., and others: Effects of caffeine on alertness in simulated automobile driving, Journal of Applied Psychology **59**:483-489, 1974.

40. Revelle, W., Amaral, P., and Turriff, S.: Introversion/extroversion, time stress, and caffeine: effect on verbal performance, Science **192**:149-150, 1976.

41. Elkins, R.N., and others: Acute effects of caffeine in normal prepubertal boys, American Journal of Psychiatry **138**(2):178-183, 1981.

42. Coffee may steady slightly tipsy drivers, Medical World News, p. 46, October 12, 1981.

CHAPTER 11

OVER-THE-COUNTER DRUGS

THIS IS THE AGE OF informed consumerism, from do-it-yourself home improvement to health care.[1,p.42] If I tell you that we Americans spend about $28 a year for each citizen on over-the-counter (OTC) drug purchases you will probably not be impressed. It's true. You might pay more attention when you realize that this is a total of $6 billion each year and that the amount increases 5% to 10% annually. To put it all in perspective—each year, for each person, we also spend: $158 on alcoholic beverages, $112 on tobacco, $84 on prescription drugs, $37 on cosmetics, $30 on candy, and . . . oh yes, $500 on education![2,3] I know there's a moral there somewhere.

Do OTC drugs help the consumer (and I use "consumer" literally—i.e., not as a synonym for "patient" but to label one who "eats, drinks, or devours")? Of course they do. Aspirin relieves headaches and musculoskeletal pains, sodium bicarbonate facilitates a good burp, and milk of magnesia moves the bowels. Nor can the placebo effects of OTC agents be discounted. But do our people really need to take OTC agents in Brobdingnagian amounts to lead more comfortable lives?[4]

Even Lemuel Gulliver and Jonathan Swift could probably agree on an answer to that question: of course not!

OTC drugs are those which are self-prescribed and self-administered for the relief of symptoms of self-diagnosed illnesses. And there surely are a lot of them. One estimate is that three out of every four individuals have the symptoms of an illness each month, but only one of those three seek professional help. The other two frequently turn to OTC drugs.

Another study showed that between the ages of 17 and 44 the average individual had almost three "acute conditions" a year (for which OTC drugs are appropriate) and the age 65 and over senior citizen averaged one a year.[1] We would all be in big trouble if even a small percentage of these people tried to see a physician for treatment. The necessary self-diagnosis, self-prescription, and self-administration of OTC compounds means they must be safe, with labels clearly spelling out how and when to use them and when not to use them.

It is probably true that most OTC users have a better knowledge of the effects and side effects of their drug than do users of prescription drugs. Only a few prescription drugs (such as oral contraceptives) currently have extensive instructions about their use and dangers. OTC packages are getting more specific and clearer in their labels, but for now they must list at least the common or generic names and quantities of their active ingredients, as well as the amount of alcohol, if any, they contain. OTC drug labels also include instructions for using the drug, including simple, direct warnings and limitations on use, such as: DISCONTINUE USE IF PAIN PERSISTS AND CONSULT A PHYSICIAN.

Sometimes the only difference between an OTC product and a prescription product is the greater amount of the active ingredient in each prescription dose.

> A drug shall be permitted for OTC sale and use by the laity unless, because of its toxicity or other potential for harmful effect or because of the method . . . necessary to its use, it may safely be sold and used only under a practitioner's prescription.[5]

In this situation the higher dose level increases the potential for harmful effects to the point where the FDA believes use should be controlled by a physician. Sometimes that's a hard decision to make.

Even more difficult decisions were put to the FDA by the Kefauver-Harris 1962 amendment to the 1938 Food, Drug, and Cosmetic Act. That act required that all drugs be evaluated for effectiveness, as well as being safe. One problem is that no one knew—and still no one knows—how many OTC products are on the market. The best estimate is about 300,000 different products. A second problem is that there is no requirement that a manufacturer tell anyone, including the FDA and the consumer, when there is a change in the ingredients, or in the amount of an ingredient, in a product. An Anacin tablet bought in 1963 contained more ingredients than the one bought in 1965 and today, but the name, and the advertising, have remained the same.

The difficulty of evaluating the effectiveness of over a quarter million OTC products was solved by the FDA decision to study only the *active* ingredients. The safety and effectiveness would be determined individually for each of the approximately 800 active ingredients. The FDA would then regulate closely the statements that would be permissible about the use and effectiveness of each ingredient. That made life much simpler for all honest men. Such a decision makes things more difficult for advertisers, though, since it severely limits the variety of statements that can be made about a product.

Since the terms *safe* and *effective* will be used repeatedly, it seems best to define them as the FDA does. Two acronyms are also important here: *GRAS, Generally Recognized as Safe*, and *GRAE, Generally Recognized As Effective*.

> Safety means a low incidence of adverse reactions or significant side effects under adequate directions for use and warnings against unsafe use as well as low potential for harm which may result from abuse. . . .
>
> Effectiveness means a reasonable expectation that, in a significant proportion of the target population, the pharmacological effect of the drug, when used under adequate directions for use and warnings against unsafe use, will provide clinically significant relief of the type claimed.[5]

Although it is not in common use, it may help also to remember *GRAHL, Generally Recognized as Honestly Labeled*. The FDA speaks to that problem as well:

> Labeling shall be clear and truthful in all respects and may not be false or misleading in any particular. It shall state the intended uses and results of the product; adequate directions for proper use; and warnings against unsafe use, side effects, and adverse reactions. . . .[5]

To evaluate the safety, effectiveness, and labeling requirements for the active ingredients in OTC products, in 1972 the FDA set up 17 advisory review panels to study the 26 classes of OTC products listed on p. 223. The panels were to review the scientific literature, solicit information and comments from manufacturers and consumer and scientific groups, and issue a tentative report. The FDA then publishes the report, requesting comments from everyone. The report is reviewed extensively by the FDA staff, revised as necessary, and then published as a regulation, unless blocked by legal action. Once the report is a regulation, manufacturers must adhere to it by removing or adding ingredients, rewriting labels, or removing the product from interstate shipping. It will still be possible to find unsafe, ineffective, and/or inadequately labeled products in your store, but these will have been manufactured in the state where they are sold. This is not a major problem, since most states have laws in this area that parallel those of the FDA.

As you can imagine this was a horrendous task. Things moved slowly—too slowly—and in 1980 the Commissioner of the FDA acted to speed up both the reviews and the effects of the reviews. Unsafe and/or ineffective drugs will be forced off the market before the final report is approved—a factor of 2 to 5 or more years—and the final report will contain rules and regulations only for the effective ingredients.[6] Once the final report is published as a regulation, all of the not-yet-proven effective or safe drugs will have to be taken off the market. They may return, of course, if research shows them to be effective. By January 1982 45 initial reports had been published and there were still 19 to go.[7] At this first level of review, the panels found that about one third of the ingredients reviewed are safe and effective, if used as directed. Additional research may push that up to about 50%.

The 26 classes of OTC products are:

1. Antacids
2. Antimicrobials
3. Sedatives and sleep aids
4. Analgesics
5. Cold remedies and antitussives
6. Antihistamines and allergy products
7. Mouthwashes
8. Topical analgesics
9. Antirheumatics
10. Hematinics
11. Vitamins and minerals
12. Antiperspirants
13. Laxatives
14. Dentifrices and dental products
15. Sunburn treatments and preventives
16. Contraceptive and vaginal products
17. Stimulants
18. Hemorrhoidals
19. Antidiarrheals
20. Dandruff and athlete's foot preparations
21. Broncodilators and antiasthmatics
22. Antiemetics
23. Ophthalmics
24. Emetics
25. Miscellaneous internal products
26. Miscellaneous external products

Each advisory panel classifies the active ingredients in its product class as being in one of the following categories:

Category I   Ingredient is GRAS and GRAE.
Category II Ingredient is not GRAS and/or GRAE; the manufacturer has 6 months from the date of the panel report to prove the ingredient should be in Category I, or it may not be shipped in interstate commerce.
Category III Data insufficient to determine safety and/or effectiveness. Manufacturers given 1 year from the date of the panel report to prove GRAS, or ingredient goes to Category II.

To summarize this in a nutshell,

the agency decided . . . to create drug category monographs that would say what active ingredients are safe and effective and what labeling would be appropriate. This means the agency will spell out what active ingredients can be used in a product.[8]

These panels did more than they had to do. In some cases they recommended that higher doses be allowed in OTC preparations—and as a result we can now buy higher strength OTC antihistamines. In other situations the suggestion was for a prescription-only ingredient to be sold as an OTC—and as a result we now have OTC hydrocortisones and fluoride mouthwashes. A panel also recommended the labeling system now found in OTC sunscreen products. Many labeling suggestions were made and most will probably be used in the final regulations. This will certainly make OTC drug advertising duller—but more specific and more honest and, everyone hopes, more informative.

A POTPOURRI OF PRODUCTS

There is a paucity of paper to present even a partial panorama of the pills that can be purchased from your pharmacist. Brief comment will be made on several of the larger categories of OTC drugs that have made a name for themselves through advertising or use. Following will be extensive discussion of the two categories of OTC products that are used most often by most people: internal analgesics and cough and cold remedies.

There are products that many people view as OTC drugs but are not part of this review process. One example is dimethyl sulfoxide (DMSO). A byproduct of the manufacture of paper and used widely as an industrial degreaser, DMSO first became famous in 1964 because of a report that it ". . . soaked through the skin like water though sand and reduced the pain and inflammation of a variety of ills."[9,p.48] "DMSO readily penetrates most biological membranes without destroying the integrity of these membranes . . . [and] has the ability to 'carry' other compounds with it through the membrane."[10,p.25] It is approved for use with animals to reduce swelling from trauma but can be used only for a rare bladder condition in humans. The FDA had issued an IND in 1963, canceled it in 1965 because of reports of damage to the eyes, allowed selective small research projects to proceed from 1966 to 1980, and in 1980 put DMSO in the same category as all other chemicals: present an acceptable IND, and you can do the research. Many studies were started and some FDA evaluations of them should appear in the mid-1980s. Preliminary results suggest that a 70% to 80% solution of DMSO is effective in treating musculoskeletal injuries.[11,p.49]

Vitamins generate a billion dollars a year in sales! Between $70 and $80 million a year is spent to advertise them! "A vitamin, if a drug at all, is not one in the ordinary sense, although vitamins may have independent pharmacologic reactions, and all may be poisons if given long enough at excessive levels."[12,p.110] Vitamins, cofactors that are essential for enzymes to function, are not produced by the body and are required only in very small amounts—maybe one-billionth of a kilogram a day. They are easily provided in the American diet, except perhaps for a pregnant woman. But people buy them by the ton. According to one survey people believe that supplemental vitamins improve energy. As far as we now know the energy would be a placebo effect.

There is no scientific evidence that in healthy people vitamins prevent infections, stimulate appetite, help to assuage neuritic pains or aid positive health in any way.[13]

Because of the possibility of adverse effects with very high intakes of some vitamins[1] the FDA tried to regulate vitamin pills that contained more than 150% of the recommended daily dietary allowance. Congress responded to the industry and its constituents by telling the FDA to leave vitamins alone!

Vitamin C requires special comment. It was the vitamin C in the limes that British sailors carried with them and ate on long ocean voyages in the eighteenth century that finally eliminated the scourge of scurvy and earned for British sailors forever the nickname "limeys." Two centuries later, in 1970, Dr. Linus Pauling published a book *Vitamin C and the Common Cold*.[14] A two-time winner of the Nobel Prize is no one to sneeze at and many people rushed to follow his prescription: 1 to 3 g of ascorbic acid (vitamin C) a day. This, he said, would reduce the incidence and severity of upper respiratory tract infections. A lot of time, money, and effort has been put forth to determine whether this is true. The research still goes on. A 1975 review and a 1979 review of the research agreed that ". . .there is no reason to accept Pauling's contention that use of vitamin C in large doses can prevent colds . . . or abort colds."[15,p.160] The cough and cold advisory panel came to the same conclusion.

There has been only a slow movement of the American public away from the excessive use of laxatives, although there has been a loosening up of attitudes in young people. Adults over 40 to 50 grew up in an era of few fresh vegetables and fruits and probably had some real problems with constipation; real or not, every year at least 50 million Americans think they have it, and they spend about $400 million annually to keep regular, whatever that means, since normal regularity ranges from three times a day to three times a week.[16] Most of what they have been buying is both safe and effective, since the review panel found 60% of the 70 ingredients evaluated to be in Category I and only 21% in Category II.

Some may believe that this "preoccupation with bowel function [is] a phenomenon explicable only by reference to Freudian hypotheses."[17] The real concern, however, is not psychological or economic, but physiological.[18] Some types of laxatives—those which are called stimulants and act to increase intestinal activity—will now have to be labeled: "Prolonged or continued use of this product can lead to laxative dependency and loss of normal bowel function."[16] It is this loss of normal functioning that makes many authorities agree "that moderate constipation constitutes a far smaller menace to health than over-enthusiastic efforts to treat it. . . ."[13]

One action taken in the category of OTC antimicrobial, or bacteria-killing, ingredients frequently found in deodorant soaps was the removal of hexachlorophene from the market in 1972. The panel report,[19] in September, 1974, stated that of hundreds of ingredients reviewed, only 19 were active, and only 5 were Category I, including tincture of iodine and hexylresorcinol. The interesting fact is that antibacterial soaps—deodorant soaps, the kind you spend $350 million a year on to take the worry out of being close—may be *too* effective. Although a 70% reduction in the normal skin flora is adequate for a deodorizing effect, most soaps remove over 90% of the gram-positive bacteria. That's bad, since

> . . . by selectively killing nonpathogenic microorganisms, an important ecological balance is upset which allows more dangerous organisms to thrive and cause potentially serious infections. . . . Although it may seem paradoxical, it is now clear that under some condition the vigorous use of antimicrobials on the skin can increase infections rather than prevent them.[19]

Fantastic. It means that you not only have to worry about the drugs you put *in* your body, but you also have to worry about the drugs you put *on* your body.

Another part of the deodorizing of America is the use of antiperspirants. "Antiperspirants are considered drugs because they affect a function of the body (reduce perspiration). Deodorants, on the other hand, only help to reduce odor and are reg-

ulated as cosmetics."[20] In your crusade against smell you will be pleased to know that nonaerosol antiperspirants were found to be effective (which means that at least 50% of users in a laboratory hot room had at least a 20% reduction in wetness!). Creams were 35% to 47% effective; roll-ons, 14% to 70%; lotions, 38% to 62%; liquids, 15% to 54%; and sticks, 35% to 40%. No one knows how they work but since we spend about $370 million a year on them—be glad they are effective.[21]

A good way to close this section is with the work of the first advisory panel, concerned with antacids. A brief comment on their activity will clarify the entire procedure as well as indicate the potential impact these OTC reviews may have when they are all completed in the mid-1980s.

When the antacid panel asked for data, 76 manufacturers submitted material on 150 products with 27 active ingredients. Interestingly, *no* consumer or consumer group submitted any comments. About 8000 antacid products are on the market today; 1972 sales were $117 million and 1982 sales were over $500 million. The June, 1974, report of the review panel listed 13 ingredients or groups of ingredients in Category I, including mother's favorite, sodium bicarbonate.

Gone forever, however, are claims of relief of "upset stomach" and "gasid indigestion." The only three therapeutic claims that can be made on the label of an antacid with active ingredients are for symptomatic relief of *heartburn, sour stomach,* and *acid indigestion*. This panel was the first of many to lament the use of multiple ingredients that are pharmacologically unrelated. Some antacid products contain both an internal analgesic and an antacid. In general this is not harmful, but the advertising and label must clearly indicate that you should use the product *only* if you have *both* acid indigestion and pain.[22]

PEOPLE AND PAIN

Pain is such a little word for such a big experience. Most people have experienced pain of varying intensities, from mild to moderate to severe to excruciating! Two classes of drugs are used to reduce pain or the awareness of pain. Anesthetics (meaning "without sensibility") have this effect by reducing awareness or by blocking consciousness completely. The barbiturates and the volatile anesthetics, such as ether, are good examples of this type of agent. Analgesics (meaning "without pain") are compounds that reduce pain without causing a loss of the senses. Narcotics are one group of drugs in this class, but this chapter will primarily discuss the OTC internal analgesics such as aspirin and acetaminophen.

One classification divides pain into two types, depending on its place of origin. Visceral pain, such as intestinal cramps, arises from nonskeletal portions of the body; narcotics are effective in reducing pain of this type. Somatic pain, arising from muscle or bone and typified by sprains, headaches, and arthritis, is reduced by salicylates (aspirin).

Another system of categorizing pain relates the type of neuron that carries the signal we call pain to the kind of pain experienced. Bright, sharp pain is mediated by large, fast neurons and seems to activate the individual, whereas dull, aching pain, which depresses the person and causes anxiety, is mediated by small, slow neurons. (To differentiate these two, hit your thumb with a hammer. The initial sensation that causes you to verbalize doubts about the hammer's ancestors is bright pain, whereas the throbbing experience that soon follows is dull pain.) A third pain experience is labeled burning pain. Neurons intermediate in size and speed produce this. Narcotics attenuate the bright pain, and salicylates the dull.

The fact that there are different types of pain—not just more or less of the same kind—should tell you that there must be different systems and mechanisms underlying them. Since 1970 major breakthroughs have occurred[23] in our understanding of these mechanisms[24] and already important new drugs are available because of our greater knowledge.[25] In our understanding of pain, and thus our ability to reduce it, this chapter and the chapter on the opiates show clearly that my daddy was right: You ain't seen nothin' yet!

Pain is unlike other sensations in many ways, mostly the result of the influence of nonspecific factors. The experience of pain varies with personality, sex, and time of day[26,27] and is increased with fatigue, anxiety, fear, boredom, and anticipation of more pain. Because pain is very susceptible to nonspecific factors, a brief comment is required on the effectiveness of a placebo in reducing pain. Classic studies have been done by Beecher, who has also summarized reports of many investigators on the effectiveness of placebos in the reduction of pain.[28] These were real situations with a variety of clinical causes ranging from postoperative pain to the aches associated with the common cold. About 35% of the patients in these studies had their pain "satisfactorily relieved" by placebos. That is, when individuals in pain were given an inactive substance along with the suggestion that it would reduce the pain, 35% of the patients obtained relief.

This 35% proportion is quite high when it is appreciated that morphine provides satisfactory relief of pain in only about 75% of patients. It was also found that placebos are most effective in reducing pain in stressful situations, whereas morphine has its smallest effect in these stressful situations. As might be expected from the last statement, placebos are more effective in real-life pain than in experimental pain. The internal analgesics mentioned in the next section have been repeatedly shown to be more effective at therapeutic doses than placebos for certain kinds of pain.

INTERNAL ANALGESICS
Aspirin

Salicylates are the most widely used class of internal analgesics. The word itself suggests their long heritage, coming from the Latin *salix*, meaning willow. Over 2400 years ago, the Greeks used extracts of willow and poplar bark in the treatment of pain, gout, and other illnesses. Aristotle commented on some of the clinical effects of similar preparations, and Galen also made good use of these formulations.

These remedies fell into disrepute, however, when St. Augustine declared that all diseases of Christians were the work of demons and thus a punishment from God. (Other effects of this edict are discussed in Chapter 13.) The American Indian, unhampered by this enlightened attitude, used a tea brewed from willow bark to reduce fever. The salicylates were not rediscovered in Europe until about 200 years ago when an Englishman, the Reverend Edward Stone, combined two bits of the best information then available and put the result to clinical test. The two pieces of data he combined were (1) listen to old wives' tales, and (2) plants acquire the characteristics of the place where they grow. The old wives kept saying willow bark is good for pain and whatever else ails you! Stone phrased the second attitude nicely:

> As this tree delights in a moist or wet soil where aches chiefly abound, the general maxim that many natural maladies carry their cures along with them, or that their remedies lie not far from their causes, was so very apposite to this particular case that I could not help applying it. That this might be the intention of Providence had some little weight with me.[29]

Stone prepared an extract of the bark and gave the same dose to 50 patients with varying illnesses and found the results to be "uniformly excellent."

In the nineteenth century the active ingredient in these preparations was isolated and identified as salicylic acid. In 1838 salicylic acid was synthesized, and in 1859 procedures were developed that made bulk production feasible. Salicylic acid and sodium salicylate were then used for many ills, especially arthritis.

In the giant Bayer Laboratories in Germany in the 1890s there worked a chemist named Hoffmann. His father had a severe case of rheumatoid arthritis, and only salicylic acid seemed to help. The major difficulty then, as today, was that the drug caused great gastric discomfort. So great was the stomach upset and nausea that Hoffmann's father frequently preferred the pain of the arthritis. Hoffmann studied the salicylates to see if he could find one with the same therapeutic effect as salicylic acid, but without the side effects.

In 1898 he synthesized acetylsalicylic acid and tried it on his father, who reported relief from pain without stomach upset. It should be noted that the same compound had been synthesized in 1853 but was apparently never tested clinically. There are conflicting stories about what happened when Hoffmann took the compound to the head of pharmacology,[30,31] but the compound was tested, patented, and released for sale in 1899 as Aspirin. Aspirin was a trademark name derived from acetyl and spiralic acid (the old name for salicylic acid).

Aspirin was marketed for physicians and sold as a white powder in individual dosage packets, available only on prescription. It was immediately popular worldwide, and the U.S. market became large enough that it was very soon manufactured in this country. In 1915 the 5-g (325 mg) white tablet stamped Bayer first appeared, and, also for the first time, Aspirin became a nonprescription item. The Bayer Company was on its way. It had an effective drug that could be sold to the public and was known by one name—Aspirin. And they had the name trademarked!

Before February, 1917, when the patent on Aspirin was to expire, Bayer started an advertising campaign to make it clear that there was only one Aspirin, and its first name was Bayer. Several companies started manufacturing and selling Aspirin as aspirin, and Bayer sued. What happened after this is a long story, but you know who lost; aspirin is aspirin—or is it?

Willow bark has come a long way! There are five major manufacturers of aspirin in the United States, and they sell bulk aspirin to many packaging companies. And sell they do—21,000 tons of acetylsalicylic acid a year, and that's only one fifth of the world's production! Quick—how many standard aspirin doses could be produced from America's production? (There are 7000 grains in a pound.) Answer next week! That answer will have to change soon: the standard dose for over 50 years—5 grains = 325 mg—is being pushed up, mostly through advertising. More is better. Big headache, big dose; extra problems, extra strength.

Therapeutic use. Say what you will, aspirin is truly a magnificent drug. It is also a drug with some serious side effects. Aspirin has three effects that are the primary basis for its clinical use. It is an analgesic that effectively blocks somatic pain in the mild to moderate range. Aspirin is also antipyretic:

it reduces body temperature when elevated by fever. Last, but not least, aspirin is an anti-inflammatory agent. It reduces the inflammation and soreness in an injured area. This action is the basis for its extensive use in arthritis. It is difficult to find another drug that has this span of effects coupled with a relatively low toxicity. It does, however, have side effects that pose problems for some people. The trend now is away from the "take-two-aspirins-and-call-me-in-the-morning" type of thinking.

These comments are true of the entire spectrum of salicylates, and there are several besides aspirin. The following comments also apply, more or less, to all agents formed from the basic chemical structure of salicylic acid, but the focus is on aspirin.

Since the action of a drug depends on its concentration at the cellular site of action, much work has been done to see how aspirin gets there, how fast it gets there, and how long it stays. Aspirin is readily absorbed from the stomach but even faster from the intestine. Thus anything that delays movement of the aspirin from the stomach should affect absorption time. The evidence is mixed[32] on whether taking aspirin with a meal, which delays emptying of the stomach, increases the time before onset of action. It is clear, however, that a water solution of aspirin is more rapidly absorbed than the tablet form and thus gives higher and earlier effective blood levels of the drug. Although the effervescent aspirins are absorbed more rapidly and result in earlier and higher blood levels of aspirin, there is no evidence that analgesia occurs sooner than with regular aspirin. Remember, too, that excessive use of these drugs disrupts the body's normal acid-base balance and creates other problems.

It is interesting that two famous compounds which the Bayer Laboratories in Germany were instrumental in introducing to the world are rapidly transformed to their original form after absorption. Both heroin and aspirin were first synthesized in the Bayer Laboratories. Heroin is more active than morphine and has morphine-like actions. Aspirin, either in the gastrointestinal tract or in the bloodstream, is converted to salicylic acid. Taken orally, aspirin is a more potent analgesic than salicylic acid,

since aspirin irritates the stomach less and is thus absorbed more rapidly.

The term *therapeutic dose* will be used repeatedly, with 600 to 1000 mg suggested as the dose range for aspirin. Most reports suggest that 300 mg is usually more effective than a placebo, while 600 mg is clearly even more effective. Many studies indicate that increasing the dose above that level does not increase aspirin's analgesic action, but some reserach indicates that 1200 mg of aspirin may provide greater relief than 600 mg.[33] In one study,[34] after ingestion of a 650-mg tablet of aspirin, headache and postpartum pain were not reduced significantly from placebo until 45 minutes had elapsed; maximum relief was obtained after 60 minutes. At 4 hours after intake, pain levels were equivalent in the drug and placebo groups, that is, the analgesia was gone. These reports agree with the salicylate blood levels measured in the same patients. At 45 minutes and at 4 hours the levels were the same. Thus it may be that a salicylate blood level of 30 μg/ml is the threshold for analgesic effect, with maximum relief at a level of 40 μg/ml.

At therapeutic doses aspirin does have analgesic actions that are fairly specific. First, and in marked contrast to narcotic analgesics, aspirin does not affect the impact of the anticipation of pain. It seems probable also that aspirin has its primary effect on the ability to withstand continuing pain. This no doubt is the basis for much of the self-medication with aspirin, since moderate, protracted pain is fairly common.

Other work suggests that aspirin is most effective as an analgesic against the middle range of pain. At low pain levels, it is difficult to show the effectiveness of any compound because of the extreme variability of patients' responses. At the level of "unbearable" pain, in experimental situations, aspirin does not increase the amount of time an individual can tolerate the high pain levels.[35] The salicylates do not block all types of pain. They are especially effective against headache and musculoskeletal aches and pains, less effective for toothache and sore throat, and almost valueless in visceral pain, as well as in traumatic (acute) pain.

The antipyretic (fever-reducing) action of aspirin does not lower temperature in an individual with normal body temperature. It has this effect only if the person has a fever. The mechanism by which the salicylates decrease body temperature is fairly well understood. They act on the temperature-regulating area of the hypothalamus to increase heat loss through peripheral mechanisms. Heat loss is primarily increased by vasodilation of peripheral blood vessels and by increased perspiration. Heat production is not changed, but heat loss is facilitated so that body temperature may go down.

More aspirin has probably been employed for its third major therapeutic use than for either of the other two. The anti-inflammatory action of the salicylates is the major basis for its use in rheumatoid arthritis. One report[31] is that 25% of all patients with rheumatoid arthritis use only aspirin, and over 50% use aspirin in addition to other compounds. These patients consume large amounts of aspirin, perhaps 3000 to 4000 mg, every day.

There are going to be some *big* changes in the marketing of internal analgesics if the advisory review panel has its way. The 1076-page tentative report was released in late 1976 and raises many important issues, but two need to be mentioned specifically. The report recommends that the only allowable therapeutic claims permitted should be "for the temporary relief of occasional minor aches, pains, headaches, and the reduction of fever." Seems reasonable—takes care of the analgesic and antipyretic effects, but what about the reduction of inflammation or the use in arthritis?

The review panel thought of that, too. It would like all salicylate products labeled, TAKE THIS PRODUCT FOR THE TREATMENT OF ARTHRITIS ONLY UNDER THE ADVICE AND SUPERVISION OF A PHYSICIAN. The panel does not believe that gout, arthritis, bursitis, and rheumatism can be self-diagnosed or self-treated. That's strong stuff, and there is no assurance that the FDA will accept that specific recommendation.

From the point of view of an occasional user, there are three other important ideas. Much work has been aimed at developing a sustained-release aspirin capsule to eliminate the need for taking medicine every 4 hours (or at night) and to maintain more constant blood levels. Usually the capsules are enteric-coated (protected with a chemical that will not be acted on by stomach juices but wil dissolve in intestinal fluids) or contain coated spheres of the drug that release it into the system slowly to maintain appropriate blood levels for 8 hours. The review panel on internal analgesics put all these products in Category III.

Another factor to be considered when buying aspirin is that most tablets, including aspirin, develop a harder external shell the longer they sit. This hardening effect does not change the amount of the active ingredient, but it does make the active ingredient less effective because disintegration time is increased by the hard exterior coating. Along the same line, moisture and heat speed the decomposition of acetylsalicylic acid into two other compounds: salicylic acid, which causes gastric distress, and acetic acid, vinegar. When the smell of vinegar is strong in your aspirin bottle, discard it!

And finally: Does buffering speed absorption of the aspirin? Does buffering speed relief? Does it act sooner but for a shorter period of time? Everyone has said the same thing for years[36]; now the review panel has said it again:

> There is no evidence that buffered aspirin preparations have a shorter duration of action than unbuffered preparations and although buffered aspirin has been shown to achieve high blood levels more rapidly than plain aspirin, there is no clinical data to confirm more rapid onset of analgesia as a result of initial early high blood levels.[37]

Various effects: adverse and otherwise

1. *Aspirin increases bleeding time by inhibiting blood platelet aggregation*. This is not an insignificant effect. Two or three aspirins can double bleeding time, the time it takes for blood to clot, and the effect may last for 4 to 7 days.[38] In one study[39] bleeding time increased 40% 2 hours after 30 mg of aspirin was administered. There are some advantages to this anticoagulant effect. The FDA[40] has found ". . . that aspirin given to men who have had minor strokes appears to help prevent some second strokes . . . The finding applies only to men—not

women—who have had minor strokes known as transient ischemic attacks . . . either two tablets twice a day or one tablet four times a day is an effective dose." The FDA has not yet approved aspirin as a treatment to reduce morbidity and deaths in men who had a recent myocardial infarction (MI), a heart attack, but the authorities in Canada did in early 1982.[41]

On the one hand the FDA is right: none of the six large studies—in the United States and Europe—on the effects of aspirin in reducing a second MI has been statistically significant. On the other hand, five of the studies showed trends favorable to aspirin—and there was good reason to believe that the doses used were too large and not started soon enough after the first MI.[42] Even the nonFDA experts can't agree.[43] The best bet that by the mid-1980s low doses (160 mg/day) of aspirin will be shown to be effective in decreasing death rates and will be approved for use in males following an MI. Note that although the media often talk about the use of aspirin prophylactically, there are no experimental data that suggest that aspirin will prevent a first MI.

There's good and bad in the anticoagulant effect of aspirin. Its use before surgery may help prevent blood clots from appearing in patients at high risk for clot formation. For many surgical patients, however, facilitation of blood clotting is desirable, and the rule is no aspirin or other salicylates for 7 to 10 days before surgery. The same principle, no aspirin, should hold for women in their last trimester of pregnancy. This may be particularly important, since aspirin does cross the placental barrier, and neither the short- nor long-term effects on the child are known.

2. *"Ingestion of aspirin, in doses of 1 to 3 gm/ day, will induce occult gastrointestinal bleeding in about 70% of normal subjects."*[44] In most cases this is only about 5 ml/day, but that is five times the normal loss. In some people the blood loss may be great enough to cause anemia. The basis for this effect is not clear but is believed to be a direct eroding of the aspirin tablets on the gastric mucosa. The rule is clear: drink lots of water when you take aspirin, or, better yet, crush the tablets and drink them in orange juice or other liquid.

3. *Aspirin use increases the number of viruses produced in sufferers of the common cold.*[45] If this result is broadly supported, it would mean that the aspirin user is more likely to "spread germs" or reinfect himself than the nonaspirin user. Fitting in with that is a report[46] showing that aspirin blocks the effect of interferon—a natural substance that makes cells resistant to viruses.

4. *Aspirin is the number one cause of accidental poisoning deaths in children under 5 years of age, as it has always been since records have been kept.*[47] Household plants and household soaps have been the first and second causes of nonfatal accidental poisonings in young children for many years, but aspirin continues to lead in mortality. Things are getting better, though. In 1966 there were 92 deaths in this age range, in 1977 only 11.

Usually (5 to 1) the poisoning agent is "baby aspirin." To decrease the seriousness of overingestion, all manufacturers of baby aspirin in this country have limited the bottles to 35 1¼-grain tablets, and a safety lid is now required to make it difficult for children to open the bottle. A far better plan is to use strip packaging, where each tablet can be obtained only by ripping open a foil container. This would decrease convenience and increase cost to the consumer, and manufacturers are resisting the move on that basis.

Some of the more incidental effects of aspirin need to be noted. At therapeutic doses these include an increase in fluid retention and blood volume, which sometimes results in a slight weight gain. Respiration is increased, as is oxygen consumption, and blood sugar levels increase in normal individuals but decrease in diabetic persons.

Mechanism of action. In 1972 it was not unreasonable to state:

> . . . the mechanisms whereby salicylates produce such diverse effects as analgesia, reduction of fever, increase in respiration and suppression of inflammation in connective tissue are not understood.[48]

Work that had been summarized in 1971[49] was already pointing the way to a better understanding of the mechanisms of pain and of aspirin's effect on the experience of pain. Aspirin is now believed to have both a central and a peripheral analgesic effect. The central effect is not clear, but the peripheral effect is well on its way to being understood; it is now known that aspirin modifies the *cause* of pain. The mechanism is really neat.

Prostaglandins are local hormones that are released when cell membranes are distorted or damaged, that is, injured. The prostaglandins then act on the endings of the neurons that mediate pain in the injured areas. The prostaglandins sensitize the neurons to mechanical stimulation and to stimulation by two other local hormones, histamine and bradykinin, which are more slowly released from the damaged tissue. Aspirin blocks the synthesis of the prostaglandins. To summarize: (1) Prostaglandins are not stored but are rapidly synthesized and released from cells when injury occurs. (2) Prostaglandins sensitize the pain neurons to other damage-released local hormones. (3) Prostaglandin synthesis is blocked by aspirin. (4) Without the prostaglandin sensitization, impulses are not initiated in the pain pathways by the other local hormones.

There is now abundant evidence to support this rough outline of the mechanism of the action of aspirin. For one, aspirin does not block the pain induced by injections of prostaglandins. Another is that aspirin has an analgesic effect only in tissues where prostaglandin formation is taking place. A similar explanation seems most reasonable and supportable as the basis for the anti-inflammatory action of aspirin.

The antipyretic action has also been spelled out: a specific prostaglandin acts on the anterior hypothalamus to decrease heat dissipation through the normal procedures of sweating and dilation of peripheral blood vessels. Aspirin blocks the synthesis of this prostaglandin in the anterior hypothalamus, and this is followed by increased heat loss. Remember well that there is a variety of different prostaglandins, and "prostaglandin . . . prepared from different tissues show different sensitivities to aspirin-like drugs. This property explains the variations in activity within the group of compounds."[50] Overall, aspirin-like drugs

inhibit prostaglandin biosynthesis, in concentrations similar to those in body fluid during therapy.

The assembled evidence, together with the actions of prostaglandins, overwhelmingly support the theory that this antienzyme effect is the mechanism of action of aspirin-like drugs.[50]

It's hard to keep from jumping up and down! In less than 10 years we have moved from knowing very little, to the marketing (as a prescription drug) of a new prostaglandin-inhibiting analgesic: zomepirac sodium (brand name, Zomax)! It's a unique drug. "With zomepirac we have the unusual situation of an analgesic that can be titrated to produce an effect that ranges from that equivalent to two aspirin tablets up to equivalency with a substantial dose of injectable morphine."[51,p.424] No one is yet sure why that is, but possibly it's because of zomepirac's high lipid solubility, which ensures its rapid and easy entrance into the brain.

Willow and poplar trees all over the world should be standing taller now. They started it and through many generations and dead-ends we have now discovered the unique importance of these hormone-like messenger chemicals.[52]

> The physiologic role of the prostaglandins is complex and not yet defined precisely . . . these ubiquitous compounds do appear important to regulation of cell function and defenses. The therapeutic potential of the prostaglandins seems to be immense, and their use in a wide variety of clinical conditions is just beginning.[53,p.80]

p-Aminophenols

There are two analgesic compounds of concern in this class: *phenacetin* and *acetaminophen*. Phenacetin was the *P* in the APC tablets your parents know about (*A* is for aspirin and *C* is for caffeine). Soldiers knew well that at sick call the APC tablets were the Army's Perfect Cure—for everything. Phenacetin has now gone to the land of dead drugs: even its best friends wouldn't tell it, but the review panel put it in Category II.

And it's about time. Phenacetin has been around since 1887 and has long been suspected of causing kidney lesions and dysfunction. In 1964, the FDA required a warning on all products containing phenacetin, which limited their use to 10 days, since the phenacetin might damage the kidneys. Anacin then dropped the *P* from its basic APC formulation, since it did not want to put the warning on the label.

The only real question is why everything took so long. Phenacetin was known to be rapidly converted to acetaminophen, which was the primary active agent. The mechanism of analgesic action of acetaminophen is not known, but it is equipotent with aspirin in its analgesic, as well as its antipyretic, effects. The antipyretic mechanism is similar to that of aspirin, but the analgesic effect may be additive to that produced by aspirin. Acetaminophen is not anti-inflammatory and thus is of minimal value in arthritis, gout, etc.

Acetaminophen has been marketed as an OTC analgesic since 1955 but it was the big advertising pushes in the 1970s for two brand name products, Tylenol and Datril, that brought acetaminophen into the bigtime. It is usually advertised as having most of the good points of "that other pain reliever" and many fewer disadvantages. To a degree this is probably true: if only analgesia and fever reduction are desired, acetaminophen is probably the drug of choice. A 1977 review of its therapeutic and other effects commented that "there is also growing concern that increasing household availability and the public's lack of recognition of acetaminophen's acute toxicity will produce a new health hazard."[54,p.126] In adults 7 g produce toxic effects, twice that in one dose causes reversible damage to the liver, and more than that may lead to hepatic coma and death. Of particular importance is the finding that chronic alcoholics and long-term heavy-alcohol users may be particularly susceptible to the damaging effects on the liver of high doses of acetaminophen.[55] In contrast to that an individual who is actually drunk at the time (or within 2 hours) of taking a high dose of acetaminophen may escape without liver damage because of some quirks in the metabolism of acetaminophen.[56]

AND THE WINNER IS . . .

It's an important battle—OTC internal analgesic sales: over $1.3 billion a year. In total sales the aspirins outsell the nonaspirins (mostly acetaminophen) by 2 to 1, but the gap is steadily closing. The aspirin whose first name is Bayer was number one for many years but it started slipping in the early 1970s and is now number four in sales. Tylenol has been king-of-the-OTC-internal-analgesics-mountain since 1978, having pushed Anacin from the top spot. Anacin still spends the most for advertising, Bayer is number two, Tylenol is third, and Bufferin fourth in advertising spending.

There has been lots of pushing and shoving and name calling among these big brand names. In the late 1970s the federal courts,[57] the FDA, and the FTC[58] all told the manufacturers that they'd better clean up their advertising or the FDA would tell the world in big headlines that they're all the same! Things quieted but Anacin keeps trying and in 1981 they had to stop using the phrase, ". . . contains the pain reliever most recommended by doctors," unless they identified it as aspirin.

There's a lot of excitement over what aspirin might be able to do, as a result of unfolding knowledge of prostaglandin effects.[59] It's used in many products—and, as plain aspirin, there are no important differences among the brands except the price—and the placebo effect that goes with the price (I paid a lot, it's got to be good!)[60] That should be important to college students since one survey found that one of every four had used aspirin within the previous 48 hours.[61]

Table 11-1 contains the better known OTC internal analgesics along with the amounts (in milligrams per tablet) of each chemical they contain. Aspirin and acetaminophen are equipotent and equieffective in their analgesic and antipyretic effects. Acetaminophen has no anti-inflammatory activity and thus, particularly in arthritis, aspirin is much more effective. The only way to select one (other than for arthritis) is on their toxic effects or side effects. "In an overdosage situation, the toxic spectrum of acetaminophen is likely to be centered around the liver, whereas aspirin's potential adverse effects mainly involve acid-balance and the gastrointestinal and hematologic systems."[62,p.20] Adverse effects with acetaminophen are rare but serious when they occur. "Overall, there can be no

TABLE 11-1 Ingredients in selected brand name OTC internal analgesics*

Brand	Aspirin	Phenacetin	Acetaminophen	Caffeine	Other
Anacin	400			32	
Bufferin	324				97 magnesium carbonate 49 aluminum glycinate
Empirin Compound	227	162		32	
Excedrin	250		250	65	
Vanquish	227		194	33	50 magnesium hydroxide 25 aluminum hydroxide gel, dried

*Numbers are milligrams in each tablet.

doubt that aspirin has a much greater potential for toxicity than [acetaminophen] and there is much to be said for restricting its use in favor of [acetaminophen] . . . ."[63,p.289]

The end of an era. But no weeping for the willows—they started a grand heritage.

THE ALL-TOO-COMMON COMMON COLD

There has to be something good about an illness that Charles Dickens could be lyrical about.

> I am at this moment
> Deaf in the ears,
> Hoarse in the throat,
> Red in the nose,
> Green in the gills,
> Damp in the eyes,
> Twitchy in the joints,
> And fractious in temper
> From a most intolerable
> And oppressive cold.[64,p.92]

The common cold is caused by a virus—well, viruses, over a hundred have been identified—but in 40% to 60% of individuals with colds researchers cannot connect the infection to a specific virus. That makes it tough to find a cure. Two groups of viruses are known to be associated with colds—the rhinovirus and the more recently identified (and less well-studied) coronaviruses. These viruses are clearly distinct from those that cause influenza, measles, and pneumonia. Success in developing vaccines against poliomyelitis and measles has made some experts optimistic about a vaccine for the common cold. Others are pessimistic because of the great variety of viruses and the fact that the rhinoviruses can apparently change their immunologic reactivity very readily. There may be hope. There are reports of two compounds that have been effective in inhibiting the growth of a high percentage (75% or more) of the strains of rhinoviruses.[65] Now known only as AR-336 and RMI-15,731 they may soon be famous.

Already famous is *interferon*. Discovered in 1957, it saved a life in a 1960 Flash Gordon comic strip episode and was the cover story of *Time* magazine March 31, 1980! Interferons are one of the body's lines of defense against infection and are naturally produced by cells attacked by viruses. "Interferons do not prevent viruses from entering cells but bind to receptors on cell surfaces and induce the synthesis of enzymes that inhibit viral replication . . . One of the most important effects of interferon . . . is its inhibition of cell division."[66,p.50] Interferon is being widely and rapidly studied—not just for the common cold but for cancer and other major infections. It has only recently been biosynthesized, through genetic engineering.

Human interferon is produced by bacteria. It's not easy or cheap but it's better than before when it had to be separated from human white blood cells and its cost was $30 to $50 billion a pound! Fortunately small amounts seem to be effective. In one study volunteers were given "a nasal spray of interferon one day before and three days after they were exposed to common cold viruses."[67,p.64] *None* of those volunteers developed symptoms while 80% of the placebo control group did! The problem? Each spray cost $700—a total of $1400 to prevent sniffles. Science is on its way—the vaccine will come.

And none too soon. Occasionally a new virus appears to which no one has developed antibodies, making some viral outbreaks quite dangerous. Influenza is a viral infection, but it is not "just a bad common cold." The 1968-1969 Hong Kong flu epidemic resulted in 51 million reported cases and 80,000 deaths in the United States.[68] Influenza outbreaks have been recorded as early as the year 1173, but the one that many people still remember occurred in 1918-1919. That post–World War I epidemic was responsible for more than 500,000 deaths in the United States and 20 million deaths worldwide!

Viruses damage or kill the cells they attack. The rhinoviruses zero in on the upper respiratory tract, at first causing irritation that may lead to reflex coughing and sneezing. Increased irritation inflames the tissue and is followed by soreness and swelling of the mucous membranes. As a defense against the infection, the mucous membranes release considerable fluid, which causes the "stuffed-up feeling."

Although the incubation period may be a week in some cases, the more common interval between infection and respiratory tract symptoms is 2 to 4 days. Prior to the onset of respiratory symptoms, the individual may just "feel bad" and develop joint aches and headaches. When fever does occur, it almost always develops early in the cold.

Most of us grew up believing that colds are passed by airborne particles, jet propelled usually through unobstructed sneezing. ("Cover your mouth! Cover your face!") The old wives—and the

old scientists—were wrong. You need to know four things so you can avoid the cold viruses of others—and avoid reinfecting yourself:

1. Up to 100 times as many viruses are produced and shed from the nasal mucosa than from the throat.
2. There are few viruses in the saliva of a person with a cold, probably no viruses at all in about half of these individuals.
3. Dried viruses survive on dry skin and nonporous surfaces—plastic, wood, etc.—for over 3 hours.
4. Most cold viruses enter the body through the nostrils and eyes.

Usually colds start by the fingers picking up viruses and then the individual rubs his eyes or picks his nose. In one study of adults with colds—40% had viruses on their hands but only 8% expelled viruses in coughs or sneezes.[69] The moral of the story is clear. To avoid colds: wash your hands frequently, and you may kiss, but not hold hands with, your sweetheart! You don't have to worry about your pets—only man and some of the higher apes are susceptible to colds.[70]

The experimental animal of choice for studying colds has to be man. In many studies with human volunteers, three types of findings seem to recur. First, not all who are directly exposed to a cold virus develop cold symptoms. In fact, only about 50% do. Second, in individuals with already existing antibodies to the virus, there may be only preliminary signs of a developing cold. These signs may last for a brief period (12 to 24 hours) and then disappear. The last finding crosses swords with the old wives, so it is best to quote:

Chilling experiments with volunteers did not show any particular influence on susceptibility to colds. Some volunteers were given an inoculation followed by a hot bath and made to stand in a draft in wet bathing suits. Some took walks in the rain and sat around in wet clothes. Other subjects were given the same chilling treatments with inoculations which contained no virus. No significant differences were found in these various well-controlled groups.[71]

The rhinoviruses discussed here seem to be the causative agent for the common cold in older children and adults. In infants and young children, however, other viruses cause most of their acute respiratory illnesses. A final comment: a cold is only a nuisance, but it can, and frequently does, develop into a serious illness. An untreated cold, if there is no new infection, will last 3 to 14 days. With proper treatment, a cold should not last more than 2 weeks.

Incidence and treatment

There have been very few large-scale long-term studies of the common cold. A 6-year study[72] of 5000 citizens of Tecumseh, Michigan, has substantiated some earlier beliefs and added some interesting new findings. The study was well done and involved a weekly phone call to determine whether any illness had occurred. If it had, detailed information was obtained, laboratory tests were done, and calls were made frequently until the illness was over. Only a few of the results can be mentioned here.

Fig. 11-1 supports the wisdom expressed some years earlier:

> Getting older would appear to be the best protection against many of the common cold viruses which attack us.[76,p.74]

Several points need emphasis. Until the age of 3, boys have more respiratory illnesses than girls, and after that age, females always have more colds. There is, in general, a decline with age in the number of colds. The increase in the number of colds reported by the 20- to 24-year-old women and 25- to 29-year-old men probably represents the influence of marriage, with the result that they are around young children, their own and others, and catch colds from them.

The study also reported that "blue Monday" was "flu Monday." Everyone above the age of 5 had the most colds on Monday and the fewest on Thursday. The effect was most dramatic in school-age chil-

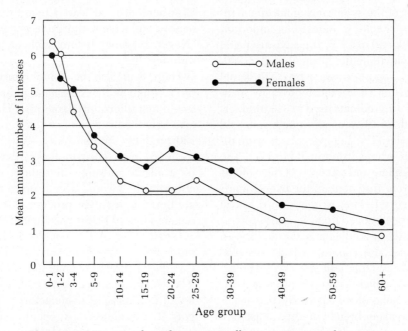

Fig. 11-1 Mean number of respiratory illnesses experienced per year.

dren, so that one would suspect that a combination of both psychological and physiological factors are involved. Another finding was a decrease in the total number of colds in the home with an increase in educational level of the head of the household. This was true even after the results were adjusted for age differences.

Since we are all getting older, we are at least doing one thing right to decrease the number of colds we have. Greater misery is hard to come by:

> Eight symptoms are usually associated with the common cold. These symptoms may occur over a period of 1 to 2 weeks. . . . The symptoms are: sore throat, sneezing, runny nose, watery eyes, aches and pains, mild fever, and congestion and coughing.
>
> These symptoms generally occur in that order, but not always. Any symptom can occur at any time during the progress of a cold. Some symptoms may even repeat. A runny nose can signal the start of a cold and occur again at the end.[73]

You should know this very well by now: no treatments are available at this time that reduce the duration or severity of the common cold infection.

Relief is just a . . . drop, swallow, poof . . . away. Treatment of the symptoms of an upper respiratory ailment, or cold, is undergoing important changes. Near the end of 1976, the advisory panel on cough and cold remedies presented its 1000-page preliminary report to the FDA. The panel reviewed information submitted by over 60 manufacturers, on 119 ingredients used in 320 products which accounted for 80% of all cough and cold (C&C) remedy sales. The 119 ingredients were divided into the six groups listed in Table 11-2. The panel took a tough line and put only 44 ingredients in Category I. Note that none of the expectorants made it to Category I. They're really hard to test and may have to be removed from the marketplace.

In addition to the ingredients in the six groups, the advisory panel also commented on miscellaneous ingredients, such as caffeine and vitamins, and found that they had no proper place in OTC C&C remedies. None of the Category II drugs is used in any of the major brands, so their departure will go almost unnoticed. It's hard to be noticed

TABLE 11-2 Number of ingredients in each category, grouped by type of drug

Type of drug	Category		
	I	II	III
Antitussives for cough relief	7	2	13
Expectorants for facilitating the removal of thick mucus from the lungs	0	10	22
Bronchodilators to ease breathing difficulties due to asthma	12	4	1
Anticholinergics for drying nasal secretions	0	2	3
Nasal decongestants for relief of swollen nasal membranes	14	2	15
Antihistamines for relief of symptoms of allergy	11	0	2

even if you are Category I, since there are between 35,000 and 50,000 C&C remedies. The number will probably increase, since the advisory panel recommended that 14 ingredients available only by prescription in 1976 should be available OTC. The FDA agreed on at least 10, so future winter cold seasons will have a multitude of new preparations: "Never available before without a doctor's prescription! Take . . . !"

There will also be some reformulations. You probably know that clinicians and scientists prefer single-ingredient preparations. That means you take only the drug you need, nothing extra. Of the 230 products studied, only 46 were single-ingredient products. The panel asked that all ingredients be available as single-ingredient products. They also said they would accept up to three active ingredients in a single product if there were a rationale for it. The advisory panel report was seen as vindication of the cough-cold industry, since most of the ingredients in wide use were put in Category I. Probably gone forever are many of the folk remedies handed down from mother to daughter to enterprising manufacturer. The only Category II ingredients most people will have heard of are the belladonna alkaloids (Chapter 18). The

C&C companies knew they were doing a good job: there was lots of customer satisfaction. A report on 32 manufacturers who sold more than 4 billion packages showed they had only one complaint for every million packages sold.

All OTC drug treatment is suppression of symptoms. To deal meaningfully with the ingredients available to reduce the misery of a cold, a quick note will be included of the basis for the more important symptoms: coughs and runny nose.

A cough is a protective reflex that keeps the lower respiratory tract clear of foreign matter. The mucous membranes in the area contain nerve endings that, if adequately stimulated, send signals to certain autonomic centers in the base of the brain. This "cough control center," when activated, does three things in sequence: causes a rapid intake of air and closing of the epiglottis; increases contraction of chest and abdominal muscles while constricting the bronchial tubes, thereby putting pressure on the epiglottis; and releases the epiglottis and expels the air at over 75 mph!

The stimulus for a cough in a cold may be an irritation resulting from a postnasal drip or from an accumulation of mucus within the bronchial tubes as a result of histamine release. Elimnination of excessive mucus facilitates the passage of air, which is usually felt to be a good thing in land animals. Because of this, it is not really desirable to completely suppress a cough that is productive, that is, producing mucus. A dry, nonproductive cough can be safely suppressed if it is the result of a cold. Coughs from smoking or emphysema or coughs that persist for more than 10 days should not be suppressed, and medical care should be sought.

Coughing caused by a cold can be reduced by making the cough control center less sensitive, reducing the sensory impulses to the center, or improving the situation in the bronchial tubes, that is, reducing the congestion. Of the three, the last is preferable, since it should facilitate the passage of air, whereas the other two methods could even impair it. Codeine is an effective narcotic depressant of the cough control center and acts at doses low enough to permit its inclusion in nonprescription cough remedies. Codeine is also a mild de-

pressant of the entire CNS, and, at higher doses than necessary to suppress coughing, it may reduce the rate of respiration. The commonly used nonnarcotic drug in OTC cough-suppressant preparations is dextromethorphan. In addition to depressing the cough center, this agent may also depress the CNS, but usually not at levels that can be reached by using OTC preparations as directed.

A cough will keep you awake at night and may be the symptom you like least in a cold. But sniffles must be the number one choice of many people for the least enjoyable symptom. To understand the treatment, it is necessary to understand the symptom.

> The nose is a common site for irritation and infection. Besides receiving abuse by rubbing, scratching, picking, blowing, and sniffing, its sensitive lining is the first tissue with which all environmental pollutants, irritants and toxicants contact before they are taken within the delicate confines of the respiratory system.[74]

The mucous membranes, the "sensitive lining," in the nose are wondrous. Under normal conditions the mucus secreted by the membranes is carried by moving cilia toward the back of the nasal cavity at a rate that replaces the mucus at least every hour and usually much more often. The mucus humidifies the air we breathe and traps small particles of dust. In a cold, the blood vessels dilate, and they, as well as the mucous membranes, release more fluid in the area of the infection. Both the capillary dilation and the mucus contribute to the nasal congestion.

The release of fluid is probably caused by histamine, which is a naturally occurring substance normally released from injured cells. Histamine has many effects, one of which was noted earlier in discussing internal analgesics. Another effect is an increase of the permeability of capillary walls, causing an increase in the amount of fluid in the injured area. This has some protective advantage for the damaged cells, but in the nose it stuffs things up.

There are two pharmacological approaches to reducing swollen membranes. One approach is to use an agent that causes vasoconstriction, since this not only reduces the size of the blood vessels but also decreases their fluid loss. The other approach is to block the action of histamine. Sympathomimetic agents, such as the amphetamine that used to be in the Benzedrine inhaler (Chapter 14), are potent vasoconstrictors and thus shrink swollen membranes. The most common sympathomimetic agent used in nasal drops is probably phenylephrine hydrochloride. When these drugs are used and the blood supply to the area reduced, there may be a decrease in the capability of the area to fight the infection and to resist new infection. Another problem is that the duration of the effect decreases each time, so that a condition of chronic congestion can result, which requires higher doses to overcome the congestion. It is possible that if sympathomimetic nose drops are used excessively, some nervousness and sweating could develop. These effects can be avoided for the most part if the directions for use are followed. Although some authorities do not sanction the oral use of sympathomimetic agents for relief of nasal congestion, they do appear in some OTC compounds. The FDA advisory panel accepted two types of oral sympathomimetics as being Category I.

> The antihistamines are widely used for symptomatic relief of upper respiratory infections caused by viruses. It is well-established that these agents have neither an antiviral effect nor shorten the duration of the common cold. A decrease in nasal congestion occurs following therapy with either an antihistamine or a combination of an antihistamine and a sympathomimetic drug.[75]

Of course, the 50- to 60-year-olds don't believe antihistamines are not anticold. Their use in the treatment of colds goes back to World War II. At that time, the antihistamines were touted as preventing and curing the common cold, not just as suppressing the symptoms. Before the FDA could step in, all America believed that antihistaminic drugs were "cold cures." Today antihistamines (usually pheniramines) are one of the many drugs in cold capsules. The advisory panel isn't too happy about that, and they would like the label to indicate

that antihistamines are "for the temporary relief of runny nose, sneezing, itching of the nose or throat, and itchy and watery eyes as may occur in hay fever, but not for the relief of nasal symptoms, such as stopped up nose, nasal stuffiness, or clogged up nose."[76] One multicenter study demonstrated ". . . that chlorpheniramine maleate . . . is clearly superior to a placebo in providing symptomatic improvement of the common cold."[77,p.2417] The greatest effect was, however, on the "wet" symptoms.

The antihistamines have one univeral side effect: sedation. The antihistamines used in antiallergy and cold tablets are chosen because they have satisfactory antihistamine actions and cause only minor sedation. Often agents in this group of drugs have greater sedating effects and are used in OTC day-time sedatives and sleep aids. Antihistamines also have some anticholinergic effects (causing dry mouth, at least).

To briefly summarize this section, the sympathomimetic agents act by causing vasoconstriction and reducing fluid loss from the capillaries. The antihistaminic drugs block histamine's effect on capillary walls, which is to increase movement of fluid from blood into tissue, and, through an anticholinergic mechanism, possibly help prevent vasodilation of the capillaries. All of this should decrease congestion in the nasal cavity, and it usually does for most people suffering from an allergy.

The misuse of these C&C remedies to produce alterations in consciousness is not uncommon. Chapters 14 and 18 give some idea of the kinds of effects obtained when high doses of sympathomimetic or anticholinergic drugs are taken. Dextromethorphan in high doses can result in sensations that some may interpret as positive feelings. Frequently these OTC compounds have a relatively high alcohol content (up to 25% [50 proof]) and, even without the addition of other psychoactive agents, can cause a high.

Last, every cloud has a silver lining. Not everyone is unhappy about the common cold. "The cold-and-cough remedy industry laughs at winter, and the extreme cold wave rolling over the nation this winter has infused it with optimism."[79,p. D4]

TABLE 11-3 Ingredients in selected brand name OTC cold and allergy products

Brand	Sympathomimetic	Antihistamine	Analgesic	Cough suppressant	Other
Comtrex*	12.5 phenylpropa-nolamine HCl	1 chlorpheniramine maleate	325 acetaminophen	10 dextromethor-phan hydro-bromide	20% alcohol (liquid)
Contac*	75 phenylpropanol-amine HCl	8 chlorpheniramine maleate			
CoTylenol*	30 pseudoephedrine HCl	2 chlorpheniramine maleate	325 acetaminophen	15 dextromethor-phan hydro-bromide	
Dristan*	20 phenylephrine HCl	4 chlorpheniramine maleate			
NyQuil†	7.9 ephedrine sul-fate	7.4 doxylamine succinate	590 acetaminophen	15 dextromethor-phan hydro-bromide	25% alcohol

*mg/tablet.
†mg/adult dose (1 ounce).

Sales have not been increasing rapidly in the early 1980s for this $1.2 billion a year industry. Even though it spends over $100 million a year on advertising, less than half of the people with colds use nonprescription cold medicines.[80] The big product is NyQuil with 25% of the market, Contac is second with 16%, and coming up fast—it's only been marketed since 1978—is Comtrex with 13% of this market. Table 11-3 lists the ingredients in some of the better known cold remedies.[81]

CONCLUDING COMMENT

The world of OTC products is bursting out all over. Prostaglandin, interferon, as-yet-unnamed drugs. What will we all do with our free time if we can't complain and comment about our minor ills, aches, and pains? There's always the weather—we know they can't control it (they can't even predict it!). These really are exciting times. With the changes in life-styles and diets acting to improve our health—and better drugs to control the minor illnesses we do have—we are having less and less disruption in our lives as a result of sickness. Maybe we're at the beginning or early stages of another

pharmacological revolution—one that has crept up on all of us, including me.

It is in the arena of OTC products that government, industry, and consumer come eyeball to eyeball and need increased interaction. The people who use OTC compounds are not sophisticated in drug use and need to be led by the hand into the land of safe, symptomatic self-treatment. This will require restraints on advertising and restraints on the proliferation of new, but not better, compounds.

With the expanding demands for better medical care and an ever-increasing patient-physician ratio, it is likely that self-medication will increase along with the potency of the drugs available and in use. It seems essential that some action must soon be taken to plan for the systematic education of everyone in the analysis of his symptoms and in the selection of the correct drug.

REFERENCES

1. Lamy, P.P.: OTC drugs and the elderly, Current Prescribing, p. 42, November 1979.
2. Gossel, T.A., and Wuest, J.R.: Over the counter, the trend to self medication, U.S. Pharmacist, p. 14, September 1981.

3. Digest of Education Statistics, National Center for Educational Statistics, Document No. ED1.113980, Washington, D.C., 1980.

4. Ingelfinger, F.J.: Editorial: Those "ingredients most used by doctors," New England Journal of Medicine **295**:616-617, 1976.

5. Edwards, C.C.: Closing the gap, FDA Papers Reprint, February 1973.

6. HHS News, p. 80-20, May 12, 1980.

7. HHS News, p. 82-2, January 5, 1982.

8. Mosley, J.H., Yingling, G.L., and Edwards, C.C.: The Food and Drug Administration's over-the-counter drug review: why review OTC drugs? Federation Proceedings **32**:1435-1437, 1973.

9. Newsweek, vol. 69, January 9, 1967.

10. Fischer, J.M.: DMSO: a review, U.S. Pharmacist, p. 25, September, 1981.

11. FDA studying results of new DMSO research, American Medical News, **24**(32):12, August 21-28, 1981.

12. Bean, W.B.: Drugs for nutritional disorders. In Modell, W., editor: Drugs of choice, 1976-1977, St. Louis, 1976, The C.V. Mosby Co.

13. Dunlop, D.: Abuse of drugs by the public and by doctors, British Medical Bulletin **26**:236-239, 1970.

14. Pauling, L.: Vitamin C and the common cold, San Francisco, 1970, W.H. Freeman & Co.

15. Coulehan, J.L.: Ascorbic acid and the common cold, Postgraduate Medicine **66**(3):153-160, 1979.

16. Beek, C.R.: Laxatives: what does regular mean? FDA Consumer, pp. 16-21, May, 1975.

17. Grollman, A.: The efficacy and therapeutic utility of home remedies, Annals of New York Academy of Sciences **120**:911-930, 1965.

18. Gossel, T.A., and Wuest, R.: Over the counter laxatives, U.S. Pharmacist, p. 20, November-December 1981.

19. Summary of report of the OTC Antimicrobial I Panel, U.S. Department of Health, Education, and Welfare, July, 1974, U.S. Government Printing Office.

20. HEW News, p. 78-83, October 6, 1978.

21. Consumer expenditure study, Product Marketing/Cosmetic and Fragrance Retailing, p. 32, August 1981.

22. Wuest, J.R., and Gossel, T.A.: Over the counter antacids, U.S. Pharmacist, p. 18, October 1981.

23. Kerr, F.W.L., and Casey, K.L.: Pain, Neurosciences Research Program Bulletin **16**(1), February 1978.

24. Bouckoms, A.J.: Analgesic adjuvants: the role of psychotropics, anticonvulsants, and prostaglandin inhibitors, Drug Therapy, **12**(1):179-186, January 1982.

25. Lewis, J.R.: Zomepirac sodium, Journal of the American Medical Association **246**(4):377-379, 1981.

26. Haslam, D.R.: Individual differences in pain threshold and level of arousal, British Journal of Psychology **58**:139-142, 1967.

27. Glynn, C.J.: Factors that influence the perception of intractable pain, Medical Times, **108**(3):11s-26s, March 1980.

28. Beecher, H.K.: Placebo effects of situations, attitudes and drugs: a quantitative study of suggestibility. In Rickels, K., editor: Non-specific factors in drug therapy, Springfield, Ill., 1968, Charles C Thomas, Publisher.

29. Smith, L.H., Jr., Chairman, Medical Staff Conference: The clinical pharmacology of salicylates, California Medicine **110**:411, 413, 1969.

30. Stevenson, J.M.: Aspirin, Journal of the Indiana State Medical Association **61**:1462-1464, 1968.

31. Salicylates, Chemical and Engineering News **46**:50, 1968.

32. Levy, G.: Aspirin: absorption rate and analgesic effect, Current Researches **44**:837, 1965.

33. Parkhouse, J., and others: The clinical dose response to aspirin, British Journal of Anaesthesiology **40**:433-441, 1968.

34. Wiseman, E.H., and Federici, N.J.: Development of a sustained-release aspirin tablet, Journal of Pharmaceutical Sciences **57**:1535-1539, 1968.

35. Wolff, B.B., and others: Response of experimental pain to analgesic drugs. III. Codeine, aspirin, secobarbital, and placebo, Clinical Pharmacology and Therapeutics **10**:217-228, 1969.

36. Moertel, C.G., and others: A comparative evaluation of marketed analgesic drugs, New England Journal of Medicine **286**:813-815, 1972.

37. Summary minutes of the OTC Panel on Internal Analgesics, Including Antirheumatic Drugs, November 19 and 20, 1973.

38. Aspirin revisited: it may lessen risk of thromboembolism, Medical World News, pp. 15-17, April 5, 1974.

39. Amrein, P.C., and others: Aspirin-induced prolongation of bleeding time and perioperative blood loss, Journal of the American Medical Association **245**(18):1825-1828, 1981.

40. HEW News, p. 80-86, February 21, 1980.

41. Canada gives one aspirin brand post-MI nod, Medical World News, **23**(3):27, February 1, 1982.

42. Kannel, W.B.: What the experts think—aspirin in prevention of cardiovascular disease, Part 1, Primary Cardiology, pp. 65-67, August 1980.

43. Phillips, J.H.: What the experts think—aspirin in prevention of cardiovascular disease, Part 2, Primary Cardiology, pp. 27-33, September 1980.

44. Weiss, H.J.: Aspirin—a dangerous drug? Journal of the American Medical Association **229**:1221-1222, 1974.

45. Stanley, E.D., and others: Increased virus shedding with aspirin treatment of rhinovirus infection, Journal of the American Medical Association **231**:1248-1251, 1975.

46. Pottathil, R., and others: Establishment of the interferon-mediated antiviral state: role of fatty acid cyclooxygenase, Proceedings of the National Academy of Sciences of the USA **77**(9):5437-5440, 1980.

47. Bulletin, National Clearinghouse for Poison Control Centers, U.S. Department of Health, Education and Welfare, Washington, D.C., September 1976, U.S. Government Printing Office.

48. Krane, S.M.: Action of salicylates, New England Journal of Medicine **286**:317-318, 1972.

49. Collier, H.O.J.: Prostaglandins and aspirin, Nature **232**:17-19, July 2, 1971.

50. Vane, J.R.: The mode of action of aspirin and similar compounds, Hospital Formulary, p. 628, November 1976.

51. Beaver, W.T.: Zomepirac: an overview—concluding remarks of the symposium chairman, Journal of Clinical Pharmacology, **20**(part 2):422-424, May-June 1980.

52. Marks, R.G., editor: Prostaglandins—from test tube to patients, Current Prescribing, pp. 15-31, October 1979.

53. Zurier, R.B.: Prostaglandins—their potential in clinical medicine, Postgraduate Medicine **68**(3):70-81, 1980.

54. Penna, R.P., project director: Handbook of nonprescription drugs, ed. 5, Project Drugs, Washington, D.C., 1977, American Pharmaceutical Association.

55. McClain, C.J., and others: Potentiation of acetaminophen hepatotoxicity by alcohol, Journal of the American Medical Association **244**(3):251-253, 1980.

56. Rumack, B.H.: Too much acetaminophen/alcohol: good or bad? Patient Care, **15**(1):165-166, January 15, 1981.

57. Sloane, L.: Pause in the battle of headaches, New York Times, August 19, 1977, p. D9.

58. Daugherty, P.H.: Anheuser-Busch names 2 to team, New York Times, December 14, 1977, p. 73.

59. Marwick, C.S.: Aspirin—new uses for an old drug, Medical World News, **20**(16):42-48, August 6, 1979.

60. Aspirin products, Medical Letter on Drugs and Therapeutics **23**(15):65-67 (Issue 588), July 24, 1981.

61. Taylor, F.: Aspirin: America's favorite drug, FDA Consumer **14**(10):12-17, December 1980-January 1981.

62. Mancini, R.E., and Yaffe, S.J.: The feverish child—aspirin or acetaminophen? Drug Therapy, **10**(5):103-114, May 1980.

63. Aspirin or paracetamol? (editoral), Lancet, **2**(8241):287, August 8, 1981.

64. Dickens, C.: The collected letters of Charles Dickens, 1880, Chapman & Hall Ltd.

65. Pramik, M.J.: The constant plague: colds and accompanying coughs, Apothecary, p. 20, November-December 1981.

66. Intriguing interferons, MD, pp. 49-52, January 1980.

67. The big IF in cancer—will the natural drug interferon fulfill its early promise, Time, pp. 60-66, March 31, 1980.

68. Maugh, T.H.: Influenza: the last of the great 68 plagues, Science **180**:1042-1044, 1973.

69. Klumpp, T.G.: The common cold—new concepts of transmission and prevention, Medical Times, **108**(11):98, 1s-3s, November 1980.

70. Tyrrell, D.A.J.: Hunting common cold viruses by some new methods, Journal of Infectious Diseases **121**:561-571, 1970.

71. Adams, J.M.: Viruses and colds, the modern plague, New York, 1967, American Elsevier Publishing Co., Inc.

72. Monto, A.S., and Ullman, B.M.: Acute respiratory illness in an American community, Journal of the American Medical Association **227**:164-169, 1974.

73. Gardner, S.: Remarks, HEW News, 76-25, pp. 1-2, September 8, 1976.

74. Gossell, T.A., and Wuest, J.R.: Common nasal disorders and their treatment, U.S. Pharmacist, pp. 27-33, January 1977.

75. Cirillo, V.J., and Tempero, K.F.: Pharmacology and therapeutic use of antihistamines, American Journal of Hospital Pharmacy **33**:1200-1207, 1976.

76. Hecht, A.: The common cold: relief but no cure, FDA Consumer, p. 9, September 1976.

77. Howard, J.C., and others: Effectiveness of antihistamines in the symptomatic management of the common cold, Journal of the American Medical Association **242**(22):2414-2417, 1979.

78. Hall, R.C.W., and others: Psychiatric and physiological reactions produced by over-the-counter medications, Journal of Psychedelic Drugs **10**(3):243-249, 1978.

79. Drug industry warms to nasty weather, New York Times, January 5, 1982, p. D4.

80. Cough/cold items, Drug Topics, p. 28, July 3, 1981.

81. Richie, E.: Over-the-counter drugs: Part 1. Preparations for coughs, colds, and allergies, Family Practice Recertification **3**(8):48-60, 1981.

CHAPTER 12

CONTRACEPTIVES

THERE'S AN AWFUL LOT OF CONFUSION about our expanding population, birth control, and the use of contraceptives, especially the oral contraceptive, the Pill. For some perspective, it may be well to remember that the original edict on which the Western world operated for many years was given to Noah: "Be fruitful, and multiply, and replenish the earth." (Gen. 9:1.) The full impact of the command came when Onan spilled his seed on the ground rather than impregnate his dead brother's wife as was required. This "displeased the Lord: wherefore he slew him also." (Gen. 38:9-10.)

As long as there was a high death rate and a need for sons and daughters to work the fields and labor for the good of the family, a high birthrate was necessary. The population of the world grew slowly for many years because infant mortality and death at an early age were facts of a very short life. Life expectancy at birth in the Roman Empire was 22 years; just over a hundred years ago it was 41. Today it is over 70 in the United States.

Until about 1750 the world population growth rate was very low. It has accelerated steadily since then, and the rate of growth is now about 30 times what it was in the mid-eighteenth century. Rate of growth, though, depends both on the birthrate and the death rate. Today's increase has come about as a result of lower death rates, not higher birthrates.

In the developed areas of the world, death rates began a gradual decline in 1750. With rapid advances in medical science, starting in the last quarter of the nineteenth century, death rates started falling rapidly and have only recently (1970) shown evidence of leveling off. Birthrates did not change much until toward the end of the nineteenth century. Since then there has been a steady decrease—with increases only during the periods after both world wars—and it still continues to drop. The most likely explanation is a combination of urbanization, the industrial revolution, and the fact that sons and daughters have become almost luxuries, rather than cheap labor to help with the family chores. You should know that in spite of the declining birthrates, "9 percent of everyone who ever lived is alive now."[1]

The foregoing is to let you appreciate that contraceptive devices, especially the Pill, only make it easier to avoid conception. They neither initiated the decline in birthrate, nor do they have a unique impact on the rate of population growth, on family planning, or on birth control. Contraceptives are probably being used by the same groups that would practice birth control in the absence of the convenience provided by today's scientists and engineers.

In the 1980s 72% of American women, ages 18

to 44, used some form of contraception. The first year "failure rates" (that is, pregnancy occurred) for the way contraceptives are used are: the Pill, 2%; IUDs, 4%; condom, 10%; diaphragm, 13%; foam, 15%; rhythm, 19%. In careful, compulsive users the failure rate is one third to one half of that listed.[2]

To keep the proper perspective for this chapter, understand that since large families are out, convenient birth control procedures are in. It is *not* true that since birth control procedures are convenient and in, large families are out. Not everyone agrees with this position.

BIRTH CONTROL AS A SOCIAL MOVEMENT

It seems to be part of the folklore in this country that in times past and among primitive peoples today there is no awareness of where babies come from. Nothing could be more wrong. The Ehrlichs, referring to the naiveté of some anthropologists, phrased it well: "If some stranger wandered up to us and asked if we knew where babies came from, we'd tell him from under cabbage leaves. Wouldn't you?" It must be admitted, however, "that contraceptive practices were rare among preliterate peoples when compared with abortion and infanticide, the chief primitive substitutes for conception control."[3,p.53]

Contraceptive devices and techniques have been known and written about for centuries. The Ebers Papyrus, which contains Egyptian medical writings from before 1550 BC, mentions the use of a "tampon" of crocodile dung to prevent conception. Aristotle described what could be relatively good contraceptive remedies: "Anoint that part of the womb on which the seed falls with oil of cedar, or with ointment of lead or with frankincense, commingled with olive oil." Such a treatment would at least be better than nothing, since oil reduces the motility of sperm and gums up the opening to the uterus. One of the more common contraceptive devices, although not in common use, in the nineteenth century was a sponge moistened with lemon juice. The citric acid worked as a spermicidal agent: "This

would seem to be one of the most effective contraceptives to be found in the whole range of literature on folk medicine."[3,p.182]

Techniques of birth control became a matter of social concern and discussion after the 1798 publication of *An Essay on Population as It Affects the Future Improvement of Society*, by Thomas Malthus. Malthus was an economist who presented the theory that population, when unchecked, increases geometrically, whereas the available food supply increases only arithmetically. The only way to avoid mass starvation was to decrease the growth of the population by "moral restraint": strict sexual continence and postponing the age of marriage. These were the only birth control methods Malthus would support.

As the motivation to decrease family size developed in the nineteenth century, the problem was *not* that people didn't know where babies came from or that abstinence would make the family smaller. The problem was *not* that there were no contraceptive devices and procedures. The problem was that very few people wanted to abstain, and only a few people knew about the contraceptive devices that were available. The question became how to solve those problems.

The answer in Britain began with a radical reformer who became an effective politician and helped start many social reforms. This man, Francis Place (1771-1854), is the father of the birth control movement, since he was the first to educate the masses about the personal, social, and economic advantages of small families. Place was a neo-Malthusian who preached in the streets (with handbills) what he believed and wrote in his 1822 book, which supported the general theory of Malthus. He not only advocated contraception, he told how to do it. One of his handbills was "To the MARRIED OF BOTH SEXES of the Working People," while another was "To THE MARRIED OF BOTH SEXES in Genteel Life."[3,pp.215-216] The differences clearly reflect the social attitudes of the era. The description of the techniques reflects the differences in the much longer handbills.

Marriage in early life, is the only truly happy state, and if the evil consequences of too large a family did not deter them, all men would marry while young, and thus would many lamentable evils be removed from society.

A simple effectual, and safe means of accomplishing these desirable results has long been known. . . . It is now made public for the benefit of every body. A piece of soft spongs about the size of a small ball attached to a very narrow ribbon and slightly moistened (when convenient) is introduced previous to sexual intercourse and is afterwards withdrawn, and thus by an easy, simple, cleanly and not indelicate method; no ways injurious to health, not only may much unhappiness and many miseries be prevented, but benefits to an incalculable amount be conferred on society.

Genteel Life, 1823

Do as other people do, to avoid having more children than they wish to have and can easily maintain.

What is done by other people is this. A piece of soft sponge is tied by a bobbin or penny ribbon, and inserted just before the sexual intercourse takes place, and is withdrawn again as soon as it has taken place. Many tie a piece of sponge to each end of the ribbon, and they take care not to use the same sponge again until it has been washed.

If the sponge be large enough, that is; as large as a green walnut, or a small apple, it will prevent conception, and thus without diminishing the pleasures of married life, or doing the least injury to the health of the most delicate woman, both the woman and her husband will be saved from all the miseries which having too many children produces.

Working People, 1823

This emphasis on the social and economic advantages of birth control began only in the nineteenth century and has continued as a primary theme even unto the present.

One indirect result of Place's work was the 1830 American publication of a book, *Moral Physiology*. This was the first book on birth control methods published in the United States. The chief method recommended was *coitus interruptus*, although it was admitted that "its practice might be impossible for some temperamental, strong-sexed men. . . ."[3,p.224]

The sale of this book in England contributed to one of the two famous trials in 1877 and 1878 that came close to completely legalizing the distribution of contraceptive information in England and gave the birth control advocates and ideas wide publicity.

In 1877 Charles Bradlaugh and Annie Besant were prosecuted for publishing and selling a pamphlet on contraception, "The Fruits of Philosophy or, The Private Companion of Young Married People," by Dr. Charles Knowlton. Because of a legal technicality, Bradlaugh and Besant were not convicted, and the right to publish contraceptive information was partially vindicated. But the battle was not yet over; the next year an elderly, quiet book publisher and bookseller, Edward Truelove, was pushed into the firing line.

Truelove had published and exhibited in his shop window the American book, *Moral Physiology*, and one other pamphlet on contraception. More than a hundred years before readers of George Orwell expected it, the Society for the Suppression of Vice was active and able to obtain the conviction of Edward Truelove for publishing and exhibiting material that would have an injurious effect on the minds of the young—4 months in prison, but without hard labor, since he was nearly 70.

That was it! The dam broke, and social protests, church groups, petitions, and newspapers called for Truelove's release from prison. He eventually was set free after serving his time. The prison stay was for a good cause, however. As happens frequently, the attempt to suppress a social trend results in more rapid spread of the ideas. The Society for the Suppression of Vice had succeeded in jailing Truelove and in destroying 200 copies of *Moral Physiology* and 1200 copies of the other pamphlet, but at what cost? National involvement by many groups of different persuasion, headlines in the newspapers of the day, and talk in the streets publicized birth control more than any advertising campaign could ever have done.

The book involved in the Bradlaugh-Besant case, *The Fruits of Philosophy*, sold about 1000 copies a year before the trial. In the 3½ years after the trial, 185,000 copies were sold in England. Many factors are involved in determining the birthrate of a country, but it should at least be noted that in England the birthrate climbed steadily until the late 1870s and then began a decline that has continued.

British birth control proponents got themselves in the thick of it again in 1971 when a drive was started to reduce the number of unwanted pregnancies and births. It was bad enough that they distributed posters of a nude male, looking very pregnant, with the caption, "Would you be more careful if it was you that got pregnant?" They outdid themselves in a marriage scene poster in which the bride, dressed in her wedding gown and looking as if she were ready to give birth any minute, is saying to the preacher, "I did."

The center of the controversy, however, was a pamphlet for high school students with a cover showing Casanova kneeling before a bare-breasted, and obviously willing, fair young maiden. The caption? "Casanova never got anybody into trouble." That's not true, but at least he did try to protect himself. The British scored another first with television ads showing a teenage couple "in love" walking, while the announcer suggests that "it's natural to worry about what might happen if you're not careful" and urges the viewer to visit a birth control center.

Where the British go, the Americans are soon to follow. Sometimes they're a little slow, however, and in the 1870s things were not too rosy in the United States.[4] The federal Comstock Act and all the state "little Comstock" laws made very tough going for those who preached birth control. The mother of the birth control movement in the United States—and later a mover worldwide—was Margaret Sanger, a New York City nurse. In 1916 in Brooklyn, Margaret Sanger opened the first contraceptive advice station in America. In 1916 in Brooklyn, the police closed the first contraceptive advice station in America and evicted Margaret Sanger as a public nuisance. She was eventually imprisoned, but she persevered. The clinic finally stayed open so that physicians could provide information for the cure and prevention of disease, but not for contraception!

The Margaret Sanger story is too involved to tell here, but it must be noted that she was the first to use the term *birth control*. In 1917 she started the National Birth Control League, which evolved into the Planned Parenthood Federation of America in 1942. Today's organization has 700 clinics in the United States and counsels over a million people a year. Partly as a response to Sanger's activity, the American Medical Association finally accepted birth control in 1937 as an integral part of medical practice and education. In the early 1950s Margaret Sanger urged a biologist friend, Gregory Pincus, to work on the development of a birth control pill. His research was partially supported by a $2,500 contribution from the Planned Parenthood Federation.

RELIGIOUS AND GOVERNMENTAL INFLUENCES ON BIRTH CONTROL

Religious beliefs and doctrines have had an important impact on sexual activity and all things associated with the biological differences between the sexes. Although the practices of individual believers do not necessarily coincide with the teachings of their churches, the general attitudes of the Protestant, Catholic, and Jewish religions need to be mentioned.

The Reform and Conservative wings of Judaism have no serious objections to the use of contraception, but the Orthodox branch condemns methods used by the male, except where the health of the female would be jeopardized by pregnancy.

The National Council of the Churches of Christ, which is a federation of the major Protestant denominations, issued a statement in 1961 that still holds true:

> Couples are free to use the gifts of science for conscientious family limitation, provided the means are mutually acceptable, non-injurious to health and appropriate to the degree of effectiveness required in the specific situation. Periodic continence (the rhythm method) is suitable for some couples, but is not inherently superior from a moral point of view. The general Protestant conviction is that motives, rather than methods, form the primary moral issue.

The position of the Roman Catholic church on birth control is based in the writings of St. Thomas Aquinas (1225-1274). Two of his statements are important:

> In so far as the generation of offspring is impeded, it is a vice against nature which happens in every carnal act from which generation cannot follow.
> *Summa Theologica*

> The inordinate omission of semen is against the good of nature, which is the conservation of the species; hence, after the sin of homicide, by which human nature actually existing is destroyed, this kind of sin, by which the generation of human nature is impeded, seems to hold second place.
> *Summa Contra Gentiles*

His work was originally interpreted to mean that sexual activity should be only for procreation. Abstinence was the only birth control method approved for Catholics until 1930. In that year Pope Pius XI, in his encyclical *On Christian Marriage*, approved the rhythm method as a way of controlling conception without severe limitations on intercourse.

National and international trends, coupled with the liberalizing effect of the 1962 Vatican Council, made the world optimistic about another change in church policy. Pope Paul VI settled that in a 1965 speech to the United Nations:

> You must strive to multiply bread so that it suffices for the tables of mankind and not rather favor an artificial control of birth . . . in order to diminish the number of guests at the banquet table.

He made it official in the 1967 encyclical, *Human Vitae:* the rhythm method was the only acceptable means of birth control. That position was strongly reaffirmed in 1981 by Pope John Paul II when he "condemned the practice of artificial birth control as a 'manipulation and degradation' of human sexuality."[5] Regardless, social trends continued, and the percentage of Roman Catholic women, ages 18 to 39, who use contraceptive methods other than rhythm increased from 30% in 1955 to 51% in 1965 to 68% in 1970 and 94% in 1975.[6]

Most countries now have as their official position something similar to the 1968 Declaration of the United Nations International Conference on Human Rights: "Couples have a basic human right to decide freely and responsibly on the number and spacing of their children and a right to adequate education and information in this respect."[7] Sometimes dealing with social trends and individual rights has interesting results.

A 1980 International Conference on World Population heard many reports that fertility is in a rapid decline in most areas of the world, especially in the more developed countries. Many European countries, such as Austria, Belgium, Britain, Denmark, Finland, France, Italy, the Netherlands, Sweden, Switzerland, and West Germany have birthrates that will not maintain their present populations. Why? "The whole system, which traditionally worked in favor of fertility, has collapsed. The Industrial Revolution, individualism, consumerism—in both Western and Eastern Europe and regardless of the political system of government—are sweeping away traditional pressures that favored the family."[8,p.C1]

India had the most controversial birth control program in recent history. It has about the worst problem and has put forth the biggest effort. From 1954 to 1976 the birthrate in India was 40/1000: 40 births occurred each year for every 1000 individuals in the population. From 1966 to 1976, 2% of the national budget was for family planning. The techniques have gradually changed over the years as one by one, information, education, and voluntary compliance failed.

An intensive campaign by Prime Minister Indira Gandhi began in April 1976 to decrease the birthrate to 25/1000 by 1984. Almost everything seemed to be fair in this total push. Both the stick and the carrot were used.[9] Vasectomy was one of the techniques that was urged for those over 25 with at least one child. The 5-minute operation earned the recipient a red printed sterilization certificate and $11, about a month's pay for an unskilled laborer. The certificate put the owner at the top of the list for public housing and farm land. Government workers had even more incentive, and after September 1977, any civil servant who increased his family above three children was to lose his job!

Phase one was working; there were 7 million vasectomies in 1976. Then a new party won the national election. The effort faltered: budgets decreased; participation was voluntary; the stick and carrot were put away; laissez-faire reigned. The program collapsed. Back in power, Prime Minister Indira Gandhi tried in 1981 to pick up the family planning momentum she had started in 1976. In March 1982, the program included birth control pills and IUDs but the emphasis was on sterilization—women received $22 for submitting to a quick surgical closing of their fallopian tubes, and men received $15 after submitting to a vasectomy. The emphasis was clearly on women. That may work because India is one of the few countries where the life expectancy of females (53 years) is less than that of males (54 years).[10] Let's hope.

FROM A LEGAL POINT OF VIEW—SHORT FORM

The thing that turned Antony Comstock (1844-1915) on was the suppression of salacious literature. He worked hard at it, organizing in 1873 the New York Society for the Suppression of Vice. In that same year he was the primary motivator behind the passage by the U.S. Congress of An Act for the Suppression of Trade in, and Circulation of, obscene Literature and Articles of Immoral Use.[11] The act said, in part, that whoever shall

> sell . . . lend . . . give away . . . exhibit . . . have in his possession . . . any drug or medicine, or any article whatever, for the prevention of conception . . . or shall write or print . . . any card, circular, book, pamphlet, advertisement . . . stating when, where, how, or of whom, or by what means, any of the articles in this section . . . can be purchased or obtained . . .

would be guilty of a misdemeanor, including manufacturers. It may seem a bit much from today's perspective, but who is in favor of immorality? Almost no one in the 1870s, and 44 states went on record by passing their own version of the "Comstock law." A hundred years after its birth, the

federal Comstock law was killed when Congress repealed it.

Between 1873 and 1973 there were some classic cases. One was in 1936, the famous *The United States* v. *One Package* trial. Dr. Hannah Stone imported a package of vaginal diaphragms from Japan, and the package was seized by the customs authorities on the basis of the Comstock law. The seizure was upheld in a lower court, but the Federal Court of Appeals supported Dr. Stone and established that it was legal to import or sell by mail things that might be used by physicians to promote the well-being of their patients.

This decision unlocked the federal door that had prevented widespread medical prescription of contraceptive devices, and the effect trickled down to the states.

The straw that broke the camel's back came in 1965 over Connecticut's 1879 little Comstock law. The law was severe (it even prevented the *use* of a device to control contraception) but could only be enforced selectively because of practical reasons. The enforcement did prevent birth control clinics from opening but allowed physicians to prescribe and druggists to stock and sell all kinds of contraceptives.

An attempt to have the law declared unconstitutional was not voted on by the U.S. Supreme Court because no one was actually enforcing the law. Since all the birth control clinics had been closed by state action 20 years before, no one had dared to open a clinic. To see if the law would be enforced, some of the Yale University faculty opened a birth control clinic in New Haven on November 2, 1961. On November 8 it was closed and the director and head physician arrested.

The U.S. Supreme Court declared the Connecticut law unconstitutional 3 years and 7 months later, and birth control clinics spread through the land. That 1965 decision by the court started the flood of states repealing their restrictive laws on birth control devices and information. The battle was not yet over; it was a 4 to 3 March 1972 decision, written by the only Catholic juror on the Supreme Court, that declared unconstitutional any law which prevented selling or giving birth control devices to unmarried individuals. This was further expanded in June 1977 when minors under the age of 16 were given the right to purchase contraceptives.

There are still problems, however. The medical director of the Planned Parenthood Federation in San Francisco made the point in 1975 that a "special program must be created for girls 9 to 12 years old who are sexually active and need advice." This is especially true, since most information pamphlets are "too complicated for a sixth-grader to understand." Still another problem exists: do you call the parents when a 9-year old comes in and asks for birth control assistance?[12] A minor problem you say. How do you define minor?

In 1978 the only age group not showing a decline in its birthrate from the previous several years was the 10 to 14 year olds. They had 12,500 births plus another 17,500 abortions. As you might expect over 90% of the mothers were unmarried.[13] Incidentally, even though it is illegal, 40% of the birth control centers require parental consent before providing abortion services to unwed mothers-to-be under the age of 15.

A February 1982 regulation requiring parents to be informed when children under 18 obtain birth control pills or IUDs from a clinic using federal funds is sure to be tested in court—and it won't stop until it reaches the Supreme Court. If the regulation stands, it means big problems. One study showed that 25% of those affected would stop applying for birth control pills or IUDs. Unfortunately, only 2% said they would stop their sexual activity.

PREVENTING CONCEPTION

> One thing this overcrowded world needs most is a perfect contraceptive—safe, effective, long-lasting but reversible in action, easy to administer, and inexpensive.[14]

Most, though not all, people agree that sexual activity is fun. The problem is how do you keep the fun but prevent pregnancy? Different ways are acceptable to different people, and there are a large number of procedures—surgical, mechanical, chemical—that prevent the union of the male sperm and the female ovum. Table 12-1 includes some of these techniques and indicates the risks associated with them and the alternative, no contraception. "With the exception of pill users who are heavy smokers in the age group 40 to 44 years, no method of contraception is associated with a higher overall mortality rate than the condition of pregnancy itself."[15] It should be noted that the safest form of interaction between members of the opposite sex is still platonic love, and the most effective oral contraceptive is "NO!"

Contributions toward the reduction of fertilization—the union of sperm and egg—by the male are few and not too effective at this time.[16] Coitus interruptus, withdrawal of the penis from the vagina before the release of sperm, is relatively ineffective, as well as unacceptable to many couples. The condom is more effective and has the great advantage, especially in today's epidemic of venereal disease, of reducing the likelihood of infection. The most effective procedure is a *vasectomy*, a form of sterilization that involves cutting and tying the tubes, the vas deferens, which carry sperm so they can be ejaculated. The operation is simple: it can be done in a physician's office in 10 to 15 minutes by making two small incisions in the scrotum, it's virtually 100% effective after 2 to 4 months, and it's permanent. There is no effect on hormone levels or any other aspect of sexual or urinary function. It is estimated that over 1 million vasectomies are performed each year.[17] In spite of early fears, there is no evidence that these males have a higher risk for any diseases.[18]

Permanent sterilization is also possible in the female. In a *tubal ligation* the physician ties off the fallopian tubes so that the mature egg is unable to reach the uterus, and sperm are unable to reach the egg. One technique that increased in popularity among the young in the late 1970s is the *diaphragm*. A diaphragm covers the end of the uterus and blocks the cervical canal through which sperm leave the vagina and enter the uterus and then the fallopian tubes. It must be fitted by a physician to ensure proper size. To obtain reasonable effective-

TABLE 12-1 Overall mortality associated with contraception per 100,000 nonsterile women

Method of contraception	Age group			
	15-29	30-34	35-39	40-44
None	6.4	13.9	20.8	22.6
Abortion only	1.5	1.7	1.9	1.2
Oral contraceptive				
Nonsmokers	1.4	2.2	4.5	7.1
Smokers	1.6	10.8	13.4	58.9
IUD	1.0	1.4	2.0	1.9
Traditional methods (diaphragm, condoms)	1.5	3.6	5.0	4.2
Traditional methods plus abortion	0.2	0.3	0.3	0.2

ness it must be used in conjunction with various jellies and foams that are spermicidal—toxic to sperm. The *oral contraceptive* acts to prevent the maturation and release of the egg from the female; it is the most effective nonpermanent contraceptive procedure now available. *Intrauterine devices (IUDs)* are nearly as effective and probably act by causing an inflammatory cell response which releases enzymes that attack the sperm and/or the fertilized egg.

Abortion has been used forever all over the world and has been important in the history of the United States.[19] It was partly abortion, as a morally and socially acceptable means of birth control, that decreased the birthrate from 7 in 1800 to 3.5 in 1900. Abortion has been in the news since 1973 when the U.S. Supreme Court ruled that during the first 3 months of pregnancy a woman had the right to obtain an abortion on request and from the third to the sixth month the state could regulate abortions on the basis of need and health of the mother and/or fetus. Fig. 12-1 shows the number of legal and illegal abortions from 1969 on.

The growing involvement of the "right of life" and the "pro-choice" groups in the late 1970s coupled with increasing political action of the religious right has put abortion back in center stage. One focus is a bill before Congress that says, "Congress finds that present day scientific evidence indicates a significant likelihood that actual human life exists from conception [and that] the fourteenth amendment . . . was intended to protect all human beings." That's a start on the road to a constitutional amendment banning abortions. "When life begins" may be a scientific question, but "when human life with rights begins" is a philosophical, religious, and social question on which reasonable people may differ. Whether abortions are outlawed or not, it seems most rational to admit that abortions will continue.[20,21]

The worldwide trend is for greater liberalization of abortions—36 nations have relaxed their laws since 1966. There are now 13 countries in which an abortion can be obtained with *no* restrictions during the first 3 months of pregnancy. As methods improve—and ease and safety increase—the incidence of abortions will probably increase. An FDA-approved prostaglandin-containing vaginal suppository for inducing abortion in the second trimester is a step in that direction.

The condom

> The condom is well on the way to becoming just another consumer product . . . bought and sold, almost as routinely and as freely as a package of cough drops or a tube of tooth paste.[22]

Condoms have burst on the marketplace with annual increases in sales of 15% for a total of $210

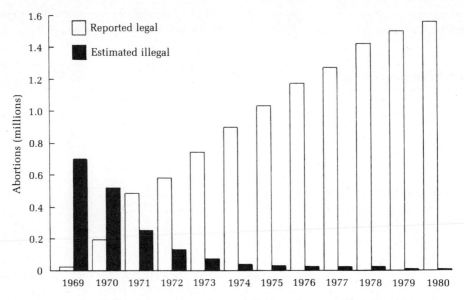

FIG. 12-1 Legal and illegal abortions in the United States from 1969 to 1980. (From Cates, W.: Legal abortion: Public Health Record, Science **215**:1586, March 26, 1982. Copyright 1982, American Association for the Advancement of Science.)

million in 1980. It's definitely a rising market and sales of condoms outstripped production in 1980![23] The condom (sheath) can not only look back on a full heritage but also forward to increased use in the 1980s. Say what you will about them, it is impossible to punch holes in the argument made by one manufacturer: "The condom is probably the only birth control device which has never been linked with side effects and the only one which guards against venereal disease."[24,p.15]

Coverings for the penis were originally used by the Egyptians,

> not for contraceptive purposes but for protection . . . against insect bites, as badges of rank or status . . . for decoration, or for modesty.[3,p.186]

> A plausible theory of the origin of the condom is that a medieval slaughterhouse worker first conceived the idea that covering the penis with the thin membranes of some animal would protect one against venereal infection. Perhaps someone tried it, found himself protected, communicated the idea to others.[3,p.191]

In 1564 the Italian scientist Falloppio (yes, he's the one who studied and named the tubes) recom-

mended a moistened linen sheath as a protection against venereal disease. The prophylactic use of the sheath has persisted throughout its history, and "prokits" became famous during World War II when the U.S. Army distributed millions to GIs all over the world.

The word "condom" first appeared in print in 1717 as *condum*. Later writers have usually attributed its invention to Dr. Condum, a physician in the court of Charles II of England (1660-1685). Unfortunately, there is no evidence that such a person ever existed; the writings of Samuel Pepys, chief chronicler of the period, do not mention anyone of that or similar name. More likely the word was derived from the Latin *condus*, a receptacle.

Casanova (1725-1798) knew and used "the English riding coat" (*redingcote anglaise*), as he called it. His memoirs are, of course, filled with his sexual exploits, and it seems clear that he used the condom against both conception and VD. Not that he liked it. As he said, "[I do not care] to shut myself up in a piece of dead skin in order to prove that I am perfectly alive."

The condom of the period was made from the cecum of a calf or sheep. The protection provided the user was not always of the highest quality. One handbill advertising condoms in 1796 spoke to that problem:

> To gard yourself from shame or fear,
> Votaires to Venus, hasten here;
> None in our wares e'er found a flaw,
> Self-preservation's nature's law.[3,p.200]

If only Casanova had lived a century later, he would have benefited from the 1839 cooking accident in America that was patented in 1844 by Charles Goodyear as the vulcanization of rubber. Rubber condoms were manufactured in the 1870s and, since they were inexpensive and reliable, sales took off and increased every year until the oral contraceptive appeared in the 1960s. The development and use of latex in the manufacture of condoms in the 1930s increased consumer acceptance, and sales reached almost a billion a year in the late 1960s. (Admittedly, hard facts about the size of the market are difficult to come by.)

Today manufacturers are trying everything: "new shapes, new textures, new lubricants, new claims for . . . sensitivity without compromising safety— and a broad spectrum of, it seems, all the colors in the rainbow."[22] Advertising has not yet reached American television, but it soon will, since the U.S. Supreme Court ruled in 1977 that it was unconstitutional to prohibit advertising or display of any form of contraception.

Condom ads have been developed for television, but the National Association of Broadcasters has not yet accepted them for national showing. They are definitely a soft sell: sex is never mentioned, and the emphasis is on romance, caring, and family planning. One ad starts with a quote from Ecclesiastes: "'To everything there is a season and a time to every purpose under the heaven . . . a time to weep, and a time to laugh; a time to mourn, and a time to dance.' The makers of Trojan Condoms believe there is a time for children. The right time. When they are wanted. And Trojans have helped people for over half a century safely practice responsible parenthood." Maybe that's better than the way most condoms are sold in Japan: door-to-door by women.

The latex in today's condom is about 0.0025 inch thick, electronically tested for holes and weaknesses before being lubricated, rolled, and packaged. Since 1938 the FDA has supervised the manufacturing and testing of condoms.[25] To this date there is no governmental group supervising their use. Forty-four states now permit condoms to be put on open display in drug stores and, in some states, supermarkets.

Intrauterine devices

IUDs have been used sporadically since Hippocrates described a device that was placed in the woman's uterus to prevent conception. Most IUDs still operate on the same principle as the smooth, round pebble that Arabian camel drivers inserted in the uteri of camels to prevent pregnancy while on long trips. The principle is simple: foreign objects in the uterus prevent the female from becoming pregnant.

Much research has been directed to discovering the mechanism by which the effect occurs. The IUD probably disrupts the physiology of the cells lining the uterus, creating a hostile environment for both the egg and the sperm. As the mechanism of action becomes clearer, IUDs should become more effective.

About 6% to 7% of women practicing birth control use an IUD; this is about 3 million American women. Worldwide probably 15 to 20 million women use the IUD.[26] In women who use an IUD, the pregnancy rate is about 6 for each 100 woman-years of use. This is second to the Pill's failure rate of less than 1 pregnancy per 100 women years of use. The superior effectiveness of the Pill, of course, depends on the woman taking it regularly and on schedule. Not every woman is able or willing to do this. Not everyone, however, can retain an IUD. Present data suggest that about 10% to 15% will spontaneously expel the IUD within the first year of use, usually during menstruation. Perhaps 10% of IUD users have side effects, such as pains and cramps similar to whose which sometimes accompany menstruation, and have the device removed. An IUD was originally recommended only for women who have had at least one child, since childbirth results in stretching of the cervix and insertion

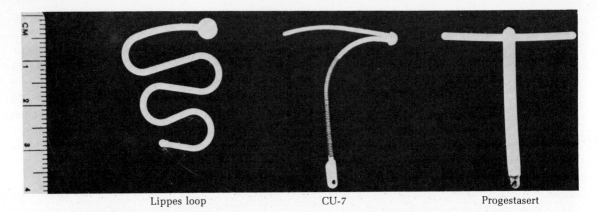

Lippes loop   CU-7   Progestasert

FIG. 12-2 *Lippes Loop* (Ortho Pharmaceutical Corp.) is probably the most widely used IUD worldwide. It is available in several width sizes, from 22.5 to 30 mm, and should be effective indefinitely. *CU-7* (Searle Laboratories) was probably the most widely used IUD in the United States in 1977. The unit is wound with copper wire weighing 89 mg and needs to be replaced every 2 years. *Progestasert* (Alza Pharmaceuticals), as of 1977 the IUD expanding most rapidly in use, has a hollow vertical stem containing 38 mg of progesterone, which is released at a rate of 65 μg a day. A Progestasert needs to be replaced every year.

of the device is easier for both physician and user. IUDs are being used increasingly in women who have not been pregnant, even though the adverse effects may be slightly higher. They should not be used by women with many sexual partners because of the increased risk of infection.[27] In all IUD users there is increased risk for pelvic infection—maybe two to four times that of nonIUD users.[28]

Although pessaries have been used since Casanova's time, today's IUDs are a direct descendant of the metal intrauterine ring that Dr. Grafenberg used in the 1920s as a contraceptive device for his German patients. His major contribution was to keep the device entirely within the uterus. The earlier devices, such as the pessary, were primarily vaginal devices that blocked the cervical canal and in some cases protruded into the uterus. This resulted in many infections as bacteria moved by way of this "ladder" from the vagina to the uterus.

World War II and a general misgiving about having foreign objects lying around inside the uterus slowed the development of IUDs until 1959, when there were two independent reports of successful contraception with Grafenberg-type devices. Many

IUDs have come and gone since that year. In 1968 the FDA removed all "closed" IUDs (for example, like the Grafenberg ring) from the market because they might obstruct the intestine if they perforated the uterine wall and entered the peritoneal cavity. Today's devices are all "open," and three brands have almost all the market: *Lippes Loop, Saf-T-Coil, CU-7*. Fig. 12-2 shows three IUDs in their actual size.

IUDs have the advantage that they do not interfere with normal body chemistry, and the IUD-related mortality rate, between 1 to 10 deaths per million users per year, is lower than that for the Pill, which is 22 to 45. The incidence of problems that require hospitalization is the same for the IUD and the Pill: less than 1 per 100 users per year. For some women the greatest advantage is that there are no pills to be taken—ever. The one *big* disadvantage is the higher pregnancy rate compared to the Pill. The greater danger to IUD users is pregnancy, since either the fetus or the IUD must be removed as early as possible. If menstruation is late in an IUD user, it is imperative that she check with her physician.

It should be noted that before May 1976 non-chemical IUDs, like the big three, did not come under FDA's jurisdiction prior to marketing. This meant manufacturers did not have to demonstrate either safety or effectiveness. If medical devices, such as IUDs, were found to be hazardous or ineffective after marketing, then the FDA could step in and regulate the sale of the device.

This is exactly what they did in 1974 with the Dalkon Shield, when it was implicated in a number of infected abortions and deaths. The problem seemed to be one that Grafenberg solved in the 1930s. Most IUDs have a nylon thread attached, which runs through the cervix and extends about an inch into the vagina. (By checking the thread each month, a woman can be sure she hasn't expelled her IUD.) All of the threads are monofilament, except the original Dalkon Shield, which had multiple strands braided together. Probably this multifilament thread provided a ladder by which bacteria could enter the uterus and cause infection.

The FDA act was amended in May 1976 to bring medical devices under the same type of control exerted over new drugs. The change came just in time, since some variations on the IUD theme were about to enter the marketplace. A few of the new devices will be impregnated with hormones. One recent IUD, Progestasert, incorporates progesterone into the device and is FDA approved for 1 year of use, after which it must be removed and replaced. The advantage is clear: it will alter the chemistry of uterine cells only, unlike the overall bodily effect of the Pill. Another recent IUD, the CU-7, is wrapped with copper wire, which alters uterine secretions and makes them toxic to sperm. IUDs such as these would always have been classed as drugs and thus needed FDA approval before marketing. They are not as effective as the Pill and retaining effectiveness requires replacing them every 1 to 2 years because of the steady loss of drug.

The menstrual cycle

In our nice, civilized, liberated, technologically advanced, low–infant mortality world, it is easy to forget that the "natural condition" of women until a century ago was to be pregnant or lactating and nursing a child. Menstruation was a relatively unique event, and it is not surprising with that history, and the experience of some women of severe discomfort during this period, that it was called "the curse." Menstruation was little understood in times past, as the fifteenth chapter of Leviticus shows clearly. Pliny[29,p.549] went overboard, however, stating that the discharge from a menstruating woman

> turns new wine sour, crops touched by it become barren, grafts die . . . the fruit of trees falls off . . . the edge of steel and the gleam of ivory are dulled . . . bronze and iron are at once seized by rust. . . .

Puberty in females is counted from the occasion of the first menstrual period, the *menarche*, and most girls achieve reproductive maturity within 3 to 6 months. In the absence of pregnancy or serious illness, most women menstruate about every 28 days until their late forties or early fifties. The time period surrounding the natural cessation of menstruation is called *menopause*. Menopause has no physiological relationship to sex drive or sexual activity; it only marks the end of fertility in the female.

The regular recurrence of menstruation about once a month from the age of 12 or 14 until 45 or 50 is a masterpiece of chemical engineering. The oral contraceptives have their effect by interfering with this normal rhythm of cycling, so it is necessary to briefly outline the process. Table 12-2 contains a summary of the time sequence and the hormones, actions, and structures involved at each point in a normal cycle in which pregnancy does not occur. Fig. 12-3 shows the sequence of events only with respect to the hormones involved.

Three structures are involved in this cycle that makes a woman fertile each month and prepares her body for pregnancy. One structure is the *hypothalamus–anterior pituitary (HY/AP)* combination in which the hypothalamus monitors blood levels of the female sex hormones, *estrogen* and *progesterone*, and regulates the output of hormones

TABLE 12-2 Structures, hormones, actions, and sequences involved in the normal monthly fertility cycle in women

Day	Hypothalamus/anterior pituitary	Ovaries	Uterus
−4	A-1 FSH output begins increasing		
−3		B-1 FSH causes egg-containing follicle to grow and begin to mature	
1 to 4			Menstruation
+5		B-2 Follicles secrete estrogen	
	A-2 Estrogen causes FSH output to decline and output of LH to increase		C-1 Estrogen causes endometrial cells lining uterus to grow in number and size
		B-3 LH causes follicles to increase output of estrogen and progesterone	
+14		B-4 Egg is released from follicle	C-2 Progesterone changes character of endometrial cells
		B-5 Follicle without egg produces high levels of progesterone and less estrogen	
	A-3 High progesterone levels suppress output of LH		C-3 Progesterone maintains these cells so they are ready for implantation of fertilized egg
		B-6 Decreasing LH levels reduce progesterone output from follicle without egg	
			C-4 Decreasing progesterone levels cannot maintain endometrial cells
+24	A-1 Low estrogen levels permit FSH to begin increasing (same as day −4)		
+28			
1 to 4			C-5 Endometrial cells die, slough off, and are discharged from body (menstruation)

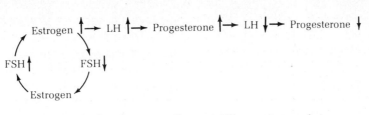

Estrogen-FSH cycle   Estrogen-LH-progesterone chain

FIG. 12-3 The interactions of anterior pituitary and ovarian hormones.

from the anterior pituitary gland. The anterior pituitary releases *follicle-stimulating hormone (FSH)* and *luteinizing hormone (LH)*.

The second structure is the pair of *ovaries*, which respond to FSH and LH by secreting estrogen and progesterone. The ovaries contain immature egg cells (ova) enclosed in special cell groups called *follicles*. When an egg cell matures, it is released from the follicle and enters one of the fallopian tubes to begin its 3-day journey to the uterus. The *uterus* is the third structure intimately involved in the monthly cycle. Under appropriate conditions a fertilized egg will embed itself and grow in the specially prepared *endometrial* cells that line the uterus.

It seems worthwhile to discuss the sequence of events in a menstrual cycle while referring to Table 12-2. About 4 days before menstruation, which marks the end of one cycle, a new cycle begins. A-1, The HY/AP begins producing and releasing ever-increasing amounts of FSH. B-1, The FSH acts on the ovaries, specifically to start the growth and maturation of cells in a follicle with immature egg. B-2, As the cells grow, they secrete more and more estrogen as well as small amounts of progesterone.

The estrogen has two functions: C-1, it causes the endometrial cells lining the uterus to increase in size and number and improves their blood supply, and A-2, it acts on the HY/AP to decrease the output of FSH and to increase the output of LH.

B-3, The LH acts on the ovaries and causes one of the follicles and its egg to mature. B-4, The egg is released from the follicle and moves into a fallopian tube. B-5, The high levels of LH change the

chemical makeup of the follicle without egg, and it is now called the *corpus luteum*, secreting high levels of progesterone but lower levels of estrogen.

Progesterone has two functions: C-2 and C-3, it acts on the estrogen-primed endometrial cells lining the uterus and prepares them for the implantation of a fertilized egg, and A-3, the high levels of progesterone also act on the HY/AP to reduce LH output.

B-6, As LH output declines, so does the amount of progesterone produced by the corpus luteum. C-4, As progesterone output decreases, the endometrial cells in the uterus break down and die. C-5, The discharge of these dead cells and some blood from the body is menstruation.

A-1, Already, before menstruation, a new cycle has started. Go back to −4.[30]

There are many reports[30] of alterations, usually decrements, in cognitive and performance functioning during the period of declining progesterone levels, the 5- to 7-day premenstrual period. Few of the studies are satisfactory from a scientific point of view; the only conclusion that seems warranted is that there may be decrements in functioning in some women in this premenstrual period.

The female sex hormones, progesterone and estrogen, have other effects on the body. Progesterone prepares the breasts for lactation. It is estrogen especially that is responsible for the development of the secondary sexual characteristics during adolescence, such as the broadening of the hips, development of the breasts, and the laying down of deposits of subcutaneous fatty tissue in the thighs and hips, which result in the typical feminine body build.

The Pill

> The oral contraceptives present society with problems unique in the history of human therapeutics. Never will so many people have taken such potent drugs voluntarily over such a protracted period for an objective other than for the control of disease.[31,p.1]

Development of oral contraceptives became possible in the late 1930s when techniques were developed to synthesize steroid hormones from plant steroids. Before then the only available sex hormones were those laboriously extracted from animal gonads; one report used over 3500 kg of sow's ovaries to obtain 25 mg of estrogen. Synthesizing the sex hormones also made it possible to make some chemical modifications so they would be effective when taken orally and be more potent than the natural hormones. This, of course, took time to accomplish.

The early 1950s brought together four individuals who started the ball rolling. Dr. Abraham Stone (husband of Hannah), Dr. Gregory Pincus (an experimental biologist), and Margaret Sanger talked about the need for an oral contraceptive. The outcome was that Dr. Pincus began work on a chemical contraceptive that at first involved only estrogen. Ideally, a combination of estrogen and progesterone would mimic pregnancy and prevent ovulation.

A Boston gynecologist, Dr. John Rock, worked with a group of "normal" women to remedy their sterility by first inducing a false pregnancy with estrogen and progesterone. A few months after treatment was stopped many of the women conceived, and the effect—cessation of artificially induced pregnancy followed by high fertility—became known as the "Rock rebound." This may happen in previously nonfertile women but the more usual effect is shown in Table 12-3.[32] For the first 3 months the probability of conception following cessation of use of the oral contraceptives is much lower than with other contraceptives, but this is not a permanent decrease—as shown by the higher conception rate beyond 1 year.

The odd couple, Pincus and Rock, met and decided to work together on the development of an oral contraceptive. The necessary breakthrough came when Searle Laboratories, a pharmaceutical house, developed a synthetic progesterone that was potent and orally effective. Early work with a synthetic progesterone-only pill was very effective. As the manufacturing procedures were improved, some of the contaminants in the early batches of hormone were removed; the pill became less effective, and "breakthrough bleeding" occurred. This minor bleeding, which occurred between menstrual periods, was stopped when one of the contaminants was put back into the pill. The "contaminant"—synthetic estrogen!

Clinical trials of the safety and effectiveness of a 45 to 1 combination of progesterone and estrogen were carried out in San Juan, Puerto Rico, with great success. Nothing is ever a total success when people and biological variability are involved. There were some pregnancies. There were some reported side effects. Overall, though, it was clear: pregnancies were reduced with only a minimum of physical and psychological discomforts. Of course, the basic trial lasted only 16 months, and only 265 women were involved! Not too overwhelming for a drug women were supposed to use almost daily for years.

But the world was waiting. *Time* magazine reported in 1957 about "hush-hush medical research" and speculated that Searle might introduce a drug that would have "a use in the field of physical birth control."[33]

Enovid was marketed in the United States by Searle in 1960, and a month's supply cost about $11. Pills were taken daily from the fifth day after the start of menstruation to the twenty-fifth day. The same schedule holds today. The price decreased to about $3 a month in the mid-1970s but was up to $15 in the early 1980s. The combination of estrogen and progesterone, both synthetics, had been standardized at 10 mg of norethynodrel (a synthetic progesterone) and 0.15 mg of mestranol (a synthetic estrogen). Today's Enovid contains half those levels.

One other historical development needs comment. You may have noticed that the *combination* pill, estrogen and progesterone, given every day

TABLE 12-3 Percent distribution of patients in time intervals to conception according to last contraceptive use

Months to conception	"Pill"	Intrauterine device	Diaphragm	All "other" methods
1-3	38.9	54.1	65.4	58.3
4-6	18.3	18.6	15.3	16.9
7-9	11.2	10.0	7.0	8.9
10-12	6.8	4.9	3.8	4.0
>13	24.8	12.4	8.5	11.9

From Linn, S., et al.: Delay in conception for former "pill" users, J.A.M.A. **247**(5):629, 1982. Copyright 1982, American Medical Association.

TABLE 12-4 Widely used progestins

Type of progestin	Classification of potency of effects		
	Progesterone	Androgen	Estrogen
Norethindrone	Strong	Mild	Weak
Norethynodrel	Mild	Weak	Mild
Norgestrel	Very, very strong	Strong	Very weak

does not follow the normal hormone pattern at all closely. Might not a pill that was more natural—estrogen in the early stages of the cycle and then progesterone added toward the end—be better? Good thinking—only too late; the first *sequential* pill was marketed in 1965. They were never big sellers: there seemed to be no advantage when compared to combination pills, and there were serious medical problems associated with the necessarily high estrogen levels. The FDA announced in February 1976 that all sequentials were voluntarily being removed from the market.

Two trends have developed over the years in the manufacturing and prescribing of oral contraceptives. One is the trend toward lower levels of progesterone and, especially, estrogen. This has paralleled the realization that most of the serious medical problems associated with the Pill have resulted from the estrogen level. As the dose levels have decreased, so have reports of the side effects that were associated with the early forms of the Pill.

The logical conclusion to the reduction of estro-

gen levels because of the side effects was reached with what are now called *minipills*—no estrogen at all, only progesterone. The minipill is taken *every* day. There is one problem though: breakthrough bleeding! The minipill also compromises effectiveness and has a failure (pregnancy) rate of 2 to 4 per 100 women-years of use.

The happy solution is the development of pills with different amounts of estrogen: 20, 30, or 35 μg of ethinyl estradiol. As the amount decreases there is an increase in the possibility of "breakthrough bleeding" but large decreases in the incidence of blood clots (thromboembolisms). It is now possible—probably in the 30- to 40 μg-range—to prevent pregnancy as effectively as with larger estrogen levels, but to decrease the risks to health.[34] The lowest effective estrogen level—as determined for each woman—should be used. Note also that here, as well as in the health-related effects of high and low tar/nicotine cigarettes, the current health statistics are based on individuals who used higher levels of the implicated drug than

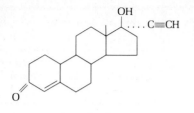

Norethindrone

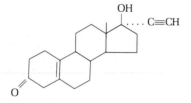

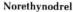

Norethynodrel

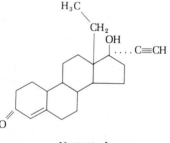

Norgestrel

FIG. 12-4 Synthetic progesterones (progestins) frequently used in oral contraceptives (see Table 12-4).

current users are receiving. Current risks should be lower.

Synthetic progesterone comes in a number of chemical formulas, and its characteristics vary as the chemical structure is changed. All synthetic progesterones are called *progestins;* three of the widely used progestins are listed in Table 12-4, and their structure are shown in Fig. 12-4. These progestins not only vary in the potency of their progesterone effects, but they also vary in the extent to which they have estrogen-like and androgen-like actions. Androgens are hormones which have effects similar to that of the male sex hormone, testosterone. Androgens, thus, are masculinizing, whereas estrogens, as mentioned earlier, are feminizing.

There are only two synthetic estrogens, and they have almost identical effects; only the potency varies. Ethinyl estradiol at a dose level of 0.05 mg has the same effect as mestranol at 0.08 mg. By varying the progestin used, it is possible to have an effective oral contraceptive that mimics closely or very poorly the effects of natural progesterone and estrogen.

Table 12-5 shows some of the side effects associated with deficient or excessive levels of progestin and estrogen. A physician will probably make the initial selection of an oral contraceptive based on examination of the patient. For example, in a female with acne, which is androgen related, the selection would probably be for a progestin with low androgenic activity combined with a moderate estrogen level. "For the less-feminine patient with acne, hirsutism, small breasts, . . . and scanty menses . . . ,"[35] an estrogen-dominant agent is the preferred choice.

The preceding has been included to help the reader appreciate that, although all of the combination oral contraceptives combine a progestin and an estrogen, fitting a specific brand to a specific patient is something of an art and makes positive use of side effects that are incidental to the purpose underlying their use: the prevention of conception.

Preventing pregnancy. The emphasis on cycles, various chemical structures, and progestagenic, estrogenic, and androgenic effects has been for a good purpose. The major mechanism by which the pill works is the prevention of ovulation.

When blood levels of FSH and LH have been monitored in women using the combination pill, the results are as you would expect. FHS output is suppressed by the estrogen component, and LH output is suppressed by the progestin in the pill. Both FSH and LH blood levels are low and consistent in users of the combination pill.

The suppression of increases in FSH prevents maturation and the follicle with egg. Indeed, examination of the ovaries of women who had been using an estrogen-containing oral contraceptive

TABLE 12-5 Effects associated with overabundance and underabundance of female sex hormones

Hormone	Effects resulting from	
	Excessive levels	**Deficient levels**
Estrogen	Nausea, bloating	Breakthrough bleeding
	Excessive menstrual flow	Irritability
	High blood pressure	Nervousness
	Uterine or leg cramps	Inadequate menstrual flow
	Breasts full and/or tender	Hot flushes
	Dizziness	
Progesterone	Persistent weight gain	No menstrual flow or excessive menstrual flow
	Fatigue, hair loss	
	Acne, abnormal hair growth	
	Depression	
	Regression of breasts	
	Inadequate menstrual flow	

showed that there were only immature follicles.

If the estrogen is effective in preventing the maturation of the egg, the suppression of ovulation by the progestin is only icing on the cake: nice but unnecessary. It may happen sometimes that a follicle does mature, and ovulation occurs. In these instances, more often when the minipills are used, a second effect of the progestins is probably important. One of the actions of estrogen is to cause the uterus to secrete much fluid through which the sperm can swim. Under normal conditions, as progesterone levels increase and estrogen decreases, the secreted fluid becomes much more viscous, and the entire uterine environment is hostile to the survival of the sperm. The level of progestin in minipills or combination pills is believed to create a continually hostile environment for the sperm: one in which they neither move far nor survive long. Still another mechanism functioning to decrease the probability of pregnancy is a change in the capacity of the endometrium to accept implantation of the fertilized egg.

If you are ever asked for a simple answer as to how the combination pills prevent conception, you will not be incorrect to answer by saying: the estrogen prevents maturation of the egg, and the progestin ensures prompt, adequate menstruation.

Physiological effects. Since the chemicals in the pill mimic several natural hormones, they have many effects, some of which we will ignore and some of which have already been mentioned. It is of interest that no one knows the fate of these synthetic estrogens and progesterones. The synthetics are active orally, in contrast to the natural hormones, because one of their chemical modifications acts to inhibit the liver enzymes that metabolize endogenous gonadal hormones.

There are some changes in carbohydrate metabolism and increases in growth hormone levels, but these are not thought to have clinically important effects. Both estrogens and progestins can cause limb deformities in the developing fetus if the mother, unaware of her pregnancy, continues to use the oral contraceptive during the early months of fetal development. Responding to increasing incidences of congenital deformities, the FDA, in September and October of 1976, placed strict new guidelines on physician instructions to patients and increased the warning on the labels of these drugs.

Brief comment must be made about the side effects (Table 12-5) of the oral contraceptive. Good evidence exists from many studies that there is both a placebo and a real component in each of these effects. It is impossible to separate these two parts in the individual patient. One reason is that users of the oral contraceptives are like the rest of us: a little bit, or very, susceptible to suggestion and anxious about trying something new. The prototype is new medical students who start to read their textbooks in clinical medicine and realize that they have every one of the diseases mentioned. By the end of the first chapter they are sure they won't live till the end of the month!

Many of the complaints about side effects diminish after a few months for a combination of both physiological and psychological reasons. It is true that some women discontinue using the Pill, but it seems that fewer beginning users are doing so now. This may be because the hormone levels are lower than before, the Pill is more an accepted part of our culture, or there are positive reasons (such as increasing opportunities for women) to tolerate mild to moderate discomfort while avoiding conception. There has been concern that the ratio of male to female offspring born after oral contraceptive use is different than the ratio in nonusers. One study found that "oral contraceptives have no bearing on the sex of subsequent offspring."[36] There is also no clearly predictable effect of the Pill on sexual response. Increases in sexual satisfaction are usually matched in studies by decreases, and by no change in enjoyment from prepill to postpill.[37,38] There is still debate over whether the use of the Pill increases the amount of sexual activity in married and other women.[39,40]

Serious medical problems. There are two approaches to the dilemma of medical problems and oral contraceptives. One is that a *very* serious medical problem, pregnancy, arises from *not* using oral contraceptives. If the decision is made to use oral contraceptives, however, is there an increased risk for any serious medical problems? The answer is clearly yes.

In the late 1960s Dr. Pincus,[41] the FDA,[42] and the AMA[43] all pooh-poohed problems resulting from use of the Pill. At the same time the British Medical Research Council was saying there were big medical risks associated with the use of the oral contraceptive. What's a person to believe? That's what Congress and the media wanted to know: hearings, articles, books—"without . . . knowing it . . . twenty million women have been taking part in an experiment and a gamble."[44,p.4] It all scared a lot of people and a 1970 Gallup Poll found that of women using the Pill, 18% had stopped and another 23% were thinking about it seriously. A lot of women never returned to the oral contraceptive after the early 1970s. Health warnings, which continue to occur on a monthly basis, it seems, made them cautious and the increased availability and ease of other forms of birth control resulted in a permanent decrease in users of the Pill—although it is still the most widely used method.[15]

The essence of all the current scientific literature is required by the FDA (as of 1977) to be included in a patient package insert (PPI), which each user is to get when she fills her prescription for an oral contraceptive. The statistics have already been presented in Tables 12-4 and 12-5, so what follows here are the major points of a PPI.

What You Should Know About Oral Contraceptives

Oral contraceptives ("the pill") are the most effective way (except for sterilization) to prevent pregnancy. They are also convenient and, for most women, free of serious or unpleasant side effects. Oral contraceptives must always be taken under the continuous supervision of a physician.

Who Should Not Use Oral Contraceptives

A. If you have now, or have had in the past, any of the following conditions you should not use the pill:
   1. Heart attack or stroke.
   2. Clots in the legs or lungs.
   3. Angina pectoris.
   4. Known or suspected cancer of the breast or sex organs.
   5. Unusual vaginal bleeding that has not yet been diagnosed.
B. If you are pregnant or suspect that you are pregnant, do not use the pill.

C. **Cigarette smoking increases the risk of serious adverse effects on the heart and blood vessels from oral contraceptive use. This risk increases with age and with heavy smoking (15 or more cigarettes per day) and is quite marked in women over 35 years of age. Women who use oral contraceptives should not smoke.**

D. If you have scanty or irregular periods or are a young woman without a regular cycle, you should use another method of contraception because, if you use the pill, you may have difficulty becoming pregnant or may fail to have menstrual periods after discontinuing the pill.

The Dangers of Oral Contraceptives

a. *Circulatory disorders (abnormal blood clotting, heart attack, and stroke due to hemorrhage).* Blood clots (in various blood vessels of the body) are the most common of the serious side effects of oral contraceptives. A clot can result in a stroke (if the clot is in the brain), a heart attack (if the clot is in a blood vessel of the heart), or a pulmonary embolus (a clot which forms in the legs or pelvis, then breaks off and travels to the lungs). Any of these can be fatal.

b. *Formation of tumors.* Studies have found that when certain animals are given the female sex hormone estrogen continuously for long periods, cancers may develop in the breast, cervix, vagina, and liver.

These findings suggest that oral contraceptives may cause cancer in humans. However, studies to date in women taking currently marketed oral contraceptives have not confirmed that oral contraceptives cause cancer in humans.

c. *Dangers to a developing child if oral contraceptives are used in or immediately preceding pregnancy.* Oral contraceptives should not be taken by pregnant women because they may damage the developing child. An increased risk of birth defects, including heart defects and limb defects, has been associated with the use of sex hormones, including oral contraceptives, in pregnancy.

d. *Gallbladder disease.* Women who use oral contraceptives have a greater risk than nonusers of having gallbladder disease requiring surgery.

The increased risk may first appear within one year of use and may double after four or five years of use.

Pregnancies Per 100 Women Per Year
Intrauterine device (IUD), less than 1-6;
Diaphragm with spermicidal products (creams or jellies), 2-20;
Condom (rubber) 3-36;
Aerosol foams, 2-29;
Jellies and creams, 4-36;
Periodic abstinence (rhythm) all types, less than 1-47;
  1. Calendar method, 14-47;
  2. Temperature method, 1-20;
  3. Temperature method—intercourse only in postovulatory phase, less than 1-7;
  4. Mucus method, 1-25;
No contraception, 60-80.
The figures (except for the IUD) vary widely because people differ in how well they use each method.

Three other comments are necessary: (1) A large prospective study, reported in 1981, found no differences in the incidence of visible birth defects between children born to oral contraceptive users and controls.[45] (2) In one 1981 report, "The findings suggest that an effect on the risk of myocardial infarction persists after the discontinuation of long-term use of oral contraceptives."[46,p.420] (3) A 10-year prospective study of over 16,000 women[47] concluded that ". . . for young, adult, healthy, white, middle-class women the risks of using oral contraceptives appear to be negligible."[15,p.40]

WHAT NEXT?

Oral contraception has come a long way in the last 20 years; where will it go in the next 20? Several directions have been pointed out in a 1981 article entitled "The brightest contraceptive hopes for the 21st century."[48] The title refers to one of the major problems in this area: the extensive and lengthy testing required by the FDA.

The requirements established for oral contraceptives are much more stringent than for any other class of drugs. High daily doses of the proposed drug must be administered for 7 years in dogs and for 10 years in monkeys to study the long-term toxicological effects. After the drug has been shown to be safe in animals—and safety in animals does not always mean safety in humans—then large-scale studies can be started in humans. Because of the use and nature of these drugs, very extensive, expensive monitoring is required on the human subjects.

From initial discovery to marketing a new oral contraceptive may take 15 years, and the patent lasts only 17 years. Two years is not a very long time in which to try to recoup the money spent on the project. Either the rules will have to be changed, the government will have to underwrite the cost, or we will give up expecting new chemical contraceptives.[49,50]

An injectable, long-term contraceptive in use in 80 countries by 10 million women and endorsed by the International Planned Parenthood Federation[51] is the focus of considerable controversy. Medraxyprogesteroneacetate (Depo-Provera) is a progestin that blocks fertility for 3 months after an intramuscular injection. The FDA has established a special committee to determine the safety and effectiveness, as well as weigh the pros and cons, of its use.[52,53] The primary disadvantage is the disruption/cessation of menstruation but that returns to normal when use ceases. The Committee on Drugs of the American Academy of Pediatrics believes it should be made available for limited use—at least with retarded adolescents.[54] If Depo-Provera doesn't make it, perhaps something will come of the World Health Organization's attempt to develop a long-term injectable contraceptive that would be a not-for-profit item[55] or maybe a once-a-month pill.[56]

Perhaps a day-after pill may emerge that does not have the possible cancer-producing side effects of diethylstilbestrol (DES), now used in emergency situations such as rape.[57] Vaccines that would stop the development of a fertilized egg and once-a-month pills that would induce menstruation even if fertilization occurred are also possibilities. These might meet with more social disapproval, since they are not truly contraceptive but, in fact, induce abortion.

Scientists are trying hard to make contraception and family planning a cooperative effort by developing a chemical contraceptive for males. The big news in the mid-1980s: a male pill. The substance is gossypol, which is derived from cottonseed, and the Chinese claim it is 99.98% effective—and without obvious side effects or reduction in male sexual drive.[58] We'll have to wait and see.

One thing is very clear and socially approved: the control of pregnancy is becoming more and more a matter of technology than of restraint. And if you needed more evidence: "Births to unwed women have increased 50 percent in the last decade and now at least one of every six American babies is born to an unmarried woman. . . ."[59,p.1] But it's everybody. Over 92% of all white, continuously married couples who want to avoid pregnancy are using some method of contraception.[60]

Whatever future birth control procedures develop, you can be sure they will be in the direction of greater effectiveness, greater safety, greater convenience. The social movement Francis Place started in the streets of London in 1822 has now become part of the mainstream of Western civilization. But I still worry about those 9-year-old girls.

REFERENCES

1. Wilford, J.N.: 9 Percent of everyone who ever lived is alive now, New York Times, October 6, 1981, p. C1.
2. Westoff, C.F.: Comparative contraceptive failure rates, Medical Aspects of Human Sexuality **15**:100, May 1981.
3. Himes, N.E.: Medical history of contraception, Baltimore, 1936, The Williams & Wilkins Co. (Reprinted by Gamut Press, New York, 1963.)
4. Kett, J.F.: The acceptance of contraception, Science **200**:645-646, May 12, 1978.
5. Tanner, H.: Pope emphasized doctrines on sex, New York Times, December 16, 1981, p. A7.
6. Westoff, C.F., and Ryder, N.B.: The secularization of U.S. Catholic birth control practices, Family Planning Perspectives, pp. 203-207, September-October 1977.
7. Callahan, D.: Ethics and population limitation, Science **175**:487-494, 1972.

8. Ibrahim, Y.M.: World fertility in rapid decline, according to vast new study, New York Times, July 15, 1980, p. C1.

9. Borders, W.: India enthusiastic about progress of its birth control programs. . . , New York Times, December 28, l976, p. 2.

10. In India, birth control focus shifts to women, New York Times, March 7, 1982, p. 6.

11. United States Statutes, 42nd Congress, 3rd Session, 1873, Chapter CCLVIII: An act for the suppression of trade in, and circulation of, obscene literature and articles of immoral use.

12. Birth control for 9-year-olds? San Francisco, 1975, Associated Press.

13. Teenage pregnancy: the problem that hasn't gone away, New York, 1981, The Alan Guttmacher Institute.

14. Culliton, B.J.: Birth control: report argues new leads are ignored, Science 194:921-922, 1976.

15. Stoehr, G.P.: Clinical complications of oral contraceptives, U.S. Pharmacist, p. 39, April 1981.

16. Jackson, H.: Chemical methods of male contraception, American Scientist 61:188-193, 1973.

17. Brodsky, S.A.: Vasectomy for elective sterilization, Family Practice Recertification 3(10):23-34, 1981.

18. Walker, A.M.; and others: Hospitalization rates in vasectomized men, Journal of the American Medical Association 245:2315, 1981.

19. Numbers, R.L.: Origins of a Prohibition, Science 202:967-968, December 1, 1978.

20. Meyer, H.S.: Science and the "human life bill," Journal of the American Medical Association 245(8):837-839, 1981.

21. Brozan, N.: Opposing sides step up efforts on abortion measure, New York Times, February 15, 1981, p. 38.

22. The condom comes out of hiding, American Druggist, pp. 26-38, January 1976.

23. Contraceptives, Drug Topics, p. 82, July 3, 1981.

24. The how-not-to book, New York, 1970, Julius Schmid, Inc.

25. Consumer Reports: Condoms, Mount Vernon, N.Y., 1979, Consumers Union of United States, Inc., pp. 583-589.

26. Ulackas, E.: Contraception: counseling yields compliance, Apothecary, p. 20, June 1981.

27. Gregg, S.R.: Tailoring contraception to patients, Medical World News, pp. 47-61, February 16, 1981.

28. Ziff, R.A.: The IUD and pelvic infection, American Family Physician 24(6):109-113, 1981.

29. Pliny: Natural history, book VII, translated by H. Rackham, Cambridge, Mass., 1942, Harvard University Press.

30. Neu, C., and DiMascio, A.: Variations in the menstrual cycle, Medical Aspects of Human Sexuality, pp. 164-180, February 1974.

31. Report on the oral contraceptives, Advisory Committee on Obstetrics and Gynecology, FDA, August 1, 1966.

32. Linn, S., and others: Delay in conception for former "pill" users, Journal of the American Medical Association 247(5):629-632, 1982.

33. Contraceptive pill? Time 69, May 6, 1957.

34. Selecting the safest oral contraceptive: is low-dose low-risk? Sexual Medicine Today, 5(9):26-31, September 1981.

35. Pattillo, R.A.: Drug and patient matching for safer oral contraception, Drug Therapy, p. 4, April 1975. (Reprint).

36. Rothman, K.J., and Liess, J.: Gender of offspring after oral-contraception use, New England Journal of Medicine 295:859-861, 1976.

37. Bragonier, J.R.: Influence of oral contraception on sexual response, Medical Aspects of Human Sexuality, pp. 130-160, October 1976.

38. Dennerstein, L., and Burrows, G.: Oral contraception and sexuality, Medical Journal of Australia, pp. 796-798, May 22, 1976.

39. James, W.H.: Coital rates and the pill, Nature 234:555-556, 1971.

40. Abramson, P.R., Repczynski, C.A., and Merrill, L.R.: The menstrual cycle and response to erotic literature, Journal of Consulting and Clinical Psychology 44:1018-1019, 1976.

41. Pincus, G.: Control of conception by hormonal steroids, Science 153:493-500, 1966.

42. Second Report on the Oral Contraceptives, Advisory Committee on Obstetrics and Gynecology, FDA, August 1, 1969.

43. Evaluation of oral contraceptives, prepared by the Council on Drugs, Journal of the American Medical Association 189:144-147, 1967.

44. Vaughn, P.: The pill on trial, New York, 1970, Coward-McCann, Inc.

45. Savolainen, E., Saksela, E., and Saxen, L.: Teratogenic hazards of oral contraceptives analyzed in a national malformation register, American Journal of Obstetrics and Gynecology 140:521-524, July 1981.

46. Slone, D., and others: Risk of myocardial infarction in relation to current and discontinued use of oral contraceptives, New England Journal of Medicine 305(8):420-424, 1981.

47. Walnut Creek contraceptive drug study: a prospective study of side effects of oral contraceptives, Journal of Reproductive Medicine 25(suppl.): 346, 1980.

48. Reproduction and human welfare, Cambridge, Mass., 1977, The M.I.T. Press.

49. Djerassi, C.: Prognosis for the development of new chemical birth-control agents, Science 166:468-473, 1969.

50. McCormack, D.: Research promising on male contraceptive pill, United Press International, December 16, 1976.

51. Anderson, S.H.: Global parenthood group backs birth-control drug U.S. restricts, New York Times, October 19, 1980, p. 56.

52. HEW News, p. 78-42, October 25, 1978.

53. HEW News, p. 79-22, July 26, 1979.

54. Medroxyprogesterone acetate (Depo-Provera), Pediatrics **56**(3):648, 1980.

55. Crabbe, P., and others: Injectable contraceptive synthesis: an example of international cooperation, Science **209**:992, August 1980.

56. Better birth control pill seen, New York Times, January 1, 1982, p. 33.

57. Dixon, G.W.: Ethinyl estradiol and conjugated estrogens as postcoital contraceptives, Journal of the American Medical Association **244**(12):1336, 1980.

58. Lilly's weapon in the cold war; a cotton-pickin male pill, Drug Topics, pp. 62-64, September 4, 1981.

59. Births to the unwed found to have risen 50% in 10 years, New York Times, October 26, 1981, p. 1.

60. Brody, J.: Study finds sterilization gains fastest of birth-curb methods, New York Times, May 5, 1976, p. C22.

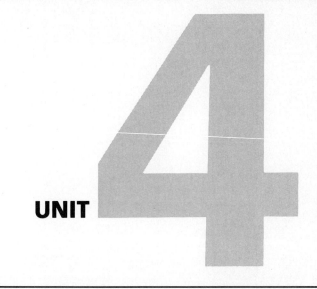

UNIT **4**

PSYCHOTHERAPEUTIC DRUGS

use and misuse

CHAPTER 13

TRANQUILIZERS AND MOOD MODIFIERS

I T WAS SAID—REMEMBER CHAPTER 5—that thoughts, feelings, and experiences were based on the interactions and activity of neurons in the brain. Changes in thinking and feeling are a result of changes in the ways neurons communicate with each other. This chapter discusses the treatment of individuals with mild, moderate, or severe disruptions in the way they think, feel, and act. But first, what is the basis for these disruptions in thinking and feeling that we call mental illness, and emotional disturbances? The changes might be a result of ghosts, death or serious damage to neurons, or changes in the biochemistry of the neurons.

Those who believe in ghosts probably aren't reading this book so I will not detail the reasons why ghosts are not the answer! Many of us do know someone whose thinking or behavior has changed as a result of damage to the brain. Perhaps it was only a minor concussion resulting in a brief loss of memory. Maybe it was a serious head injury that resulted in coma. Most of us know someone's grandparent who has had a stroke with a loss of some function or an elderly person whose memory and judgment have declined to such a level that they need to be continually watched. The thought, feeling, and behavior disorders that are the result of structural damage are called *organic disorders;*

their physical base is obvious. They will not be discussed further.

If mental illness is not a result of ghosts or structural damage to the brain, then it must result from alterations in the way the nervous system functions. The disorders discussed in this chapter are called *functional disorders:* there is a disruption in the normal functioning of the brain and there is no known organic basis. What might cause a nonstructural disruption of function? Right! A change in the biochemistry of the neurons. Why would there be differences in the behavior, thoughts, and feelings among groups? Correct again—there must be different biochemical changes or the changes must occur in different systems or parts of the brain. One last question: If differences in brain biochemistry underlie the differences experienced by emotionally disturbed people, what does that suggest? (Think a minute.) You are so good! Of course: (1) maybe there are ways to assess and evaluate brain chemistry by analyzing its waste products as they appear in blood or urine, (2) maybe we can develop a way of testing the chemistry of the brain to see if it's working okay, and (3) maybe we can correct the impaired functions by administering drugs that alter brain chemistry!

Perfect. That's exactly the line of thought that is revolutionizing the treatment of the mentally ill.[1]

It's exciting and fast moving. This chapter can only present a single picture from the ongoing and still incomplete series. But, as of now . . .

The drugs described in this chapter are in part very unlike those previously described. The effects of caffeine, nicotine, and alcohol have been repeatedly experienced, through choice, by a majority of adults in this country. In the case of the over-the-counter agents, a symptom or group of symptoms is identified by an individual, and he then prescribes and treats himself and monitors the decline of symptoms. Even though the oral contraceptives are so potent that they require a prescription, they are actually selected by the user and do not treat any symptoms or prevent any illnesses in the usual sense. Previously discussed drugs, then, are self-selected and self-administered, and their effects personally evaluated. The antipsychosis, antianxiety, antidepression, and antimania drugs outlined here are available only by prescription and are used in the treatment of major illnesses.

CLASSIFICATION OF THE MENTALLY ILL

Only some broad guidelines for the functional disorders can be laid down here but these will be adequate for present purposes. Historically the more severe disorders are called the *psychoses*, suggesting that the illness affected the psyche (the mind). The less disruptive mental disorders were called *neuroses* since it was believed that only neurons (the brain) were impaired. As will be elaborated, the psychoses are a disorder of thinking coupled with a blunting of affect. The neuroses are best viewed as life-adjustment problems.

In 1899 the great German psychiatrist, Emil Kraepelin, was the first to point out that within the psychoses there are two dimensions of behavior that must be considered in diagnosis. One dimension refers to the degree of disorganization of thought processes, while the second dimension is concerned with disturbances of mood. Most psychotics differ from nonpsychotics on both these dimensions, and their actual classification is still a problem. In the United States, if a patient has some

disorganization of thought, he is usually classed as a schizophrenic, even if there is a mood disruption. In Great Britain the emphasis is on the mood, and the same patient would most likely be classified as a depressive.[2]

Organization was brought to the thinking-disorder psychoses by the 1924 work of a Swiss psychiatrist, Eugen Bleuler. He termed one large group of psychotics as schizophrenics and emphasized the splitting of thinking from reality as basic in their illness. The major relevance of Bleuler is that he was the first to separate *fundamental symptoms*, those existing in every schizophrenic, from *accessory symptoms*, which were of far less importance and occurred with greater variability.

The fundamental symptoms were primarily disordered associations in thinking and a blunting or loss of affect or feeling, which are reflected well in the apathy and low level of responsiveness of the schizophrenic.

The accessory symptoms are usually the more dramatic ones. Hallucinations, delusions, and ideas of persecution are examples. These symptoms sometimes come and go in the same patient and certainly do not appear in all patients.

The distinction between fundamental and accessory symptoms is still used, but few authorities believe that schizophrenia is really a single entity. Some people, including Bleuler, even talk of the schizophrenia*s*. Many schizophrenics also differ from normal on the mood disturbance dimension. So common is this that many schizophrenics are labeled schizoaffective, or schizophrenic with affective disorder.

There are a number of psychotic patients (and many neurotic patients) who suffer severe disruptions in their mood. Take special note that many of these individuals have thinking *patterns* that are basically normal; it is the affect, the *emotional tone*, of the thoughts that is disturbed. At one end of the continuum the general characteristics of the depressed patients have been well described as a "temporary, severe lack of present or anticipated satisfaction associated with the conviction that one cannot perform adequately."[3,p.175] The depressed patient may be further classed as a retarded depressive in whom there is a slowing and a deterioration of behavior and thought. This is the type of patient one usually thinks of as a depressed patient. The agitated depressive has the general characteristics mentioned previously, but the manifestation may be through hyperactivity.

As might be expected, at the other end of the mood continuum is the manic individual.

> The hallmark of the manic episode is psychomotor acceleration, coupled with an ease of enjoyment and an unrealistically optimistic attitude toward achievement and the possibility of future enjoyment.[3,p.185.]

HISTORY

A brief history is helpful to appreciate the use of drugs in the treatment of these illnesses and to understand the impact of these psychoactive agents on the field of psychiatry. It is meaningful to divide the history of the treatment of the mentally ill into four eras: pre-Pinel, Pinel to custodial hospitals, custodial hospitals to 1950, and 1950 to present.

Pre-Pinel treatment

Before Pinel's influence began in the last decade of the eighteenth century, there were many different beliefs about the causes of mental illness, and they all shared the premise that the mentally ill could not be cured or helped in any way. The ancient belief that the mentally ill were possessed by demons and evil spirits was part of St. Augustine's dictum: "There are no diseases that do not arise from witchery and hence from the mind." This idea persisted and was reaffirmed as late as 1489 in the publication of *Malleus maleficarum* (Witch Hammer), which described many symptoms of mental illness and attributed that behavior to witchcraft. This book was widely used in various inquisitions and witch hunts for almost 300 years.

The attitude of society about what should be done with the mentally ill changed gradually in the western world from one of ignoring them, in the hope that they would go away, to a concern for public safety. This concern initially resulted in the

mentally ill being chained in dungeons, but it gradually moved to an enlightened management policy that paralleled the growth of asylums. The asylums were very clearly custodial, and the mentally ill, the mentally retarded, and the paupers were all carefully isolated from the sane, normal, moral members of the community.

The famous Bethlehem Hospital (Bedlam) was started in London in 1553 by Henry VIII. The treatment offered the "patients" in asylums and the loss of personal identify reflected the state of the art of medicine as well as society's attitude toward these individuals. A good idea of the general approach to the treatment of the mentally ill is given by the following description.

> About the last of May or the first of June, depending on the weather, they were all bled. Following this, they were given weekly vomits, and after that they were purged. The violent were confined in chains, or caged, or encased in muffs, leggins, or straight-jackets. They snapped and snarled, and tore and tugged at their chains like wild beasts. In the seventeenth century a man might take his entire family on a holiday outing through this chamber of horrors for a sixpence. . . .[4,p.66.]

Pinel to custodial hospitals

All reforms move slowly in historical perspective, and, when the history is long enough, it can be seen that changes occur only through a series of advances and setbacks. Philippe Pinel was trained as a physician in Paris and studied methods of treatment of the insane at the Gheel colony in Belgium. The Gheel community was very much like some of the most modern treatment centers in Europe today. The entire village was devoted to the care of the mentally ill, and most of the patients lived in the villagers' homes and worked at jobs on farms. Only a few were held in the hospital. Treatment consisted of the proper diet, some work, love, and kindness. No restraints or punishments were used.

Pinel published his essay on the diseases of the mind in 1791 and was placed in charge of Paris's

Saltpetriere Hospital for Men in 1792.[5] Conditions were really bad. The inspector general of French hospitals had reported in 1785:

> Thousands of lunatics are locked up in prisons without anyone ever thinking of administering the slightest remedy. The half-mad are mingled with those who are totally deranged, those who rage with those who are quiet; some are in chains . . . the duration of their misery is lifelong, for unfortunately the illness does not improve but only grows worse.[6,p.31]

Pinel quite literally cast off the chains of the inmates. He liberated them, and the newspapers of the day were quick to point out the common basis between the French Revolution and the removal of restraints from the mentally ill (that is, the liberation of the individual). It wasn't a statistically significant double-blind study, and less than a hundred patients lost their chains, but Pinel wrote: "I have examined with scrupulous care the effects which the iron chains had on the insane and afterward the comparative results of their removal and I cannot help favoring a wiser and more moderate restraint."[6,p.32] In 1793 restraints were considerably reduced in the women's hospital for the mentally ill in Paris, but little was accomplished outside the capital city for 50 years.

Word of Pinel's reforms as well as those instituted by others spread to many medical centers, and at the turn of the century *the* mode of treatment was "Moral Treatment." Moral Treatment was primarily respect for the individual, concern for his problems, work for his hands, and a calm environment. This treatment increased discharge rates to levels that have only recently been reattained. Wherever Moral Treatment was tried it seemed to be effective. Within 80 to 100 years of its formulation, however, such treatment vanished. Its use decreased partly because of changes in the attitude of the medical scientists and partly because of the effectiveness of the pioneers in the field of mental health such as Dorothea Dix.

In the United States there were no great medical centers. The asylums in this country contained a varied collection of mentally ill individuals without professional treatment or supervision. One of the pioneers in the treatment of the mentally ill in the United States was Dr. Benjamin Rush. He had good credentials: in addition to medical training in this country and in Europe, he was a signer of the Declaration of Independence, director of the Philadelphia Mint, and physician-general of the mid-Atlantic portion of the Continental Army. Later he was Professor of Medicine at the University of Pennsylvania, then the leading medical school in the country.

As an influential physician in this new country, he was effective in instituting some reforms in the treatment of the mentally ill. Unfortunately, Rush strongly believed in the influence of physical factors on the functioning of the psyche, and his treatment procedures frequently innvolved inducing great pain, fear of death, and the letting of 20 to 40 ounces of blood, which he found "wonderful for calming mad people"! Because of Rush's prestige, these treatment methods prevailed and prevented the concepts of Moral Treatment from being widely applied in the United States.

In addition to Rush's influence, treatment of the mentally ill was, in part, determined by the still-persisting common feeling that it was a disgrace to be mentally ill. Many disturbed family members were in fact skeletons-in-the-closet when guests came. With most people abhorring the mentally ill, one could not expect that much would be done to assist them. As a result they were at various times assigned to poorhouses, jails, and county homes. Not only the attitudes of society toward the mentally ill but also attitudes toward hospitals help hospitals from being built. Medical hospitals were dangerous places in those days; Lister, germ theory, and aseptic conditions were still in the future. If hospitals were bad, and they also cost money, it seemed silly to construct them for people you didn't really care about!

In 1840 the United States government for the first time counted the number of "insane" in the census. A total was reported of 17,434 out of a population of over 23 million, a little less than 1 in 1000. By this date there was institutional care for mentally ill only in 11 of the 26 states, and a total of 14 hospitals for mental disease with a capacity of less than 2500 beds. Conditions were appalling: the mentally ill, the poor, the criminal, the mentally retarded were all housed indiscriminately wherever they could be placed. Usually poorhouses and prisons were used and filled two to three times normal capacity. Once institutionalized, these people were forgotten—out of sight, out of mind.

Onto this scene came Dorothea Dix. Her career is an interesting story and a milestone in mental health history, but unfortunately we must emphasize here only a negative outcome of her efforts. Miss Dix devoted her life to the separation of the mentally ill from the retarded, the poor, and the criminal and was responsible for the construction of hospitals in many parts of the country for the treatment of the mentally ill. Dorothea Dix concentrated on getting the states to assume responsibility from the local communities. She was responsible for moving the mentally ill out of other institutions into mental hospitals and for dispelling some of the negative attitudes people had about the illness so that family members were hospitalized instead of hidden. However, the construction of hospitals and the commitment of more people to them operated to assure the general neglect of the mentally ill.

The hospitals gradually grew larger and larger, to the point where no treatment could be given because there were not enough professional and other personnel. The hospitals were built away from crowded cities, and the patients became more isolated from the community. The isolation and overcrowding made the hospital role more and more custodial, and discharge rates went down. The few private hospitals that had been able to earlier implement Moral Treatment had to relinquish it for a custodial role.

Not all of the blame for the failure of Moral Treatment to triumph as a treatment for the mentally ill can be attributed to Dorothea Dix. One factor was the developing attitude in the late nineteenth century in some influential scientists that mental illness was a brain disorder and as such should be treated by physical and physiological methods. The

fact that the physiological methods available did not work was unimportant; clearly, Moral Treatment was not consistent with this attitude. A second factor, which appealed more to another group of physicians, was culminating in the work of Freud in Vienna. The psychoanalytic emphasis on the unconscious dynamics underlying symptoms was not easily translated into treatment methods for large numbers of patients. Neither of these important developments can be traced here, but, combined with overcrowded and understaffed hospitals, they seemed to provide adequate justification for "locking up the loonies" and waiting for an effective treatment to appear.

Custodial hospitals to 1950

There is no clear line dividing this period from the preceding one. In 1860, though, mental hospital discharge rates began to decrease. The trend toward lower discharge rates, and thus longer periods of hospitalization, continued from 1860 to 1920. There was no increase in the patient discharge rate, and decrease in duration of hospitalization, until the mid-1950s.

The effective use of malaria-induced fever for the treatment of general paresis in 1917 renewed hope for a physical treatment of the mentally ill. The 1920s had their narcosis therapy, which consisted of long periods of almost continuous drug-induced sleep, up to a week or 10 days in some cases. The first of the old modern physical therapies was developed by Manfred Sakel in Vienna in the late 1920s. Sakel, in 1933, induced coma in schizophrenics by the administration of insulin. The resulting drop in blood glucose level caused the brain neurons to first increase their activity and cause convulsions and then to decrease their activity and leave the patient in a coma. From 30 to 50 of these treatments over a 2- to 3-month period was said to be highly effective, and discharge rates of 90% were reported in the early years of use.

In 1954 a standard text in psychiatry could describe insulin shock therapy as "the only effective method of treating early schizophrenia." A 1957 survey of the literature found, however, that even when initial treatment was reported to be effective, relapse rate was high, and recovery following insulin shock treatment was actually no higher than the rate of spontaneous remission.[7]

Ladislas von Meduna believed strongly that epilepsy and schizophrenia were mutually exclusive illnesses. He had observed, incorrectly, that no epileptic was schizophrenic, and no schizophrenic ever had epilepsy. Reasoning that the epileptic convulsions prevented the development of schizophrenia, he felt that inducing convulsions might have therapeutic value for these patients. His first convulsant drug was camphor, but it had disadvantages, the major one being a time lag of hours between injection and the convulsions. In 1934 he started injecting Metrazol (pentylenetetrazol), which induced convulsions in less than 30 seconds, and reported improvement rates in schizophrenics of 50% to 60%.

The use of a drug was not ideal for inducing convulsions, since the 30-second interval between injection and loss of consciousness (with the convulsion) produced much anguish in the patient. Ugo Cerletti used pigs in a slaughterhouse to develop the technique for the use of electric shock to induce convulsions. This method has the advantage of inducing loss of consciousness and convulsion at the moment the electric shock is applied. Although originally using mouth and rectum electrodes, he changed to brain electrode placement in 1938 and found it safer and more effective.

Electroconvulsive therapy (ECT) is only rarely used now with schizophrenics. Although early studies in 1943 suggested that almost 70% of the treated schizophrenics showed marked improvement, more recent reports in 1957 are in the neighborhood of 50%. Electroconvulsive therapy, however, is still used with severely depressed patients with good effect.[7]

Throughout the early part of this history of treatment methods, reference was made only to the mentally ill, the insane, the psychotics. As treatments became more specific, so did the need for a careful classification system. As we will see, that need continues.

The group of emotionally disturbed individuals classed as neurotics are not as severely disrupted in their interactions with the world as the psychotics. Rarely are neurotics hospitalized for prolonged periods. Their general characteristics are much anxiety (which may be directly experienced or partially expressed in various symptoms), dissatisfaction, and unhappiness. There is no gross deficit in reality testing, but neurosis is always accompanied by some decrease in efficiency and effectiveness. This decrease occurs typically without a major deficit in thinking and has led one writer to comment: "Neurosis consists of stupid behavior by an unstupid person."

Neurotic behavior can perhaps best be understood as maladaptive solutions to life-adjustment problems. Neurotic symptoms are behavior that provides short-term relief from anxiety, feelings of inferiority, and other similar negative feelings. They become self-defeating when used frequently, and at that point the symptoms cause more problems than they solve. Inability to solve these self-caused problems results in frustration, increased feelings of inadequacy, and anxiety. When the discomfort becomes unbearable, the individual seeks help in solving his problems in living. As of 1981 individuals are no longer classified as "neurotic." Use of the term will persist for many years, and it is still an excellent term for the group of individuals just described. We will use it here.

These, then, are the four large classes of emotionally disturbed individuals for which psychotherapeutic agents have been sought and found: the schizophrenics, the depressives, the manics, and the neurotics. The next section traces the history of the treatment of the seriously mentally ill and provides a background for modern approaches.

TREATMENT OF SCHIZOPHRENIA

From 1945 to 1955 there was an average increase each year of 13,000 patients residing in state mental hospitals. This was a continuation of a long-term trend and the result of a dedicated effort to move mentally ill individuals into hospitals so that treatment could be provided and the community protected. Because of these increases, although the

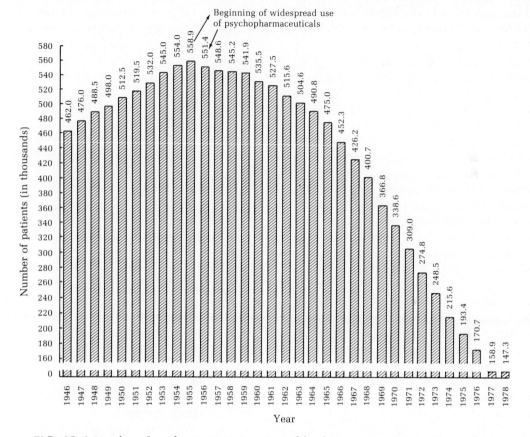

FIG. 13-1 Number of resident patients in state and local governmental mental hospitals in the United States. (Based on U.S. Public Health Service Data.)

population of the United States doubled from 1903 to 1952, the population of state mental hospitals quadrupled from 133,000 to over half a million.

The year 1955 was the high water mark of residents in mental hospitals. If the 1945 to 1955 rate of increase had continued, there would have been over 923,000 patients in state mental hospitals by 1983. Instead, though, the number has decreased each year since 1955, so that in 1978 there were 400,000 fewer patients in those hospitals than in 1955. The 1946 to 1978 mental hospital population changes are clearly seen in Fig. 13-1. This decline in the resident population has occurred in spite of a large increase in the number of admissions to state hospitals. In 1955 there were 178,000 patients admitted to state and local mental hospitals. By

1966 there were over 330,000, and in 1976 there were over 435,000 admissions to these non-federal government hospitals. By 1978 this had dropped to 390,000. One crucial factor is that the average period of hospitalization in 1955 was 6 months, whereas in 1966 it was about 2 months. The length of stay dropped to even briefer durations, and in 1971 the median hospitalization stay for new admissions to mental hospitals was 41 days, and in 1975, 26 days. A large study compared 3- to 4-month and 3- to 4-week hospitalization for schizophrenics. The result: there is no advantage on any measure for hospitalization longer than 4 weeks. Parallel with this increasing discharge rate from hospitals has been an increase in aftercare facilities. In 1970 there were 185 operating community mental health centers, and in 1978 there were 600. And these 600 centers treated over 2.1 million people in 1978!

Many authorities feel that the primary factor underlying the decline in mental hospital population in the United States can be identified as the introduction of new psychoactive agents into treatment programs in 1954 and 1955. There are three basic questions to be answered when considering any class of drugs used in the treatment of a behavioral disturbance. The first is, as a result of the drug treatment, is there a decrease in the frequency of the behaviors that brought the individual to, and keeps him in, the hospital? That is, are the drugs effective? Do they reduce symptoms? Second, are there adverse side effects that inevitably occur when the individual is receiving a therapeutic dose? Phrased differently, how safe is the drug? Can it be used without harm to the patient? The last question is, if an individual is released from the hospital while still under medication, can he function adequately in the community? To what extent is the medicated psychotic patient who is free of major symptoms different from nonpsychotic, nonmedicated individuals?

Background

Of individuals in mental hospitals the largest group, about 50%, are diagnosed as schizophrenic. It is estimated that signs of schizophrenia are shown by 2% of the population at some time in their life.[3]

The major class of drugs to be considered in treatment of schizophrenia is the phenothiazines. Three other classes of drugs have been used minimally: reserpine and similar drugs, which were used briefly in the early 1950s; the butyrophenones, which were introduced into the United States in the sixties, and the dibenzodiazepines, which are not yet marketed.

Although a phenothiazine was first synthesized in 1883, and one was tried as an insecticide in 1934, the present story will be brief and begins in 1950 in France with promethazine. Promethazine was used to potentiate surgical anesthesia and was successful enough to start a search for other pheno-

thiazines. In 1950 chlorpromazine was synthesized, and in 1952 its use to potentiate anesthesia had been described. In addition, reports were that, by itself, chlorpromazine did not induce a loss of consciousness, although it did decrease the interest of the patient in what was going on around him.

As a result of this last characteristic, chlorpromazine was tried in France in the treatment of the mentally ill. The very first report of this work, in 1952, mentioned that not only was anxiety reduced but also the drug acted on the psychotic process itself. Chlorpromazine was first used in the United States in 1954 for the treatment of psychomotor excitement and manic states. The use of chlorpromazine and other phenothiazines with similar actions had expanded dramatically, and in 1982 there were 14 antipsychotic phenothiazines available in the United States under 18 brand names and several generic brands. No one attempts to estimate the number of individuals who have received phenothiazines but they are widely used. A 1976 report by the Veterans Administration[9] indicated that of their then hospitalized psychotic patients, 74% received antipsychotic medication. Of those, 78% were receiving a phenothiazine, and 16% a butyrophenone.

The chemical structure of some of the phenothiazines is indicated in Fig. 13-2. These agents dffer in their potency, as indicated, but at therapeutic doses have essentially the same effect on the schizophrenic symptoms. Side effects do vary from one compound to another, and frequently the therapeutic use of a specific agent is determined by how well the patient tolerates a particular side effect.[10]

One of the early reports (1955) dealing with the side effects of chlorpromazine on a large number of hospitalized psychotic patients stated that:

> . . . [it] produces marked quieting of the motor manifestations. Patients cease to be loud and profane, the tendency to hyperbolic associations diminished, and the patients can sit still long enough to eat and to take care of normal physiological needs. . . .
>
> In the more chronic psychotic states, the effect of the drug is much less immediately dramatic,

Phenothiazine
nucleus

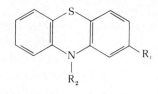

Generic name	Brand name	Clinical potency	R_1	R_2
Chlorpromazine*	Thorazine	7	$-Cl$	$-CH_2-,CH_2-CH_2-N\begin{smallmatrix}CH_3\\CH_3\end{smallmatrix}$
Triflupromazine	Vesprin	5	$-CF_3$	Same as above
Prochlorperazine	Compazine	4	$-Cl$	$-CH_2-CH_2-CH_2-N\underset{}{\bigcirc}N-CH_3$
Trifluoperazine	Stelazine	1	$-CF_3$	Same as above
Perphenazine	Trilafon	2	$-Cl$	$-CH_2-CH_2-CH_2-N\underset{}{\bigcirc}N-CH_2-CH_2OH$
Thiopropazate	Dartal	3	$-Cl$	$-CH_2-CH_2-CH_2-N\underset{}{\bigcirc}N-CH_2-CH_2-O-\overset{O}{\underset{\parallel}{C}}-CH_3$
Thioridazine	Mellaril	_ 6 _	$-SCH_3$	$-CH_2-CH_2-\underset{\underset{CH_3}{\mid}}{\overset{}{\bigcirc}}_N$

*Chemical name for chlorpromazine is 2-chloro-10-(3-dimethylaminopropyl)-phenothiazine.

FIG. 13-2 Phenothiazines.

but, for those experienced with the relief of psychotic symptoms from other measures, the use of the drug produces results that are equally gratifying when compared with results in the more acute situations.[11]

This early evaluation was well founded, as suggested by the following statement made in 1976:

Since chlorpromazine . . . and . . . subsequent antipsychotic drugs . . . have had profound effects on . . . psychiatry, reducing the lengths of hospitalization for schizophrenic patients and permit-

ting many patients to be handled in the community in ways not heretofore even anticipated, it is remarkable that no Nobel Prize in medicine has been awarded to the discoverers of chlorpromazine.[12,p.13]

The tremendous impact of phenothiazine treatment on the management of hospitalized psychotics is clear from a 1955 statement by the director of the Delaware State Hospital:

We have now achieved . . . the reorganization of the management of disturbed patients. With rare exceptions, all restraints have been discontinued.

The hydro-therapy department, formerly active on all admission services and routinely used on wards with disturbed patients, has ceased to be in operation. Maintenance EST [electroshock treatment] for disturbed patients has been discontinued. . . . There has been a record increase in participation by these patients in social and occupational activities.

These developments have vast sociological implications. I believe it is fair to state that pharmacology promises to accomplish what other measures have failed to bring about—the social emancipation of the mental hospital.[13,pp.83-84]

Treatment effects and considerations

Paralleling an increase in the use of phenothiazines in the treatment of the mentally ill was the increase in the sophistication of experimental programs that evaluate the effectiveness of various drugs. Results from these studies show clearly that phenothiazine-treated patients improve more than patients receiving placebo or no treatments. In an NIMH study after 6 weeks, 75% of acute schizophrenics receiving phenothiazines showed either moderate or marked improvement, whereas of those receiving placebos only 23% improved. One summary of the double-blind, controlled studies found that 106 studies reported that phenothiazine treatment of psychotics was more effective than placebo treatment, while only 24 found it to be no better than placebo treatment.[3] In each of the 24 studies where phenothiazines were not shown to be significantly better treatment than placebo, low doses of the drug were used. Even then there were nonsignificant trends favoring phenothiazine treatment.

"Ninety-five percent of acute schizophrenic patients treated with a drug given in an adequate dose will show some improvement within 6 to 8 weeks. More than 50% . . . will improve moderately to markedly. . . ."[14,p.203] From the sixth to twelfth week some improvement is still occurring, but beyond that there is little if any change. As might be expected, motor effects are usually the first to manifest themselves, whereas the psychological symptoms show a more gradual decline. It is true that

improvement is sometimes seen with placebo treatment but the effects of the phenothiazines are quite different. The phenothiazines primarily reduce the intensity of the fundamental symptoms but also act on the accessory symptoms; placebos have their only effect on the accessory symptoms[15], which is what Chapter 6 would have led you to predict. It is important to remember that the actions of the phenothiazines are much more specific than the term "tranquilizer" implies.

> The inappropriateness of the term "tranquilizer" is evident when the pattern of response produced by antipsychotic drugs is examined. They certainly do more than simply calm patients or put them in a "chemical straitjacket." The core symptoms of schizophrenia are consistently improved: emotional withdrawal, hallucinations, delusions and other disturbed thinking, paranoid projection, belligerence, hostility and blunted affect. On the other hand, somatic complaints, anxiety and tension, symptoms which might ordinarily be favorably affected by a "tranquilizer," are not much changed. . . .[16,p.4]

Another aspect of evaluating the effectiveness of drug treatment is determining the incidence of relapse or symptom recurrence when treatment is discontinued. A good summary of the state of the art was made by one of the leading workers in this area:

> There are 25 controlled studies, essentially all of which find that any antipsychotic drug prevents relapse. A total of 377 out of 1884 patients on drugs relapsed (20%) in comparison to 705 out of 1346 patients on placebo (52%).[17]

It is most likely that discontinuation of drug therapy will lead to relapse in 75% to 95% of patients within a year and in more than 50% of patients in 6 months.[18] Almost all studies report that when medication is resumed, there is again a reduction in symptoms.[19] It has been shown that antipsychotic medication can be withdrawn 2 or 3 days a week without relapse occurring in "chronic schizophrenics on maintenance chemotherapy" in mental hospitals.[20]

Some patients respond to one phenothiazine and

not to another, a few don't respond to any of them. No one is quite sure why. It may be that the phenothiazine does not get absorbed and thus does not get into the bloodstream and then into the brain. Blood levels of the phenothiazines are difficult to do but a majority of the few studies that have been done show a relationship between blood levels and clinical effectiveness.[21] One review phrased the problem of "no effect with treatment" very briefly: "The most common cause of treatment failure in acute psychosis is an inadequate dose, and the most common cause of relapse is patient noncompliance."[14,p.202]

Many physicians will prescribe low doses of two or more phenothiazines rather than an adequate dose of a single drug. There is *no* evidence that the use of more than one antipsychotic agent is advantageous, and it complicates handling of side effects and increases the probability of patient noncompliance with the medication regimen. Another problem is the failure to reduce the daily dosage after the patient's behavior has been stabilized on the drug. It is now clear that adequate symptom control can be maintained by drug administration once or twice a day or every other day, rather than the more common three or four times each day.

One study[22] is of particular interest, since within a single hospital, using five wards, it compared the effectiveness *and the cost* of each of five treatment methods in first-admission schizophrenics. The five methods were (1) individual psychotherapy, (2) phenothiazine medication, (3) methods 1 and 2, (4) electroshock, and (5) milieu, in which social interactions and support and understanding are the keystones. Effectiveness was measured by the release rate within a year of admission. The percent of patients discharged in each of the five groups was 64%, 95%, 96%, 79%, and 59%, respectively. Clearly medication was the most significant factor. The cost to treat each patient until discharge or for 1 year if not released is given here in rounded figures (the costs are for 1965): (1) $7,200, (2) $3,000, (3) $3,600, (4) $4,400, and (5) $6,200. All mental health workers know generally this state of affairs, but it seems important to emphasize it. The use of antipsychotic drugs in the treatment of schizophrenics is not only the most effective treatment, it is also the least expensive. One study[23] has shown that a *very* intensive (and thereby expensive) psychotherapy and psychosocial hospital treatment program can perhaps provide even more effective treatment than a program based on medication. The program unfortunately cannot be widely adopted because of its high requirement of professional time.

In evaluating antipsychotic drugs, the concern is not only the decrease in symptoms and the patient's release from the hospital, but also his adjustment to the community. Three large studies in the 1950s and 1960s told the same story. "Most (89%) of all patients still in the community after one year were judged to be functioning less well than the average person at their general social level and many were clearly not without psychopathology."[24,p.124] "Few patients who have been hospitalized for any appreciable period as schizophrenics ever function in a completely 'normal' way thereafter, probably less than 15 percent. Accordingly, realistic efforts must be made to help the patient so that he can live in the community despite his handicap."[25] "These patients manifested a rather marginal level of community adjustment."[26]

Those results aren't the most encouraging in the world to someone who hasn't worked with the emotionally ill. Compared to what the choices are drug treatment is still preferable: patients leave the hospital sooner, function better, and stay out longer with drug treatment than with any other treatment.[27] The debate is certainly not over[28] and as better drug and nondrug treatments develop the balance may shift either way. For now, "Drugs may be helpful in promoting restitution and restoring perceptual control [but] treatment of the schizophrenic person will always need people and the kind of things that only persons can do."[29,p.689]

Finally, you must appreciate that proper medication and professional treatment can only do so much. The rest is up to the community and the family. "The schizophrenic walks a tight rope: too much stimulation precipitates the florid symptoms (hallucinations, delusions, excitement), whereas a barren environment promotes the negative symptoms of withdrawal, apathy, and blunted affect."[30] One study[31] showed that schizophrenics who returned to homes in which there were critical, hostile relatives required rehospitalization sooner than those released to homes not showing those attitudes. Even though antipsychotic medication decreases the vulnerability of the schizophrenic to the slings and arrows of the world, it cannot shield him completely.[32] Remember, moral treatment worked before.

A 1970 statement is still valid as a summary of the treatment effect:

> Chlorpromazine and other phenothiazines are not considered truly curative in psychotic disorders since most patients usually display some residual psychotic symptomatology, even following considerable improvement. Individual patients may require phenothiazine medication for years, perhaps for a lifetime. It must be pointed out, however, that some patients are so benefited by the drugs that psychopathology is not detectable even by highly skilled observers.[33,p.167]

Side effects to phenothiazine treatment

Two very positive aspects of the phenothiazines are that they are not addictive and it is extremely difficult to use them to commit suicide. A few deaths have been reported following ingestion of high doses. In the early stage of phenothiazine treatment some allergic reactions may be noted, such as jaundice, photosensitivity of the skin, and skin rashes. These reactions have a low incidence and with a reduction in dose level decrease and/or disappear. Agranulocytosis, low white blood cell count of unknown origin, can develop in the early stages of treatment. It is extremely rare but has a high mortality, perhaps 50%. The anticholinergic and antiadrenergic actions have such side effects as dry mouth, nasal congestion, and constipation. These can usually be satisfactorily controlled by reducing the dose of the drug.

Tardive dyskinesia is the most serious complication of antipsychotic drug treatment and its prevalence among inpatients treated with antipsychotic drugs is now about 25%. Although first observed in the late 1950s, it was not viewed as a major problem until the mid-seventies, 20 years after these drugs were introduced.[35] The term *tardive dyskinesia* means "late-appearing abnormal movements" and refers primarily to "slow, rhythmical movements in the region of the mouth with protrusion of the tongue, smacking of the lips, blowing of the cheeks, and side-to-side movements of the chin, as well as other bizarre muscular activity."[36,pp.126-127] The fact that this syndrome usually occurs only after years of antipsychotic drug treatment and that the symptoms persist and sometimes increase when medication is stopped raised the possibility of irreversible changes. The current belief is that tardive dyskinesia is the result of supersensitivity of the dopaminergic receptors.[37] Although reversal of the symptoms seems possible, the best treatment is prevention, which can be accomplished through early detection and an immediate lowering of the level of medication.[38,39] There is still debate over the relative importance of age, dosage level, and years on medication in the onset of tardive dyskinesia.[40]

The more familiar side effects of antipsychotic medication are the extrapyramidal symptoms. The major extrapyramidal effects include a wide range of signs from facial tics to the usual symptoms reported in Parkinson's syndrome, such as passive tremors, rigidity, and a shuffling walk. All can usually be controlled by the use of antiparkinsonian drugs, which typically are anticholinergics.[41] It has been suggested that there is no antipsychotic effect of the phenothiazines without accompanying extrapyramidal effects. In fact, some individuals do not show even minimal extrapyramidal signs but are helped by the drugs. The mechanims underlying these side effects are discussed in the next section.

Although there is no experimental basis for believing that one phenothiazine is more effective than another in controlling psychotic symptoms, there are some rather clear differences in the side effects common to the various drugs. One general rule is that the more potent phenothiazines result more often in the appearance of extrapyramidal symptoms than do the less potent agents, even though both are administered at doses equally effective against the schizophrenic behavior. The basis for this will be clear in the next section.

Pharmacology of phenothiazines

The phenothiazines are antieverything. They are antiadrenergic, antidopaminergic, anticholinergic, antihistaminic, and antiserotonergic. Their effects on these compounds vary, however, being strong adrenergic and dopaminergic blockers, mild to moderate cholinergic, and weak histaminic blockers. Two more general effects are probably also of crucial importance in their antipsychotic actions: depression of the hypothalamus and depression of input to the reticular activating system.

The reticular activating system, which controls cortical arousal, receives inputs from each of the sensory systems. The primary sensory pathways travel to the thalamus but send collaterals (branches) to the reticular system. Impulses through these collaterals activate the reticular system, which in turn sends alerting impulses to the cortex. The phenothiazines act to diminish activity in these collaterals, and this decreases the ability of sensory input to arouse the reticular system and the cortex.

This action is probably the basis for the observation by an early worker that with chlorpromazine "there is not any loss in consciousness nor any change in the patient's mentality but a slight tendency to sleep and above all 'disinterest' for all that goes on around him." Following phenothiazine administration, there is a slowing of the electroencephalogram, which may reflect the lowered arousal level of the individual. One group of scientists suggested that schizophrenics are normally overaroused and that phenothiazines return them to the normal range of reactivity.

The effects of the phenothiazines on the hypothalamus are ubiquitous and result in many minor changes in autonomic activities that are only incidental to the antipsychotic actions. One effect that may well be fundamental in this respect is the action on the reward system. There is good behavioral evidence that the phenothiazines diminish the ef-

fectiveness of the reward system. This is consonant with the finding that the neurotransmitter in the system is noradrenaline, which is blocked by the phenothiazines.

A decrease in the functioning of the reward system would agree with a decline in motor agitation, while the decrease in responsiveness to external stimuli may explain in part the decrease in hallucinations and confused thought that occurs after phenothiazine treatment. Blocking off minimal, irrelevant, sensory stimuli, which may be misinterpreted as voices, may be the basis for part of the antipsychotic action of these drugs. Until the mid-1970s, there was little agreement on the biochemical, neurophysiological, or neuroanatomical basis for the symptoms of schizophrenia and no agreement on which action or set of actions of the phenothiazines were producing *the* antipsychotic effect. There now seems to be a growing consensus, and the pieces are more and more falling into place.

Biochemical mechanisms. Explanations are never complete in science, so remember that this "explanation" is the best bet for the state of the art. In the beginning the best bet was that the phenothiazines had their antischizophrenic effect by blocking noradrenergic receptors.[42] The next best bet was that they acted by occupying and blocking dopaminergic receptors.[43] In the center ring today . . . we now know that there are two types of dopamine receptors, DA-1 and DA-2, and that only the DA-2 receptors are involved in the antischizophrenic action. This set of receptors is also involved in the extrapyramidal effects. It seems unlikely that it will ever be possible to have an antischizophrenic agent that does not also cause extrapyramidal symptoms. Unless, of course, additional work shows that there are two or more types of DA-2 receptors! The phenothiazines occupy both the DA-1 and DA-2 receptors, while the butyrophenones block only the DA-2 receptor.[44] The correlation between the clinical potency for antipsychotic action and the effectiveness of these drugs in occupying dopamine receptors is very high $(+0.87)$.[45] Dopaminergic systems are involved in the control of motor activity (extrapyramidal system), autonomic processes (hypothalamus), and emotional behavior (limbic system).

Effective motor function and control are the results of a delicate balance in the extrapyramidal system between the activity of dopamine and of acetylcholine. When the action of dopamine is blocked, the balance shifts in favor of acetylcholine activity and extrapyramidal symptoms occur. In the clinical situation these symptoms are reduced by the administration of anticholinergic drugs, which restores the proper balance between acetylcholine and dopamine.[46] (For the purist who knows there are two types of acetylcholine receptors [nicotinic and muscarinic], it is only the muscarinic receptor that is involved here.)

Phenothiazines are anticholinergic as well as antidopaminergic. To make a long story very short: drugs that produce few extrapyramidal side effects at antipsychotic dose levels are those which also have strong anticholinergic actions. Thioridazine (Mellaril), which produces very few extrapyramidal effects, is about seven times as potent as an anticholinergic as cholorpromazine (Thorazine), which is about nine times as anticholinergic as trifluoperazine (Stelazine),[47] which produces many extrapyramidal effects. A new drug, clozapine (which is an antipsychotic of the dibenzodiazepine class), is not available in the United States. It is a potent anticholinergic agent and produces few if any extrapyramidal effects at clinically effective dosages. Haloperidol, a butyrophenone, is a very potent antipsychotic drug but is only weakly anticholinergic and thus produces many extrapyramidal side effects. Do not forget that there are other side effects of these drugs, and to avoid certain of these other effects it may sometimes be necessary to use a drug that produces extrapyramidal effects.[48]

Interestingly, tardive dyskinesia probably results from receptor actions on the other side of the scale. Most experts believe that this syndrome is the result of an increase in the sensitivity of the dopamine receptors to dopamine as a result of prolonged administration of dopamine blockers, the antipsychotic agents. In 1977 it was shown in animals that chronic treatment with antischizophrenic drugs increases the dopamine receptor sites in the extra-

pyramidal system.[49] This increase in receptor activity also upsets the balance in the extrapyramidal system. The resulting symptoms can be blocked by even larger doses of the antipsychotic drugs.

In quick summary: the antipsychotic action of the clinically effective drugs seems to be most related to their ability to block dopaminergic neurons. The number and severity of the extrapyramidal side effects of these drugs, at equally effective dose levels, are related to their anticholinergic activity. As the anticholinergic activity goes up, extrapyramidal effects go down. The development of tardive dyskinesia is a result of hypersensitivity of the extrapyramidal dopamine receptors. This is the result of prolonged blockage of these receptors by antipsychotic medication.

Metabolism. The metabolism of the phenothiazines is not known, but at least 168 breakdown metabolites of chlorpromazine have been proposed, and many of them are already identified in the urine. The liver is the primary organ of detoxification and usually contains the highest drug level of any structure in the body after the administration of these drugs. The rate at which chlorpromazine leaves the body is extremely slow, and some investigators have reported breakdown products of chlorpromazine in the urine several months after termination of medication. These data are still debated, but they do agree with the general finding that when medication is stopped, symptoms only slowly recur, perhaps not until 3 months after the last drug administration.

TREATMENT OF MOOD DISORDERS

Mood fluctuations are probably more common in the general population than is disordered thinking. They are also tolerated more: in 1976 only about 125,000 individuals entered mental hospitals for the treatment of depression. Since most patients have recurrent episodes of illness throughout life, possibly fewer than one fourth of these admissions are new patients. Approximately 250,000 patients are treated annually for depression on an outpatient basis. Treatment is important, since it may be that 15% of patients with only mood disorders commit suicide each year.[50] Depression is probably the basis for the fact that suicide is the second largest killer of indivduals 15 to 19 years old. What is perhaps most discouraging here is the fact that family physicians—general practitioners—recognize depression less than 10% of the time in their first contact with a depressed patient.[51] Hospitalization for mania is rare, partly as a result of the low incidence of mania in the general population. A good guesstimate is that there are less than 10% as many manics as depressives.

There is some agreement that the disorders considered as mood disorders are closely related to impaired functioning of central adrenergic and serotonergic systems. The two systems that would seem a priori to be most relevant are the medial forebrain bundle and the periventricular system. As will be seen, the drugs that act to diminish the symptoms of mania and depression also have specific effects on these reward and punishment systems.

Depression

Everyone seems to have their own way to classify depressions: retarded or agitated; anxious, retarded, or hostile. Most of the traditional classifications are being replaced by systems that have importance for treatment and that make sense biochemically.[52] Major depression can be divided into *unipolar* or *bipolar* depression. Unipolar depressed patients are those who never show symptoms of mania but may vary between normality and depression. The bipolar depressed patient cycles across three mood states: depression, a normal mood state, and mania. There is evidence that mood swings have a strong genetic component, whether unipolar or bipolar.[53] Another helpful way to classify depressions is: *primary (endogenous)* and *secondary (reactive)*. The secondary depressions are just that—secondary to something else (for example, sexual dysfunction, alcohol or drug abuse, a medical illness). The secondary depressions are reactions to another event or situation. As such they are frequently time-limited and diminish when the event or situation goes away. Primary depressions do not have a clear pre-cipitating event and more than likely arise as a result of changes within the individual. There are some meaningful subclasses of depressed patients within the larger category of primary depression.

There is much excitement among those working in laboratories and hospitals about a diagnostic laboratory test for primary unipolar depression: the dexamethasone suppression test (DST). The basis for this test was discovered, doubted, and denied in the 1950s but in the early 1980s it is well on its way to being an essential part of the clinical diagnosis of primary unipolar depression.[54] The details need not concern us here but you should know that the test is only about 50% accurate in identifying those patients who are primary unipolar depressives. However, it eliminates about 90% of those who are not.[52] That is, there are few false positive results but false negative results still exist.[55] Other tests are equally or more promising.[54]

Probably the single most effective treatment for the depressed patient is electroconvulsive therapy (ECT). One report[3] summarized the available good studies and showed that in seven of eight studies ECT was more effective in relieving the symptoms of depression than was placebo. Further, in four studies ECT was more effective than the most effective class of antidepressant drugs, and in three other studies the two treatments were equal. One factor that makes ECT sometimes the clear treatment of choice is its more rapid effect than that found with current antidepressant drugs. Reversal of the depression may not occur for 2 or 3 weeks with drug treatment, but with ECT results sometimes are noticed almost immediately. When there is a possibility of suicide, ECT is thus the obvious choice, and there is no danger in pursuing both drug and ECT treatment simultaneously.[56]

Drug treatment. The story of the antidepressant drugs starts with the fact that tuberculosis was a major chronic illness until about 1955. In 1952 preliminary reports suggested that a new drug, isoniazid, was effective in treating tuberculosis; isoniazid and similar drugs that followed were responsible for the emptying of hospital beds. One of these antituberculosis drugs was iproniazid, which was introduced simultaneously with isonia-

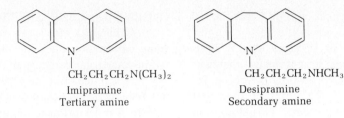

FIG. 13-3 Tricyclic antidepressants. Imipramine:(5-[3-dimethylaminopropyl]-10,11-dihydro-5H-dibenz [b,f] azepine).

zid but was withdrawn as too toxic. Clinical reports on its use in tuberculosis hospitals emphasized that there was considerable elevation of mood in the patients receiving iproniazid. These reports were followed up, and the drug was reintroduced as an antidepressant agent in 1955 on the basis of early promising studies with depressed patients.

Iproniazid is a monoamine oxidase inhibitor (as well as many other things), and its discovery opened up a whole new class of compounds for investigation. As was mentioned in Chapter 7, monoamine oxidase is the only enzyme involved in the deactivation of serotonin and is also responsible for the deactivation of free noradrenaline within the neuron. Inhibition of these enzyme results in high levels of functional serotonin, but the importance of the noradrenaline increase is not clear.

Despite the promise monoamine oxidase inhibitors held as antidepressant drugs, the number and severity of their side effects led to their demise. Iproniazid itself was removed from sale in 1961 after being implicated in at least 54 fatalities. Furthermore, a recent compilation of studies showed that in 15 of 31 well-controlled studies, the monoamine oxidase inhibitors were no more effective than placebo. Therefore, because of their dangerous side effects and their relative ineffectiveness, this group of agents has been dropped out of use. In the late 1970s the monoamine oxidase inhibitors increased in popularity and in use for the treatment of some subgroups of depressed patients—the "atypical depressives"—as well as for the treatment of patients with extreme anxiety and certain phobias.[57] Maybe these drugs will have a second chance.

Chlorpromazine had been used and studied as an antihistaminic before its potential as an antipsychotic agent was appreciated. Imipramine, the next antidepressant to be discussed, left the animal testing laboratory as a phenothiazine-like antipsychotic. The similarity of the imipramine structure to that of the phenothiazines is clearly seen by comparing Figs. 13-2 and 13-3. In clinical tests, though, its outstanding characteristic was that it reduced the depression of depressed schizophrenics. Imipramine was the first of a series of compounds called *tricyclics* because of their chemical structure.

Tricyclic compounds have been shown to reduce depression better than placebo treatment in about 65% to 75% of the controlled studies. This class of drugs is closely related to the phenothiazines but has weaker antiadrenergic and more potent anticholinergic properties than the phenothiazines.

A major effect of the tricyclics is the blocking of the presynaptic reuptake of noradrenaline and serotonin that is released into the synaptic gap. This increases the amount of neurotransmitter available to act postsynaptically, thereby increasing the activity of the systems involved. From the start of tricyclic treatment it may take 2 to 3 weeks before improvement is obtained.

That 2- to 3-week delay used to mean that the clinician was running blind—giving a drug but not getting any feedback from changes in the patient that said either too much or too little drug was being given. This is a particular problem with these drugs since the side effects of large doses are severe enough to considerably reduce patient compliance and since there is great variability in the bioavailability of the drug in different patients given the same amount of the drug. The tricyclics are unusual

TABLE 13-1 A summary of tricyclics

Type of tricyclic	Possible deficiency	Blockade effectiveness	Best clinical effect in
Tertiary	Serotonin	Serotonin > Noradrenaline	Anxious, agitated
Secondary	Noradrenaline	Noradrenaline > Serotonin	Psychomotor retardation

in two ways that are helpful here. One is that it is not difficult to determine their blood levels—and thus their bioavailability. Second, the tricyclics have a "therapeutic window"—a blood level range in which the therapeutic effect occurs. This means that the drug dose can be adjusted to the correct blood level even though the symptoms have not yet changed.[58,59]

Since the late 1970s there have been dramatic increases in our understanding of how tricyclics work.[60,61] We needed it. Until recently it was true that "Many early publications provided enthusiastic testimonials for the efficacy of antidepressants, but the few controlled studies by the VA and others have provided only lukewarm support for belief in their effectiveness.[62,p.19] The problem was that a variety of subgroups were lumped together in one big bag called depression and clinicians were trying to affect just one of those groups with a chemical that is not very specific. Things have changed. The subgroups are being taken out of the bag and identified so that specific drugs can be used to treat specific subgroups—and with good results.

The more we learn, the better our treatment is, and the better able we are to develop more effective drugs with fewer side effects. It became clear in the clinic that the *tertiary amine tricyclics* (see Fig. 13-3) were most effective in depressives with certain symptoms: for example, high levels of anxiety and psychomotor agitation. The *secondary amine tricyclics* were most effective in depressed patients with, among other symptoms, psychomotor retardation. You also need to know that the agitated, anxious depressives have low levels of the final metabolite (5HIAA) of brain serotonin—which suggested a deficiency of serotonin. The slowed down, less anxious depressives have lower than normal levels of the major metabolite (MHPG) of

brain noradrenaline—which suggested a deficiency of noradrenaline. It all becomes clear when you know that the tertiary amine tricyclics are more potent in blocking serotonin reuptake than in blocking noradrenaline reuptake. The secondary amine tricyclics are just the opposite—more potent in blocking noradrenaline. MHPG (methoxyhydroxyphenylglycol), the metabolite of noradrenaline, can be measured in the urine. If the MHPG level in the urine is low in a depressed patient, a secondary amine tricyclic is probably the first type of antidepressant to try. A summary of the discussion of tricyclics is presented in Table 13-1. These results have not gone unnoticed by pharmaceutical houses and, through chemical modifications, they are beginning to market tricyclics that selectively block only one of these transmitters.

You may have wondered why it takes 2 to 3 weeks of tricyclic administration to produce a clinical effect. It is not because it takes that long to block reuptake—that is fairly rapid. The answer is really neat: (1) Remember homeostasis. (2) There are neuronal mechanisms that operate to control the amount of serotonin and noradrenaline released into the synaptic gap. (3) With high levels of noradrenaline (for example) already in the synaptic gap (because reuptake is blocked) the homeostatic mechanism decreases the amount that is released with each nerve impulse! (4) It takes 2 to 3 weeks to desensitize the controlling mechanism (the presynaptic alpha-adrenergic receptor) so that normal amounts of the transmitter are released with each nerve impulse. (5) This means that it takes 2 to 3 weeks before there are significant increases in the amount of neurotransmitter acting on the receptors—and that is what is necessary for clinical improvement! Think a minute—what is a good idea? Right—produce a drug that blocks the reuptake *and* inhibits the homeostatic mechanism. It's been done—they're called tetracyclics. They work faster and they will really hit the U.S. market in the mid-eighties! It's *so* exciting![54]

A few final comments. These antidepressant drugs are not stimulants and at clinical dose levels have little effect on normal individuals. Animal studies[63] show that long-term administration of an antidepressant increases the sensitivity of the reward systems in the brain. Whether enhancement of reward systems in humans would occur is not known but the mechanisms that have been described for the control of the release and reuptake of noradrenaline may underlie the variability among people in their sensitivity to rewards, as well as set the level of their general affective mood.

Well over half of the prescriptions written for antidepressants are written by nonpsychiatrists. This is unfortunate since they frequently prescribe too little for too short a time to decrease the depression. It is understandable though since the tricyclics can cause severe side effects: about one user in 20 will have disorientation, hallucinations, or other anticholinergic effects (see Chapter 18). Large doses (several grams) can be lethal so quantities prescribed to suicidal patients need to be restricted. A 1980 alert to physicians by the FDA[64] pointed out how dangerous the tricyclics can be when accidentally taken by children: 1000 emergency room visits a year, resulting in 500 hospitalizations and 10 deaths. Caution is certainly the watchword, but it is still true that until the late 1980s the tricyclics are the drug of choice for the treatment of unipolar depression.

Mania

The core symptoms of mania are an elated mood and hyperactivity. The manic person feels absolutely marvelous mentally and physically, but his normal judgments about the world and his own capabilities have disappeared. . . .

Although chlorpromazine and other antipsychotic drugs are not sedatives . . . they effectively suppress . . . mania by wrapping the patient's entire mind in a cocoon of stupefaction. . . .

Lithium, on the contrary . . . is as if the manic symptoms were veins of porous limestone in a block of granite and lithium were water cascading through the block: Only the symptoms are leached out while the rest of the personality remains unaffected.[65]

Lithium is unlike any other drug discussed in this chapter. It is an element (but is administered as a salt), cannot be patented, and has been approved by the Food and Drug Administration for use in the treatment of mania only since April 1970. Since the 1960s there has been considerable research. As you might suspect, these results are not quite as glowing as the early reports. A 1976 article by one of the major workers in this area stated:

During the past 25 years, the practice of psychiatry has been revolutionized by the introduction of psychoactive drugs, and none has been so potentially revolutionary as lithium. It has been firmly established that lithium is a specific and effective antimanic agent, capable of controlling and preventing recurrence of episodes of mania. . . . Although definitely not the panacea some supporters claim, lithium has become established as the first prophylactic drug in psychiatric history.[66,p.193]

A 1980 authoritative review of lithium concluded: "Of all the drugs used in psychiatry today, lithium carbonate . . . offers the closest approximation to a pharmacological cure."[67,p.17] Well-controlled studies show that lithium controls acute mania in about 70% of the cases. Blood levels of the lithium ion can easily be monitored to ensure a level high enough to yield a therapeutic effect but low enough to avoid the toxic side effects. Interestingly, its medical use may reach back to the fifth century in Greece where the use of alkaline mineral spring water was suggested for the treatment of mania! Lithium was used about 100 years ago in the treatment of gout, but in the early part of the twentieth century its use was discontinued because of the side effects.

In the late 1940s two medical uses and their results were reported almost simultaneously and in the United States very nicely canceled each other out. Lithium chloride had been suggested and used with patients on low-sodium diets. Unfortunately this use caused some fatalities, so no one was very interested in following up a report on lithium use that came out of Australia in 1949. The Australian report suggested strongly that mania and excitement were reduced when patients were given lithium carbonate. The lithium ion had been stumbled onto quite by accident, but it seemed to work well, and some research programs on it began even before chlorpromazine was used with schizophrenics. The most comprehensive program is one still continuing in Denmark, where in a well-controlled double-blind study good antimania effects were obtained in 80% of the cases.[68]

Treatment with lithium requires 10 to 15 days before symptoms begin to change. Lithium is both safe and toxic. It is safe because the blood level can be monitored routinely and the dose administered adjusted to ensure therapeutic but not excessive blood levels. It is a toxic agent but may be used with caution with patients with a kidney or cardiovascular disorder. The more minor side effects of gastrointestinal disturbances and tremor do not seem to persist with continued treatment. If excessively high blood levels persist, central nervous system and neuromuscular symptoms appear; these can progress to coma, convulsions, and death if lithium is not stopped and appropriate treatment instituted.

The clinical use and effectiveness of lithium has had some interesting effects in several areas. The mechanism of action is still not clear, but one biochemical effect is that lithium increases the synthesis of serotonin in the brain. This, of course, is compatible with the theory that mood reflects a balance between the adrenergic and serotonergic.[69] One report[70] found that lithium is antieuphoric in normal individuals, and its subjective effects are much like that experienced from a small dose of chlorpromazine. This article reported that lithium did not block a narcotic-induced euphoria, which suggests that at least two biochemical mechanisms exist for the experience of euphoria. Of primary importance in the therapeutic use of lithium is the realization that lithium acts as a mood-normalizing

TABLE 13-2 Drug treatment 2-year outcome in unipolar and bipolar patients

	Percent of patients with relapses during treatment for	
	First 4 months	Next 20 months
Unipolar subjects		
Lithium	30%	41%
Imipramine	32%	29%
Placebo	73%	85%
Bipolar subjects		
Lithium	22%	18%
Imipramine	46%	67%
Placebo	54%	67%

agent in individuals with bipolar manic-depressive illness. Lithium will block both the manic state and the depressed state. Lithium has only moderate effects on unipolar depressions.

These very selective clinical effects of lithium have forced better diagnostic decisions and have given a new basis for the belief that unipolar and bipolar mood disorders are not the same illness. This fact is most clearly seen in Table 13-2, which contains the treatment outcome of one study.[71] Either lithium, placebo, or imipramine (a tricyclic) was given to hospitalized patients, who were later discharged and observed for a prolonged period. For patients diagnosed as unipolar, a relapse means an episode of depression, whereas for the bipolar patients relapse can mean either a depressed or manic period.

The results are relatively clear: lithium is very effective in preventing relapses in biopolar subjects, whereas imipramine treatment showed no clinical improvement compared to placebo. With unipolar subjects imipramine was superior to lithium, but both drugs were superior to placebo treatment. It is of interest to note one major difference between the unipolar and bipolar patients: 55% of next-of-kin relatives of bipolar patients had some type of psychiatric illness, compared to only 28% of the unipolar patients. This suggests that there may be a stronger genetic component in bipolar mood disorders than in unipolar disorders. Research continues, and additional chemical elements are being studied for possible effectiveness in the treatment of other psychiatric disorders.[66]

TREATMENT OF NEUROSES

The neuroses are the most pervasive of the emotional disorders. The actual classifying of an individual as neurotic is interesting in its own right, since for the most part it is a label that a person seeks for himself.

An individual is put into the large group of people society calls the emotionally disturbed under one of two conditions. His behavior may be disturbing or disruptive to others, and society then takes the responsibility for classifying, hospitalizing, and treating the individual. This is what is typically done with the psychotic, manic, and depressed individuals already mentioned.

Relatively few neurotics show behavior, thinking, or mood disorders of sufficient magnitude to require society's intervention. Usually an individual is labeled neurotic when he presents himself to a mental health professional and states directly or indirectly: "Help me, I'm unhappy, nothing seems right in my life, there must be some way in which you can make me feel more comfortable."

Interestingly, Galen, the second-century Greek physician, estimated that about 60% of the patients he saw had emotional and psychological rather than physical illnesses. This is remarkably close to the present estimates of 50% to 60%. Treatments change, but patients don't. Perhaps though, treatments don't change much either, just brand names!

The treatment of neurosis, or of emotional problems, has never been shown to be very effective with any procedure. Psychotherapy seems to reduce symptoms more rapidly in some cases than no treatment but after 6 to 12 months there is no difference in symptom reduction. About 60% of patients report improvement, that is, reduction in the aversive symptoms whether treated or not. These facts are important because they make clear the base rate against which the effects of drugs must be measured. Also, most of the antianxiety drugs used by neurotics are used in situations and for symptoms that are very susceptible to influence by the nonspecific factors mentioned in Chapter 6.

Drug treatment

This section is labeled "Drug Treatment" for want of a better term or the use of 6 to 10 pages listing the symptoms the drugs included here are supposed to control. At the base of all of them is anxiety, but a better description of the kind of problem and their chemical solution are given by Shakespeare in *Macbeth*:

> Raze out the written troubles of the brain,
> and with some sweet oblivious antidote
> Cleanse the stuff'd bosom of that perilous stuff
> Which weighs upon the heart?

We don't have a "sweet oblivious antidote" and, unlike William, we have to worry about side effects. Since the early decades of the twentieth century, the drugs used routinely with anxious individuals were the barbiturates (see Chapter 14), excluding, of course, alcohol, which has always been effective in the short-term control of anxiety.

The modern antianxiety agents, *anxiolytics*, developed from a muscle relaxant called mephenesin, which was patented in 1946 and was a commercial success but had a short duration of action. One compound patented in 1952 was not only longer lasting but believed to be a unique type of CNS depressant. Clinical trials in 1953 supported this belief and the compound was approved by the FDA and released for prescription use in 1955. Meprobamate, the generic name, became Miltown to the public, and it represented the drug revolution of the 1950s to most people. Fig. 13-4 shows the chemical structure of meprobamate, the first of several drugs of this type.

The boom in meprobamate use is difficult to see in perspective. In the year it was introduced, sales of Miltown went from $7,500 in May to over $500,000 in December. The happy pills had arrived! A publicity agency and excessive prescribing by physicians combined to make Miltown a public nuisance as well as the unnamed object of comment

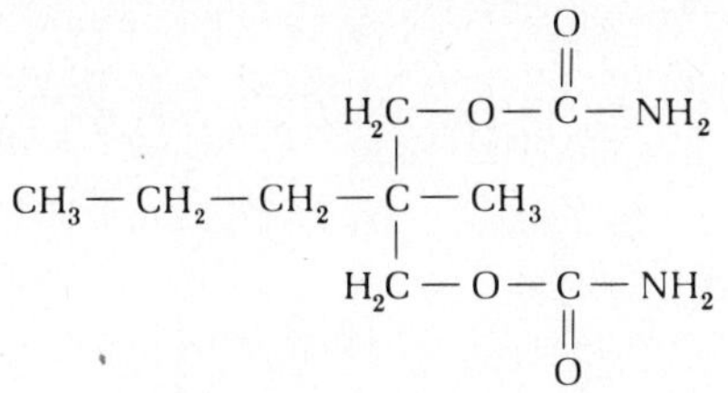

$$
\begin{array}{c}
\text{O} \\
\| \\
\text{H}_2\text{C} - \text{O} - \text{C} - \text{NH}_2 \\
| \\
\text{CH}_3 - \text{CH}_2 - \text{CH}_2 - \text{C} - \text{CH}_3 \\
| \\
\text{H}_2\text{C} - \text{O} - \text{C} - \text{NH}_2 \\
\| \\
\text{O}
\end{array}
$$

Meprobamate
Miltown (Wallace), Equanil (Wyeth)
(2,2-di [carbamoyloxymethyl] pentane)

FIG. 13-4 Meprobamate.

concerning overuse by the American Psychiatric Association and the World Health Organization in 1957. Miltown became such a common word that physicians began prescribing meprobamate under its other brand name, Equanil.

It gradually became clear that meprobamate, like the barbiturates, is an addicting drug, but only if taken at several times the normally prescribed therapeutic dose. One review suggests that daily doses above 3200 mg for over 2 months can result in addiction in many people.[72] Given that, considerable care had to be used in prescribing it. In June 1970, the Bureau of Narcotics and Dangerous Drugs brought meprobamate under the drug abuse control laws, which limited the number of times a prescription for it can be refilled. The real irony came in late 1970, however, when the NAS-NRC reported to the FDA that meprobamate was effective for the relief of anxiety and tension but was not effective as a muscle relaxant! Meprobamate has come a long way from its parent, mephenesin.

Another class of compounds, the benzodiazepines, includes the drugs that most people think of as antianxiety agents. The first of this class was chlordiazepoxide, which is marketed under the trade name Librium. (With a name like that it was very easy to write ads directed toward physicians.) Chlordiazepoxide was synthesized in 1947, but it was 10 years before its value in reducing anxiety was suggested, and it was not sold commercially until 1960. Fig. 13-5 contains chemical structures for several of benzodiazepines in use today. They are arranged so that you can appreciate the

differences in their metabolic pathways. Many of the breakdown products—metabolites—have long half-lifes and are pharmacologically active as antianxiety agents (Table 13-3) (not all metabolites are shown). Note particularly that one of the breakdown products (in the body) of Librium and Valium is oxazepam, which is sold under the trade name of Serax. Flurazepam is the number one nonbarbiturate prescription "sleeping pill" in the United States. You should know that there are at least two benzodiazepine receptors.[73]

Knowing all of the above you might be chomping at the bit: Do they work? Are they better than the less expensive barbiturates? Are they abused, dangerous? Are they the drug of choice for the control of anxiety? For those of you who have to run off somewhere (to the library I'm sure) the answers are: yes, no, yes, yes.

One summary[3] of the studies, in which the three groups of drugs (meprobamate, benzodiazepines, and barbiturates) were compared separately to the effectiveness of placebo treatment, showed that each class was usually significantly better than placebo. When studies were summarized in which the two classes of minor tranquilizers were compared to the barbiturates, a predominance of results showed the minor tranquilizers were not more effective than the barbiturates.[74]

A good summary of the clinical usefulness of the benzodiazepine class of drugs was made in 1969. Its still true today:

> Librium and Valium are effective sedatives, but, except in potentially suicidal patients, it is still not clear that they have any important advantages over the barbiturates.[75]

This was echoed in 1975 when a review stated that "there is no evidence at present that benzodiazepines are more efficacious than phenobarbital in reducing anxiety."[76] It must be noted, however, that "many authorities now advise against prescribing barbiturates as sedatives or hypnotics; tolerance develops quickly, overdosage is often lethal, withdrawl symptoms can be severe, and interactions occur with many other drugs."[77] Because the benzodiazepines are safer (more difficult to use for sui-

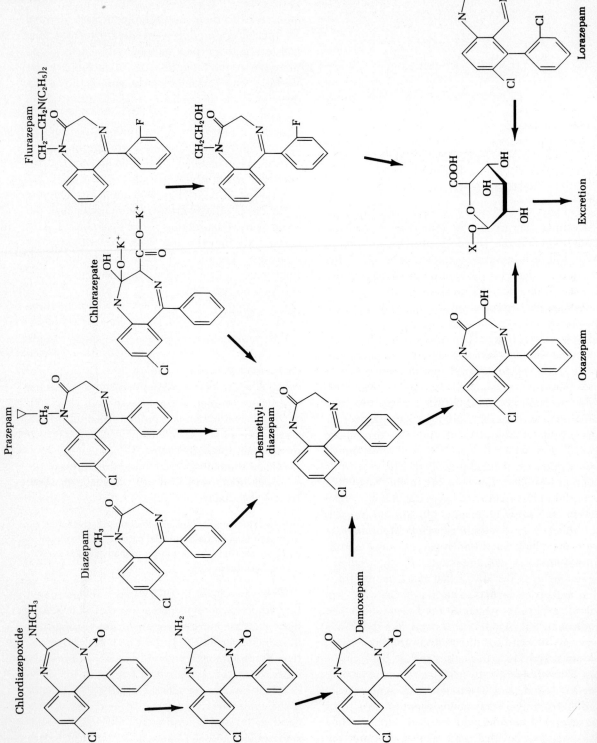

FIG. 13-5 Benzodiazepine metabolism in man. (Adapted from Vacik, J.P., and Palmer, G.C.: The pharmacological basis for rational clinical appreciation of benzodiazepines, Continuing Education, pp. 34-44, December 1980.

TABLE 13-3 Benzodiazepines: generic name, brand name, and half-life of structures in Fig. 13-5

Generic name	Brand name	Half-life (hours)
Chlordiazepoxide	Librium	10
Demoxepam	—	14-46
Diazepam	Valium	31
Prazepam	Verstran	36-200
Chlorazepate	—	—
Desmethyl diazepam	—	51
Flurazepam	Dalmane	short
Oxazepam	Serax	7
Lorazepam	Ativan	14

Adapted from Vacik, J.P., and Palmer, G.C.: The pharmacological basis for rational clinical appreciation of benzodiazepines, Continuing Education for the Family Physician, 13(6):34-44, December 1980.

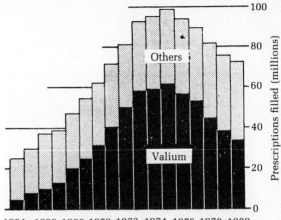

FIG. 13-6 Prescriptions for minor tranquilizers filled annually in the United States, 1964 to 1980. Copyright © 1981 by The New York Times Company. Reprinted by permission.

cide), have only minimal side effects at therapeutic doses, are potent anticonvulsants, reduce anxiety, and produce muscle relaxation, they became the number one class of psychoactive drugs prescribed by American physicians. From 1972 to 1978 Valium was *the* number one drug, with over three times as many prescriptions in 1974 as the number two drug, Librium. Fig. 13-6 shows the yearly number of prescriptions written for the minor tranquilizers and for Valium from 1964 through 1980. Valium is from the Latin, meaning "to be strong and well!"

This is a good place to pause and comment on the prescribing of psychoactive drugs. The benzodiazepines are of particular concern because (1) some are abusable and (2) they are frequently given for symptoms in situations where their use is debatable. The man who started it all by discovering meprobamate, Dr. Frank Berger, comments that; The effectiveness of antianxiety drugs in reducing anxiety and inducing a measure of tranquility in persons suffering from certain forms of anxiety disorders has been documented. . . . They are effective primarily in . . . neurasthenia, hypochondriasis, and anxiety neuroses . . . but are ineffective in . . . phobias, hysteria, and obsessive neu-

roses. . . . [They] are also widely prescribed to ease problems of living. They may be effective for this purpose to the extent that they dull sensibility to the knocks, annoyances, and frustrations of everyday life. When used in this manner, they are being used as sedatives and not as antianxiety drugs. . . . I find it difficult to believe that the insight and self-confidence needed to understand and cope with one's problems can be acquired by the use of any medication.[78]

That really says it all: the minor tranquilizers work well against certain types of symptoms—but they are used, improperly, for so much more. Some believe they are much overprescribed. Most of the minor tranquilizers are prescribed by general practitioners and internists; psychiatrists who are more aware of the misuse potential write fewer than 10% of the prescriptions. You have to sympathize somewhat with the average physician—confronted with patients with a variety of real and imaginary illnesses, most of which give rise to anxiety and depression, what do you do? You try to make the patient as comfortable as possible with the least dangerous drug at the lowest cost. Valium might not be the optimal drug for this, but it is at least one of the top few. One problem is that an individual can go to a dozen different doctors in one day with the same complaint and get a dozen prescriptions for Valium. Those you don't use or misuse yourself are easily sold—and sometimes are.

However, the worldwide data suggest that Americans are middle-of-the-road with respect to antianxiety drug use—about 15% of the population used them. Some countries are higher, some lower. The Ralph Nader Health Research Group has long been critical of the high levels of Valium use and other anxiolytic drug use—pointing particularly to the fact that maybe 1.5 million Americans have used Valium long enough to be addicted. How long is that? One report suggests that individuals using more than 300 mg a day of chlordiazepoxide or 120 mg a day of diazepam for over 2 months may be addicted. In the usual dose range, 30 to 40 mg of diazepam a day, there was no evidence of addiction, if duration of use was less than 4 months. Abrupt stoppage of the drug may result in seizures, sometimes occurring as late as the twelfth day after the drug is stopped.[73] Some severe withdrawal episodes have been reported in the literature,[79] but the confirmed reports are miniscule compared to the high level of use.[80,81] The primary concern is the casual street and home use of the drug.[82] Valium is today's barbiturate (see Chapter 14) or, as someone has termed it, Valium is dehydrated gin.

Just as with the question of the number of angels that can fit on the head of a pin, the debate over whether the minor tranquilizers are over- or underprescribed can go on indefinitely. Everyone agrees on the facts. The question is: What do the facts mean? Two more points. One study identified individuals who were suffering from "high psychic distress" and found that only one third were taking some psychotropic medication. An important and influential researcher-clinician has asked ". . . whether it is better for society to excessively smoke, eat, or drink, use illicit drugs, self-medicate, and so on, or to use a psychotherapeutic agent under the control of a responsible and caring physician?"[83,p.735]

On July 10, 1980 the Commissioner of the FDA announced that the manufacturers of the minor tranquilizers agreed to tell physicians that the products are not for "everyday" use: "Anxiety or tension associated with the stress of everyday life usually does not require treatment with an anxiolytic (antianxiety) drug."[84]

Side effects. Only a few additional comments will be made here. The most frequently reported side effect of benzodiazepine therapy is CNS depression, which usually expresses itself as drowsiness. This effect is reported by only 1 in 25 patients, so it is not a major problem. In some cases when the drug is taken before bedtime, this side effect may be helpful in assisting the anxious and depressed individual in falling asleep. In July 1976 the FDA issued a warning that all minor tranquilizers, meprobamate and the benzodiazepines, should be avoided by women in the first 3 months of pregnancy. "Three recent studies indicate there may be an association between use of the tranquilizers in early pregnancy, and malformations such as cleft lip in babies."[85] You should take special note that this warning was first issued 21 years after meprobamate was placed on the market—how many more surprises are in store for us? The evidence is overwhelming; it sometimes takes a long time to clearly establish a danger from the use of a drug. At the very least, avoid all recreational and nonessential drugs during pregnancy.

Mechanism of action

Soon after they were first introduced into clinical medicine in the early 1960s, the benzodiazepines leaped into an easy first place in the world's tranquilizer field. And yet, despite vast research endeavor, we do not know how they work.[86,p.i]

That statement is from the preface of a 1975 book that includes chapters by almost all the major teams of scientists working on this problem. There have been some giant steps, though, and the late 1980s will probably tie the multiple mechanisms up in a reasonably neat package. Early biochemical work began to center on one of the little known, but probably true, neurotransmitters: gamma-aminobutyric acid (GABA). GABA is primarily an inhibitory transmitter located in selected parts of the brain. One series of studies suggests that the ". . . depression of [central nervous system] excitability by benzodiazepines is a result of an increase in γ-aminobutyric acid (GABA) mediated inhibition."[87,p.3016] It's exciting to be able to pin down the neurotransmitters involved. Even more exciting, however, is that there is now good evidence for two or more benzodiazepine receptors in the brain! The endogenous substances that normally act to reduce anxiety by occupying the receptors have not yet been identified, but it seems reasonable to believe that they exist and are part of the body's normal coping systems. A benzodiazepine receptor! Work is going on right now all around the world to develop blocking agents for the receptors, new molecules to occupy and activate the receptors. In short, now the biochemists have some guidelines and some information that will make it possible for them to build new molecules that are more specific in their actions and that have fewer side effects![88,89]

Evidence is accumulating that the reason why diazepam—particularly—gives a euphoric feeling when taken is that its lipid solubility is very high and it is absorbed and taken up in the brain much more rapidly than the other benzodiazepines. Similarly, the probability of discomfort (withdrawal effects) on abruptly stopping use of a benzodiazepine seems to be related to the absence of long-acting metabolites. Last, but not least, the potency of the benzodiazepines correlates highly with the affinity of the various molecules for the benzodiazepine receptor.

Other levels of explanation are also meaningful, and research at present suggests that both classes of the minor tranquilizers seem to have their primary action on the limbic system. The limbic system is seen as the intermediary between the hypothalamus, which controls changes in the the autonomic nervous system, and the cerebral cortex, which is responsible for the experience of emotion. The important action of antianxiety drugs may be the result of depressing information exchange between two levels of emotional reaction. In this way experiences would elicit fewer body changes, and, also, body changes would not be experienced with as great impact. By blunting this circle of action and reaction, there may be a decrease in both the experience of emotion as well as the body changes that occur in emotional situations. This would certainly fit with the colloquial expression that these minor tranquilizers are the "I don't care" pills. Recent work[90] supports this colloquialism, since the benzodiazepines block the increase in noradrenaline turnover that usually accompanies stress. In fact, this may be part of the critical antianxiety action of these drugs.

Meprobamate and the barbiturates act on the liver microsomal enzymes to increase their activity. This will then increase the rate at which most drugs in the body are deactivated. There has been identification of the breakdown products, and, using radioactively labeled meprobamate, it has been shown that some breakdown products appear in the urine about 30 minutes after oral intake and almost all within 24 hours. Peak blood levels are obtained 1 to 2 hours after intake, and, with a single administration, almost all the meprobamate has left the bloodstream within 10 hours.

CONCLUDING COMMENT

This has been a varied chapter beginning with an understanding of the various classes of mental illness and moving on to the drug treatments that are used to control the symptoms of these illnesses. With the possible exception of lithium, none of these drugs is seen as cures or even prophylactics for the illnesses mentioned—only symptoms are affected.

But things may change very rapidly. In each of the four classes of drugs—antischizophrenic, antidepressant, antimania, and antianxiety—there have been giant steps of understanding since the late 1970s. Trying to shoot down illness depends on having both an accurate and specific tool as well as a fairly clear idea of the important mechanisms that underlie the illness. Psychotherapeutics have advanced fast and far in recent years. No one should be foolish enough to think that soon all emotional problems and mental illness can be washed away with drugs—but we are getting closer to that day.

REFERENCES

1. Maugh, T.H.: Biochemical markers identify mental states, Science **214**:39, October 1981.
2. Mosher, L.R., and others: Special report on schizophrenia, U.S. Department of Health, Education and Welfare, National Institute of Mental Health, April 1970.
3. Klein, D.F., and Davis, J.M.: Diagnosis and drug treatment of psychiatric disorders, Baltimore, 1969, The Williams & Wilkins Co.
4. Marshall, H.E.: Dorothea Dix—forgotten Samaritan, Chapel Hill, N.C., 1937, The University of North Carolina Press.
5. Weiner, D.B.: The apprenticeship of Philippe Pinel: a new document, "observations of Citizen Pussin on the insane," American Journal of Psychiatry **136**(9):1128-1134, 1979.
6. The history of depression, Psychiatric Annals, New York, 1977, Pfizer, Inc.
7. Tourney, G.: A history of therapeutic fashions in psychiatry, 1800-1966, American Journal of Psychiatry **124**:784-796, 1967.
8. Glick, I.D., and Hargreaves, W.A.: Psychiatric hospital treatment for the 1980s: a controlled study of short versus long hospitalization, Lexington, Mass., 1979, Lexington Books.
9. Mesard, L., Wrigley, A., and Gee, S.: The ordering of antipsychotic drugs for the treatment of psychotic patients in V.A. hospitals, Biometrics Division, Veterans Administration Central Office, Washington, D.C., August 1976.
10. Appleton, W.S.: Fourth psychoactive drug usage guide, Journal of Clinical Psychiatry, **43**(1):12, January 1982.
11. Goldman, D.: Treatment of psychotic states with chlorpromazine, Journal of the American Medical Association **157**:1274-1278, 1955.
12. Cole, J.O.: Phenothiazines. In Simpson, L.L., editor: Drug treatment of mental disorders, New York, 1976, Raven Press.
13. Freyhan, F.A.: The immediate and long range effects of chlorpromazine on the mental hospital. In Chlorpromazine and mental health, proceedings of a symposium under the auspices of Smith, Kline and French Laboratories, Philadelphia, 1955, Lea & Febiger.
14. Kessler, K.A., and Waletzky, J.P.: Clinical use of the antipsychotics, American Journal of Psychiatry, **138**(2):202, February 1981.
15. Goldberg, S.C., Klerman, G.L., and Cole, J.O.: Changes in schizophrenic psychopathology and ward behavior as a function of phenothiazine treatment, British Journal of Psychiatry **111**:120-133, 1965.
16. Veterans Administration: Drug treatment in psychiatry, Washington, D.C., 1970, U.S. Government Printing Office.
17. Davis, J.M., Gosenfeld, L., and Tsai, C.C.: Maintenance antipsychotic drugs do prevent relapse: a reply to Tobias and MacDonald, Psychological Bulletin **83**:431-447, 1976.
18. Prien, R.F., Caffey, E.M., Jr., and Klett, C.J.: Pharmacotherapy in chronic schizophrenia, Department of Medicine and Surgery, Veterans Administration, May 1973.
19. Prien, R.F., and Klett, C.J.: An appraisal of the long-term use of tranquilizing medication with hospitalized chronic schizophrenics, Schizophrenia Bulletin No. 5, pp. 64-73, 1972.
20. Prien, R.F., Gillis, R.D., and Caffey, E.M., Jr.: Intermittent pharmacotherapy in chronic schizophrenia, Hospital and Community Psychiatry **24**:317-322, 1973.
21. Rivera-Calemlim, L., and others: Correlation between plasma concentrations of chlorpromazine and clinical response, Communications in Psychopharmacology **2**:215, 1978.
22. May, P.R.A.: Cost efficiency of treatments for the schizophrenic patient, American Journal of Psychiatry **127**:1382-1385, 1971.
23. Carpenter, W.T., Jr., McGlashan, T.H., and Strauss, J.S.: The treatment of acute schizophrenia without drugs: an investigation of some current assumptions, American Journal of Psychiatry **134**:14-20, 1977.
24. Cole, J.O., Bonato, R., and Goldberg, S.C.: Nonspecific factors in the drug therapy of schizophrenic patients. In Rickels, K., editor: Non-specific factors in drug therapy, Springfield, Ill., 1968, Charles C Thomas, Publisher.
25. Veterans Administration: Drug treatment in psychiatry, Washington, D.C., 1970, U.S. Government Printing Office.
26. Gurel, L.: A ten year perspective on outcome in functional psychosis, Highlights of the Fifteenth Annual Conference, Veterans Administration Cooperative Studies in Psychiatry, Houston, Texas, April 2-4, 1970.
27. May, P.R.A., and others: Schizophrenia—a follow-up study of results of treatment, Archives of General Psychiatry **33**:481, April 1976.
28. Braun, P., and others: Overview: deinstitutionalization of psychiatric patients, a critical review of outcome studies, American Journal of Psychiatry, **138**(6):736, June 1981.
29. May, P.R.A.: When, what and why?: psychopharmacotherapy and other treatments in schizophrenia, Comprehensive Psychiatry **17**(6):683, 1976.
30. Custer, R., editor: Draft of a publication on the use of psychotropic medication, Veterans Administration, May 1977.
31. Leff, J.: Schizophrenia and sensitivity to the family environment, Schizophrenia Bulletin **2**(4):566-574, 1976.
32. Mosher, L.R., and Keith, S.J.: Research on the psychosocial treatment of schizophrenia: a summary report, American Journal of Psychiatry, **136**(5):623, May 1979.
33. Jarvik, M.: Drugs used in the treatment of psychiatric disorders. In Goodman, L., and Gilman, A., editors: The pharmacological basis of therapeutics, New York, 1970, The MacMillan Co.
34. Jeste, D.V., and Wyatt, R.J.: Changing epidemiology of tardive dyskinesia: an overview, American Journal of Psychiatry, **138**(3):297, March 1981.

35. Tardive dyskinesia: summary of a task force report of the American Psychiatric Association, Task Force on late neurological effects of antipsychotic drugs, American Journal of Psychiatry, **137**(10):1163, October 1980.

36. Tarsy, D., and Baldessarini, R.J.: The tardive dyskinesia syndrome. In Klawans, H.L., editor: Clinical Neuropharmacology, 1, New York, 1976, Raven Press.

37. Donlon, P.T., and Stenson, R.L.: Neuroleptic induced extrapyramidal symptoms, Diseases of the Nervous System **37**:629-635, 1976.

38. Quitkin, F., Rifkin, A., Gochfeld, L., and Klein, D.F.: Tardive dyskinesia: are first signs reversible? American Journal of Psychiatry **134**(1):84-87, 1977.

39. Ayd, F.: Sodium valproate therapy for tardive dyskinesia (editorial), International Drug Therapy Newsletter **11**(9), 1976.

40. Jus, A., and others: Epidemiology of tardive dyskinesia. Part II, Diseases of the Nervous System **37**:257-261, 1976.

41. Snyder, S., Greenberg, D., and Yamamura, H.I.: Antischizophrenic drugs and brain cholinergic receptors, Archives of General Psychiatry **31**:58-61, 1974.

42. Ray, O.: Drugs, society, and human behavior, ed. 1, St. Louis, 1972, The C.V. Mosby Co.

43. Ray, O.: Drugs, society, and human behavior, ed. 2, St. Louis, 1978, The C.V. Mosby Co.

44. Snyder, S.H.: Dopamine receptors, neuroleptics and schizophrenia, American Journal of Psychiatry, **138**(4):460, April 1981.

45. Meltzer, H.Y.: Dopamine receptors and average clinical doses, Science **194**:545-546, 1976.

46. Stimmel, G.L.: Neuroleptics and the corpus striatum: clinical implications, Diseases of the Nervous System **37**:219-224, 1976.

47. Iversen, L.L.: Dopamine receptors in the brain, Science **188**:1084-1089, 1975.

48. Appleton, W.S.: Third psychoactive drug usage guide, Diseases of the Nervous System **37**:39-51, 1976.

49. Burt, D.R., Creese, I., and Snyder, S.H.: Antischizophrenic drugs: chronic treatment elevates dopamine receptor binding in brain, Science **196**:326-327, 1977.

50. The history of depression, Psychiatric Annals, New York, 1977, Pfizer, Inc.

51. Kraft, D.P., and Babigian, H.M.: Suicide by persons with and without psychiatric contacts, Archives of General Psychiatry **33**:209-215, 1976.

52. Gold, M.A., and others: Diagnosis of depression in the 1980s, Journal of the American Medical Association **245**(15):1562, 1981.

53. Goodwin, F.K., and Bunney, W.E., Jr.: A psychobiological approach to affective illness, Psychiatric Annals **3**:19-56, February 1973.

54. Brown, W.A.: The dexamethasone suppression test: a potential tool in the management of depression, Behavioral Medicine, p. 22, September 1981.

55. Carroll, B.J., and others: A specific laboratory test for the diagnosis of melancholia, Archives of General Psychiatry **38**:15, January 1981.

56. Small, J.G., and Small, I.F.: Electroconvulsive therapy update, review, Psychopharmacology Bulletin **17**(4):27, 1981.

57. Gonzalez, E.R.: New studies confirm MAO inhibitors efficacy in treating severe anxiety, Medical News **245** (18):1799, 1981.

58. Reed, K.: Tricyclic antidepressant blood level, Postgraduate Medicine **70**(5):81, 1981.

59. Amsterdam, J., and others: The clinical application of tricyclic antidepressant pharmacokinetics and plasma levels, American Journal of Psychiatry, **137**(6):653, June 1980.

60. U'Prichard, D.C., and others: Tricyclic antidepressants: therapeutic properties and affinity for α-noradrenergic receptor binding sites in the brain, Science **199**:197, January 1978.

61. DeMontigny, C., and Aghajanian, G.K.: Tricyclic antidepressants: long-term treatment increases responsivity of rat forebrain neurons to serotonin, Science **202**:1303, December 1978.

62. Veterans Administration: Drug treatment in psychiatry, Washington, D.C., 1970, U.S. Government Printing Office.

63. Fibiger, H.C., and Phillips, A.G.: Increased intracranial self stimulation in rats after long-term administration of desipramine, Science **214**:683, November 1981.

64. HHS News P80-56, November 18, 1980.

65. Gattozzi, A.: Lithium in the treatment of mood disorders, National Clearinghouse for Mental Health Information, Publication No. 5033, 1970.

66. Fieve, R.R.: Therapeutic uses of lithium and rubidium. In Simpson, L.L., editor: Drug treatment of mental disorders, New York, 1976, Raven Press.

67. Another look at lithium, The Medical Letter **22**(4):17, 1980.

68. Schou, M.: New evidence on the prophylactic value of lithium carbonate. In Highlights of the Fifteenth Annual Conference, Veterans Administration Cooperative Studies in Psychiatry, Houston, Tex., April 1970.

69. Tosteson, D.C.: Lithium and mania, Scientific American **244**(4):164, 1981.

70. Jasinski, P.R., Nutt, J.G., Haertzen, C.A., and Griffith, J.D.: Lithium: effects on subjective functioning and morphine-induced euphoria, Science **195**:582-584, 1977.

71. Pokorny, A.D., and Prien, R.F.: Lithium in treatment and prevention of affective disorder, Diseases of the Nervous System **35**(7):327-333, 1974.

72. Berger, P.A., and Tinklenberg, J.R.: Treatment of abuses of alcohol and other addictive drugs. In Psychopharmacology from theory to practice, 1977, Oxford University Press.

73. Sepinwall, J., and Cook, L.: Relationship of γ-aminobutyric acid (GABA) to antianxiety effects of benzodiazepines, Brain Research Bulletin **5**:839, 1980.

74. Miller, R.R., and Greenblatt, D.J.: Drug effects in hospitalized patients, New York, 1976, John Wiley & Sons, Inc.

75. Librium and Valium, Medical Letter on Drugs and Therapeutics 11(20):81-84, 1969.

76. Goodwin, D.W.: Psychopharmacology, Psychiatry Digest, pp. 39-48, May 1975.

77. Drugs for psychiatric disorders, Medical Letter on Drugs and Therapeutics 18(22):89-93, 1976.

78. Berger, F.M.: The use of antianxiety drugs, Clinical Pharmacology and Therapeutics 29(3):291, 1981.

79. Preskorn, S.H., and Denner, L.J.: Benzodiazepines and withdrawal psychosis, Journal of the American Medical Association 237:36-38, 1977.

80. Tyrer, P., and others: Benzodiazepine withdrawal symptoms and propranolol, Lancet, 1(8219):520, March 7, 1981.

81. Hollister, L.E., and others: Long-term use of diazepam, Journal of the American Medical Association 245(14):1568, 1981.

82. Woody, G.E., O Brien, C.P., and Greenstein, R.: Misuse and abuse of diazepam: an increasingly common medical problem, International Journal of the Addictions 10:843-848, 1975.

83. Rickels, K.: Are benzodiazepines overused and abused?, British Journal of Clinical Pharmacology 11:71, 1981.

84. HHS News P80-30, July 10, 1980.

85. HEW News 76-20, July 22, 1976.

86. Sandler, M.: Preface. In Costa, E., and Greengard, P., editors: Mechanism of action of benzodiazepines, advances in biochemical psychopharmacology, vol. 14, New York, 1975, Raven Press.

87. Geller, H.M., and others: Electrophysiological actions of benzodiazepines, Federation Proceedings 39(12):3016, 1980.

88. Snyder, S.H.: Benzodiazepine receptors, Proceedings of symposium—anxiety: the therapeutic dilemma, p. 1, February 1981.

89. Tallman, J.F., and others: Receptors for the age of anxiety: pharmacology of the benzodiazepines, Science 207:274, January 1980.

90. Costa, E., and Greengard, P., editors: Mechanism of action of benzodiazepines, advances in biochemical psychopharmacology, vol. 14, New York, 1975, Raven Press.

CHAPTER 14

STIMULANTS AND DEPRESSANTS

UPPERS AND DOWNERS. Drugs that can light a "fire in your brain" and drugs that can put you down—*hard*. Drugs that make you feel good! Not just good, but *really* good! Drugs that can—and sometimes do—kill. The "in" drug of the early seventies—the "in" drug of the eighties. These are the elevator drugs—the ones that alter an individual's level of arousal or behavioral activity. We all have undergone large changes in arousal level: from deep sleep to a highly charged emotional situation. For most activities there seems to be an optimal level of activation. If the level is too low, then we will neither be aware of changes in the environment nor can we respond to them. When arousal is too high, the nervous system fails to filter out irrelevant signals. As a result the information processing system is overloaded and unable to discriminate multiple inputs or to integrate them. Too much or too little arousal has the same effect: an inability to identify or respond to significant signals.

Arousal level is primarily controlled by the reticular activating system. The cortex and other parts of the brain and body, as well as the external environment, send information to the reticular system to regulate it. The drugs considered here have been grouped as stimulants and depressants. The stimulants at proper dose levels increase the activity of the activating system as well as responsiveness to sensory input. The depressants are compounds that decrease activity level and sensitivity to the environment, usually through their actions on the reticular system.

Classically, stimulants are considered agents that improve mental and physical performance when they are impaired because of fatigue. There are three broad groups of stimulants, one of which, the xanthines, was discussed in Chapter 10. Cocaine, a naturally occurring stimulant, is in a class by itself. The amphetamines are the best-known stimulants and will serve as the prototype of the third group of agents.

Depressants are drugs that decrease the activity of the reticular activating system and other areas of the brain, causing a reduction in behavioral output and in the level of awareness. Sometimes a differentiation is made among agents used as sedatives, hypnotics, and anesthetics, but these distinctions are only meaningful in a clinical sense. A sedative causes a mild depression of the central nervous system and decreases excitability and anxiety. Usually these effects can occur without excessive drowsiness or inefficiency. A larger dose of a sedative turns it into a hypnotic, that is, a drug used to induce sleep. By increasing the dose to still higher levels, an anesthetic state can be reached, and with more drug and consequently greater depression of the CNS, death can occur. One experiment studying the effects of barbiturates given orally to dogs reported that sedative, hypnotic, and anesthetic effects were obtained at dose levels that were roughly one-eighth, one-sixth, and one-half the lethal dose.[1]

Usually no distinction other than dosage is made between sedatives and hypnotics. Rarely, though, is a compound used as both a hypnotic and an anesthetic. Hypnotic (sleep-inducing) drugs are typically poor choices as anesthetic agents, since they usually have a slow rate of elimination from the body with a long and not easily controlled duration of action. As with alcohol, some depressants have only a narrow safety margin between the anesthetic and the lethal doses. Alcohol is one type of CNS depressant; its use and misuse are discussed in Chapter 8. The remaining agents in this group are classed here as barbiturates and nonbarbiturates.

STIMULANTS
Coca and cocaine

History. A grave in Peru dating from about 500 AD contains an early record of use of coca leaves. Included along with other necessities for the afterlife were several bags of the leaves. Use of coca in this way gives no hint of the extent of cultivation or general use of the leaf at that time, but it certainly must have produced "exaltation of spirit, freedom from fatigue, and a sense of well being."[2,p.12] even as it does today. By 1000 AD the coca shrub was extensively cultivated in Peru; today approximately 50 million kg of coca leaves are produced each year. Less than 5 million kg are exported for legal use or consumed by the 2 million Peruvians who live in the highlands. Simple and inexpensive processing of 500 kg of coca leaves yields 1 kg of cocaine.

Growing coca is illegal in Bolivia and Colombia, and no new plantings have been authorized by the government of Peru since 1964. The terrain of the Andes in Bolivia and Peru is poorly suited for growing almost everything. *Erythroxylon coca,* however, seems to thrive at elevations of 2000 to 8000 feet on the Amazon slope of the mountains, where there is over 100 inches of rain a year. The shrub is pruned to prevent it from reaching the normal height of 6 to 8 feet, so that the picking, which is done three or four times a year, is easier to accomplish. The shrubs are grown in small, 2- to 3-acre patches called *cocals,* some of which are known to have been under cultivation for over 800 years.

Before the sixteenth-century invasion by Pizarro, the Incas had built a well-developed civilization in Peru. The cocoa leaf was an important part of the culture, and, although earlier use was primarily in religious ceremonies, it was treated as money by the time the conquistadors arrived. The Spanish adopted this custom and paid coca leaves to the native laborers for mining and transporting gold and silver.

The mountain natives at that time, as today, chewed coca leaves almost continually, keeping a ball of them tucked in their cheek as they went about their business. The habit was so common that distances were measured by how far one could travel before it became necessary to stop and replenish the leaves. Even then, the leaf was recognized as increasing strength and endurance while decreasing the need for food. Early European chroniclers of the Inca civilization recorded and reported on the unique qualities of this plant, but it never interested Europeans until the last half of the nineteenth century.[3] At that time the coca leaf contributed to the economic well-being and fame of three individuals. They, in turn, brought the Peruvian shrub to the notice of the world.

One of these men was Angelo Mariani, a French chemist. His contribution was to introduce the coca leaf indirectly to the general public. Mariani imported tons of coca leaves and used an extract from them in many products. The quid of leaves was gone, but you could suck on a coca lozenge, drink coca tea, or obtain the coca leaf extract in any of a large number of products. It was Mariani's coca wine, though, that made him rich and famous. Assuredly, it had to be the coca leaf extract in the wine that prompted the pope to present a medal of appreciation to Mariani. Not only the pope but royalty and the man in the street benefited from the Andean plant. For them, as it had for the Incas for 1000 years and was to do for Americans who drank Coca-Cola (Chapter 10), the extract of the coca leaf lifted their spirits, freed them from fatigue, and gave them a general good feeling.

It was these three characteristics that led to the use of cocaine by Sherlock Holmes and Sigmund Freud. Coca leaves can contain a considerable amount (up to almost 2%) of the active ingredient, cocaine. Cocaine was isolated before 1860, but there is still debate over who did it and exactly when. An available supply of pure cocaine and the newly developed hypodermic syringe improved the drug delivery system, so that the following scene was easily conceived by Arthur Conan Doyle in 1890:

> Sherlock Holmes took his bottle from the corner of the mantelpiece, and his hypodermic syringe from its neat morocco case. With his long, white nervous fingers, he adjusted the delicate needle and rolled back his left shirtcuff. For some little time his eyes rested thoughtfully upon the sinewy forearm and wrist, all dotted and scarred with innumerable puncture-marks. Finally, he thrust the sharp point home, pressed down the tiny piston, and sank back into the velvet-lined armchair with a long sigh of satisfaction.
>
> Three times a day for many months I had witnessed this performance, but custom had not reconciled my mind to it. . . .
>
> "Which is it today," I asked, "Morphine or cocaine?"
>
> He raised his eyes languidly from the old black-letter volume which he had opened.
>
> "It is cocaine," he said, "a seven-per-cent solution. Would you care to try it?"
>
> "No, indeed, " I answered brusquely. "My constitution has not got over the Afghan campaign yet. I cannot afford to throw any extra strain upon it."
>
> He smiled at my vehemence. "Perhaps you are right, Watson," he said. "I suppose that its influence is physically a bad one. I find it, however, so transcendently stimulating and clarifying to the mind that its secondary action is a matter of small moment."
>
> "But consider!" I said earnestly. "Count the cost! Your brain may, as you say, be roused and excited, but it is a pathological and morbid process which involves increased tissue-change and may at least have a permanent weakness. You know, too, what a black reaction comes upon you. Surely the game is hardly worth the candle. Why should you, for a mere passing pleasure, risk the loss of those great powers with which you have been endowed? Remember that I speak not only as one comrade to another but as a medical man to one for whose constitution he is to some extent answerable."
>
> He did not seem offended. On the contrary, he put his finger-tips together, and leaned his elbows on the arms of his chair, like one who has a relish for conversation.
>
> "My mind," he said, "rebels at stagnation. Give me problems, give me work, give me the most abstruse cryptogram, or the most intricate analysis, and I am in my own proper atmosphere. I can dispense then with artificial stimulants. But I abhor the dull routine of existence. I crave for mental exaltation."[4,pp.91-92]

Sherlock Holmes! Perhaps even more surprising is the fact that the use of cocaine for these same purposes had been advocated 6 years earlier by the father of psychoanalysis.

> In 1884 Sigmund Freud wrote to his fiancée that he had been experimenting with "a magical drug". After dazzling success in treatment of a case of gastric catarrh he continues "If it goes well I will write an essay on it and I expect it will win its place in therapeutics by the side of morphium, and superior to it. . . . I take very small doses of it regularly against depression and against indigestion, and with the most brilliant success." He urged his fiancée, his sisters, his colleagues, and his friends to try it . . . extolled the drug as a safe exhilarant which he himself used and recommended as a treatment for morphine addiction. For emphasis he stated, in italics, that "Inebriate asylums can be entirely dispensed with". . . .[3,p.17]

In an 1885 lecture before a group of psychiatrists, Freud commented on the use of cocaine as a stimulant, saying, "On the whole it must be said that the value of cocaine in psychiatric practice remains to be demonstrated, and it will probably be worthwhile to make a thorough trial as soon as the currently exorbitant price of the drug becomes more reasonable." The first of the consumer advocates!

Freud was more convinced about another use of the drug, however, and in the same lecture said:

> We can speak more definitely about another use of cocaine by the psychiatrist. It was first discovered in America that cocaine is capable of alleviating the serious withdrawal symptoms observed in subjects who are abstaining from morphine and of suppressing their craving for morphine. . . . On the basis of my experiences with the effects of cocaine, I have no hesitation in recommending the administration of cocaine for such withdrawal cures in subcutaneous injections of 0.03-0.05 g per dose, without any fear of increasing the dose. On several occasions, I have even seen cocaine quickly eliminate the manifestations of intolerance that appeared after a rather large dose of morphine, as if it had a specific ability to counteract morphine.[5]

Even great men make mistakes. The realities of life were harshly brought home to Freud when he used cocaine to treat a close friend, Fleischl, to remove his addiction to morphine. Increasingly larger doses were needed, and "Freud spent one frightful night nursing Fleischl through an episode of cocaine psychosis and thereafter was bitterly against drugs. . . ."[6,p.17]

Even before Freud became aware of the problems with cocaine, Louis Lewin had attacked his proposal to use cocaine to cure morphine addiction and referred to Freud as "Joseph, the dream interpreter"!

Although physicians were well aware of the dangers of using cocaine regularly, nonmedical as well as quasimedical use of cocaine was widespread in the United States around the turn of the century. It was one of the secret ingredients in many patent medicines and elixirs but was also openly advertised as having beneficial effects. The Parke-Davis Pharmaceutical Company noted in 1885 that cocaine "can supply the place of food, make the coward brave, and silent eloquent . . ." and called it a "wonder drug."[7] With so much going for the drug, and its availability in a large number of products for drinking, snorting, or injection, it may seem strange that between 1887 and 1914 46 states passed laws to regulate the use and distribution of cocaine. One author[8,p.89] provided extensive documentation and concluded:

> All the elements needed to insure cocaine's outlaw status were present by the first years of the twentieth century: it had become widely used as a pleasure drug, and doctors warned of the dangers attendant on indiscriminate sale and use; it had become identified with despised or poorly regarded groups—blacks, lower-class whites, and criminals; it had not been long enough established in the culture to insure its survival; and it had not, though used by them, become identified with the elite, thus losing what little chance it had of weathering the storm of criticism.

Cocaine was included but unlabeled in all sorts of nerve tonics, patent medicine, and home remedies until the 1906 Pure Food and Drugs Act was passed. It went underground with the Harrison Act of 1914 and pretty much stayed there until the late 1960s. It did come to the surface often enough to let America know that it was around and still being used. "Cocaine Lil," a song written in the 1920s, included the line, "Lil went to a 'snow' party one cold night, and the way she sniffed was sure a fright." Cole Porter's "I Get a Kick out of You" in 1934 originally contained the verse:

> I get no kick from cocaine
> I'm sure that if
> I took even one sniff
> It would bore me terifically too
> But I get a kick out of you.

The very late sixties and early seventies showed a rapid resurgence of cocaine as a recreational drug. One reason for this increase may be that:

> For its devotees, cocaine epitomizes the best of the drug culture—which is to say, a good high is achieved without the forbiddingly dangerous needle and addiction of heroin, or the mindtwisting wrench of LSD and the hallucinogens.[9]

Therapeutic use and mechanism of action

Cocaine is a unique drug in that it is both a local anesthetic and a sympathomimetic with powerful central nervous system stimulant effects. Like other psychomotor stimulant drugs, such as the

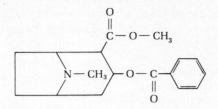

Cocaine
(3β-hydroxy-1αH,5αH-tropane-2β-carboxylic acid, methyl ester, benzoate [ester])

FIG. 14-1 Cocaine.

amphetamines, it can produce psychological dependence, but does not appear to cause any physical dependence.[10]

The local anesthetic properties of cocaine, that is, the ability to numb the area to which it is applied, were discovered in 1860 soon after its isolation from coca leaves. It was not until 1884 that this characteristic was used medically; the early applications were in eye surgery and dentistry. The use of cocaine spread rapidly, since it apparently was a safe and effective drug. The potential for misuse soon became clear, and a search began for synthetic agents with similar anesthetic characteristics but little or no potential for misuse. This work was rewarded in 1905 with the discovery of procaine (Novocain), which is still widely used. Many similar drugs have been synthesized since 1905 that have local anesthetic actions similar to that of cocaine but that do not have stimulatory effects on the CNS. Because these drugs have more specific effects, they have replaced cocaine for medical usage.

Local anesthetics probably block pain by preventing the generation and conduction of nerve impulses. They seem to act quite specifically on the cell membrane. By disrupting the membrane processes necessary for the initiation and generation of electrical impulses, impulse conduction and information processing are stopped.[11]

Cocaine, compared to the other local anesthetics, is much more potent in causing increased activation and arousal of the CNS. The evidence suggests that the initial effect is on the cerebral cortex (although perhaps through action elsewhere). Motor activity increases at low doses; with higher doses convulsions may occur. At still higher dose levels, the respiration centers of the brain are affected, and the breathing rate will increase. Moderate doses also increase heart rate, but high levels of the drug delivered intravenously may stop the heart because of a direct action of cocaine on the heart muscle.

The central activation and the sympathomimetic actions are correlated with the action of cocaine at adrenergic synapses. Cocaine induces the release of noradrenaline from presynaptic axon terminals. It also prevents reuptake of the released noradrenaline. The noradrenaline continues to act postsynaptically for an extended period and causes an enhancement of all adrenergic neurons and sympathetic nervous system effects. Fig. 14-1 shows the chemical structure of cocaine.

Cocaine and amphetamine. The perennial debate has been: Does cocaine give the same effect as amphetamine, differing only in having a shorter duration of action? What we know of their mechanisms of action suggest that they are the same. However, there is one report of lithium (used for the treatment of bipolar depression) blocking the effects of cocaine but not the effects of amphetamine. This needs to be followed up.[12] What about the similarity or difference of the experienced effects of cocaine and amphetamine? Some say, "The 'high' produced by cocaine is similar to that produced by a large dose of amphetamines except that cocaine's effect lasts a very short time."[13] Others say:[8,p.179]

. . . pharmacologically, cocaine and the amphetamines are very similar. Their subjective effects are, however, quite different. And this is not simply a difference in *duration*, it is a difference in *kind*. Cocaine is a subtle drug when ingested in the usual manner, i.e. by snorting; so subtle that naive users frequently need to have its effects pointed out to them before they can recognize them. . . . The amphetamines on the other hand are anything but subtle. . . . Indeed persons who have thought they were using cocaine but were in fact using cocaine heavily cut with speed—a common street product these days—often charge a dealer with cheating them after he has sold them high-quality cocaine.

It has been known for many years that prolonged high doses of either cocaine or amphetamine produce the same toxic syndrome: enhanced sense of physical and mental capacity, loss of appetite, grinding of teeth, stereotyped, repetitious behavior, and paranoia. One particularly interesting common effect is the appearance of "cocaine bugs" (technically called *formication*). The user feels something like bugs crawling under his skin, and the sensation may become so great that he will use a knife to cut them out. Even without this extreme reaction the heavy cocaine or amphetamine user may have many open sores as a result of his scratching and picking at the "bugs." The basis for this experience is probably a drug-induced stimulation of nerve endings in the skin, but how the mechanism operates is not yet clear.[14] One report[15] gives evidence that these tactile hallucinations are the final stage of a series of hallucinations, the first of which are visual: "snow lights."

A study[10] of volunteers who had previously used street cocaine intravenously reported that 10 mg of dextroamphetamine intravenously had a subjective effect the same as 12 to 16 mg of cocaine. In fact, these regular intravenous cocaine users frequently identified dextroamphetamine as cocaine—"the same kind of cocaine that I'm used to shooting up." Amphetamine is frequently used to adulterate cocaine sold on the street. This may mean that very few cocaine users know what effects

pure cocaine will produce. One other aspect is also of interest: 16 mg of intravenous cocaine were rated as similar to the average dose these individuals were self-injecting on the street, and 24 to 32 mg of cocaine were rated as the highest they had ever used.

The first controlled study of the psychological effects of cocaine administered intranasally appeared in 1977.[16] Doses of 0, 10, 25, and 100 mg were administered either intravenously or intranasally to volunteers who had regularly administered cocaine to themselves. When the 10 and 25 mg doses were injected, they increased heart rate and blood pressure as well as producing a "high." Ratings of "pleasantness" began to increase within 2 minutes, peaked in 5 minutes, and returned to normal in 15 to 25 minutes. A dose of 10 mg intranasally had no effect, but both the 25 and 100 mg doses were followed by increased heart rate, blood pressure, and feelings of a "high" and "pleasantness." This time the "high" reached a maximum 10 minutes after administration and persisted for over 60 minutes.

The study also questioned the subjects using a true-false inventory on drug effects. The four items most often marked "true" following use of cocaine were "(i) I feel as if something pleasant had just happened to me, (ii) I am in the mood to talk about the feeling I have, (iii) a thrill has gone through me one or more times, since I started the test, (iv) I feel like joking with someone."[16] Very interesting was the frequent spontaneous remark, "I feel more relaxed,"—not what most people would expect, although some intravenous amphetamine users give the same response. This research also found:

A biphasic effect from cocaine consisting of an initial euphoria followed by dysphoric effects was reported by four subjects 20 to 30 minutes after the 25-mg intravenous dose, and by two subjects 45 to 60 minutes after the 100-mg intranasal dose. This dysphoria, referred to as "post-coke blues" or "crashing," was characterized by feelings of anxiety, depression, fatigue, and wanting more cocaine.[16]

It probably is true that cocaine and amphetamine have similar physiological and psychological effects when given intravenously in equipotent doses. When cocaine is sniffed, the dose and rate of absorption possibly provide a qualitatively different psychological experience from the usual intravenous amphetamine effect. In large enough doses it seems likely that both amphetamine and cocaine—no matter how administered—can produce a post-high dysphoria.[17]

Cocaine use today. Coke *is* it! In the senior class of the high schools of America the percent who report ever having tried cocaine increased from 9% in 1975 to 17% in 1981. The number reporting use "in the last 30 days" tripled—to 6%. In the "young adult" group, 18 to 25, 20% report having tried cocaine. The percentages will certainly increase—what no one knows is how high they'll get. It's fairly clear though that cocaine is not a drug of the downtrodden, the poor, the weak, the uneducated. At $100 a gram, and rising regularly, it seems to have settled in along with $10 wines as one of the luxuries of the upper-middle class. The market is increasing every year.

The best guesstimate is that in 1980 40 metric tons of illegal cocaine entered this country and sold for an estimated $30 billion.[18] The coca grower gets about $2.50 for each kilo of leaves. Five hundred kilo of leaves makes up 2.5 kilo of coca paste, which makes 1 kilo of cocaine hydrocholoride, which gets cut to about 10% to 15% purity. The dealer sells 6 to 10 kilo on the street, "Real thing, very pure," for which he gets between $500,000 and $1 million—in cash.

It used to be said that "in the heroin trade, the users die; in the cocaine trade, the dealers die." It's believable. Miami probably averages one cocaine-dealing–related death a week. The Miami banks are the only ones in the country with a surplus of cash. Miami, as you may have guessed, is the center for the illegal entry and distribution of cocaine to the United States.

On March 10, 1982, U.S. Customs seized one shipment of 3748 pounds of cocaine—the largest ever—at the Miami Airport. Using the estimates just mentioned it would have been worth about $1 billion on the street. One thing that didn't make the papers: officials believe that a shipment this size arrives every 2 weeks! That's in addition to all the other, smaller, amounts of cocaine being smuggled in regularly. Grown in Peru and Bolivia, refined in Colombia, and shipped in every possible way, cocaine arrives in South Florida. It's like shipping cash—very dangerous to the transporters and to the dealers. A basic rule students need to learn: high profits also mean high risk! In the cocaine trade the government is the least of your worries. The battle for the cocaine business is just like the battles in the twenties during prohibition for the booze business—lots of shooting.

Cocaine is getting more dangerous to the users. In the mid-seventies there were fewer people using cocaine and those who were using it were using it smarter. A mid-1981 report to the National Institute on Drug Abuse puts cocaine twelfth in drug-related deaths (up from eighteenth in 1978). About 1.4 g is lethal in the hypothetical 150 pound person. From 1979 to 1980 there was a 40% increase in cocaine-related admissions to emergency rooms and that increased by 50% in 1981. The head of the Haight-Ashbury Free Clinic in San Francisco said, "Heavy cocaine users exhibit symptoms similar to those of the 'speed freak'. Continued high doses result in irritability, suspicion, paranoia, nervousness and unrelieved fatigue, lapses in attention, inability to concentrate, and hallucinations. Intensified use leads to exhaustion and eventual collapse. . . ."[19]

Quite probably it's just beginning. If we could all follow the example of the Peruvian Indians, or Angelo Mariani, or Dr. Andy Weil we might be okay:

> My personal experiences with coca leave me convinced that the leaf is pleasant to consume and moderately stimulating in a useful way. It does not appear to be associated with dependent behavior or to provoke development of tolerance. It can be left alone if one chooses.
>
> By contrast, cocaine is much less pleasant to consume, easily becomes associated with depen-

dent behavior, is not very useful, and is very hard to leave alone. Yet in our society a great many people are using cocaine, and hardly anyone has seen a coca leaf. How have we managed to create such a situation?[19a]

Never content to let bad enough alone—the mid-eighties will show a great increase in freebasing. That will mean real problems. Take note that people can, and do, use cocaine in many ways. Chewing and sucking the leaves and slowly absorbing the cocaine through the mucous membranes, which is very reminiscent of tobacco chewing or snuff dipping, are two of the many ways cocaine is used. The blood levels of cocaine obtained by chewing or sucking the leaves are only about half of that obtained through snorting.[20,21]

In snorting the attempt is to get the very fine cocaine hydrochloride powder high into the nasal passages—right on the nasal mucosa. This is where it's rapidly absorbed. The less you get on the septum the less likely you are to cause tissue damage there. But you still get the hallmark of a snorter—a perpetually runny nose. The intravenous use of cocaine delivers a very high concentration to the brain and gives the most powerful and brief result. You probably remember that inhalation is a very effective and fast way to deliver a drug. That's where freebasing comes in.

Cocaine hydrochloride is a nice stable compound—great for shipping, lousy for smoking. The solution is to turn the cocaine hydrochloride into basic cocaine (freebase), which melts at body temperature and is quite volatile. Cocaine freebase can readily be smoked—the rapid speed and amount of cocaine that reaches the brain is the same as using cocaine intravenously. The effects?

> . . . tachycardia, increased blood pressure and respiration rate are the autonomic effects. The 'rush' is sudden and intense. Feelings of energy, power and competency are described. The euphoric high subsides after a few minutes into a restless irritability. . . . Sleep is impossible during a freebase binge, but exhaustion eventually supervenes. Enormous weight loss takes place in heavy users due to the anorectic action of cocaine. Manic, paranoid or depressive psychoses have

been seen. Overdoses can cause death due to cardiorespiratory arrest.[22]

Four things need to be mentioned. First, the "restless irritability" is one of the reasons that, in the early years of this century and again recently, intravenous cocaine users injected "speedballs," a combination of cocaine *and* heroin. Freeebasers also sometimes use heroin to take the edge off the post-high down. Second, that down is really bad—many use the term *anguish* to describe it. To remove it they use more cocaine—frequently continuing until the supply is gone. True, cocaine is not addicting—but not too many users stop when there is still cocaine available. Third, even as the high is leaving and the anguish grows, the blood levels of cocaine are unchanged from those measured at the peak of the high.[23] The critical factor for the effect of many psychoactive drugs seems to be the rate at which the drug enters the brain, not just the steady state level. (The same is true with alcohol—people report, and behavioral measurements show, more effect at a given blood alcohol level on the increasing side of the curve than on the decreasing side.) Fourth, and last: Why freebase at all? The preparation takes time and is dangerous since it involves volatile, explosive solvents. Why hasn't the smoking of coca paste caught on? It will, it just hasn't been available in the United States. The coca paste—maybe 80% cocaine sulfate—is just as effective when smoked as freebase.

The fact that emergency room visits and deaths resulting from cocaine use are increasing and that freebasing is accelerating may make you nervous (at least, it makes *me* nervous). It was only in 1974 that a respected psychiatrist, who went on to work in the White House and became the number one person in the federal government's drug abuse prevention program, said: "Cocaine . . . is probably the most benign of illicit drugs currently in widespread use."[24] It was only in 1977, proposing to Congress the decriminalization of marijuana, that this authority said that the Carter administration was considering a similar move on cocaine!

Smoke it, shoot it, snort it, swallow it. Any way

you use it, from here it looks like in the 1980s: Coke *is* it!

A last thought. How pleasurable is the cocaine experience? There *is* some variability among people (as there is with heroin) and certainly there are great differences among the many ways in which cocaine is used.[25] In one study: "Rhesus monkeys were allowed to choose between intravenous injections of cocaine and food reinforcement for lever pressing. . . . The animals chose cocaine almost exclusively, which resulted in . . . weight loss. . . ."[26] The experiment was stopped, but . . . even unto death.

Amphetamines

History. Amphetamine is a Johnny-come-lately in the stimulant world. The story of this stimulant starts with the search for a substitute for the naturally occurring sympathomimetic ephedrine. In the late 1920s researchers synthesized and studied the effects of the amphetamine salts and received the patent for them in 1932.

All major effects of amphetamine were discovered in the 1930s, although some of the uses developed later. Quite early it was shown that amphetamine was a potent dilator of the bronchial tubes and could be efficiently delivered through inhalation. To capitalize on this effect of amphetamine, the Benzedrine (brand name) inhaler was introduced as an over-the-counter product in 1932. Some of the early work with amphetamine showed that the drug would awaken anesthetized dogs. As one writer put it, amphetamine is the drug that won't let sleeping dogs lie!

Amphetamine, a CNS stimulant, seemed to be effective for the tratment of narcolepsy in 1935. Narcolepsy is a condition in which the individual spontaneously falls asleep, five, ten, fifty times a day (even outside the classroom). Amphetamine enables these patients to remain awake and function almost normally. In 1938, however, two narcolepsy patients treated with amphetamine developed acute paranoid psychotic reactions. The paranoid reaction to amphetamine has reappeared regularly and has been studied (as will be seen later).

In 1937 amphetamine became available as a prescription tablet, and a report appeared in the literature suggesting that amphetamine, a stimulant, was effective in reducing activity in hyperactive children. Two years later, in 1939, notice was taken of a report by amphetamine-treated narcolepsy patients that they were not hungry when taking the drug. This appetite depressant effect became the major clinical use of amphetamine. The drug is now viewed as an effective but trivial short-term anorexiant. Both the effect on hyperactive children and the appetite suppressant effect are discussed later.

In 1939 amphetamine went to war. There were many reports that Germany was using stimulants to increase the efficiency of their soldiers. A 1944 report in the *Air Surgeon's Bulletin* titled "Benzedrine Alert"[27] stated that "this drug is the most satisfactory of any available in temporarily postponing sleep when desire to sleep endangers the security of a mission." Some studies were reported, including one in which

> one hundred Marines were kept active continuously for sixty hours in range firing, a twenty-five mile forced march, a field problem, calisthenics, close-order drill, games, fatigue detail and bivouac alerts. Fifty men received seven 10-milligram tablets of benzedrine at six hour intervals following the first day's activity. Meanwhile, the other fifty were given placebo (milk sugar) tablets. None knew what he was receiving. Participating officers concluded that the benzedrine definitely "pepped up" the subjects, improved their morale, reduced sleepiness and increased confidence in shooting ability. . . . It was observed that men receiving benzedrine tended to lead the march, tolerate their sore feet and blisters more cheerfully, and remain wide awake during "breaks," whereas members of the control group had to be shaken to keep them from sleeping.[27]

Although the blisters may have been in a different place, it was the same desire for increased alertness that resulted in the order in 1969 to astronaut Gordon Cooper to take an amphetamine prior to his manual control of reentry of his space capsule. These alerting characteristics had already been well noted by truck drivers and college students. A group of psychology students at the University of Minnesota began experimenting with various drugs in 1937 and found that amphetamine was ideal for "cramming." (This experiment has probably been informally replicated more times than any other, except perhaps the one mentioned by Shakespeare in Chapter 4!) College kids will try anything once (or twice, or . . .), but no real concern over nonmedical use of amphetamine developed until after World War II. A 1946 article, "On a Bender with Benzedrine," appeared in a popular national magazine. It made explicit just how one could get his amphetamine without a prescription.

> After I bought an inhaler, Hal worked off the perforated cap and pulled out the medicated paper, folded accordion-wise. . . . "Like this—" Hall took the innocent looking scrap of paper he had torn away and held it between thumb and finger. He alternately dunked and squeezed this paper into his glass of beer.[28]

Some of the medical and psychiatric problems that occurred when the contents of the Benzedrine inhaler were used were discussed in a 1947 report[29] in the *Journal of the American Medical Association* titled "Oral Use of Stimulants Obtained from Inhalers." Since each inhaler contained 250 mg of amphetamine, a considerable dose could be obtained if taken all at once. Of 15 army prisoners using inhaler amphetamine, hallucinations and the feeling that others were talking about them were observed in four.

Misuse of oral amphetamine was widespread and common knowledge. This was the period of charm bracelets with an attached pillbox and the advertisement: FOR "BENZEDRINE" IF YOU'RE HAVING FUN AND GOING ON FOREVER; "ASPIRIN" IF IT'S ALL A HEADACHE. Wearing your bracelet and singing one of the recently current pop tunes. "Who Put the Benzedrine in Mrs. Murphy's Ovaltine," who could care about inhaler eaters?

It was not until 1959 that the FDA banned the use of amphetamine in inhalers. Because of a loophole in the law, one inhaler by another company, containing 250 mg of mephentermine, also a stimulant, was available as an OTC item until 1971.[30]

The problem of the misuse of the inhalers was actually a minor one compared to the amphetamine problem that began during World War II in Japan. Amphetamines were widely used in Japan to maintain production on the homefront and to keep the fighting men going. To reduce large stockpiles of methamphetamine after the war, the drug was sold without prescription, and the drug companies advertised them for "elimination of drowsiness and repletion of the spirit." As a result, "drug abuse grew as furiously as a storm."[31,p.138]

Medical problems developed, and in 1948 stricter controls on amphetamine were put into force. Although they were tightened each year, the problem increased, and in 1954 the Japanese Pharmacists Association estimated that 1.5 million people (about 2% of the population) were abusing the amphetamines. In that year the penal provisions were strengthened and treatment facilities expanded, and a year later, 1955, production was very tightly controlled. A massive public education program in 1954 to 1955 completed the triad of treatment, education, and penalties. These three factors eliminated the amphetamine abuse problem in Japan within 3 years.

In Sweden the amphetamine and stimulant misuse problem was probably greater than in any other country. In 1965 that country experimented with giving legal prescriptions for narcotics and stimulants to some users. The plan was disastrous and was stopped in 1967. CNS stimulants are now forbidden in Sweden except by special license for very selected medical cases.

Most of the misuse of amphetamines until the 1960s was through the legally manufactured, and sometimes legally purchased, oral preparation. Even today most amphetamine misusers take the drug orally. Those called "speed freaks," heavy users of the amphetamines intravenously, usually start with large oral doses. As recently as 1963 the AMA Council on Drugs could state: "At this time, compulsive abuse of the amphetamines [is] a small problem. . . ." As the later section on misuse will show, times changed.

Therapeutic use. Until mid-1970, amphetamines had been prescibed for a large number of conditions, including depression, fatigue, and long-term weight reduction. Acting on the recommendation of the NAS-NRC, the FDA in 1970 restricted the legal use of the amphetamines to three types of conditions: narcolepsy, hyperkinetic behavior, and short-term weight reduction programs.[32] Although the Kefauver Act of 1962 only mandated a reexamination of drugs introduced between 1938 and 1962 (amphetamine was introduced prior to 1938), the FDA felt it could evaluate and require changes in the approved uses for amphetamines because new uses for the drug had been added since 1938.

The use of amphetamine for the treatment of narcolepsy will not be discussed, since its use for this condition is extremely infrequent. The value of amphetamine in the treatment of hyperkinetic children and in short-term weight reduction deserves comment for several reasons. There is dispute over the effectiveness of the amphetamines in *any* weight-control program, and there is considerable concern over the increasing tendency to routinely medicate the so-called hyperactive child.

Hyperactive children. Hyperactive children aren't called hyperactive children by professionals anymore. Nor do they call them minimal brain damage children. Research, careful observations, and a need to quantify the disorder, has evolved a new—and much more accurate—name: attention deficit disorder (ADD). Children with ADD may or may not be hyperactive, the critical factor is the deficit in attention. The items listed in the boxed material give the criteria for diagnosing ADD (with or without hyperactivity).[33]

The cause (or causes) of the attention deficit disorder is not known. One idea that attracted a lot of attention suggested that it was the additives in the foods we eat that were the basis for ADD with hyperactivity.[34] Many studies were done and in 1982 a Blue Ribbon Panel handed down the verdict on diets without food additives: ". . . there is no firm evidence that the diets work. Claims that the diets produce dramatic effects simply did not hold up in well-designed clinical trials."[35,p.958]

Some hyperactive children have histories of difficult births or contracting encephalitis when very young. Some reports indicate a higher incidence of abnormal electroencephalograms (EEGs) in

---

Criteria for diagnosing attention deficit disorder (ADD)

1. Onset before age 7
2. Duration of at least 6 months
3. Not a result of mental retardation or psychosis
4. Inattention (at least three of the following are presented)
   a. Often fails to finish things that he or she starts
   b. Often doesn't seem to listen
   c. Is easily distracted
   d. Has difficulty concentrating on tasks requiring sustained attention
   e. Has difficulty sticking to a play activity
5. Impulsivity (at least three of the following are presented)
   a. Often acts before thinking
   b. Shifts excessively from one activity to another
   c. Has difficulty organizing work
   d. Needs lots of supervision
   e. Frequently calls out in class
   f. Has difficulty in waiting his or her turn
6. Hyperactivity
   a. Runs about or climbs on things excessively
   b. Fidgets excessively
   c. Has difficulty staying seated
   d. Moves excessively in his or her sleep
   e. Is always "on the go"

---

these children than in nonADD children. There are as many children, however, who do not show abnormal EEGs or medical histories, so the importance of these factors is not clear. There is also no evidence that a large percentage are mentally retarded, although school achievement is usually quite poor. Some believe[36] that these ADD children suffer only from a maturational lag: they are exhibiting behavior that is typical of children several years younger. There is some debate over whether the symptoms continue into adulthood or decline soon after puberty, ages 16 to 17.

Animal research suggests that stimulants direct, or channel, behavior during the early developmental stages when cortical control of behavior is not yet complete. The mechanism underlying this effect is not known. One study [39] of lead-induced hyperactivity in rats reported a 20% reduction in brain dopamine but normal noradrenaline levels in these animals. It may be that stimulants reduce hyperactivity by restoring the effectiveness of certain dopaminergic neural pathways. The stimulants *are* effective in at least two out of three cases, as far as decreasing the behavioral problems these children pose to their parents and teachers.

There is some debate as to whether stimulants "calm" ADD children. It is clear, however, that vigilance, persistence, and impulse control increase following the use of stimulants in these children. Focused, goal-directed behavior also increases, which results in "a reduction in motor activity . . . in the context of task performance."[38] "Recent studies strongly suggest that methylphenidate and *d*-amphetamine 'normalize' the hyperkinetic child by improving or sustaining attention rather than by sedating the child."[36]

In one review[39] of studies reporting on the use of drugs in the treatment of the hyperactive child, it was found that methylphenidate (Ritalin) could be considered the drug of choice. Methylphenidate is a mild stimulant of the CNS that counteracts physical and mental fatigue while having only slight effect on blood pressure or respiration. In potency it is intermediate between the amphetamines and caffeine. When methylphenidate was used, 84% of the patients showed improvement (reduction of the hyperactive symptoms), whereas only 69% of the patients improved with amphetamine. There were annoying side effects in almost 15% of the patients regardless of which drug was used.

One of the more disturbing side effects of stimulant therapy is a suppression of height and weight increases during drug treatment.[40] Amphetamine has the greater effect compared to equally effective but higher daily doses of methylphenidate. Amphetamine reduced the average growth to 70% to 80% of normal, whereas methylphenidate reduced growth to 80% to 90% of normal. In children in whom drug treatment was stopped over the summer vacation, there was a rebound and a growth spurt 15% to 68% greater than the growth rate shown by nondrug-using children. The indications

are that this accelerated rate of growth diminishes after 2 to 3 months.

The seemingly indiscriminate but medically prescribed use of stimulant drugs to influence the behavior of school-age children has evoked much social protest[41] and commentary. The problem is no one knows the underlying cause of the hyperactivity, the mechanism whereby amphetamine acts, or the long-term effects of daily stimulant use in children ages 6 to 14 or 16. Until some of these questions are answered, it seems a bit much to allow stimulant drugs to be widely used for behavioral control, no matter how good the intentions are. There are a considerable number of children categorized as having attention deficit disorder: 3% to 4% of all grade school students; of these, 40% are referred to mental hygiene clinics for behavior problems. Most of these students are boys.[42,43] Maybe up to half a million of these children are receiving drugs as part of their treatment. It should be emphasized that whenever drug therapy is used, it should be only one component of an effective treatment program.[44]

Obesity. Why are one third of Americans overweight? How can they lose weight or stay slim? Just as to the question of how to reduce the number of colds you have, science gives a hard, no-nonsense answer: eat less, or work more! With the exception of thyroid compounds there are no drugs that appreciably increase the rate at which we burn calories. Thyroid agents, by affecting the metabolic rate, will increase the rate at which our bodies use energy—but these have serious side effects. Americans spend hundreds of millions of dollars each year on appetite suppressants—both prescription and OTC. Their story weaves an interesting tale of the interactions among professionals, the FDA, and the public.

One pound of body weight equals 3500 calories. If you believe you are—and maybe actually are—underweight, you can "easily" add on pounds. Three dozen plain cake doughnuts, 18 large glazed doughnuts, or a double helping of my mother's apple pie a la mode equal 3500 calories! Losing weight is even easier. To use 3500 calories—and lose 1 pound (if everything else stays the same)—

all you need to do is jog for 6 hours and 6 minutes! Best you check with your physician first, and work up to it slowly—and don't stop at those fast food places!

Eating is so much fun! It may be that everything that's fun is fattening, illegal, or immoral but here we are concerned only with the first of the three. Are there pharmacological aids to help decrease the desire to eat? "Obesity is frequently defined [as] . . . actual body weight . . . greater by 20% of ideal weight. . . . It is estimated that 35% of *all* ages are obese, and over 50% of all *adult population.* . . . Harmful effects . . . include an increased incidence of cardiovascular disease, adult-onset diabetes, and an overall increase in morbidity and mortality. . . . Hypertension in overweight patients [aged 20 to 39 years] is double that of normal-weight [patients] . . . ."[45,p.90-91]

In 1979 the FDA proposed to withdraw its approval for the use of amphetamines for weight reduction.[46] The DEA permits less than 6000 pounds of amphetamines to be produced each year[47] and since almost 90% is used for weight reduction, production could be greatly reduced when amphetamine becomes illegal for use in weight control programs.[48] The State of New York banned amphetamines for weight control in 1981.[49]

OTC appetite suppressants must be mentioned here as an aside because: (1) they constitute a $200 million plus a year market (in 1980, and growing rapidly), (2) in 1979 an FDA OTC advisory panel concluded that two ingredients were safe and effective for use in weight reduction programs: benzocaine (which acts by numbing the oral cavity) and phenylpropanolamine (PPA), (3) the FDA has not approved or endorsed that conclusion but in February 1982 it did publish the advisory panel's report and ask for public comment and (4) serious side effects can accompany use of PPA, especially at levels above the 75 mg a day recommended level—nervousness, increased heart rate and blood pressure, and some deaths have occurred.[51-53]

PPA is a mild stimulant, a sympathomimetic that has been widely used in OTC drugs and *is* approved by the FDA for use as a nasal decongestant (for example, Contac contains 50 mg of PPA, the same amount as found in many appetite supression products!).[54] The problem with all of this is that they *do* work—but marginally, maybe 2 pounds a week more than a placebo—but most of the effect is gone after 2 weeks of use. Also, individuals who use appetite suppressants regain their lost weight faster than those who learned new eating habits via behavioral control techniques to lose weight.

There is one more problem. To capitalize on the recreational use of stimulants some manufacturers have been putting their PPA in capsules and tablets that are virtually identical in color, shape, and markings to marketed amphetamines. The greatest difficulty with these "look-alike" capsules and tablets is that if an individual has been using them and then unintentionally gets some of the undistinguishable real amphetamines, they will have a serious overdose reaction, and deaths have occurred in this way.[55] In the fall of 1981 the U.S. Department of Justice moved to close down some of the manufacturers and packagers of "look-alike" drugs. About 15 states had outlawed them by 1982.[56,57]

Amphetamine, as well as a number of similar compounds, is used for appetite control because it does decrease hunger. The drug does this in animals and in humans by a variety of mechanisms that have not yet been clearly specified. One partial basis is that amphetamine acts to suppress the appetite centers in the hypothalamus.[58] Amphetamine does not affect blood sugar levels, but it does decrease food intake. Use of this drug for some weight-loss programs was banned in Canada as of 1973.

Many authorities believe that the euphoric effect of the amphetamines is the real basis for their continued use in weight-reduction programs. As one physician phrased this attitude:

> There is very strong evidence, for example, that although they are effective in the short-term treatment of obesity, their effectiveness here relates not to a depression of the appetite control center but to the stimulant effect that they provide. In other words, fat people may be taking the drug for just the same reasons that the young teenage speed-freak takes the drug—the stimulant effect, the euphoria effect.[59,p.44]

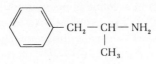

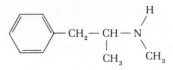

dl-amphetamine
Benzedrine (SKF)
(1-phenyl-2-aminopropane)

Methamphetamine
Methedrine (Burroughs Wellcome)
(1-phenyl-2-methylaminopropane)

FIG. 14-2 Amphetamines.

Two factors argue against the widespread, prolonged use of amphetamines for weight control. One is that tolerance develops rapidly to the apetite depressant characteristics of the drug. Even with moderate dosage increases, 4 to 6 weeks seems to be the limit before tolerance occurs to this effect of the drug. (With high doses tolerance can be overcome, and, frequently, the speed freaks report little or no appetite and even an inability to swallow!)

The second reason for not relying on amphetamine-like drugs for long-term weight reduction is that overeating seems to be primarily controlled by psychological-behavioral factors, not by the physiology of the body. Overeating is a habit; unless the habit patterns are changed, overeating will occur as soon as the appetite-suppressing effects of the drug disappear.[60]

The NAS-NRC review of the prescription antiappetite drugs, anorectics, concluded in 1972 that all the single-ingredient anorectic drugs should stay on the market for use in obesity but insisted that "the clinically trivial contribution of these drugs to the overall weight reduction is properly emphasized."[61] Other people had worried about the abuse potential of the amphetamines. As a result they were placed on Schedule II by the Controlled Substance Act of 1970. Concern over misuse and trivial effects on weight reduction reduced the number of prescriptions for amphetamine from 24.5 million in the peak year of 1965 to 3.3 million in 1978. Over the same time span the prescriptions of non-amphetamine anorectic drugs increased from 9.5 to 16 million.

These anorectics might work if 4- to 6-week drug periods were alternated with similar no-drug periods (to reduce tolerance); a meaningful weight reduction program might then be established. Drug periods could be used to teach new patterns of food intake. These new eating habits could be tested in the no-drug period before moving to more severe dietary restrictions in the next drug period. One major problem is that overweight individuals do not like the on-again, off-again schedule because the euphoria the amphetamines produce shows little tolerance. The amphetamine user would like to continue obtaining the euphoriagenic effect even though there is no suppression of food intake.

Basic pharmacology and mechanism of action. There are three amphetamines, all of which have as a basic chemical structure the phenethylamine nucleus. Two of these are optical isomers of each other, while the third is a methylated form of either or both of the isomers. These two forms of amphetamines are shown in Fig. 14-2.

Amphetamine is usually manufactured as the sulfate salt, and the chemical synthesized in 1927 was dl-amphetamine, a combination of both the d and l isomers in a 1 to 1 ratio. In amphetamine the d form is more active (three to four times) than the l isomer as a stimulant on the CNS. d-Amphetamine was first marketed in 1945 as Dexedrine for use as an antiappetite drug. The l form, however, is slightly more active than the d form as a sympathomimetic and in its actions on the cardiovascular system.

Methamphetamine, which has a methyl group added to the basic amphetamine structure, was previously marketed as Methedrine and in illegal use is called Meth, crystal, or speed. It has CNS stimulant effects about equal to *d*-amphetamine but is the drug of choice for euphoric effects. Perhaps the basis for intravenous users reports that methamphetamine is smoother than *d*-amphetamine is that it has fewer peripheral effects than the other amphetamines.

Amphetamine is rapidly absorbed when taken orally, and, with the usual therapeutic dose of 10 mg, peak effects are found 2 to 3 hours after ingestion or sooner on an empty stomach. There is a report that has not been followed up of a "paradoxical drowsiness" in 60% of the subjects in the first hour after 10 mg of dextroamphetamine taken orally. This "was accompanied by depressed brain activity and subjective reports of a dysphoric mood. . . ."[62] These reports are similar to those with cocaine use. Tolerance to the cardiovascular effects and increased heart rate and blood pressure develop much more rapidly than tolerance to the CNS effects of arousal and euphoria.

The amphetamines have major effects on two brain systems that seem particularly relevant to their clinical use as well as their misuse. It should be clear, however, that no one can state for any psychoactive drug just which action is crucial in its effect. The reticular activating system is responsible for controlling the level of activation of the brain and is itself regulated by inputs from many areas of the brain as well as by sensory inputs. The reticular system in turn arouses the brain to prepare it to receive and process these sensory inputs. The degree of arousal is thus related to the amount of stimulus input and its meaning.

Amphetamine causes a biochemical arousal of the reticular activation system in the absence of sensory input. The activation is transmitted to all parts of the brain: the individual is aroused, alert, hypersensitive. Literally, the individual is "turned on." All circuits are go, even in the absence of external input. This activation may be itself a very pleasant experience, but there is some evidence that a continual high level of activation by itself may be anxiety arousing.

The other system on which amphetamines have potent effects is the medial forebrain bundle, the reward system. Increases in activity in this system are experienced as pleasurable—it feels good! This is, no doubt, the basis for the euphoria experienced even by individuals who take only low doses of the amphetamines. The "flash" or sudden feeling of intense pleasure that is experienced when amphetamine is taken intravenously probably represents only the delivery of a very high blood concentration of the drug to the reward area of the brain. There are many other effects reported and sought by intravenous amphetamine users that are difficult to understand, let alone accept as pleasurable. One user reported that it "freezes my brain."

The pleasurable, rewarding characteristics of amphetamine, as well as of cocaine, have been shown in monkeys. These animals were given the opportunity to work (press a lever) to have amphetamines injected intravenously. When the chemical injected was amphetamine or cocaine, they worked cyclically for the drug just as human users inject at intervals. Data such as these support the idea that the drug itself has an action directly on the reward system.[63]

Until recently it was felt that amphetamine had its action at adrenergic sites by mimicking the neurotransmitters. That is, it was believed that amphetamine occupied and activated the receptor sites. Few authorities believe this today; the story is much more complicated.[64]

Amphetamine seems to have its adrenergic effects by acting on the axon terminal presynaptically. Three major actions form the basis for the effects of amphetamine as well as for the development of tolerance, which is regularly observed. First, amphetamine causes adrenergic neurotransmitters to leak spontaneously from the presynaptic sites. Such leakage will result in stimulation of the postsynaptic fiber in the same way as if normal information processing were occurring. It is quite important fundamentally, but of little significance here, that amphetamine has its action by causing the release of newly synthesized noradrenaline and not by emptying any of the storage depots of this compound.

Second, amphetamine enhances its own effects as well as those resulting from electrical stimulation by blocking the presynaptic reuptake of noradrenaline and dopamine so that the neurotransmitter will continue to act postsynaptically.

A third action of amphetamine is probably one mechanism for tolerance. Amphetamine is metabolized by liver-microsomal enzymes into p-hydroxynorephedrine. This metabolite, at least in the peripheral nervous system, functions as a false adrenergic transmitter. A false transmitter (see Chapter 6) is not as effective postsynpatically as the normal neurotransmitters, but it occupies space normally filled by the endogenous neurohumor. To offset this decrease in effectiveness of the released transmitter, larger doses of amphetamine would be needed to block more of the reuptake of the transmitter substance released into the synaptic space.

Both in understanding how the brain works and in appreciating the different effects of the two isomers of amphetamine, you should know

that d- and l-amphetamine have differential effects on the uptake of dopamine and noradrenaline in the brain, the levo isomer being approximately ten times less potent in blocking catecholamine uptake into noradrenergic neurons, but being equally efficient in blocking uptake into striatal dopaminergic neurons.[65]

Behavioral effects: use, misuse, and abuse

The psychologic effects of amphetamines usually include a general increase in alertness, wakefulness and sense of well-being; however, increased irritability, tension and tremors may also occur. Amphetamines can counteract the impairing effects of fatigue, boredom and depressant drugs on the performance of many mental and physical tasks. However, contrary to widespread belief, complex intellectual functioning (involving comprehension, problem solving and judgment) is not improved by amphetamines in normal rested people.

The somatic effects of amphetamines include improvements in motor coordination and performance in activities requiring sustained physical exertion. . . ."[66]

The effects of low, moderate, and high doses will be discussed here. (See also Chapter 4 for a discussion of drugs and sports.) In terms of CNS potency, 5 mg of dl-amphetamine is about the equivalent of 150 mg of caffeine, that is, one strong cup of coffee. Amphetamine has several actions that may influence behavior. The clearest effect is the prevention of the performance decrement caused by fatigue or boredom; "amelioration of the feeling of fatigue developed by prolonged work is perhaps the most fully documented subjective affect of the amphetamines."[67,p.54]

The abuse of the central nervous system stimulants known as amphetamines has dropped since "speed" had its heyday in the 1960s. But amphetamine abuse is still a major problem in terms of physical damage and emotional dependency. And despite the fact that manufacture and distribution of the most dangerous varieties of the drug have been under strict federal controls since 1971, it still seems to be available to anyone who wants it.[68]

In the bad old days—the late sixties—speed was methamphetamine put into liquid for injection and used intravenously. Two common slogans of that period, "speed kills" and "meth is death," contained enough truth to make them debatable. The two points of view are succinctly phrased in the preface to an excellent series of papers entitled *Speed Kills*. One author

takes issue with the term "speed kills" indicating very few people die from direct overdosage of high dose amphetamine.

The editor, however, points out that the secondary morbidity and mortality resulting from the use of amphetamines, including those deaths that occur from hepatitis, infection and violence certainly make the title *Speed Kills* appropriate.[69]

Intravenous amphetamine use may begin with only (!) 30 mg. In a long run (speed binge) of 3 or 4 days with injections occurring every 2 or 3 hours, tolerance develops rapidly, and 500 to 1000 mg may be injected at one time. The peripheral effects show greater tolerance than those of the CNS, so only moderate cardiovascular effects may occur even with high doses that still yield the euphoria. The effects of single and repeated doses have been well described:

The physical effects of methamphetamine are quite variable depending on dose, duration of drug use, mental state and drug environment of the individual user. In general, however, after the intra-venous user injects the drug in sufficient quantity he experiences a "flash or rush" which he describes as orgasmic in nature. After this initial experience he usually becomes euphoric, with an increase in motor and speech activity. The individual may stay hyperactive for many hours with no signs of fatigue. . . .

The action phase of the "speed binge" is in effect repeated injection of the drug from one to ten times per day. With each "hit," the individual experiences the desired "flash" which the user often describes as a "full-body orgasm." Between "hits" the user is euphoric, hyperactive and hyperexcitable. This action phase of stimulation may last for several days in which the individual does not sleep and rarely eats.

For a variety of reasons this action phase terminates, however. The user may stop voluntarily because of fatigue, he may become confused, paranoid or panic-stricken and stop "shooting," or he may simply run out of drug.[70,p.2]

The "flash" or "splash" from amphetamine is difficult to differentiate from that of cocaine, but both are uniquely distinct from that induced by heroin. The amphetamine rush produces "an abrupt awakening feeling as opposed to the drowsy, drifting effect of heroin."[71] Some individuals inject "speed balls" to obtain both effects. It is a little disconcerting to realize that this use has been around long enough so there are classic speed balls, cocaine and heroin, as well as modern speed balls, amphetamine and heroin. In both cases *some* people report the same effect: a brief period of intense pleasure followed by a longer, more moderate, good feeling.

If euphoria and orgasms followed by depression and hunger were the total story on the intravenous use of methamphetamine, it would not be more disturbing than other forms of drug misuse. Two additional interrelated factors make intravenous use of methamphetamine particularly noteworthy. Some users develop a paranoid psychosis, so called because of the presence of hallucinations. Other heavy users only become suspicious and hostile, feelings that can lead to aggressive behavior. Because of this great potential for violence when speed users move into communes or into hallucinogen-using groups, the nonspeed users move out. As Allen Ginsberg put it:

Let's issue a general declaration to all the underground community *contra speedamos ex cathedra*. Speed is anti-social, paranoid making, it's a drag, bad for your body, bad for your mind, generally speaking, in the long run uncreative and it's a plague in the whole dope industry. All the nice gentle dope fiends are getting screwed up by the real horror monster Frankenstein speedfreaks who are going around stealing and bad-mouthing everybody.[72]

The development of a paranoid psychosis has been long known to be one of the effects of sustained cocaine use. The first amphetamine psychosis was described in 1938, but little attention was given this syndrome until the late 1950s. There have been many suggestions as to the reason for the psychosis: that heavy methamphetamine users have schizoid personalities[73] or that the psychosis is really caused by sleep deprivation, particularly dream-sleep deprivation. The question of the basis for the amphetamine psychosis was resolved by the demonstration that it could be elicited in the laboratory in individuals who clearly were not prepsychotic and who did not experience great sleep deprivation.[74] It seems, then, that the paranoid psychosis following high dose intravenous use of amphetamine is primarily the result of the drug and not the personality predisposition of the user.

The amphetamine psychosis has been studied many times.[75] both in and out of the laboratory. One researcher[76] commented about his results:

The psychosis was the facsimile of the disorder observed during drug abuse—a schizophrenic-like state of paranoia in a setting of clear consciousness accompanied by auditory or visual hallucinations, or both, but without thought disorder . . . in some cases the onset of the psychosis was sudden and occurred within one hour of commencing the intravenous injection. . . .

There is another behavior induced by high doses of amphetamine: compulsive and repetitive actions. The behavior may be acceptable (the individual may compulsively clean a room over and over) or it may be bizarre (one student spent a night counting cornflakes). There is a precedent for this stereotyped behavior in animal studies using high doses of amphetamine; it probably results from an effect of amphetamine on dopaminergic systems in the basal ganglia.[77] A 1971 report[78] showed that it is the dopaminergic system that is primarily involved in the amphetamine psychosis. A 1980 review of this topic suggested that "behaviors that involve noradrenaline activity are stimulus bound and are related to attentional processes, whereas behaviors primarily subserved by [dopamine] appear to be motorically based."[79,p.551;80] Remember that it is *l*-amphetamine that is most active in dopaminergic systems. The entire package of stereotyped behavior, hyperactive children, and amphetamine psychosis may all tie together as an impairment of goal-directed behavior.

Still debatable is the evidence that the use of intravenous amphetamines may be related to constriction of arteries in the brain, possibly causing strokes even in teenagers.[81,82] Also unsettled is the question of physical addiction to amphetamines. Certain regular features occur in abstinence, such as depression, overeating, and extreme fatigue, but usually go away in a week. Importantly, abrupt cessation of regular high doses of amphetamine is not life threatening, and convulsions rarely occur. In some instances the depression may persist; it is not clear whether this is a result of the amphetamine abstinence or a part of the personality of the individual that led him initially to use stimulants.[83]

The speed scene was one of the motivating factors behind passage of the Controlled Substance Act of 1970. This law allowed the government to put restrictions on the production and distribution of amphetamines. As you know, there are still problems; delays in removing amphetamine use as treatment of obesity may go on for years! If removal of treatment of obesity is accomplished use will certainly decrease a bit, but some users will move to illegal amphetamine and others to nonamphetamine stimulants and appetite suppressants. For these nonmedical oral stimulant users there are two primary patterns, intermittent and sustained low-dose use.

Many individuals occasionally take 5 to 20 mg of amphetamines orally to allay fatigue, elevate mood while doing an unpleasant task, produce prolonged wakefulness, help recover from a hangover, or to "get high."

In this pattern, the individual obtains amphetamine pills from the doctor for weight control, but takes the pills 3 to 4 times a day for the stimulation and euphoria produced by the drug. He may develop a strong psychological dependence on the pills and feel that he cannot get along without them. If he stops taking daily amphetamines, withdrawal depression occurs.[84]

Summary. Amphetamine can be misused and abused in many ways, and it is. These different forms of misuse are not very closely related; the housewife using amphetamine regularly for "weight control" is as far from the speed freak as a heavy coffee drinker is from a cocaine user. The motivations, dosage form, social atmosphere, and end result are different. There is not an amphetamine problem, there are several amphetamine problems; the answer to one is not the answer to the others.[85]

DEPRESSANT DRUGS

As mentioned at the beginning of this chapter, "Sedatives and hypnotics are both depressants of the central nervous system, but in one case the intention is to relieve anxiety or restlessness and in the other it is to induce sleep. Many drugs may therefore be used in either capacity, depending upon the dose and the time of day that they are given."[86] The most widely used drug in this general category is alcohol. The second most commonly used depressant drugs are the barbiturates.

Nonbarbiturates

There are three CNS depressants with a longer history than the barbiturates that are rarely prescribed today. Chloral hydrate and paraldehyde have chemical and pharmacological characteristics much like alcohol, while the bromides are different.

Chloral hydrate was synthesized in 1832 but was

not used clinically until about 1870.[87] It is rapidly metabolized to trichloroethanol, which is the active hypnotic agent. When taken orally, chloral hydrate has a short onset period (30 minutes), and 1 to 2 g will induce sleep in less than an hour. This agent does not cause as much depression of the respiratory and cardiovascular systems as a comparable dose of the barbiturates and has fewer aftereffects.

In 1869 Dr. Benjamine Richardson introduced chloral hydrate to Great Britain. Ten years later he called it "in one sense a beneficient, and in another sense a maleficient substance, I almost feel a regret that I took any part whatever in the introduction of the agent into the practice of healing. . . ."[88] He had learned that what man can misuse, some men will abuse. As early as 1871 he referred to its non-therapeutic use as "toxical luxury" and lamented that chloral hydrate addicts had to be added to "alcohol intemperants and opium-eaters."[89] Chloral hydrate addiction is a tough way to go, since its major disadvantage is that it is a gastric irritant, and repeated use causes considerable stomach upset. A solution of chloral hydrate was used before 1900 as the famous "knockout drops" or "Mickey Finn"—a "few" drops in a sailor's drink, and before he woke up, he was shanghaied onto a boat at sea for a long trip to the Orient.

No such use ever occurred with paraldehyde, which was synthesized in 1829 and introduced clinically in 1882. Paraldehyde would probably be in great use today because of its effectiveness as a CNS depressant with little respiratory depression and a wide safety margin, except for one characteristic. It has a most noxious taste and odor that permeates the breath of the user.

The bromides are little used today, now that they have been removed from OTC sleep preparations. Bromides accumulate in the body, and the depression they cause builds up over several days of regular use. There are serious toxic effects with repeated hypnotic doses of these agents. Dermatitis and constipation are minor accompaniments; with increased intake, motor disturbances, delirium, and psychosis develop.

Methaqualone. My daddy was right: If you miss a streetcar, don't worry, another one just like it will be along in a little while. That seems also to be true of drug use crises. Illegal use of methaqualone hit a peak in the early seventies and then declined. From 1978 to 1979 it increased again and has persisted into the early 1980s. New generations of drug users have to rediscover the wheel and see for themselves! In 1980 about 4 tons of methaqualone was made and distributed legally in the United States. One guesstimate was that 100 million tons were smuggled in during that year. And that must not be enough. There may be honor among thieves, but there is none between an illegal drug producer and those who buy the product: there are an increasing number of tablets that look like legal methaqualone being sold on the street that contain OTC sedatives![90] The legal but unethical distribution of methaqualone is under attack but difficult to stop.[91] Some believe the only step now is to make the drug Schedule I—since it really isn't a unique contribution to the therapeutic armamentarium. Maybe we got ourselves into this mess because of sloppy thinking and action.

> The methaqualone boom should make an interesting case study in future medical textbooks: How skillful public relations and advertising created a best seller—and helped cause a medical crisis in the process.[92]

The methaqualone story is one where everyone was wrong—the pharmaceutical industry, the FDA, the DEA, the press, the physicians. No one can say he was without sin. Methaqualone was originally synthesized in India, tested and found to be ineffective as an antimalaria drug. But it was a good sedative, so in 1959 it was introduced as a prescription drug in Great Britain. It never sold well, but after the thalidomide disaster there was increased interest in a "safe" nonbarbiturate sleeping pill. Mandrax, 250 mg methaqualone and 25 mg of an antihistamine, promised to be that when it was introduced in 1965 in a massive advertising campaign to physicians. The campaign worked, and there were 2 million prescriptions issued for Mandrax in 1971 in Great Britain. Even before that the drug had found its way into the street where it was widely abused: by heroin users, by high school students, by anyone who wanted a cheap but potent down. Misuse was so great by 1968 that Great Britain tightened controls on it in 1970 and then again in 1973. After that the methaqualone problems subsided as other drugs came to prominence.

Germany introduced methaqualone in 1960 as a nonprescription drug, had its first methaqualone suicide in 1962, and discovered that 10% to 22% of the drug overdoses treated in this period were a result of this drug. In 1963 Germany reduced the problem by making methaqualone a prescription drug. In this 1960-1964 period Japan experienced a major epidemic of methaqualone abuse, causing over 40% of all overdoses admitted to mental hospitals. Japan tightened controls almost to the maximum possible on methaqualone and stemmed the tide. This happened even though they never took the final step of making it a prescription drug!

The same kinds of incidents followed around the world. By 1965 both Germany and Japan had experienced some very traumatic times with methaqualone. In 1965, after 3 years of testing, Quaalude and Sopors, brand names for methaqualone, were introduced in the United States as prescription drugs with the package insert, "Addiction potential not established." Methaqualone was *not* a scheduled drug: there were no monitoring rules or restrictions on the number of times the prescription could be refilled. In June 1966, the FDA Committee on the Abuse Potential of Drugs decided that there was no need to monitor methaqualone, since there was no evidence of abuse potential! Thus, from 1967 to 1973, the package insert read, "Physical dependence has not clearly been demonstrated," although by 1969 the evidence was very clear that methaqualone was an addicting drug.

In the early 1970s in this country, "ludes" and "sopors" (from *Quaaludes* and *Sopors*) were familiar terms in the drug culture and in drug treatment centers. Physicians were overprescribing what they believed to be a drug that was safer than the barbiturates as well as nonaddicting. Most of the methaqualone sold on the street was legally manufactured and then either stolen or obtained through prescriptions. At any rate, sales zoomed, and front-page reporting of its effects when misused helped build it as a drug of abuse.

Finally, 8 years after it was introduced into this

country, 4 years after American scientists were saying it was addicting, 11 years after the first suicide, methaqualone was put on Schedule II October 4, 1973: quite a jump from not being scheduled to Schedule II. Really stupid. Maybe someday someone will write a more comprehensive report on this tale of bureaucratic boondoggling, but the one published in 1975 by the Drug Abuse Council[93] suffices for now.

Addiction can develop to methaqualone as easily and rapidly as with the other barbiturates. The "high" or "down" you get with methaqualone is very similar to that obtained with all other sedative-hypnotics. There is, possibly, one difference: loss of motor coordination seems to be greater with this drug; the resulting loss of control, including walking into walls, is why one of the slang terms for methaqualone is "wallbanger." Methaqualone has had a better press than the other drugs in this class, and it was called "heroin for lovers," an aphrodisiac. Hardly. As the director of Clinical Activities of the Haight-Ashbury Clinic[94] said in 1973:

> What a drug to take. It has all the possible disadvantages a drug can have. It's a garbage drug, a real drug of abuse.

Barbiturates

History may not be strange, but records of history frequently are. On the fourth of December, 1862, one of the following things occurred in Munich, Germany. Dr. A. Bayer (yes, it's that Bayer) left the laboratory early to visit a tavern because he had successfully combined urea with malonic acid and made a new compound. A compound must have a name, and perhaps "Barbara's urates" were so named by Bayer

> because he wished to commemorate Barbara, a person he held in affectionate regard—a Munich waitress perhaps?—who gave him samples of urine for research purposes.[95,p.118]

> Bayer celebrated the occasion of the synthesis of the new compound by visiting a nearby tavern frequented by artillery officers. It happened that it was the Day of St. Barbara, the patron saint of

artillery officers, and in the ensuing festivities *Barbara* was amalgamated with *urea* to give the new compound its name.[96, p. 98]

The new compound was barbituric acid, which is *not* a CNS depressant. The barbiturates, which are derived from it, are excellent CNS depressants. Over 2500 barbiturates have been synthesized. Some of the best are among the oldest, although barbital (Veronal), the first to be used clinically in 1903, is little used today. It did start the practice of giving barbiturates names ending in *-al*. The second barbiturate in clinical use, phenobarbital (Luminal), was introduced in 1912 and is still one of the widest used and best compounds in this class. Amobarbital (Amytal) in 1923, as well as pentobarbital (Nembutal) and secobarbital (Seconal),

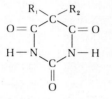

Generic name	Brand name	R_1	R_2
		Long-acting	
Barbital	Veronal	$-CH_2-CH_3$	$-CH_2-CH_3$
Phenobarbital*	Luminal	$-CH_2-CH_3$	⟨⟩
		Intermediate-acting	
Amobarbital	Amytal	$-CH_2-CH_3$	$-CH_2-CH_2-CH-CH_3$ $\quad\quad\quad\quad\quad\quad CH_3$
		Short-acting	
Pentobarbital	Nembutal	$-CH_2-CH_3$	$-CH-CH_2-CH_2-CH_3$ $\;\; CH_3$
Secobarbital	Seconal	$-CH_2-CH=CH_2$	$-CH-CH_2-CH_2-CH_3$ $\;\; CH_3$

*Chemical name is 5-ethyl-5-phenylmalonylurea.

FIG. 14-3 Barbiturates.

both introduced in 1930, are well-established and widely used examples of the barbiturates.

As Fig. 14-3 indicates, barbiturates are typically grouped on the basis of the duration of their activity. Some researchers do not feel that this categorization can be validated experimentally,[97] but other authorities report that the classification is meaningful. A standard reference book[98] indicates differences between the short, intermediate, and long-acting agents in both the delay to onset of action and the duration of action. The approximate time intervals are given in Table 14-1. The grouping of these agents on the basis of their duration of action is supported by their rate of metabolism. The short-acting barbiturates are very lipid soluble and are deactivated at a rate of about 2.5% per hour. Deactivation of the long-acting agents is at about one-third or one-fourth that rate (0.7% per hour).[99]

Deactivation occurs in the liver, although some of the drug is excreted essentially unchanged. The barbiturates are one of the classes of drugs that stimulate the activity of the microsomal enzymes of the liver. Perhaps some of the tolerance that develops to the barbiturates is the result of an increased rate of deactivation caused by this stimulation of microsomal enzymes.[100] Tolerance does develop gradually, and the dosage must be increased periodically to maintain a constant effect. Physical addiction, dependence, also occurs, and when the daily dose rises about 400 mg, some major withdrawal symptoms will occur after abrupt termination of use. Addiction and withdrawal will be discussed in the next section.

The barbiturates have their primary effect on chemical transmission at the synapse, not on conduction in the neuron. The best guess now is that the barbiturates decrease the release of excitatory neurotransmitters from the axon terminals. The basic mechanism in the CNS has not yet been determined, but it is probably related to the depression of oxidative metabolism, which is one of the primary biochemical effects of these agents. A general lowering of brain excitability, as in the case of alcohol, sometimes releases behavior from inhibition. The actual mechanisms that underlie the ef-

TABLE 14-1

	Time to onset (hours)	Duration of action (hours)
Long	1	6 to 10
Intermediate	½	5 to 6
Short	¼	2 to 3

fects of barbiturates are not known but approaches are being made in this area.[101,102] In the initial stages of these drugs' effects there may be some loss of inhibition, euphoria, and behavioral stimulation. The multisynaptic pathways such as the reticular system are among the first to be depressed. This occurs before the primary sensory or motor pathways are affected. At clinical doses

the CNS is exquisitely sensitive to the barbiturates, so that, when the drugs are given in sedative or hypnotic doses, direct actions on peripheral structures are absent or negligible.[96]

In normal therapeutic use, the barbiturates are not particularly toxic agents, but they have additive CNS effects with other depressants such as alcohol. There are many reported cases of death caused by respiratory failure resulting from the use of barbiturates as a sleeping aid at the end of an evening of alcohol intake.

Use and misuse. Barbiturates and other depressants account for 25% of mood-changing prescriptions and are used for anxiety, insomnia, anesthesia, and epilepsy. Barbiturates for the treatment of anxiety have been in large part replaced by the antianxiety agents, even though there is no good evidence that they are more effective. As mentioned in Chapter 13, the benzodiazepines are safer. For this antianxiety, sedative purpose secobarbital or pentobarbital is prescribed at a dosage level of 25 to 35 mg three times a day.

The barbiturates are losing ground as the number one drug prescribed as a hypnotic, that is, to induce sleep. Concern over the wide use of hypnotics and better education of physicians are decreasing the total number of hypnotic prescriptions written each year.[103] Additionally, prescribing patterns have changed and since 1976 one of the benzodiazepines, flurazepam, has been the number one hypnotic drug (over 50% of sleeping pill prescriptions). Two benzodiazepines, triazolam and temazepam, introduced in the early eighties will soon change that—they both have shorter half-lives than previous benzodiazepines; triazolam's is less than 3 hours.

Insomnia. Insomnia is a symptom, not a disease, and it is fairly common. The fact that it's a symptom of many diseases and responses to life situations tells you that it is not a problem that should be treated pharmacologically for long periods. From 2 to 6 weeks of treatment with hypnotics—sleeping pills—is considered long-term treatment.[104] Nonpharmacological treatments should be tried[105,106] as well as every effort being made to identify and treat the situation or disease that is producing the insomnia. First, though, you have to be sure there's a real problem. Insomniacs are very poor at estimating their sleep patterns: "Most insomniacs consistently *under* estimated the amount of time they slept and *over* estimated how long it took them to get to sleep."[107,p.28] Most insomniacs report difficulty falling asleep as well as remaining asleep throughout the night. A dose of 100 or, at the most, 200 mg of secobarbital or pentobarbital before bed is usually effective in helping the insomniac get to sleep and stay asleep. Some problems do occur, however. One is the barbiturate hangover, the residual sedation that exists after the drug-assisted sleep ends. Even routine users sometimes require so great a dosage of a bartiturate to get and stay asleep that the drug effects are not gone in the morning. One study showed performance decrements 22 hours after 200 mg of secobarbital prior to bedtime, that is, the sedative effects were still measurable almost at bedtime the next evening.[96] As a result, an amphetamine or other stimulant is frequently used in the morning to counteract the remaining sedative effects.

Another problem may be that the barbiturates decrease the amount of sleep time spent in dreaming. This can be easily monitored, since rapid eye movements (REM) are highly related to dreaming.

The scientific study of dreaming behavior is just beginning, but some evidence suggests that it is psychologically healthy to dream three to six times each night. In addition, when an individual who has been using barbiturates regularly as a sleeping pill suddenly stops using them, he may overdream or even have nightmares. Because of the "hangover" and the decrease in REM sleep, drugs that hope to replace the barbiturates will have to have less effect in these areas. They do—but they are far from ideal.[108,109]

A report by the National Academy of Science[110] entitled *Sleeping Pills, Insomnia, and Medical Practice* put it all in perspective. It reported that (1) sleeping pills are prescribed more often and with less care than they should be, (2) the barbiturates are addictive and readily lethal—still responsible for more drug-related suicides than any other class of drugs, (3) hypnotic drugs reduce the time to fall asleep, on the average of 10 to 20 minutes, and (4) hypnotic drugs add 20 to 40 minutes to a total night's sleep. That's not much but, as noted, insomnia is a very subjective symptom. If the insomniac believes it's a lot and performance and attitude improve, then it may be worth it.

Misuse. The evidence is difficult to obtain, but the problem of accidental fatalities may also develop with the barbiturates or any hypnotic. After the regular sleeping dose has been taken, the individual may doze briefly and then awaken slightly sedated. In this condition he may be confused about whether he has taken his medication and may then take a second dose or even more—sometimes a fatal amount.

The barbiturates are one of the few drugs that bridge the generation gap; everyone abuses them. Used for nonmedical purposes, they provide an alcohol-like experience without the alcohol taste, breath, or expense. A top authority in the area of drug abuse, Dr. Sidney Cohen,[111] told a U.S. Senate investigating committee:

> For the youngster barbiturates are a more reliable "high" and less detectable than "pot." They are less strenuous than LSD, less "freaky" than amphetamines, and less expensive than heroin. A

school boy can "drop a red" and spend the day in a dreamy, floating state of awayness untroubled by reality. It is drunkenness without the odor of alcohol. It is escape for the price of one's lunch money.

Many of the older abusers, 40 to 60, would probably deny that they were abusing the drug and would be quite indignant if they were labeled as addicts.

> These individuals usually obtain their supply of barbiturates from physicians rather than from "street dealers." They visit many different physicians with the same complaint, usually difficulty in sleeping, in order to obtain several prescriptions for barbiturates. Sometimes it is also possible to refill the prescriptions without the physicians knowledge.
> Confusion, decreased ability to work and episodes of acute intoxication with slurred speech and staggering finally draws attention to their addiction. Intentional (suicide attempt) . . . unintentional (due to confusion) overdose and accidents are the major medical hazard in this type of abuse pattern.[112]

Between these two age groups and distinct patterns of abuse there are several other frequently occurring methods of recreational use. Some individuals do mainline barbiturates—alone or with heroin—but this is not a usual mode of use. The drugs most frequently used are those with short duration of effect, such as secobarbital and pentobarbital, agents which are likely to produce the disinhibition euphoria, the "alcohol high." One pattern has been described thus:

> When 200 mg of secobarbital are taken with the expectation of going to sleep in a suitable sleeping environment, most indivduals will respond in the predicted way. When the same amount of secobarbital is taken in a stimulating environment with the expectation of "having a good time," many individuals will experience intoxication and excitement.[112]

It is of more than passing interest that secobarbital has been implicated in drug-related aggressive behavior, almost as if these users were fighting to stay awake.

Higher levels of the barbiturates produce an intoxication characterized by "confusion, intellectual impairment, personality change, emotional lability, motor incoordination, staggering gait, slurred speech and nystagmus."[113] Higher doses cause death; the barbiturates are the drug of choice by those commiting suicide.

> A federal study estimates that . . . nearly 5000 deaths occurred each year that were either directly related to barbiturates or in which barbiturates were involved . . . users . . . made 25,000 trips to hospital emergency rooms each year, and about the same number entered drug abuse treatment annually.[114]

When a lethal dose is taken, there is little opportunity to change one's mind, since loss of consciousness occurs within a few minutes.

Although the clinical use of the barbiturates began in 1903, and the first reference to barbiturate intoxication and withdrawal convulsions was in 1905, it was not until 1950 that a controlled study was published that conclusively showed physical dependency to the barbiturates.[115] There may be some anxiety and slight muscle twitches that develop when even a daily dose of 200 to 300 mg of pentobarbital or secobarbital is abruptly terminated. A level of 400 mg per day seems to be crucial for the development of convulsions and/or psychosis on withdrawal. As the daily dose increases above that amount, the probability of these symptoms increases. One important danger is that the difference between the lethal dose and the effective dose decreases as tolerance develops. This means that an overdose can occur more easily in the addicted individual than in the low dose–level, therapeutic user. The basis for this is the fact that tolerance to the cardiorespiratory effects develops much more slowly than tolerance to the sedative effects. Enough communality exists between alcohol addiction and barbiturate addiction that taking one drug can prevent the occurrence of withdrawal effects to the other agent.

Although it is probably more socially acceptable to be addicted to the oral use of the barbiturates than to require narcotics intravenously, the barbiturate addiction is medically more serious, as can be seen from the effects of abstinence. Death may occur in 5% of addicted individuals who abruptly stop using barbiturates. The barbiturate abstinence syndrome has been repeatedly described, but none has done better in summarizing the effects than one of the first American reports in 1953.

> Upon abrupt withdrawal of barbiturates from individuals who have been ingesting 0.8 gm. or more daily of one of the potent barbiturates (secobarbital, pentobarbital, amobarbital), signs of barbiturate intoxication disappear in the first 8-12 hours of abstinence, and, clinically, the patient seems to improve. Thereafter, increasing anxiety, insomnia, tremulousness, weakness, difficulty in making cardiovascular adjustments on standing, anorexia, nausea and vomiting appear. One or more convulsions of grand mal type usually occur during the second or third day of abstinence. Following the seizures, a psychosis characterized by confusion, disorientation in time and place, agitation, tremulousness, insomnia, delusions and visual and auditory hallucinations may supervene. The psychosis clinically resembles alcoholic delirium tremens, usually begins and is worse at night, and terminates abruptly with a critical sleep.[116]

Rarely today does anyone go through the agony just described. The preferred mode of treatment for the withdrawal of a barbiturate-addicted individual involves substituting a long-acting barbiturate, such as phenobarbital, for the addicting agent. The individual is then withdrawn slowly and with greater safety from the phenobarbital.

Summary

Methaqualone and the barbiturates are being used and misused greatly in the United States. From the antianxiety-pill popper to the heavy user for the induction of sleep, legal barbiturate misuse is second only to alcohol. Alcohol and the barbiturates are difficult drugs to use if one wishes to maintain a euphoric mood, since generally the user slips into sedation. In spite of the dangers and problems, depressant drug use by the young increased rapidly in the early 1970s, until 1972 was labeled the year of the "barbs." Hopefully, we will never have that again.

CONCLUDING COMMENT

The uppers and the downers. It is perhaps worthwhile to reemphasize here that these drugs, especially the amphetamines and the barbiturates, are primarily misused by older individuals. Their misuse is not as spectacular as that of the speed freak, but the misuse is more consistent and more widespread. It is reassuring to know that all is not a series of fads in the world of drug misuse—there are some groups you can count on to misuse drugs: overweight and fatigued matrons and hyperexcitable and anxious housewives and businessmen. The increasing use of cocaine marks the return of "a golden oldie"—it's been misused before. The question is whether it is now here to stay.

REFERENCES

1. Chen, K.K.: In Symposium on sedative and hypnotic drugs, Baltimore, 1954, The Williams & Williams Co.
2. Taylor, N.: Plant drugs that changed the world, New York, 1965, Dodd, Mead & Co.
3. Taylor, N.: Flight from reality, New York, 1949, Duell, Sloan & Pearce.
4. Doyle, A.C.: The sign of the four. In The complete Sherlock Holmes, New York, 1938, Garden City Publishing Co.
5. Freud, S.: On the general effect of cocaine, lecture before the Psychiatric Union on March 5, 1885. (Reprinted in Drug Dependence 5:17, 1970.)
6. Holmstedt, B.: Historical survey. In Efron, D.H., editor: Ethnopharmacologic search for psychoactive drugs, Public Health Service Publication No. 1645, Washington, D.C., 1967, U.S. Government Printing Office.
7. Perry, C.: The star-spangled powder, Rolling Stone, p. 26, August 17, 1972.
8. Ashley, R.: Cocaine: its history, uses and effects, New York, 1976, Warner Books, Inc.
9. Crittendon, A., and Ruby, M.: Cocaine: the champagne of drugs, New York Times Magazine, p. 14, September 1, 1973.
10. Fischman, M.W., and others: Cardiovascular and subjective effects of intravenous cocaine administration in humans, Archives of General Psychiatry 33:983-989, 1976.
11. Van Dyke, C., and Byck, R.: Cocaine, Scientific American 246(3):128, 1982.
12. Cronson, A.J., and Flemenbaum, A.: Antagonism of cocaine highs by lithium, American Journal of Psychiatry, 135(7):856, July 1978.
13. Heroin problem, Drugs and Drug Abuse Education Newsletter 7(5):1-3, 1976.

14. Ellinwood, E.H.: Amphetamine psychosis: a multi-dimensional process, Seminars in Psychiatry **6**:208-226, 1969.

15. Siegel, R.K.: Cocaine hallucinations, American Journal of Psychiatry, **135**(3):309, March 1978.

16. Resnick, R.B., Kestenbaum, R.S., and Schwartz, L.K.: Acute systemic effects of cocaine in man: a controlled study by intranasal and intravenous routes of administration, Science **195**:696-698, 1977.

17. Post, R.M.: Psychomotor stimulants as activators of normal and pathological implications for the excesses in mania. In Mulbe, S.J., editor: Behavior in excess, New York, 1981, Free Press.

18. Demarest, M., and others: Cocaine: middle class high, Time, p. 56, July 6, 1981.

19. Cocaine deaths and illness rising, Physicians Washington Report, vol. 4, no. 2, 1980.

19a. Weil, A.: The green and white, Journal of Psychedelic Drugs **7**(4):401-413, 1975.

20. Wilkinson, P., and others: Intranasal and oral cocaine kinetics, Clinical Pharmacology and Therapeutics **27**(3):386, 1980.

21. Holmstedt, B., and others: Cocaine in blood of coca chewers, Journal of Ethnopharmacology, p. 69, 1979.

22. Cohen, S.: Coca paste and freebase: new fashions in cocaine use, Drug Abuse and Alcoholism Newsletter, vol. 9, no. 3, 1980.

23. Jaraid, J.I.: Cocaine plasma concentration: relation to physiological and subjective effects in humans, Science **202**:227, October 1978.

24. Bourne, P.G.: The great cocaine myth, Drugs and Drug Abuse Education Newsletter **5**(8):5, l974.

25. Gottlieb, A.: The pleasures of cocaine, The Twentieth Century Alchemist, 1976.

26. Aigner, F.G., and Balster, R.L.: Choice behavior in rhesus monkeys: cocaine versus food, Science **201**:534, August 1978.

27. Benzedrine alert, Air Surgeon's Bulletin **1**(2):19-21, 1944.

28. On a bender with Benzedrine, Everybody's Digest **5**(2):50, 1946.

29. Monroe, R.R., and Drell, H.J.: Oral use of stimulants obtained from inhalers, Journal of the American Medical Association **135**:909-915, 1947.

30. Grinspoon, L., and Hedblom, P.: Amphetamines reconsidered, Saturday Review, pp. 33-46, July 8, 1972.

31. Hemmi, T.: How we have handled the problem of drug abuse in Japan. In Sjöqvist, F., and Tottie, M., editors: Abuse of central stimulants, New York, 1969, Raven Press.

32. FDA orders curbs on amphetamine claims, American Druggist **162**:16, August 24, 1970.

33. Jellinek, M.S.: Current perspectives on hyperactivity, Drug Therapy **11**(10):77-82, October 1981.

34. Thompson, D.D., and Trinkaus, E.: Food colors and behavior, Science **212**:578, May 1981.

35. Kolata, G.: Consensus on diets and hyperactivity, Science **215**:958, February 19, 1982.

36. Cole, S.O.: Hyperkinetic children: the use of stimulant drugs evaluated, American Journal of Orthopsychiatry **45**(1):28-37, 1975.

37. Sauerhoff, M.W., and Michaelson, I.A.: Hyperactivity and brain catecholamines in lead-exposed developing rats, Science **182**:1022-1024, 1973.

38. Stroufe, L.A., and Stewart, M.A.: Treating problem children with stimulant drugs, New England Journal of Medicine **289**:407-413, 1973.

39. Millichap, J.G., and Fowler, G.W.: Treatment of "minimal brain dysfunction" syndromes: selection of drugs for children with hyperactivity and learning disabilities, Pediatric Clinics of North America **14**(4):767-777, 1967.

40. Safer, D.J., Allen, R.P. and Barr, E.: Growth rebound after termination of stimulant drugs, Journal of Pediatrics **86**:113-116, 1975.

41. MBD, drug research and the schools, Institute of Society, Ethics, and the Life Sciences (Special suppl.), June 1976.

42. Millichap, J.G.: Drugs in management of hyperkinetic and perceptually handicapped children, Journal of the American Medical Association **206**:1527-1530, 1968.

43. Sprague, R.L., and Sleater, E.K.: Methylphenidate in hyperkinetic children: differences in dose effects on learning and social behavior, Science **198**:1274-1276, 1977.

44. Gradow, K.D., and Lorey, J.: Psychosocial aspects of drug treatment for hyperactivity AAAS Symposium No. 44, Boulder, CO 1981, Westview Press Inc.

45. House, M.L.: Obesity control with OTC products, Pharmacy Times, p. 90, July 1981.

46. HEW News, p. 79-21, July 16, 1979.

47. Drug enforcement administration, Federal Register **45** (92):30732, 1980.

48. Treffert, D.A., and Joranson, D.: Restricting amphetamines, Journal of the American Medical Association, **245**(13):1336, 1981.

49. Dionne, E.J.: New York bans amphetamines as obesity cure, New York Times, August 4, 1981, p. B1.

50. The new diet pills, Consumer Reports **47**(1):14, 1982.

51. Dietz, A.J.: Amphetamine-like reactions to phenylpropanolamine, Journal of the American Medical Association **245**(6):601, 1981.

52. Blum, A.: Phenylpropanolamine: an over-the-counter amphetamine? Journal of the American Medical Association **245**(13):1346, 1981.

53. Silverman, H., and Lewis, G.: Phenylpropanolamine, Journal of the American Medical Association **247**(4):460, 1982.

54. HEW News, P80-17, April 28, 1980.

55. Pietrusko, R.G., and Anderer, T.J.: Drug information forum, U.S. Pharmacist, p. 8, September 1981.

56. HHS News, P81-14, September 30, 1981.

57. Gruson, L.: A controversy over illegally sold diet pills, New York Times, February 13, 1982, p. 52.

58. Cole, S.: Hypothalamic feeding mechanisms and amphetamine anorexia, Psychological Bulletin **79**(1):13-20, 1973.

59. Crime in America—why eight billion amphetamines? Hearings before the Select Committee on Crime, House of Representatives, Ninety-first Congress, First Session, Washington, D.C., 1970, U.S. Government Printing office.

60. Schachter, S.: Some extraordinary facts about obese humans and rats, American Psychologist 26(2):129-144, 1971.

61. Crout, J.R.: Statement before U.S. Senate Subcommittee on Monopoly, Select Committee on Small Business, November 19, 1976.

62. Tecce, J.J., and Cole, J.O.: Amphetamine effects in man: paradoxical drowsiness and lowered electrical brain activity (CNV), Science 185:451-453, 1974.

63. Thompson, T., and Pickens, R.: Stimulant self-administration by animals: some comparisons with opiate self-administration, Federation Proceedings 29(1):6-12, 1970.

64. Sulser, F., and Sanders-Bush, E.: Biochemical and metabolic considerations concerning the mechanism of action of amphetamine and related compounds. In Efron, D.H., editor: Psychotomimetic drugs, New York, 1970, Raven Press.

65. Phillips, A.G., and Fibiger, H.C.: Dopaminergic and noradrenergic substrates of positive reinforcement: differential effects of d- and l-amphetamine, Science 179:575-577, 1973.

66. Tinklenberg, J.R.: A clinical view of the amphetamines, American Family Physician 4(5):82-86, 1971.

67. Weiss, B.: Enhancement of performance by amphetamine-like drugs. In Sjöqvist, F., and Tottie, M., editors: Abuse of central stimulants, New York, 1969, Raven Press.

68. Holden, C.: Amphetamines: tighter controls on the horizon, Science 194:1027-1028, 1976.

69. Smith, D.E.: Speed kills, Journal of Psychedelic Drugs 2(2):ii, 1969.

70. Smith, D.E., and Fischer, C.M.: High dose methamphetamine abuse in the Haight-Ashbury, Section 4: Drug abuse of the stimulant type. In Smith, D.E., editor: Drug abuse papers 1969, ed. 2, Berkeley, Calif., 1969, University of California Press.

71. Kramer, J.C., Fischman, V., and Littlefield, D.C.: Amphetamine abuse, Journal of the American Medical Association 201:305-309, 1967.

72. Pittel, S.M., and Hofer, R.: The transition to amphetamine abuse, Journal of Psychedelic Drugs 5(2):105-111, 1972.

73. Ellinwood, E.H., Jr.: Amphetamine psychosis, I. Description of the individuals and process, Journal of Nervous and Mental Disease 144:273-283, 1967.

74. Griffith, J.D., and others: Experimental psychosis induced by the administration of d-amphetamine. In Costa, E., and Garattini, S., editors: Amphetamines and related compounds, Proceedings of the Mario Negri Institute for Pharmacological research, Milan, Italy, New York, 1970, Raven Press.

75. Bell, D.S.: Comparison of amphetamine psychosis and schizophrenia, British Journal of Psychiatry 111:701-707, 1965.

76. Bell, D.S.: The experimental reproduction of amphetamine psychosis, Archives of General Psychiatry 29:35-40, 1973.

77. Ellinwood, E.H., and Cohen, S.: Amphetamine abuse, Science 171:420-421, 1971.

78. Comparative psychotomimetic effects of stereoisomers of amphetamine, Nature 234:152-153, 1971.

79. Kokkinidis, L., and Anisman, H.: Amphetamine models of paranoid schizophrenia: an overview and elaboration of animal experimentation, Psychological Bulletin 88(3):551, 1980.

80. Haber, S., and others: A primate analogue of amphetamine-induced behaviors in humans, Biological Psychiatry 16(2):181, 1981.

81. Rumbaugh, C.L., Bergerton, R.T., Fang, H.C., and McCormick, R.: Cerebral angiographic changes in the drug abuse patient, Radiology 101:335-344, 1971.

82. Rumbaugh, C.L., and others: Cerebral vascular changes secondary to amphetamine abuse in the experimental animal, Radiology 101:345-351, 1971.

83. Connell, P.H.: The use and abuse of amphetamines, The Practitioner 200:234-243, 1968.

84. Amphetamine, Drug Enforcement 2(1):26-29, 1975.

85. The politics of uppers and downers, Journal of Psychedelic Drugs 5(2), Winter 1972. (Entire issue.)

86. Hinton, J.: Sedatives and hypnotics, The Practitioner 200:92-101, 1968.

87. Butler, T.C.: The introduction of chloral hydrate into medical practice, Bulletin of the History of Medicine 44:168-172, 1970.

88. Richardson, B.W.: Chloral and other narcotics, I., Popular Science Monthly 15:492, 1879.

89. Richardson, B.W.: Chloral and other narcotics, II., Popular Science Monthly 15:647, 1879.

90. Gonzales, E.R.: Methaqualone abuse implicated in injuries, deaths nationwide, Medical News 246(8):813, 1981.

91. The Quaalude scam, Newsweek, p. 93, September 28, 1981.

92. Zwerdling, D.: Methaqualone: the "safe" drug that isn't very, Washington Post, November 12, 1972, p. B3.

93. Falco, M.: Methaqualone: a study of drug control, Washington, D.C., 1975, Drug Abuse Council, Inc.

94. Perry, C.: Unconsciousness expansion: the sopor story, Rolling Stone, p. 8, March 29, 1973.

95. Hordern, A.: The barbiturates. In Joyce, C.R.B., editor: Psychopharmacology: dimensions and perspectives, Philadelphia, 1968, J.B. Lippincott Co.

96. Sharpless, S.K.: Hypnotics and sedatives. In Goodman, L., and Gilman, A., editors: The pharmacological basis of therapeutics, New York, 1970, The Macmillan Co.

97. Hinton, J.M.: A comparison of the effects of six barbiturates and a placebo on insomnia and motility in psychiatric patients, British Journal of Pharmacology 20:319-325, 1963.

98. Martindale, W.: Extra pharmacopoeia, ed. 25, London, 1967, The Pharmaceutical Press.

99. Haddon, J., and others: Acute barbiturate intoxication: concepts of management, Journal of the American Medical Association **209**:893-900, 1969.

100. Brown, S.R., and Hartshorn, E.A.: Interactions of CNS drugs—hypnotics and sedatives, Drug Intelligence and Clinical Pharmacy **10**:579-587, October 1976.

101. Tabakoff, B., and others: Brain noradrenergic systems as a prerequisite for developing tolerance to barbiturates, Science **200**:449, April 1978.

102. Skolnick, P., and others: Pentobarbital: dual actions to increase brain benzodiazepine receptor affinity, Science **211**:1448, March 1981.

103. Cohen, S., and Blutt, M.J.: Hypnotic drug therapy, Drug Abuse and Alcoholism Review **1**(2):1, 1978.

104. Hypnotic drugs and treatment of insomnia, Journal of the American Medical Association **245**(7):749, 1981.

105. Hauri, P.: Behavioral treatment of insomnia, Medical Times **107**(6):36, 1979.

106. Coates, T.T., and Thoresen, C.E.: What to use instead of sleeping pills, Journal of the American Medical Association **240**(21):2311, 1978.

107. Miller, R.R.: A guide to the use of hypnotic drugs, Medical Times **107**(6):28, 1979.

108. Church, M.W., and Johnson, L.C.: Mood and performance of poor sleepers during repeated use of flurazepam, Psychopharmacology **61**(3):309, 1979.

109. Gillin, J.C., and others: Flurazepam and insomnia, Science **205**:954, September 1979.

110. Sleeping pills, insomnia, and medical practice, National Academy of Sciences, Washington, D.C., 1979.

111. Cohen, S.: Statement before the Subcommittee to Investigate Juvenile Delinquency of the U.S. Senate Committee on the Judiciary on Drug Abuse, December 15, 1971.

112. Wesson, D.R., and Smith, D.E.: Barbiturate use as an intoxicant, presented to the Subcommittee to Investigate Juvenile Delinquency, December 15, 1971.

113. Bakewell, W.E., Jr., and Ewing, J.A.: Therapy of nonnarcotic psychoactive drug dependence, Current Psychiatric Therapies **9**:136-143, 1969.

114. Federal study links sleeping pills to 5000 deaths yearly in U.S., New York Times, November 28, 1977, p. C18.

115. Essig, C.: Drug dependence of the barbiturate type, Drug Dependence **5**:24-27, 1970.

116. Fraser, H.F., Shaver, M.R., Maxwell, E.S., and Isbell, H.: Death due to withdrawal of barbiturates, Annals of Internal Medicine **38**:1319-1325, 1953.

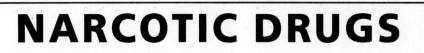

UNIT **5**

NARCOTIC DRUGS

CHAPTER 15

OPIATES THROUGH THE AGES

And soon they found themselves in the midst of a great meadow of poppies. Now it is well known that when there are many of these flowers together their odor is so powerful that anyone who breathes it falls asleep, and if the sleeper is not carried away from the scent of the flowers he sleeps on and on forever. But Dorothy did not know this, nor could she get away from the bright red flowers that were everywhere about; so presently her eyes grew heavy and she felt she must sit down to rest and to sleep. . . . Her eyes closed in spite of herself and she forgot where she was and fell among the poppies, fast asleep. . . . They carried the sleeping girl to a pretty spot beside the river, far enough from the poppy field to prevent her breathing any more of the poison of the flowers, and here they laid her gently on the soft grass and waited for the fresh breeze to waken her. [1,pp.69,70,72]

From the land of Oz to the streets of Harlem the poppy has caused much grief—and much joy. Opium is a truly unique compound. This juice from the plant *Papaver somniferum* has a history of medical use, perhaps 6000 years long. Except for the last century and a half, opium stood alone as the one agent physicians could use and obtain sure results. Compounds containing opium solved several of the recurring problems for medical science wherever used. Opium relieved pain and suffering magnificently. Just as important in the years gone by was its ability to correct dysentery, the resulting constipation being one of the regular problems of opiate users today. Its reputation and use as an aphrodisiac have persisted through the ages, but the real effect of opium and its friends is to suppress sexuality: desire, activity, and pleasure. Male narcotic users often report frequent impotence[2] and that the "time to ejaculation was long."[3] The aphrodisiac claims probably result from both the prolongation of performance in the male and the narcotic-induced loss of inhibitions.

Parallel with the medical use of opium was its use as a deliverer of pleasure and relief from anxiety. Because of these effects, extensive recreational use of opium also occurred. Soon after 1800 Frederich Sertürner opened the alkaloid century by isolating morphine, the primary psychoactive agent in opium. The use of opium, smoked or eaten, and morphine, injected or oral, increased over the nineteenth century, and there was widespread and frequent use of narcotics by 1890. This was probably the peak period of use in the United States. Heroin, which became available only three generations ago, is a more active form of morphine and, used by injection, has been the illegal narcotic drug of choice in recent years.

With a history longer than that of most other

psychoactive agents, it should not be surprising that opium and the drugs related to it have been important in the medical and social history of the world.[4] As the complexity of opium becomes apparent in the following pages, it will also be understandable that the actions it and its derivatives have on the brain have only recently become partially known.[5]

EARLY HISTORY

Some believe that the written story of opium begins 4000 years before the birth of Christ with a reference to the "joy plant" on a Sumerian tablet. The same symbol appears 3300 years later along with a description of the method used to harvest the opium: "Early in the morning old women, boys and girls collect the juice by scraping it off the wounds [of the poppy capsule] with a small iron scoope, and deposit the whole in an earthen pot."[6]

The most likely origin of opium is in a hot, dry, Middle East country several millennia ago when some unknown native discovered that for 7 to 10 days of its year-long life *Papaver somniferum* produced a substance that, when eaten, would ease pain and suffering. The opium poppy is an annual plant 3 to 4 feet high with large flowers 4 to 5 inches in diameter. The flowers may be white, pink, red, purple, or violet; "legend ascribes particular potency to plants distinguished by white seeds and flowers; fact is that all varieties of *P. somniferum* are similar in opium yield. . . ."[7]

Opium is produced and available for collection for only a few days, between the time the petals drop and before the seed pod matures. Today, as before, to harvest the opium, workers move through the fields toward evening and use a sharp multiclawed tool to make shallow cuts into, but not through, the unripe seed pod. During the night a white substance oozes from the cuts, oxidizes to a red-brown color, and becomes gummy. In the morning the resinous substance is carefully scraped from the pod and collected in small balls. This raw opium forms the basis for the opium medicines

used through history and is the substance from which morphine is extracted and then heroin is derived.

The importance and extent of use of the opium poppy in the early Egyptian and Greek cultures are still under debate, but in the Ebers papyrus (circa 1500 BC) a remedy is mentioned "to prevent the excessive crying of children." Since a later Egyptian remedy for the same purpose clearly contained opium (as well as fly excrement), as does the western culture's remedy for this problem, paregoric (opium and alcohol), many writers report the first specific medical use of opium as dating from the Ebers papyrus.

Homer's *Odyssey* (1000 BC) contains a passage that some authors believe refers to the use of opium. A party was about to become a real drag because everyone was sad thinking about Ulysses and the deaths of their friends, when:

> Helen, daughter of Zeus, poured into the wine they were drinking a drug, nepenthes, which gave forgetfulness of evil. Those who had drunk of this mixture did not shed a tear the whole day long, even though their mother or father were dead, even though a brother or beloved son had been killed before their eyes. . . .[8,p.6]

The drug could only have been opium.

The classical literature of Virgil and Ovid contains references to the sleep-producing poppy. The Greek god of sleep, Hypnos, as well as the Roman god of sleep, Somnus, was usually adorned with or carried poppies and sometimes an opium container. Unlike the sandman of today pouring sand into the eyes of children, Somnus was frequently pictured pouring juice from the container into the eyes of the sleeper. Greek mythology suggests that Ceres created the poppy so she could sleep and thus forget that her daughter had been given to Pluto. The Chinese legend has the poppy plant springing up from the earth where Buddha's eyelids fell when he cut them off to prevent sleep. Since seeds of the opium plant were carried to China only about 600 to 700 AD, it would seem that the Greek legend has more validity!

Although Hippocrates was not an advocate of opium or the poppy, one of his remedies probably referred to it. A hundred years later, about 300 BC, a Greek physician provided a method for extracting poppy juice (meconium) by grinding the entire plant, but not until the first century AD was the extraction of opium clearly differentiated from meconium in Greek writings. Beginning around this period, the spread of opium use and poppy cultivation grew rapidly, and the Greek word *opius*, meaning "little juice," came into written records. Derivations and modifications of *opius* have been used as the term for the poppy sap in Arabic, Chinese, and English.

Opium was important in Greek medicine. Galen, the last of the great Greek physicians, emphasized caution in the use of opium but felt that it was almost a cure-all, since it

> resists poison and venomous bites, cures chronic headache, vertigo, deafness, epilepsy, apoplexy, dimness of sight, loss of voice, asthma, coughs of all kinds, spitting of blood, tightness of breath, colic, the iliac poison, jaundice, hardness of the spleen, stone, urinary complaints, fevers, dropsies, leprosies, the troubles to which women are subject, melancholy and all pestilences.[8,p.111]

Recreational use even then must have been extensive, since Galen commented on the opium cakes and candies that were being sold everywhere in the streets. The medical use of opium was common in this period. Although the concepts of addiction and withdrawal had not yet been established, a recent writer suggests that the reports on the behavior and health of the Roman emperor in this period, Marcus Aurelius, clearly indicate that he was addicted to opium and occasionally suffered withdrawal symptoms.[9]

Greek knowledge of opium use in medicine died with the decline of the Roman Empire and thus had little influence on the world's use of opium for the next 1000 years. To the south in North Africa, though, the Arabic world clutched opium (and hashish) to its breast, since the Koran forbade the use of alcohol in any form. Opium and hashish became the primary social drugs wherever the Islam culture moved, and it did move. The Mohammedans were active fighters, explorers, and traders. While Europe rested through the Dark Ages, the Arabian world reached out and made contact with India and China. Opium was one of the products they traded, but they also sold the seeds of the opium poppy, and home cultivation began in these countries. By the tenth century AD, opium was referred to in Chinese medical writings.

During this period when the Arabian civilization flourished, two Arabian physicians made substantial contributions to medicine and to the history of opium. Shortly after 1000 AD, Biruni composed a pharmacology book. In his descriptions of opium was what some believe to be the first written description of addiction.[10] In this same period, the best-known Arabian physician, Avicenna, was using opium preparations very effectively and extensively in his medical practice. His writings, along with those of Galen, formed the basis of medical education in Europe as the Renaissance dawned, and thus the glories of opium were advanced. (Strange but true that a physician as knowledgeable as Avicenna, and a believer in the tenets of Mohammedanism, should die as a result of drinking too much of a mixture of opium and wine. Perhaps, as some suggest, he has been overrated as a physician.)

Early in the sixteenth century, European medicine had a phenomenon by the name of Paracelsus. A true iconoclast and Renaissance man, he denounced all the famous medics of history—Hippocrates, Galen, Avicenna—as well as his contemporaries. He apparently was a successful clinician and accomplished some wondrous cures for the day. One of the secrets of Paracelsus was a potion called laudanum. Although it is not clear that his laudanum contained opium, he did use opium very extensively in his treatment of patients. Paracelsus was one of the early Renaissance supporters of opium as a panacea and referred to it as the "stone of immortality." According to a later writer (1701), Paracelsus believed that opium "will dissolve Diseases, as Fire does Snow. . . ."[6]

To this point in history there is no clear evidence that the regular use of opium was recognized as producing changes in the body that required continued use of the drug for normal functioning. Since the Roman period, there had been incidental reports of tolerance to the drug so that larger and larger quantities were needed to obtain the same effect. There were also reports of discomfort at times in habitual opium users that could be relieved by the ingestion of more opium, but the concept of addiction was not delineated. Not until the last half of the sixteenth century was a clear association formed between discontinuing regular use of opium and the appearance of certain symptoms we now call the withdrawal syndrome.

The first report of clearly addicted individuals appeared in 1563 when a Portuguese explorer, Garcia de Orta, commented on the use of opium in India. A better description, however, is from the German physician Rauwolf, who reported on his travels in the 1570s in the Middle East.

> Not least of all one finds there (namely in the bazaar of Aleppo) also a trade by pharmacists in opium (the inhabitants call it 'Ofinn'), which the Turks, Moors, Persians, and still other peoples are in the habit of taking—not alone during wars, to make them of good heart and strong courage at the time when they are to fight the enemy—but also at times of peace, to take away troubles and deliriums, or at least to alleviate them. Also their men of religion eat this, but particularly among others, the Dervishes; and they take so much of it that they thereupon immediately become sleepy and go out of their senses, so that when they, in their mad habit, cut, hack or burn themselves, they find the pains and sufferings much less. When now one or more thereby have thus begun (they in the habit of taking as much of it as the size of a pea without danger), then can they never more leave off therefrom, it being as if they sink into a sickness, or at least other new hazards are ready to excite them, as they themselves confess, if they leave off somewhat taking it, so that then they feel physically ill.[6]

Because of the increasing awareness of the broad effectiveness of opium as a result of Paracelsus and

his followers, a variety of new opium preparations was developed in the sixteenth, seventeenth, and eighteenth centuries. Only two will be mentioned, partly because of their importance in medical history and partly because they are still available today by the same names in many places. The first compound is laudanum, as prepared by Dr. Thomas Sydenham, the father of clinical medicine. (Although the name is the same as Paracelsus' compound, this seems to be the only similarity.) Sydenham's general contributions to English medicine are so great that he has been called the English Hippocrates. He spoke more highly of opium than did Paracelsus, saying that "without opium the healing art would cease to exist." His laudanum contained 2 ounces of strained opium, 1 ounce of saffron, and a dram of cinnamon and of cloves dissolved in 1 pint of Canary wine and taken in small quantities.

Thomas Dover, a resident of Sydenham's house and possibly his student, concocted an even more potent preparation of opium. Dover never did complete medical training, but he practiced medicine for 24 years before kicking over the traces in 1708 and commanding a ship on an around-the-world voyage. During his medical career, Dover made his claim to fame and fortune with Dover's Powder. Originally, it contained 1 ounce each of opium, ipecac, and licorice and 4 ounces each of saltpeter and tartar. The dose was about 100 grains of this mixture taken in wine. This quantity was so potent that even Dover admitted that the apothecaries wanted the patients to make their wills before taking the medicine. But it did provide relief from pain.

Thomas Dover can mark the end of an era. In the nineteenth century, big things happened to opium in the hands of the chemist that began to change the nature of the story. Also in the nineteenth century, opium and hashish became the touchstones for a number of famous writers in England and France. In this same period, Britain became the opium pusher for China and indirectly set the stage for the opiate addiction problem of today.

Writers and opium: liquid sky and the keys of paradise

In a momentous year for opium, 1805, Thomas De Quincey, a 20-year-old English youth who had run away from home at 17, purchased some laudanum for a toothache and received change for his shilling from the apothecary. His response to this dose was described:

> I took it: and in an hour, O heavens! what a revulsion! what a resurrection, from its lowest depths, of the inner spirit! what an apocalypse of the world within me! That my pains had vanished was now a trifle in my eyes; this negative effect was swallowed up in the immensity of those positive effects which had opened before me, in the abyss of divine enjoyment thus suddenly revealed. Here was a panacea . . . for all human woes; here was the secret of happiness, about which philosophers had disputed for so many ages, at once discovered; happiness might now be bought for a penny, and carried in the waistcoat-pocket; portable ecstasies might be had corked up in a pint-bottle; and peace of mind could be sent down by the mail.[11,p.179]

For the rest of his life De Quincey used laudanum, although he possibly was no longer addicted at his death. He did not try to conceal the extent of his addiction. Rather, his writings are replete with insight into the opiate-hazed world, particularly his article "The Confessions of an English Opium-Eater," which was published in 1821 (and in book form in 1823). ("Opium eating" throughout this period was the phrase generally used to refer to laudanum drinking.)

Several other famous English authors were also addicted to laudanum, including Elizabeth Barrett Browning and Samuel Taylor Coleridge.[12-15] Coleridge's magnificently beautiful "Kubla Khan" was probably conceived and composed in an opium reverie and then written down as best he could remember it. However, De Quincey is of primary interest here, as Baudelaire will be with hashish. His emphasis was on understanding the effects that opium has on consciousness, experience, and feeling, and as such he provided some of the most vivid accounts of the power of opium.

Opium does not produce new worlds for the user.

> If a man, "whose talk is of oxen," should become an opium-eater, the probability is, that (if he is not too dull to dream at all)—he will dream about oxen; whereas, in the case before him [De Quincey], the reader will find that the opium-eater boasteth himself to be a philosopher; and accordingly, that the phantasmagoria of *his* dreams (waking or sleeping, day-dreams or night-dreams) is suitable to one [of] that character. . . .[16,p.156]

Opium does, however, change the way the world is perceived. For example, "an opium eater is too happy to observe the motion of time."[11] De Quincey wrote about the added dimensions to sounds and music that occurred when he attended the opera while using opium:

> it is by the reaction of the mind upon the notices of the ear (the *matter* coming by the senses, the *form* from the mind) that the pleasure is constructed. . . . Now opium, by greatly increasing the activity of the mind, generally increases . . . its activity by which we are able to construct out of the raw material of organic sound an elaborate intellectual pleasure.[11,p.189]

The contrast between the feelings, effects, and experiences that result from alcohol were discussed extensively and sharply contrasted with those accompanying the use of opium:

> crude opium . . . is incapable of producing any state of body at all resembling that which is produced by alcohol. . . . It is not in the quantity of its effects merely, but in the quality, that it differs altogether. The pleasure given by wine is always rapidly mounting, and tending to a crisis, after which as rapidly it declines; that from opium, when once generated, is stationary for eight or ten hours. . . . The one is a flickering flame, the other a steady and equable glow. But the main distinction lies in this—that, whereas wine disorders the mental faculties, opium, on the contrary (if taken in a proper manner), introduces amongst them the most exquisite order, legislation, and harmony. Wine robs a man of his self-possession; opium sustains and reinforces it. Wine unsettles the judgment. . . . Opium, on the contrary, communicates serenity and equipoise to all the faculties. . . .[11,pp.180-181]

In spite of all the good things De Quincey said about opium and the effects it had on him, he suffered from its use. For long periods in his life he was unable to write as a result of his addiction. As with most things: "Opium gives and takes away. It defeats the *steady* habit of exertion; but it creates spasms of irregular exertion. It ruins the natural power of life; but it develops preternatural paroxysms of intermitting power."[17,p.424]

Publication of De Quincey's book in 1823 and its first translation into French in 1828 were events that spurred the French Romantic writers into exploration with opium and hashish in the 1840s and later. Baudelaire's famous book *The Artificial Paradises*[18] was composed of two parts, the first being an original account of the effects of hashish and the second his translation of *The Confessions of an English Opium-Eater*. Baudelaire was to repeatedly comment that much of what he wrote at various times about the effects of opium could equally be said about hashish.[19] The only associated American article of note in this period, "An Opium Eater in America,"[20] appeared in an American magazine in 1842.

An 1854 article in *The Journal of Psychological Medicine* on the addiction of Coleridge and De Quincey was at times almost as lyrical in describing the effects of opium eating as were the writers of this period. The paper also clearly indicated the difficulty of dealing with the problem of opiate addiction, a difficulty that existed then as well as now, over a hundred years later.

> How extraordinary is the human mind! how elevated in comprehension—how god-like in sympathy—and yet the human mind may be rendered joyous or fierce, wild or torpid—foolish or entranced, by such agents as alcohol or opium! Spiritual, indeed, we are, but how curiously is our spirituality mixed up with the gross and material. A miserable and despairing being, shall, under the influence of such an agent, be transferred to a paradise of joy, and yet his real condition be not a whit the less destitute. After all, there is something more in this than our philosophy can reach, but it teaches one piece of philosophy, that it is the state of mind, rather than external circumstances, which constitutes happiness.[21]

The Opium Wars

While literary figures experimented, merchants made money with opium. Although opium and the opium poppy had been introduced to China well before the year 1000, there was only a moderate level of use by a select, elite group. Spreading much more rapidly after its introduction was tobacco smoking. It is not clear when tobacco was introduced to the Chinese, but its use had spread and become so offensive that in 1644 the Emperor forbade tobacco smoking in China. The edict did not last long (as is to be expected), but it was in part responsible for the development of opium smoking.

Up to this period the smoking of tobacco and the eating of opium had existed side by side. The restriction on the use of tobacco and the population's appreciation of the pleasures of smoking led to the subterfuge of combining opium and tobacco for smoking. The amount of tobacco used was gradually reduced and soon omitted altogether. Very rapidly the smoking of opium spread, although opium eating had never been very attractive to most Chinese,[22] perhaps, at least partly, because smoking results in a rapid effect compared to oral use of opium.

In 1729 China's first law against opium smoking mandated that opium shopowners were to be strangled. Once opium for nonmedical purposes was outlawed, it was necessary for the drug to be smuggled in from India, where poppy plantations were abundant. Smuggling opium was so profitable for everyone—the growers, the shippers, and the customs officers—that unofficial and illegal, but formal and binding, rules were gradually developed for the game.[8] The background to the Opium Wars is too lengthy and complex to even attempt to sketch adequately. However, some points must be made to explain why the British went to war so they could continue pouring opium into China against the wishes of the Chinese national government.

Since before 1557, when the Portuguese were allowed to develop the small and remote trading post of Macao, pressure had been increasing on the Chinese emperors to open the country up to trade with the "barbarians from the West." Not only the

Portuguese but the Dutch and the English repeatedly knocked on the closed door of the Chinese. Near the end of the seventeenth century the port of Canton was opened under very strict rules to foreigners. Tea was the major export, and the British shipped out huge amounts. There was little that the Chinese were interested in importing from the "barbarians," but opium could be smuggled so profitably that it soon became the primary import. The profit the British made from selling opium paid for the tea they shipped to England.[23]

In the early nineteenth century the government of India was actually the British East India Company. As such it had a monopoly on opium, which was legal in India. Each year agents of the government contracted with farmers for the cultivation of poppies; in the spring they received the raw opium and prepared it into cakes. The production of opium was legal in India, under the auspices of the government, but smuggling it into China was not. That posed a problem for the government of India, that is, the East India Company. They auctioned chests of opium cakes to private merchants, who gave the chests to selected British firms, who sold it for a commission to Chinese merchants. In this way the British were able to have the Chinese "smuggle" the opium into China! No matter who was responsible, everyone made much money. The number of chests of opium, each with about 120 pounds of smokable opium, that were annually imported to China increased from 200 in 1729 to about 5000 at the century's end to 25,000 chests in 1838.

The following year, 1839, the emperor of China made a fatal mistake—he sent an honest man to Canton to suppress the opium smuggling. Commissioner Lin made everyone nervous. He demanded that the barbarians deliver all their opium supplies to him and subjected the dealers to confinement in their houses. After some haggling, the representative of the British government ordered the merchants to deliver the opium—20,000 chests worth about $6 million—which was then destroyed and everyone set free. Pressures mounted, though, and an incident involving drunken American and British sailors killing a Chinese started the Opium War in 1839. The British army arrived 10 months

later, and in 2 years, largely by avoiding land battles and by using the superior artillery of the royal navy ships, won a victory over a country of more than 350 million citizens. As victors, the British were given the island of Hong Kong, broad trading rights, and $6 million to reimburse the merchants whose opium had been destroyed.

Through it all, the smuggling of opium continued. There was another Opium War in the 1850s, but the British imports of illegal opium continued and increased until 1908, when Britain and China agreed to limit imports of opium from India.

The Chinese opium trade posed a great moral dilemma for Britain.[24-26] The East India Company protested until its end that it was not smuggling opium into China, and technically it was not. Although the 1839 Opium War was precipitated by opium-related incidents, the primary British motivation in both wars was to open the vast country of China to world, and especially British, trade. From 1870 to 1893 motions in Parliament to end the extremely profitable opium commerce failed to pass but did cause a decline in the opium trade. In 1893 a moral protest against the trade was supported, but not until 1906 did the government support and pass a bill that started the process which ended the opium trade by 1913.[27]

MIDDLE HISTORY

In 1805 in London, England, a 20-year-old eased a toothache and fell into the abyss of divine enjoyment. In Hanover, Germany, a 20-year-old worked on the experiments that were to have great impact on science, medicine, and the pleasure seekers. In 1806, this German youth, Frederich Sertürner, published his report of over 50 experiments, which clearly showed that he had isolated the primary active ingredient in opium. In doing this he also opened the door to the new field of alkaloidal chemistry, actually an even more important and amazing achievement.

The active agent was ten times as potent as opium. Sertürner named it *morphium* after Morpheus, the god of dreams. Use of the new agent developed slowly, but by 1831 the implications of his chemical work and the medical value of morphine were so overwhelming that this pharmacist's assistant was given the French equivalent of the Nobel Prize. Later work into the mysteries of opium found over 30 different alkaloids, with the second most important one being isolated in 1832 and named *codeine*, the Greek word for poppy head.

The availability of a clinically valuable, pure chemical of known potency is always capitalized on in medicine. The major increase in the use of morphine came as a result of two nondrug developments, one technological and one political. The technological development was the perfection of the hypodermic syringe in 1853 by Dr. Alexander Wood. This made it possible to rapidly deliver morphine directly into the blood or tissue rather than the much slower process of eating opium or morphine and waiting for absorption to occur from the gastrointestinal tract. A further advantage of injecting morphine was thought to exist. Originally it was felt that morphine by injection would not be as addicting as the oral use of the drug. This belief was later found to be false.

The political events that sped the drug of sleep and dreams into the veins of people worldwide were the American Civil War (1861 to 1865), the Prussian-Austrian War (1866), and the Franco-Prussian War (1870). Military medicine was, and to some extent still is, characterized by the dictum "first provide relief." Morphine given by injection did work rapidly and well, and it was administered regularly in large doses to many soldiers for the reduction of pain and relief from dysentery. The percentage of returning veterans from these wars who were addicted to morphine was high enough that the illness was later called the "soldier's disease" or the "army disease."

In this second half of the nineteenth century three forms of opiate addiction were developing in the United States. The long-useful oral intake of opium, and now morphine, increased greatly as patent medicines became a standard form of self-medication. After 1850 Chinese laborers were imported in large numbers to the west coast, and they introduced opium smoking to this country. The last form, medically the most dangerous and ultimately

the most disruptive socially, was the injection of morphine.

Around the turn of the century the percentage (and perhaps the absolute number) of Americans addicted to one of the opiates was very probably greater than at any other time before or since. Several authorities, both then[28] and more recently,[29] agree that no less than 1% of the population was addicted to opium, although accurate statistics are not available. In spite of the high level of addiction, it was not a major social problem. In this period:

> Little emphasis was placed on the effects of evil association, and dope peddlers were not mentioned because they were rare or nonexistent.
>
> The public then had an altogether different conception of drug addiction from that which prevails today. The habit was not approved, but neither was it regarded as criminal or monstrous. It was usually looked upon as a vice or personal misfortune, or much as alcoholism is viewed today. Narcotics users were pitied rather than loathed as criminals or degenerates—an attitude which still prevails in Europe.[30,p.211]

The opium smoking the Chinese brought to this country never became widely popular, although around the turn of the century about one fourth of the opium imported was smoking opium. Perhaps it was because the smoking itself only occupies about a minute and is then followed by a dreamlike state of reverie that may last 2 or 3 hours, hardly behavior that is conducive to a continuation of daily activities or consonant with the outward, active orientation of most Americans in that period. Another reason why opium smoking did not spread was that it originated with Orientals, who were scorned by whites. Similarly, the opium smoking that did occur among whites was found within the asocial and antisocial elements of this culture.[30] Amusingly, even the underworld has its standards of morality, and opium smokers looked down on those who used their drugs by injection. In a New York opium-smoking den early in this century "one of the smokers discovered a hypodermic user in the bathroom giving himself an injection. He immediately reported to the proprietor that there was a 'Goddamned dope fiend in the can'. The offender was promptly ejected."[30] Those who used morphine, and later heroin, by injection will be reported later, but brief mention must be made of one of the major sources of addiction in this period, patent medicines.

The growth of the patent medicine industry after the Civil War has been well documented.[31-33] Everything seemed to be favorable for the industry, and it took advantage of each opportunity. There were few government regulations on the industry, and as a result addicting drugs were an important part of many tonics and remedies, although this fact did not have to be indicated on the label. Since labeling of ingredients was not required, a user who had become aware that he was addicted and who wanted to purchase a cure could be sold a remedy labeled as a cure that contained almost as much of the addicting drug as he had been receiving in the original tonic.

The generally poor level of health care in the country and a large number of maimed and diseased veterans created a need for considerable medical treatment. Patent medicines promised, and in part delivered, the perfect self-medication. They were easily available, not too expensive, socially acceptable, and, miracle of miracles, they did work. The amount of alcohol and/or opiates in many of the nostrums was cetain to relieve the user's aches, pains, and anxieties.

Two other points help explain the increase in the sales of patent medicines. One was the lack of sophistication and education of most Americans during this period, and the other was the use of fantastic advertising campaigns. The two elements worked together, the first explaining the great appeal and effectiveness the active advertising campaigns had in selling the merchandise. Medicine shows, testimonials, songs, newspaper and magazine ads all said the same thing: "You feel ill! *This* product will cure." People believed and bought!

Gradually some medical concern developed over the number of people who were addicted to opiates, and this concern was a part of the motivation that led to the passage of the 1906 Pure Food and Drugs Act. In 1910 a government expert in this area made clear that this law was only a beginning.

The thoughtful and foremost medical men have been and are cautioning against the free use of morphine and opium, particularly in recurring pain. The amount they are using is decreasing yearly. Notwithstanding this fact, and the fact that legislation, federal, state and territorial, adverse to the indiscriminate use and sale of opium and morphine, their derivatives and preparations, has been enacted during the past few decades, the amount of opium per capita imported and consumed in the United States has doubled during the last forty years. . . . It is well known that there are many factors at work tending to drug enslavement, among them being the host of soothing syrups, medicated soft drinks containing cocaine, asthma remedies, catarrh remedies, consumption remedies, cough and cold remedies, and the more notorious so-called "drug addiction cures." It is often stated that medical men are frequently the chief factors in causing drug addiction.[28,pp.105-106]

Data were presented in this paper that tended to support the belief that medical use of opiates initiated by a physician was one, if not *the*, major cause of addiction in this country at that time. A 1918 government report clearly indicted the physician as the major cause of addiction in addicts of "good social standing."

That physicians widely used opiates as drugs in treatment is understandable in light of articles that had been published, such as one in 1889 titled "Advantages of Substituting the Morphia Habit for the Incurably Alcoholic." The author stated:

The only grounds on which opium in lieu of alcohol can be claimed as reformatory are, that it is less inimical to healthy life than alcohol, that it calms in place of exciting the baser passions, and hence is less productive of acts of violence and crime; in short, that as a whole the use of morphine in place of alcohol is but a choice of evils, and by far the lesser. . . . If a person has got to the stage of abnormity that he cannot do without a pathological nutrient, particularly of the alcoholic kind, is it better to allow him to go on, or to endeavor to have him substitute morphine for it? After years of experimental trial and observation I have arrived at the conclusion that the latter is immeasurably the best, or by far the least of the two evils.[34]

The author justifies at length the exchange of oral morphine addiction for alcohol addiction since:

> In this way have I been able to bring peacefulness and quiet to many disturbed and distracted homes, to keep the head of a family out of the gutter and out of the lock-up, to keep him from scandalous misbehavior and neglect of his affairs, to keep him from the verges and actualities of delirium tremens horrors, and above all, to save him from committing, as I veritably believe, some terrible crime.[34]

Besides all those good things, morphine addiction was cheap: by one estimate it was ten times as expensive to be an alcoholic, all of 25 cents a day. The article concludes:

> I might, had I time and you space, enlarge by statistics to prove the law-abiding qualities of opium-eating peoples, but of this any one can perceive somewhat for himself, if he carefully watches and reflects on the quiet, introspective gaze of the morphine habitue, and compares it to the riotous, devil-may-care leer of the drunkard.[34]

This middle history period, 1806 to 1914, is rich in material on the use of opiates that gives background to the thesis that if drugs are widely used, it is because they meet the needs of a culture. An 1880 report called addiction a "vice of middle life."[35] The typical opiate addict of this period was a 30- to 50-year-old white woman who functioned well and was adjusted to her life as a wife and mother. She bought opium or morphine legally at the local store, used it orally, and caused few, if any, social problems. She may have ordered her "family remedy" through the mail from Sears, Roebuck—two ounces of laudanum for 18 cents or 1½ pints for $2. She may even have decided to make Dr. Pierce's Golden Medical Discovery at home:

> Fifteen grains pure honey, one grain extract of poisonous or acrid lettuce (bot.: *herba lactucae virosae*), two grains laudanum, 100 grains dilute alcohol (64 per cent), tasting like fusel oil and wood spirit, with 100 grains of water.[36]

Do not be misled. There *were* problems associated with addiction during this period. There are always individuals who are unable to control drug intake, whether the drug is used for self-medication or recreation. Because of the high opiate content of patent medicines and the ready availability of addicting drugs for drinking and/or injecting, very high levels of drug were frequently used. As a result, the symptoms of withdrawal were very severe—much worse than today—and there were no medications or treatment programs to reduce the pain or anxiety.

The picture changed with the passage of the Harrison Act in 1914, which virtually removed opiates from the nonprescription market. One other factor helped change the opiate addiction scene to the one we have today. Toward the end of this period, a chemical transformation of the morphine molecule was put on the market. In 1874 two acetyl groups were attached to morphine, yielding heroin, which was placed on the market in 1898 by Bayer Laboratories as a nonaddicting substitute for codeine. The chemical change was important because heroin is about three times as potent as morphine. The pharmacology of heroin and morphine are identical except that the two acetyl groups increase the lipid solubility of the molecule, and thus the molecule enters the brain more rapidly. The additional groups are detached, yielding monoacetylmorphine, which is then converted to morphine. Therefore, effects of morphine and heroin are identical except that heroin is more potent and acts faster.[37]

The history of heroin is interesting in that it provides strong support for those who argue for extended experimental study of new therapeutic agents before they are marketed. Heroin was originally marketed as a nonaddicting substitute for codeine.[38] It seemed to be the perfect drug, more potent yet less harmful. Although not introduced commercially until 1898, heroin had been studied, and many of its pharmacological actions were reported in 1890.[39] By January 1900 a comprehensive review article began with the statement:

> A sufficiently long period having elapsed since the introduction of heroine, the new substitution product for codeine, during which it has been used very extensively, we are now enabled to pass judg-

ment upon its real value, and to definitely determine in what manner this drug has fulfilled the expectations raised in its behalf.[40]

The author then proceeded to extensively survey the pharmacological and clinical literature, after which he concluded that tolerance and addiction (habituation) to heroin were only minor problems.

> Habituation has been noted in a small percentage . . . of the cases. . . . All observers are agreed, however, that none of the patients suffer in any way from this habituation, and that none of the symptoms which are so characteristic of chronic morphinism have ever been observed. On the other hand, a large number of the reports refer to the fact that the same dose may be used for a long time without any habituation.[40]

Many other articles and letters expressed the same attitude. They generally echoed the following sentiment: "he finds heroine an excellent sedative for the respiratory tract, devoid of the narcotic effect of codeine and morphine, and therefore in physiological doses entirely uninjurious."[41] The basis for the failure to find addiction and the resulting attitudes probably was the fact that heroin was primarily used as a substitute for codeine, which meant oral doses of 3 to 5 mg used for brief periods of time. Slowly the situation changed, and a 1905 text on *Pharmacology and Therapeutics* took a middle ground on heroin by saying that it "is stated not to give rise to habituation. A more extended knowledge of the drug, however, would seem to indicate that the latter assertion is not entirely correct."[42,p.860] In a few more years everyone knew that heroin was the most addicting of the opiates.

Toward the end of this era the 1906 Pure Food and Drugs Act made it necessary for manufacturers to place on the label of their products the kind and amount of opiates the compound contained. The 1909 Exclusion Act restricted the importation of opium for nonmedical purposes, but it was the Harrison Narcotic Act of 1914 that finally resulted in a decrease in the percentage of people addicted to the opiates. However, this same act produced the conditions that led to opiate addiction becoming an increasing social problem.

PHARMACODYNAMICS

Pain has long been one of society's and medicine's primary concerns. Second only to curing an illness or preventing death and disability has been the reduction of pain. Opium, its constituents such as morphine and codeine, its semisynthetics such as heroin, and the purely synthetic opiate-like agents such as methadone and meperidine (Demerol) are the most effective analgesics known today (Figs. 15-1 and 15-2).

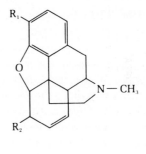

	R_1	R_2
Morphine	— OH	— OH
Codeine	— O — CH₃	— OH
Heroin	— O — C — CH₃ (=O)	— O — C — CH₃ (=O)

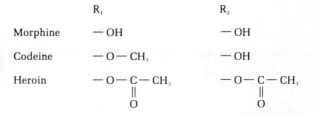

FIG. 15-1 Narcotic agents isolated or derived from opium.

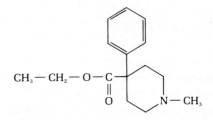

Meperidine
Demerol (Winthrop)
(1-methyl-4-phenyl-4-carbethoxypiperidine)

FIG. 15-2 Meperidine.

In spite of considerable research effort, it was only in the mid-seventies that the mechanism by which these drugs reduce pain started to become clear. Collectively, the opiates and the synthetic compounds with similar activity are classed as narcotic analgesics.

Tolerance develops to most of the effects of these drugs, which means the dose must be regularly increased to maintain a constant effect. Concomitant with tolerance is the establishment of physiological dependency, which is manifested as a consistent pattern of physiological responses when regular drug use is discontinued. These agents also have the capability to induce a sense of euphoria in many people. The euphoria seems to be more than just the reduction of tension and suffering. For years pharmacologists and biochemists have sought to develop compounds that would make possible a separation of analgesia, tolerance, physiological dependency, and euphoria. To date there has been little success. For most compounds there is a high correlation between analgesic potency and the euphoriant effects the agent elicits. In some synthetic narcotics, however, analgesia, euphoria, and physical dependency have been dissociated. Considering the many narcotic agents in the marketplace, they offer little advantage for the most part over the primary active ingredient in *Papaver somniferum*, and so morphine remains the standard against which other narcotics are judged.[43] For this reason, the pharmacological and physiological effects of morphine in humans will be emphasized.

Pharmacological effects

The major therapeutic indication for morphine is the reduction of pain, whereas codeine is used widely and effectively as a cough suppressant. Both of these therapeutic effects are CNS actions. At therapeutic doses morphine has little effect on conduction in the peripheral nerves of the sensory systems; the results are mixed as to whether morphine raises the threshold to pain.

After the administration of an analgesic dose of morphine some patients report that they are still aware of the pain, but the pain is no longer aversive. Frequently, though, the pain stimulus is not attended to by the drug user. He is not aware of the pain stimulus until it is pointed out to him, and when made aware of the stimulus, he does not perceive it as aversive. The narcotic agents seem to have their effect in part by diminishing the awareness the individual has of the aversive stimulus and in part on his response to the stimulus. Morphine, then, primarily reduces the emotional response to pain, the suffering, and to some extent also decreases knowledge of the pain stimulus. The effect of narcotics is relatively specific to pain. Fewer effects on mental and motor ability accompany analgesic doses of these agents than with equipotent doses of other analgesic and depressant drugs. "Continuous dull pain is relieved more effectively than sharp intermittent pain . . . ,"[44,p.248] but, most types of pain are reduced following administration of narcotic agents. Although one of the characteristics of these drugs is their ability to reduce pain without inducing sleep, drowsiness is not uncommon after a therapeutic dose. (In the addicts' vernacular, the patient is "on the nod.") The patient is readily awakened if he sleeps, and dreams during the sleep period are frequent.

Another very specific effect of morphine is to depress the respiratory centers in the brain so that respiration slows and becomes shallow. This is perhaps the major side effect of the narcotic agents and one of the most dangerous, since death resulting from respiratory arrest can easily follow an excessive dose of these drugs. The basis for this effect is that the respiratory centers become less responsive to carbon dioxide levels in the blood, but again the mechanism of morphine is not known. Not nearly so dangerous but almost as common is another effect of the narcotics: constriction of the pupils of the eyes. The pinpoint pupils that everyone talks about are seen only in overdoses. Opiate users have a hypersensitive pupillary response to light, so their pupils are always more narrowed than nonusers'. Tolerance to this pupillary response is minimal.

Morphine also stimulates the brain area controlling nausea and vomiting, which are other frequent side effects. Usually, nausea occurs in about

TABLE 15-1 Partial comparison of some characteristics of frequently used narcotic analgesics

	Equianalgesic doses (milligrams)	Time to peak action (subcutaneous injection)	Duration of analgesic action (hours)
Morphine	10	30-60 minutes	4-5
Codeine	120		2-4
Heroin	3-4	15 minutes	4-5
Methadone	8-10	30 minutes	4-6
Meperidine	80-100	10 minutes	2-4

half of the ambulatory patients given a 15-mg dose of morphine. Still other side effects result from morphine-induced decreases in the response of the hypothalamus to external input, which impairs its regulation of many homeostatic functions. For example, body temperature decreases slightly, and fluid is retained in the body. In addition, the hormonal output from the pituitary gland is generally depressed.

To summarize the CNS effects of therapeutic levels of morphine: sensory pathways function normally, but the response to pain stimuli is diminished; respiration is depressed, and nausea is induced by effects on lower brain centers; the hypothalamic response to external input is decreased, and pituitary gland functioning is depressed. In spite of these seemingly selective actions, work with radioactively labeled narcotics does not show specific localization of the drug anywhere in the CNS.

The effects of morphine on the gastrointestinal system have been well studied, although, again, the mechanisms remain elusive. Morphine impairs digestion by decreasing the secretion of essential digestive juices. The narcotic agents also slow the passage of food through the gastrointestinal tract by decreasing the number of peristaltic contractions. At the same time, however, there may be an increase in other gastrointestinal contractions, with the result that there is much activity but little movement of the material in the intestines. Considerable water is absorbed from from the intestinal material; this fact, plus the near absence of contractions to move material through the intestine,

results in constipation. Tolerance to these effects develops very slowly.

Both the central and the peripheral effects described are generally true for all narcotic agents. Differences between these compounds are primarily in their speed and duration of action and their potency. When given intravenously, the latency to onset of action of most of the narcotics is about the same. Since 10 mg of morphine is effective in providing relief to about 70% of patients with moderate to severe pain (such as postoperative pain), that dose is generally used as the standard. The data in Table 15-1 present a partial comparison of some characteristics of the most frequently used narcotic analgesics. These data are only approximations, since many factors determine the effects in a particular person.[45]

Mechanism of action

The 1970s will be long remembered in pharmacology as the decade in which the interaction between the narcotics and the central nervous system was finally glimpsed—but far from understood. An excellent 1971 article provides the background for the breakthroughs that were soon to come.[46] Many studies had suggested that the opiates act through very specific sites, receptors, in the brain. One fact pointing to an opiate receptor is the finding that usually it is only the *l*-form which is effective, that is, the action of the drug is very dependent on the shape of the molecule. Adding weight to this result is an appreciation that all effective opiate analgesics have very similar molecular structures. Much like the analogy with the neurotransmitters and their receptors (Chapter 5), only the opiate structure can serve as the key to open (activate) the lock (receptor).

A pharmacologist at Stanford University, Avram Goldstein, was the first to really identify the narcotic receptor in the brain, but it was a young research physician at Johns Hopkins University, Sol Snyder, and his graduate student who provided the technological giant step leading to the rapid advances of the mid- and late seventies. The work of Snyder and collaborators made it possible to identify brain areas that contain many narcotic receptors.[47]

Some parts of the limbic system are also packed with opiate receptors, and one part, the *amygdala*, has the greatest abundance of opiate receptors in the brain. It seems likely that the euphoric effects of narcotics are mediated by the limbic system, since this system is not associated with analgesia.[48-51]

A really fantastic breakthrough. You may be wondering, what are opiate receptors doing sitting around in the brain? Waiting for someone to discover opium? Hardly, and scientists know that the presence of an "opiate receptor" means that there must be a naturally occurring molecule with the same basic structure and effects as those of morphine. Everyone knew that this field was ripe for a Nobel Prize, and research activity and paper publication in this area became "the hottest growth industry in the neurosciences. . . ."[49]

The story is far from complete and there *are* conflicting data. Because information is published almost daily, things may change rapidly.[52] As of now, we know of at least two major opiate peptide systems in the brain. The molecules involved may function as neurotransmitters, hormones, or both—this is not yet clear. One system involves a molecule called β-endorphin (meaning "the morphin within"). This molecule is associated primarily with long axon neurons that interconnect the hypothalamus, the limbic system, and the medial thalamus. "the medial thalamic nuclei mediate poorly localized and emotionally influenced deep pain, the type that is best affected by opiates. Op-

iate receptor density is much greater in the medial than in the lateral thalamus."[53] The second opiate peptide system involves the enkephalins (meaning "in the head"), which are located in short axon neurons located throughout the central nervous system. The possibility certainly exists that these short-axon interneurons are primarily modulator neurons—and that the longer axon, β-endorphin, neurons primarily mediate euphoric/emotional components.[54,55] This separation of pain intensity and pain unpleasantness is in keeping with existing research and differential effects of some narcotics.[56]

There are many theories about how opiate tolerance, addiction, and withdrawal can be explained now that some pathways and mechanisms are beginning to unfold.[57] There may only be two opiate systems but the fact that there is reasonably good evidence, as of 1981, for at least five distinct opiate receptors[58] should make you cautious about accepting any of this material on the enkephalins, endorphins, and "brain opiates" as anything more than a comment at the quarter-mile in a 3-mile race! A 1981 report that alcohol, at appropriately low doses, selectively inhibits one of the five receptors (an enkephalin receptor) may develop into a link between alcohol use and effects and actions of the endogenous opioid system.[59] The role that these endogenous opiates may have in mental illness will be discussed and widely debated through the 1980s, but as of the mid-1980s there is no answer.[60] This summary is only a brief and simplified version of the complex problem of identifying and characterizing the opiate receptor and the actions and effects of the opioid systems.

There are still many unexplained effects of the opiates on brain biochemistry. Whether they will turn out to be incidental or critical cannot be answered. The effects are real, however, and may mediate some of the actions of morphine and similar agents. Serotonin, for example, is implicated in the action of morphine, since as tolerance develops, the synthesis, but not the accumulation, of serotonin doubles. Relevant also is the finding that a decrease in brain serotonin level increases the sensitivity of the animal to painful stimuli and decreases the analgesic effect of morphine. Noradrenaline and dopamine show an increase in release, synthesis, and turnover in the CNS following the administration of morphine. Narcotic administration also decreases the release of acetylcholine from neurons and increases brain levels of this neurotransmitter. These data on the neurotransmitters, when combined with other information, suggest that serotonin is in some way involved in the analgesic and sedative effects of morphine, whereas the euphoria and excitation are related to noradrenergic processes.

Work with protein synthesis inhibitors has made possible a separation of the analgesic effects and the development of tolerance. The protein synthesis inhibitors modify the metabolism of the neurons by preventing the building of proteins. These inhibitors do not affect the analgesic potency of morphine or similar compounds, but they do prevent tolerance. A possibility, then, is that an alteration in general neuronal metabolism is directly responsible for tolerance and physiological addiction but not analgesia.

Narcotic antagonists. The hypothesis of specific narcotic receptors fits with the fact that there are narcotic antagonists, drugs that specifically block the effects of a narcotic drug when given to an individual. Most investigators now believe that these drugs compete with the narcotic agents for the opiate receptor. The antagonists have two important characteristics. They have a greater affinity for the receptor site than do the narcotics, that is, they combine with, but do not initiate a response in, the receptor.

> Narcotic antagonists are capable of reversing effects such as analgesia, sedation, euphoria, gastrointestinal effects, and the frequently lethal respiratory depression caused by morphine and its surrogates. These antagonists are specific in that they will not reverse depression resulting from other classes of drugs such as barbiturates.[50]

There are two types of narcotic antagonists. One is the pure antagonists; naloxone (Narcan) and naltrexone are good examples of this group. These drugs do not produce any morphinelike effects, which makes them valuable drugs in clinical use.

The only significant effect naloxone has is to reverse the effects of a narcotic already in the individual. It is the drug of choice and is commonly used in emergency rooms to reverse the effects of a narcotic overdose.

The second group, the partial antagonists such as nalorphine (Nalline) and cyclazocine, are just that: they only partially antagonize the narcotic already in the system. When administered to an individual who is addicted to a narcotic, the partial antagonists do induce withdrawal symptoms. Because they have some narcotic-like effects, partial antagonists are not now used in emergency rooms. If they were administered incorrectly to an individual with barbiturate-induced respiratory depression, the partial antagonists would increase the depression. This cannot happen with naloxone. The partial antagonists have found some use in experimental programs for the treatment of addicts (see Chapter 16).

To summarize the actions of the narcotic antagonists briefly, they have a greater affinity than do the narcotic drugs for the narcotic receptor site.[51] They therefore will displace the narcotic drug at the receptor or prevent its combination with the receptor. Because of the much lower (or absence of) activity of the antagonist at this receptor, narcotic effects will greatly diminish if they are present or, with the partial antagonists, will appear only minimally if not already present.

THE NEXT FEW YEARS

The story of "The Brain's Own Opiates"[61] is exciting and represents a major breakthrough that will have scientific and therapeutic effects for many years to come. A major impact of this work is that it has helped to open the area of brain peptides— a field of probable great importance. The next big story in the field of opiates, however, will probably come from one of our old friends: heroin. In the late 1970s the U.S. government finally authorized an American research institute to begin studying the effectiveness of heroin (orally and intramuscularly) in the reduction of pain in terminal cancer patients. England has long used a "heroin cocktail" for terminal patients and has reported considerable success in easing cancer pain.[62] Interestingly, in spite of all the noise about the superior pain-reducing effectiveness of heroin compared to morphine, the data do not support the publicity, and neither do the biochemical facts. Heroin taken orally is transformed into morphine in the digestive system, and, when used in this manner, both drugs are equivalent in every way and equipotent in reducing pain. (Given intramuscularly or intravenously, heroin is about three times as potent as morphine.) The important thing, though, is that the enlightened attitude of the federal government—viewing heroin as a potential therapeutic agent and not just a drug of abuse—coupled with the public focusing on problems of the reduction of pain in the terminally ill may result in dramatic changes in the attitudes of physicians and patients about the pharmacological management of pain.[63] As noted earlier (Chapter 1) it's about time.

REFERENCES

1. Baum, L.F.: The new wizard of Oz, New York, 1944, Grosset & Dunlap, Inc.
2. Mintz, J., and others: Sexual problems of heroin addicts, Archives of General Psychiatry 31:700-703, 1974.
3. DeLeon, G., and Wexler, H.K.: Heroin addiction: its relation to sexual behavior and sexual experience, Journal of Abnormal Psychology 81(1):36-38, 1973.
4. Halper, S.C.: The heroin trade: from poppies to Peoria, Drug Abuse Council, 1975, U.S. Government Printing Office.
5. Kramer, J.C.: The opiates: two centuries of scientific study, Journal of Psychedelic Drugs 12:89, April-June 1980.
6. Sonnedecker, G.: Emergence of the concept of opiate addiction, Journal Mondial de Pharmacie; Federation Internationale Pharmaceutique 3:275-290, 1962; 1:27-34, 1963.
7. Poppy of perdition, MD, pp. 306-313, June 1965.
8. Scott, J.M.: The white poppy; a history of opium, New York, 1969, Funk & Wagnalls.
9. Africa, T.W.: The opium addiction of Marcus Aurelius, Journal of the History of Ideas 22:97-102, 1961.
10. Hamarneh, S.: Sources and development of Arabic medical therapy and pharmacology, Sudhoffs Archiv fur Geschichte der Medizin und der Naturwissenschaften 54:34, 1970.
11. De Quincey, T.: Confessions of an English opium-eater, New York, 1907, E.P. Dutton & Co., Inc.
12. Abrams, M.H.: The milk of paradise, Cambridge, Mass., 1934, Harvard University Press.
13. Lowes, J.L.: The road of Xanadu, Boston, 1927, Houghton Mifflin Co.
14. Ober, W.B.: Drowsed with the fume of poppies: opium and John Keats, Bulletin of the New York Academy of Medicine 44:862-881, 1968.
15. Hayter, A.: Opium and the Romantic imagination, Berkeley, Calif., 1970, University of California Press.
16. Turk, M.H.: Selections from De Quincey, Boston, 1902, Ginn & Co.
17. De Quincey works, vol. 206. Quoted in Lowes, J.L.: The road to Xanadu, Boston, 1927, Houghton Mifflin Co.
18. Baudelaire, C.: Les paradis artificiels, Paris, 1961, Le Club du Meilleur Livre.
19. Mickel, E.J.: The artificial paradises in French literature, Chapel Hill, N.C., 1969, The University of North Carolina.
20. Blair, W.: An opium-eater in America, The Knickerbocker (New York Monthly Magazine) 20:47-57, 1842.
21. Harrison, J.B.: The psychology of opium eating, The Journal of Psychological Medicine 7:240, 1854.
22. Hahn, E.: The big smoke, The New Yorker, pp. 35-43, February 15, 1969.
23. Kramer, J.C.: Opium rampant: medical use, misuse and abuse in Britain and the West in the 17th and 18th centuries, British Journal of Addiction, p. 377, 1979.
24. Fry, E.: China, England, and opium, Contemporary Review 27:447-459, 1876.
25. Fry, E.: China, England, and opium, Contemporary Review 30:1-10, 1877.
26. Fry, E.: China, England and opium, Contemporary Review 31:313-321, 1878.
27. Edwards, G.: Opium and after, Lancet 1(8164):351, February 16, 1980.
28. Kebler, L.F.: The present status of drug addiction in the United States. In Transactions of the American Therapeutic Society, Philadelphia, 1910, F.A. Davis Co.
29. Seevers, M.H.: Drug addiction problems, Sigma XI Quarterly 27(1):91-102, 1939.
30. Lindesmith, A.R.: Addiction and opiates, Chicago, 1968, Aldine Publishing Co.
31. Cook, J.G.: Remedies and rackets, New York, 1958, W.W. Norton & Co., Inc.
32. Holbrook, S.H.: The golden age of quackery, New York, 1959, The Macmillan Co.
33. Young, H.H.: The toadstool millionaires, Princeton, New Jersey, 1961, Princeton University Press.
34. Black, J.R.: Advantages of substituting the morphia habit for the incurably alcoholic, The Cincinnati Lancet—Clinic 22:538-541, 1889.
35. Lindesmith, A.R.: The addict and the law, Bloomington, 1965, Indiana University Press.
36. Simmons, C.: The standard cyclopedia of recipes, 1901 (How to make Dr. Pierce's Golden Medical Discovery), New York Times Magazine, p. 71, January 23, 1977.
37. Bassett, C.A., and Pawluk, R.J.: Blood-brain barrier: penetration of morphine codeine, heroin and methadone after carotid injection, Science 178:984-986, 1972.
38. Kramer, J.C.: Heroin in the treatment of morphine addiction, Journal of Psychedelic Drugs 9(3):193-197, 1977.

39. Dott, D.B., and Stockman, R.: Proceedings of the Royal Society of Edinburgh, p. 321, 1890.

40. Manges, M.: A second report on the therapeutics of heroine, New York Medical Journal **71**:51, 82-83, 1900.

41. Floeckinger, F.C.: Clinical observations on heroin and heroin hydrochloride as compared with codeine and morphine, New York Medical Journal **71**:970, 1900.

42. Wilcox, R.W.: Pharmacology and therapeutics, ed. 6, Philadelphia, 1905, P. Blakiston's Son & Co.

43. Eddy, N.B., and May, E.L.: The search for a better analgesic, Science **181**:407-414, 1973.

44. Jaffe, J.H., and Martin, W.R.: Narcotic analgesic and antagonists. In Goodman, L.S., and Gilman, A., editors: The pharmacological basis of therapeutics, ed. 5, New York, 1975, Macmillan Publishing Co., Inc.

45. Osol, A., Pratt, R., and Altschule, M.D., editors: The United States dispensatory and physician's pharmacology, ed. 26, Philadelphia, 1967, J.B. Lippincott Co.

46. Exploring the nature of heroin addiction, Medical World News, pp. 57-66, September 10, 1971.

47. Snyder, S.H.: Opiate receptors and internal opiates, Scientific American, pp. 44-56, March 1977.

48. Goldstein, A.: Opioids peptides (endorphins) in pituitary and brain, Science **193**:1081-1086, 1976.

49. Marx, J.L.: Neurobiology: researchers high on endogenous opiates, Science **193**:1227-1229, 1976.

50. Brown, J.K., and Malone, M.H., editors: Pacific Information Service on Street-Drugs **5**(1), May 1976. (Entire newsletter.)

51. Snyder, S.H., Pert, C.B., and Pasternak, G.W.: The opiate receptor, Annals of Internal Medicine **81**:534-540, 1974.

52. Bloom, F.E.: Neuropeptides, Scientific American **245**(4):148, 1981.

53. Snyder, S.H.: Opiate receptors in the brain, New England Journal of Medicine **296**:266-271, 1977.

54. Akil, H., and Watson, S.: Endorphins: basic science issues. In Pickens, R.W., anhd Heston, L.L., editors: Psychiatric factors in drug abuse, New York, 1979, Grune & Stratton, Inc.

55. Akil, H., and Watson, S.: Endorphins: clinical issues. In Pickens, R.W., and Heston, L.L., editors: Psychiatric factors in drug abuse, New York, 1979, Grune & Stratton, Inc.

56. Gracely, R.H., and others: Narcotic analgesia: fentanyl reduces the intensity but not the unpleasantness of painful tooth pulp sensations, Science **203**:1261-1263, March 23, 1979.

57. Simon, E.J.: Opiate receptors and endorphins: possible relevance to narcotic addiction. In Stimmel, B., editor: Advances in alcohol and substance abuse, vol. 1, no. 1, New York, Fall 1981, The Haworth Press.

58. Chang, K., and Cuatrecasas, P.: Heterogeneity and properties of opiate receptors, Federation Proceedings **40**(13):2729-2730, 1981.

59. Hiller, J.M., and others: Multiple opiate receptors: alcohol selectively inhibits binding to delta receptors, Science **214**:468, October 1981.

60. Check, W.A.: Endorphin-mental illness link far from proved, Medical News **247**(5):570, 1982.

61. Snyder, S.H.: The brain's own opiates, Chemical and Engineering News **55**(48):26-35, 1977.

62. Pietrusko, R.G.: Brompton's mixture: a re-evaluation, U.S. Pharmacist, p. 32, April 1981.

63. Holden, C.: New look at heroin could spur better medical use of narcotics, Science **198**:807-809, 1977.

CHAPTER 16

ILLEGAL NARCOTIC USE AND TREATMENT: TODAY AND TOMORROW

ABRIEF REVIEW MAY HELP in appreciating the changes that have taken place between 1850 and the present. Opium smoking always stayed out of the mainstream of American life.[1] The use of patent medicines containing opiates increased greatly during the period from 1850 to 1906, when the labeling requirements of the Pure Food and Drugs Act caused many preparations to be withdrawn. The individuals addicted to these medicines were primarily middle aged and female, rural as well as urban dwellers. In general they carried out their normal duties even though addicted. After 1906 many of these users switched to prescriptions from physicians or to opiate-containing medicines that were freely available from the druggist. There seems to be no general picture of the addict who used the hypodermic in this period, but many of these had apparently been introduced to the drug through a physician's treatment of an illness.

In 1908 Great Britain and China agreed to stop the importation of opium into China. At the time about 25% of the Chinese population were estimated to be intermittent opium smokers. President Theodore Roosevelt recognized that no single country could control its internal use of these drugs without some international regulations. To that end President Roosevelt called the First Opium Con-ference in 1909. By 1912 some agreements had been reached, and, in part, it was to honor and support the international commitments that the Harrison Narcotic Act was passed in 1914.[2,3] Appreciate, though, that the primary pressure for the Harrison Act was internal, not international. To clarify the discussion of our present situation in illegal narcotics use, the years between 1914 and the present have been divided into six stages.

STAGE ONE

The Harrison Act was a regulatory and revenue measure. As is true of most laws, it is not the law itself that becomes important in the ensuing years, but the court decisions and government regulations that evolve around the law.

The passing of the Harrison Act in 1914 left the status of the addict almost completely indeterminate. The Act did not make addiction illegal and it neither authorized nor forbade doctors to prescribe drugs regularly for addicts. All that it clearly and unequivocally did require was that whatever drugs addicts obtained were to be secured from physicians registered under the act and that the fact of securing drugs be made a matter of record. While some drug users had obtained supplies from physicians before 1914, it was not necessary for them to do so since drugs were available for purchase in pharmacies and even from mail-order houses.[2,p.5]

In 1915 the United States Supreme Court decided that possession of smuggled opiates was a crime, and thus users not obtaining the drug from a physician became criminals with the stroke of a pen. An addict could still obtain his supply of drugs on a prescription from a physician until this avenue was removed by the 1920 Webb and the 1922 Behrman Supreme Court decisions. The ruling in these cases prevented the prescribing of drugs to an addict unless he was institutionalized and the daily dose gradually decreased, that is, withdrawal initiated. Even though the Lindner case in 1925 reversed these earlier decisions and stated that a physician could prescribe drugs to a nonhospitalized addict just to maintain him, the doctors had been harassed and arrested enough. Though it was legal to prescribe drugs to an addict, few physicians would do so. Attempts in the early 1920s to maintain clinics for the treatment of opiate addicts failed for a number of reasons, including poor management and disapproval by law enforcement officials.

The oral opiate users began to decline after the Harrison Law was passed, and the primary remaining group were those who injected morphine or heroin. That has stayed true up to the present. By 1920, about the only source of opiates for a nonhospitalized addict was an illegal dealer. The cost through this source was 30 to 50 times the price of the same drug through legitimate sources, which no longer were available to the addict. As a consequence, then, of the 1914 law and the Supreme Court decisions in the early 1920s, the opiate user was forced to either stop using the drug or buy from an illegal dealer. To maintain a supply of the drug in this way was expensive. Many addicts resorted to criminal activity, primarily burglary and other crimes against property, to finance their addiction.[4-6]

During this period, law enforcement agencies and the popular press brought about a change in the attitudes of society toward the addict. Thus in the 1920s

the addict was no longer seen as a victim of drugs, an unfortunate with no place to turn and deserving of society's sympathy and help. He became instead a base, vile, degenerate who was weak and self-indulgent, who contaminated all he came in contact with and who deserved nothing short of condemnation and society's moral outrage and legal sanction. The law enforcement approach was accepted as the only workable solution to the problem of addiction.[1]

STAGE TWO

The change in the type of addict population in the United States from the 1920s to the 1970s is easier to specify than the number of addicts in this country after 1914. After the Harrison Act, there almost certainly was a decline in the number of addicts using opiates orally and thus a drop in white middle-aged users. One paper comments that between World War I and World War II heroin received little publicity and was primarily used by "people in *the life*—show people, entertainers and musicians; racketeers and gangsters; thieves and pickpockets; prostitutes and pimps."[7] The transition from the 1930s to the 1950s in the United States has been best described by an internationally recognized expert who worked in the area of drug addiction through this period.

If you go back to 1935 the other problems, apart from alcohol, were primarily the opiates and cocaine, usually taken together in the form of the so-called "speed-ball" and then as now . . . drug use was multiple. These individuals that I know used morphine, cocaine, heroin, bromides, phenobarbital or whatever happened to come along but they preferred the opiates and cocaine. The people of those days were really predominantly white individuals, they were on the whole members of various criminal trades, pickpockets and so on, and in fact most of them had been involved in these criminal trades either before or after their onset of their career of using drugs. These people more or less disappeared during the Second World War which practically made these drugs unavailable . . . the old fashioned addict, the expert pickpocket, the short change artist couldn't get drugs.

This group was succeeded, after the war was over, by a new kind of opiate taker. These were primarily individuals from the minority groups in the big city slums and in contrast to the older addicts who got good drugs, who knew good stuff when they got it, this new group were getting drugs extremely diluted, full of all kinds of other poisons and were a very different kind of people. They were not expert thieves, in fact very inexpert.[8,p.32]

STAGE THREE

In the early years after World War II heroin use slowly increased in the lower-class, slum areas of the large cities. Heroin was inexpensive in this period; a dollar would buy enough for a good high for three to six people; $2-a-day habits were real and not uncommon. As the fifties passed by, heroin use spread rapidly. Some authorities believe that it was increasing heroin use as much as anything else that removed the street gangs and their wars from city streets by the end of the decade. As demand increased, so did the price and the amount of adulteration.

STAGE FOUR

A brief summary of heroin use from 1940 to 1970 suggests that all rules changed in November 1961.[7] A critical shortage of heroin developed, prices tripled, and adulteration was carried to new heights. Since this increased profits, the price and adulteration level stayed the same when heroin was again in good supply. This article suggested that it was the large increase in price that disrupted the previous social cohesiveness among addicts, increased considerably the amount of crime, and contributed to the general social disorganization of the ghettos, where most addicts lived.

By the 1960s the use of heroin and other drugs skyrocketed. Flower children, hippies, Tim Leary, and LSD received most of the media attention, but within the central core of the large American cities the number of regular and irregular heroin users increased daily. As you might expect, mainstream

U.S.A. gradually became concerned with the heroin problem of the large cities. The increase in crime was the key, since most addicts were black or Latin, and the white majority saw little relevance of the addiction to their own personal, family, and social problems. What the man in the street didn't appreciate was that the young criminal population—both addicted and nonaddicted—was becoming increasingly non-white, meaning it wasn't just drugs that were involved. Of more interest perhaps is the report that among youthful offenders in the period from 1968 to 1972 "heroin addicts . . . were found to be older, better educated, and more intelligent than nonaddicts."[9,p.222] This agrees with other studies indicating that heroin addicts, since the mid-sixties, are not usually from the bottom rung of the social ladder.

STAGE FIVE

The attitude of the man in the street toward the relevance of addiction to his personal life changed rapidly with the reports that began to filter out of Southeast Asia toward the end of the 1960s. Public anxiety increased dramatically with the possibility that the Vietnam conflict might produce thousands of white middle-class addicts among the soldiers stationed there.

> It is ironic indeed that in the last two years of the war our biggest casualty figures will come from heroin addiction, not from combat.[10,p.18]

A replay of the Civil War and its aftermath (Chapter 2)? Read on and see.

The Department of Defense established a Task Force on Drug Abuse in 1967; initial reports emphasized concern over the widespread use of marijuana by troops in combat zones as well as in rest and rehabilitation areas. In 1970 public and federal concern began to focus on the problem of heroin addiction among service personnel stationed in Southeast Asia.[11]

Opium poppies grow widely in Burma, Laos, and Thailand in areas far removed from governmental control. It is estimated that these three countries produce about 1000 tons of opium each year—over half of the world's illegal production. Much of this is consumed as opium, but the available evidence indicates that the amount converted to heroin was increased as the demand for heroin increased among Americans in South Vietnam. Although the governments of these countries verbalized willingness to fight the illegal production of opium and heroin with American money, no realist expected that a significant impact could be made on such an excellent money crop. And none was.

Heroin was about 95% pure and almost openly sold in South Vietnam, whereas purity in the United States was about 5% in 1969. Not only was the Southeast Asia heroin undiluted, it was inexpensive. Ten dollars would buy about 250 mg, an amount that would cost over $500 in the United States. The high purity of the heroin made it possible to obtain psychological effects by smoking or sniffing the drug. This fact, coupled with the completely wrong belief that addiction occurs only when the drug is used intravenously, resulted in about 40% of the users sniffing, about half smoking, and only 10% mainlining their heroin.[10] An addict accustomed to sniffing heroin in Vietnam would be forced to inject the diluted United States drug to obtain the same effects.

Some early 1971 reports estimated that 10% to 15% of the American troops in Vietnam were addicted to heroin. As a result of the increased magnitude and visibility of the heroin problem, the U.S. government took several rapid steps in mid-1971. One step was to initiate Operation Golden Flow, a urine testing program for opiates in servicemen ready to leave Vietnam. The testing program, which tested *only* for opiates, was later expanded to include other American personnel.

As the result of the poor facilities and the speed with which the testing program was initiated, there were varied reports. In October 1971, the Pentagon released figures for the first 3 months of testing, which showed that 5.1% of the 100,000 servicemen tested showed traces of opiates in their urine. The Army had a higher incidence of users (6.4%) than either the Air Force (1.3%) or the Navy (1.7%), and most of the opiate users were concentrated in the lower ranks.

In July 1971, the Department of Defense made mandatory an amnesty program that held that if a drug user turned himself in for treatment, he would be placed in a rehabilitation program, retained in the service for his normal tour of duty, and not be given a less than honorable discharge on the basis of illegal drug use by itself. The amnesty program was later made retroactive, so that any veteran given a dishonorable discharge because of drug use could have his case reviewed and possibly changed to an honorable discharge.

In retrospect the Vietnam drug use situation was "making a mountain out of a molehill," but much was learned. An excellent follow-up study[12] of veterans who returned from Vietnam in September 1971 showed that most of the Vietnam heroin users did *not* continue heroin use in this country. Only 1% to 2% were using narcotics 8 to 12 months after returning from Vietnam and being released from the service, approximately the same percentage of individuals found to be using narcotics when examined for induction into the service. Although the emphasis—in 1971 and in this discussion—is on heroin, there is ample evidence for other drug use by American personnel in Vietnam. Approximate rates for use (*ever* used in Vietnam) were:

Alcohol	92%
Marijuana	69%
Opium	38%
Heroin	34%
Amphetamines	25%
Barbiturates	23%

One of the important things learned from the Southeast Asia caper was that narcotic addiction and compulsive use is *not* inevitable among occasional users. The pattern of drug use in Vietnam also supports the belief that under certain conditions—availability and low cost of the drug, boredom, unhappiness—there is a relatively high percentage of individuals who will use narcotic drugs recreationally.

There was considerable action on the home front in this period; the developing storm was chronicled in July 1969:

> Within the last decade, the abuse of drugs has grown from essentially a local police problem into a serious national threat to the personal health and safety of millions of Americans.[13]

Street crime increased, and bad (but incorrect) news kept coming from the drug scene in Vietnam. In June 1971 the president declared a "national emergency . . ." and asserted that "America's Public Enemy No. 1 is drug abuse."[14]

All fairy tales have happy endings (remember that when Snow White was drugged—in the apple!—by the queen, she was finally awakened by Prince Charming), and 1973 was the happy year for heroin.

> Can that really be a ray of light, shining faintly way down there at the end of the heroin-addiction tunnel? It can, it is, and it's getting brighter every minute . . .[15]
>
> As far as heroin is concerned, the worst is over.[16]

STAGE SIX

One thing you may not remember from your childhood is that all fairy tales have sequels; they don't get published because they usually aren't happy. We are now living in the sequel to the heroin story of stage five. It didn't take long for the honeymoon to end. In 1974, "gov't indicators of heroin use on upswing again . . ."[17] By 1976, "the trend is now for a worsening situation in heroin abuse."[18] In 1981, "federal monitoring systems show heroin at new epidemic levels."[19] There is one bright spot, however; government officials are beginning to appreciate what by now should be apparent to you: drug use or misuse never goes away. Sooner or later it becomes acculturated and institutionalized, and we worry about it less. In April 1976 at a drug abuse symposium on National Issues and Strategies, the director of the National Institute on Drug Abuse[20] said:

The major lesson we have learned these past few years is that the drug abuse problem will not go away. But, for most of us, the idea that we are going to wage a war on drugs and someday be able to declare a victory has gone away. Drug abuse prevention, like the nurturing of a garden, requires constant attention.

ADDICTIVE AND WITHDRAWAL PROCESSES

> Addiction is a unique symptom in medicine. It is a symptom of comfort rather than discomfort, providing relief from emotional as well as physical pain. Its comfort goes even further by lessening the tensions of psychic and biologic drives.[21]

Addiction to a drug is more than a habit of regularly using a drug. The term *addiction* is restricted to conditions where physiological symptoms occur when the regular use of the drug is discontinued. The evidence is clear that addiction can occur to alcohol, the barbiturates, the antianxiety agents, and the opiates. These are all depressant drugs. The evidence is still debated as to whether addiction can occur to stimulant drugs.

Some writers feel that addiction should be defined as a personal and social concept rather than a biomedical one. In such a definition, addiction includes recognition by the individual that the physical symptoms he is experiencing are caused by a low level of the drug in the body and that he must take steps to correct the situation.

> One can only be addicted when he experiences physiological withdrawal symptoms, recognizes them as due to a need for drugs, and relieves them by taking another dose. The crucial step of recognition is most likely to occur when the user participates in a culture in which the signs of withdrawal are interpreted for what they are. When a person is ignorant of the nature of withdrawal sickness, and has some other cause to which he can attribute his discomfort (such as a medical problem), he may misinterpret the symptoms and thus escape addiction. . . .[22]

Such an explanation is offered for why hospitalized patients can receive large doses of morphine regularly without showing drug-seeking behavior after the drug is stopped.

Addiction to a drug is characterized by three features: a tendency to increase the dose (since tolerance occurs); appearance of physiological changes when drug use is discontinued (withdrawal symptoms develop); and a strong desire to continue taking the drug, frequently stronger than any other desire the addict has known. One article states: "In susceptible persons they [narcotics] produce a pathological hunger of such intensity that the drive for narcotics displaces all other responsibilities."[23]

Still not resolved is the basis for the "pathological hunger." There are two basic positions.[24] One is that the primary drive is euphoria.

> The primacy of euphoria, as asserted by the addict, is central to the elaboration of addiction. The addict seeks to limit tolerance and avoid abstinence, but he also urgently demands the recovery of his capacity for the "high."[25]

The other point of view holds that avoidance of withdrawal is fundamental.

> The hook in addiction arises, not from the euphoria which the drug initially produces, but from the beginner's realization that the discomfort and misery of withdrawal is caused by the absence of the drug and can be dispelled almost magically by another dose of it. [26,pp.73-74]

Neither theory is complete. One study[27] indicates that addicts who can afford it always go for the euphoria. Those who work primarily to avoid withdrawal are less adept at hustling on the street.

The middle ground presented here suggests (1) learning to be an addict is a separate and distinct stage from being an addict, (2) learning to be an addict can result from either an approach to pleasure or an escape from discomfort, (3) being an addict has multiple motivations and rewards, and (4) the same nonspecific factors that help determine other forms of drug taking operate in addiction.

It has been suggested that becoming and staying an addict are separate stages. The acquisition of addiction requires some steady behavior on the part of the individual. It seems clear that the behavior in this initial stage is maintained either by the delivery of positive feelings or the reduction of unpleasant feelings. Some individuals probably persist in the use of the drug for one reason, some for the other, and a third group for a combination of the reasons. It seems meaningless to look for a single type of individual who is susceptible to heroin addiction.

In the second stage of use of the opiates, the individual acquires an additional motivation for using the drug. No longer is he only looking for pleasure or to decrease the tensions and stresses of his nondrug life. This stage is marked by the clear development of withdrawal symptoms when the drug level in the body drops too low. It is at this stage that the behavior of the addict becomes truly routinized. The drug-taking behavior becomes very closely and directly tied to the removal of specific symptoms. The regularity of drug use is no doubt controlled by the appearance of withdrawal symptoms. The amount of drug used is probably related to the positive pleasure it delivers, since usually much lower doses, or doses taken orally, would be adequate to prevent withdrawal discomfort.

Misconceptions and preconceptions

There has been so much written in the popular press about heroin use and heroin users that readers may believe that they know enough about it. This section deals with some of the major misconceptions most people, including many professionals, have about nonmedical use and misuse of narcotics. One of the most common is that mainlining heroin or morphine induces in everyone an intense pleasure unequaled by any other experience. Addicts talk in glowing terms of the "rush" or "kick" they frequently experience.[28] Often it is described as similar to a whole-body orgasm that persists up to 5 or more minutes. Some addicts report that they try with every injection to reexperience the extreme euphoria of the first injection, but they always have a lesser effect. There are studies, however, as well as clinical and street reports, that some people experience only nausea and discomfort following the initial intravenous administration of morphine or heroin.[29] For whatever reasons, some of these users persist and the discomfort decreases, that is, shows tolerance more rapidly than the euphoric effects. Under these conditions the injections soon result primarily in pleasant effects. To maintain these pleasurable feelings, though, the dose level must gradually be increased. There is no resolution of what type of individual—socially, psychologically, or biochemically—readily experiences pleasure in contrast to those whose initial symptoms are unpleasant.[30] It is true, however, that even with the narcotics some addicts must partially learn which experiences are defined as pleasurable.[31,32] There are other points of view and other sets of data. One author[33] has referred to the two "powerfully pleasurable effects"—the initial brief rush and then the longer tranquility—and then commented:

> This sequence of events occurs with virtually every nontolerant person, although the first few experiences may be accompanied by vomiting. Even so, the sensations are often pleasurable ("You don't mind vomiting behind smack").

Another misconception has to do with the development of withdrawal symptoms. The addict undergoing withdrawal without medication is always portrayed as being in excruciating pain, truly suffering. It depends. With a large habit, withdrawal without medication is truly hell. The opiate addiction scene is changing too rapidly to be definite about today's user, but most addicts of the 1960s and 1970s are described as having "ice cream habits," that is, they use a low daily drug dose. That may change in the mid-1980s but it's doubtful. High purity—90% pure—Persian heroin was available in the United States from 1981 to 1982 but what usually happens is that as the demand goes up, the purity goes down. Keep checking it—if purity stays high and the users don't kill themselves with it, withdrawal will be *very* bad and *very* hard.

Perhaps the most common misconception about

heroin is that after one shot, you are hooked for life. None of the narcotics, or any other drug, fits into that fantasized category. Becoming addicted takes some time, perhaps a week, and persistence on the part of a beginner. Regular use of the drug seems to be more important in establishing physiological addition that the size of the dose used. Becoming physiologically addicted is possible on a weekend, but it frequently requires a longer period with three or four injections a day.[34]

The evidence on this point has been around for a long time, even before the heroin users in Vietnam proved it again, but it is still not accepted by most people. There is much talk, discussion, and disagreement among the experts[35] but there are probably about 500,000 narcotic addicts in the United States. There may be two to three times as many heroin *chippers*—occasional users. Several reports and studies have appeared on the characteristics of these occasional users, but no consistent differences, compared to addicts, have yet been found other than the pattern of use. One review of this topic contains several case histories, and you must appreciate that there are no "typical" chippers, but Arthur D. is representative.

> Arthur D. is a forty-year-old white male with a wife and three children who works regularly as a union carpenter. He has no family history of alcoholism or drug dependency.
> Drug use began with occasional marijuana use at age sixteen, which became daily use by age eighteen. By nineteen he had stopped his heavy drinking though he continued regular marijuana use, which included some dealing in marijuana. For about one and a half years from ages twenty to twenty-two he experimented with psychedelics, and for two years from ages twenty-one to twenty-three he used amphetamines with some frequency.
> Mr. D. first used heroin at age twenty-four. He used it sporadically for two years, but with growing frequency, until at age twenty-seven he recognized that he had a habit. He was married at age thirty-two to a woman who disapproved of his use of narcotics in particular and of drugs in general. Although his drug use had sharply decreased, it never ceased. For the last ten years his use of heroin has been confined to weekends, with an occasional

shot during the week. For the last five years, however, this occasional "extra" shot has virtually ceased. His wife does not use heroin at all but will smoke marijuana with him occasionally. As a result of her disapproval of his drug use and the people with whom he uses drugs, on almost every weekend he will select a time to go to a using friend's home and get high there.[36,p.10]

A fairly common misconception that rises to the surface every once in a while is that you do not become addicted to heroin, morphine, or any narcotic if you don't inject it intravenously. You should know by now that this is not true—it is the physiological-pharmacological action of the drug that can lead to the development of tolerance and addiction. The amount and regularity of use are the important factors in addiction and they determine the strength of the withdrawal effects when drug use is stopped. At a given dose level the euphoria depends on how rapidly the drug enters the brain. Similar effects can thus be obtained using the drug intravenously or by smoking it (smoking if the heroin is at very high purity). *Whether you smoke it, chip it, shoot it, or drink it—all the narcotics are addicting.*

The final misconception to be discussed is the belief that "it can't happen to me"—you've got to be weird or something to become addicted to heroin. In fact, environmental and peer pressures are probably more important than personality. Some experts strongly disagree[37] and believe that addicts do have a constitutional predisposition to addiction.

One study[38] of heroin and nonheroin users concluded that "results did not support interpretations that predisposing personality features contribute to compulsive drug use." Another report compared heroin users to delinquents, psychiatric patients, college undergraduates, and police officers.

> The results suggested that the heroin users were relatively normal in terms of social poise and self-esteem; however, they were significantly more hostile, rebellious, and irresponsible. . . . The addicts seemed relatively well adjusted, suggesting that their drug use is symptomatic not of neurosis but of a generalized antisocial disposition.[39]

Much the same thing was said in 1943[40] when the narcotic addict was described as "an inadequately adjusted individual, not radically different from his non-addicted fellows." Although the search for unique personality differences in the heroin addict will doubtless continue, you have to agree that "further search for the 'addictive personality' would be a less than profitable venture."[41]

Conditioning, addiction, and withdrawal

A very powerful process is at work throughout the entire process of learning to be an addict and unlearning it. Each drug administration is followed by a decrease in discomfort, an increase in pleasure, or both. As a result, the behavior itself of preparing and injecting the drug and the setting in which it occurs acquire pleasurable, positive associations through learning mechanisms. Because of this conditioning, the *process of using* heroin becomes rewarding as well as the *use* of heroin. One occasional user commented on the ritual of heroin use:

> Once you decide to get off it's very exciting. It really is. Getting some friends together and some money, copping, deciding where you're going to do it, getting the needles out and sterilizing them, cooking up the stuff, tying off, then the whole thing with the needle, booting, and the rush, that's all part of it. . . . Sometimes I think that if I just shot water I'd enjoy it as much.[34]

Perhaps strangely to the reader, that last statement is true for some individuals who label themselves "addicts." Things aren't always what they seem to be. One out of five individuals who apply for treatment in one large city center is clearly not physically dependent: they show *no* response to a narcotic antagonist. Another 15% to 20% show only "a very mild reaction to a large naloxone injection. . . ."[44,p.35] These individuals have been called "needle freaks"—they are psychologically dependent on shooting up and may or may not be physiologically dependent on the drug.

The heroin addict of today is very different from the addicts we saw ten years ago. We've seen an evolution of drug-taking patterns during the time we've been involved—from the "Aquarian Age junkie," as we call them, through the "Nixon Era junky," the transitional junky, to a new and extremely different group. . . .

This new junkie is not a true heroin addict. There will be needle marks all over him, he may have abscesses, but upon testing you will find that he is not truly addicted.[45]

A research team headed by a psychiatrist, Charles O'Brien, has studied the process of eliminating (extinguishing) the needle habit. A long-acting, experimental narcotic antagonist was administered and the patients allowed to shoot up, using their own equipment and rituals. Since most addicts usually shoot up in a bathroom, the researchers used a special bathroom where the patients could inject their drugs. Under double-blind conditions the users injected saline or a high or low dose of a narcotic. No matter which he used, there was no effect because of the administration of the antagonist. Both objective and subjective measures were used, and "all of the self-injections are rated by the patients as pleasurable at first"[44,p.36] Only after 3 to 5 injections were the subjective reports neutral. Continued self-injections under these conditions resulted in the patients reporting that they hated the whole process. Remember always that there is variability in any biological system: one patient continued to report euphoria after each injection for 26 trials, and he regularly showed the pupillary constriction that accompanies the injection of a narcotic! That patient was one of those receiving saline, so it was not a question of the narcotic dose being high or the antagonist dose being low.

This same research group showed that the subjective *and* physiological manifestation of withdrawal from narcotics could also easily be conditioned.[46] The withdrawal syndrome resulting from the administration of the narcotic antagonist, naloxone, was associated with a sound and odor stimulus. Later presentation of the sound and odor elicited the withdrawal reaction even in the absence

of the narcotic antagonist. The authors concluded: "These data support clinical anecdotes of withdrawal symptoms occurring in former addicts when they return to their drug-related environment." Earlier work with animals supports and complements these results and conclusions.[47]

Since many individuals who have been labeled as addicts use only low daily drug doses, and another group may not use any narcotic on a regular basis, some hospitals provide no medication during withdrawal. Other hospitals operate on the assumption that if the individual expresses discomfort, it should be relieved. The American Medical Association has stated that:

Abrupt, untreated, complete withdrawal ("cold turkey") as routine "treatment" is inhumane, unnecessary, and distinctly contraindicated, even if the patient is in jail[48]

Researchers at the NIMH Addiction Research Center in Lexington were able to differentiate between symptoms that appeared during withdrawal as a function of the level of the addiction.

Physical illness, tension, worry, dysphoria, insomnia, poor cognitive and social efficiency, loss of sense of humor, and a feeling of subjective need for the drug of choice characterize some of the common symptoms for weak and strong withdrawal. Symptoms such as goose pimples, hot and cold spells, sweating, watering eyes, difficulty in movement, cramps, and yawning are more common during strong opiate withdrawal.[49]

Some professionals working in this area will label as addicted only those individuals who show at least two of these four symptoms—chills, stomach cramps, insomnia, muscle pain—lasting over 2 days. The experience of the withdrawal syndrome from even a small habit (such as 60 mg of morphine per day) can be very uncomfortable. It is probably true, however, that the amount of withdrawal discomfort from small habits depends to a considerable degree on the attitude, personality, and other characteristics of the individual. The actual intensity of the symptoms, however, is directly related to the daily dose of the drug. One ex-addict described his withdrawal from a moderate habit. "Re-

TABLE 16-1 Sequence of appearance of some of the abstinence syndrome symptoms

Signs	Approximate hours after last dose	
	Heroin and/or morphine	**Methadone**
Craving for drugs, anxiety	6	24
Yawning, perspiration, running nose, teary eyes	14	34 to 48
Increase in above signs plus pupil dilation, goose bumps (piloerection), tremors (muscle twitches), hot and cold flashes, aching bones and muscles, loss of appetite	16	48 to 72
Increased intensity of above, plus insomnia; raised blood pressure; increased temperature, pulse rate, respiratory rate and depth; restlessness; nausea	24 to 36	
Increased intensity of above, plus curled-up position, vomiting, diarrhea, weight loss, spontaneous ejaculation or orgasm, hemoconcentration, increased blood sugar	36 to 48	

member when you had a bad case of the 24-hour virus. You're coming out both ends—vomiting and diarrhea—and every joint in your body hurts. You wish you could die but feel too badly to do anything about it. Take that, double it, and spread it over 4 or 5 days. That's cold turkey." (Cold turkey because the goose bumps that occur in abrupt withdrawal resemble a plucked turkey.)

The sequence of appearance of some of the abstinence syndrome symptoms are included in Table 16-1 along with the time of their appearance after the last dose of the indicated drugs.[50,51] In general, the longer it takes for the initial symptoms to develop, the less intense the withdrawal effects will be. The muscle twitches appearing about 12 hours after the last dose of heroin are primarily in the legs and feet and increase in intensity over the next day or so. The foot twitches are particularly severe and are the basis for the phrase "kicking the habit."

Only the drug-centered bases for addiction have been mentioned. The addict lives, however, in a heroin-centered subculture that provides support for his behavior and the means and opportunity to engage in drug-taking behavior. All three factors—drug, individual, and setting—contribute to making an addict. This has been convincingly demonstrated with animals as well.

Two brief points will close this section. One deals with the 4- to 6-hour period between the possible euphoria of the injection and the beginning of withdrawal signs. The effects will vary. Some addicts report that all drives feel satisfied: sex, hunger, aggression. These feelings are muted to the point where they no longer cause anxiety. Anxiety and stresses from other sources also diminish into nothing, as does any physical pain the individual may have. In other addicted individuals these drives are not blunted at all, and they continue without change. For this 4 to 8 hours heroin acts as the perfect tranquilizer for some chronic users.[52] If the dose is correct, the individual is able to function well in a job; many addicts, however, do as little as possible for a large portion of this interval.[53]

The second point follows from the previous one but also expands the idea. There is nothing in the drug or the addiction processs itself to prevent a controlled addict (one whose dosage is carefully adjusted to the appropriate level) from working normally. Neither are there any necessary negative physiological or medical effects from heroin or being addicted. The usual medical and vocational problems that are correctly associated with opiate addiction today stem neither from the drug nor from its regular use but from the drug delivery system and the subculture that surrounds this illegal drug use. Many physicians and other biomedical people become addicted and continue their normal activities for years. Physicians have a high addiction rate, 1% or 2%, compared to the general population.[54,55]

PRODUCTION AND DELIVERY OF OPIATES TO THE UNITED STATES

Around the world the pattern of opium poppy growing regularly shifts, sometimes because of the United States, sometimes in spite of it. With respect to this country's handling of illegal opium production, Shakespeare had a title for it: either *A Comedy of Errors* or *Much Ado About Nothing*. Throughout this section, keep one thing in mind: anytime there is a demand for anything, you can find someone to supply it—at a price. As the world turns in these days of our lives and we search for tomorrow, the guiding light of the young and the restless is that with one life to live they look for another world—and sometimes end in a general hospital, cared for by the doctors. Only by decreasing demand will production and supply decrease.

Background

Opium use for legal purposes has been increasing gradually and in 1980 the amount produced for medical purposes was estimated at 1,756,227 kg. To have it delivered to you in New York City it would have cost then about $125 per kilogram—a four-fold increase from the early seventies. This is opium with a 10% morphine base. Converted to heroin the kilo of opium would have sold on the street for *$1 to $2 a milligram*. (There's a slight markup!) Although use increased, production of legal opium in the 1960s decreased each year, and there were shortages. Production expanded in the seventies and now can easily match medical needs and can also permit countries to replenish stockpiles of medicinal opium necessary to offset disruption of supplies and/or large increases in need, as in war. It is estimated that the United States uses about 60,000 kg of opium a year—most of it for the production of codeine.

Until 1972, most of the world's opium, 1500 to 2000 tons a year, was grown by three countries: India, Russia, and Turkey. India produced about 70% of the total, Russia 15%, Turkey only 9%, and Iran a very small amount. Concern over adequate opium for medical use led the French government to encourage the cultivation of opium poppies in the Loire Valley, Yugoslavia to increase its opium production four-fold, and Australia to grow opium for its own use. India had, and still has, the best system in the world for paying its over 200,000 poppy farmers. The more opium a farmer produces from his land, the more he is paid for each kilogram. The system encourages a high yield per acre and also rewards putting all of the opium crop into legal channels, since the more the farmer sells legally, the more he gets for each kilogram. Not so in Turkey in the 1960s and up to 1972, and that was *part* of the problem.

The French connection

Prior to 1973, 1 kg of legal opium yielded about $10 to the Turkish farmer. Temptation was great, since the same amount sold illegally for three times as much.[56] Many farmers grew extra poppies just for the illegal market and in 1970 at least 60 tons of Turkish opium were sold illegally. Illegal opium is converted to its primary active ingredient, morphine. This relatively simple chemical procedure reduces the bulk by 90% without losing any pharmacological activity.

Changing 10 kg of opium worth $300 into 1 kg of morphine increased its value to $500. Delivery to the contact in southern France doubled the value of the kilogram of morphine. At this stage the morphine was converted to heroin, which is about three times as potent as morphine. This is a more sophisticated technique and requires some chemical expertise. There is little change in the bulk when the morphine is transformed to heroin, but the appearance changes from the light fluffy powder of morphine to the crystal-like form of heroin.

The kilogram of heroin was worth $4,000 to $6,000 in France and $10,000 to $15,000 delivered to the United States. It was then sold to distributors who paid $30,000 to $40,000 for the heroin, mixed it with milk sugar or quinine, and sold small amounts to street dealers. The dealers adulterated the drug still more so that a user might pay $5 for a bag containing 2 to 50 mg of heroin. The dilution was so great that a kilogram of heroin sold at the street level might retail for a half million dollars, $300 of which was received by the farmer in Turkey. It was estimated that organized crime took in over $2 billion a year from the illegal narcotic trade. Clearly there is money to be made in illegal opiate traffic.

Until 1973 about 80% of the 5000 to 8000 kg of illegal heroin entering the United States originated in the poppy fields of Turkey and was delivered here by way of the French connection in Marseilles. It must have seemed easy to the American officials: cooperate with and partially fund the French police drive to break the French connection and get the Turkish government to eliminate the cultivation of poppies. Do those two things, and Shazam! The heroin problem will go away.

Much arm twisting and international diplomacy did in fact eliminate the morphine-to-heroin laboratories in southern France and banned poppy growing in Turkey. In June 1971, the government of Turkey announced: "ALL OPIUM cultivation and production throughout Turkey will be banned by the end of the Fall, 1972, definitely and totally." In return for this action the United States agreed to give $35 million to the poppy farmers and their government for their financial loss and to help develop new crops.[57-59]

The decision to ban a cash crop, even though part of the cash received was illegal, was not well loved in Turkey. The agitation of the farmers there, plus the fact that the world shortage of opium led the United States to encourage India to grow *more* opium, plus the fact that the United States was thinking about growing its own poppies resulted in both Turkish political parties advocating the return of poppy growing. In July 1974, over American protests Turkey announced that the ban against opium poppy cultivation was abolished! The sojourn into the domestic affairs of Turkey was, in one sense, not completely lost: the present method

of harvesting is technologically advanced compared to the lancing of the poppy bud. It is also mundane. The "poppy straw" method involves leaving the poppy plant in the field to dry, and the farmer delivers unlanced poppy pods to the government station. By drying, no opium is produced, and morphine and codeine are extracted from the total plant material without going through the opium stage. On no more that 1.27 acres each, 90,000 farmers were licensed by the government to grow and harvest poppies in this way. Their chances for big money are over for now, anyway.

With the closing of the poppy fields in Turkey in 1972, there were two expectations in this country: the optimists hoped that heroin supplies would dry up on the street and send the addicts running for treatment programs. In fact, for a brief period in 1973 heroin *was* in short supply on the streets of New York, but it was not a prolonged shortage and did not have any significant impact. The pessimists expected that the Golden Triangle of Southeast Asia—Burma, Laos, and Thailand, which produces more than half the world's illicit opium, mostly for home use—would step in and flood the country with heroin marked MADE IN ASIA. The pessimists were wrong too, and that is most unfortunate.

Mexican brown

In 1972 only about 40% of the heroin in this country was produced in Mexico, and its distribution was mostly in the West and Southwest. By 1975 the Drug Enforcement Administration could support its statement that 80% to 90% of all the heroin in this country was brown heroin from Mexico. The Mexican connection was much easier for the traffickers and tougher for the enforcers than the French connection: there are 2000 miles of border between the United States and Mexico, as well as many miles of easily accessible coastline.

The opium poppy can grow almost anywhere at moderate altitudes in the Sierra Madre mountains. The greater profit from opium has led to the growing of poppies rather than marijuana, although there is plenty of room for both. Part of the problem is that poppy growing is so lucrative that it is worthwhile to plant poppy plants almost anywhere they will grow—and the Mexicans do just that. As an example, in 1977 70,800 fields covering 32,700 acres were destroyed, in 1978 33,400 fields in 8200 acres, and in 1979 28,180 fields in 3700 acres. Each "field" was about one eighth of an acre! City slickers should remember that a football field is about 1$\frac{1}{10}$ acres.

The Mexicans harvest opium in the traditional Turkish way; each acre yields about 8 kg of opium, and there are two crops a year. Mexican heroin is brown because of the method used to process the opium, not as a result of impurities. Morphine hydrochloride rather than morphine base is the starting point for brown heroin.

The Mexican government requested assistance from the United States in 1974 in stemming the heroin growth industry. Cooperation between the governments has mostly been excellent but the task is one that would have frustrated Sisyphus. Even with the use of herbicides sprayed from the air, spy satellites, and multifilter photographs from NASA to locate opium fields, the job of eradicating the poppies in Mexico seems hopeless.[60] A congressional committee reported in April 1977 that the flow of narcotics into the United States from Mexico is "almost entirely out of control. . . ."[61] Not quite. Pressure on the poppy growers had some impact: in 1980 only about 35% of the heroin in the United States was the distinctive brown of Mexican mud.[62]

Even if the poppy population of Mexico could be eliminated without poisoning the countryside with chemicals or requiring the entire federal budget of Mexico, so what? As one official put it, "The heroin market abhors a vacuum." There are individuals in many countries who would love to get a piece of the American heroin action.

TODAY AND TOMORROW

Moving into the 1980s, the United States has a bigger heroin use and antinarcotic law enforcement problem than it has ever had. As has been hinted, most of it is our own fault. We need to talk about

it a little. Some terms and a review will help you be *in*, as well as help you understand the size of the problem.

Three countries in Southeast Asia have common borders and are called the Golden Triangle. The Golden Triangle consists of Laos, which produces 70 metric tons per year of opium for illegal sale, Burma, which produces 350 metric tons per year, and Thailand, which produces 70 metric tons per year. There is an area in Southwest Asia where three countries form what is called the Golden Crescent. These three countries are Iran, Afghanistan, and Pakistan. Together they produced 1600 metric tons of opium for illegal sale in 1980. In the mid-seventies Mexico supplied about 10 metric tons of illegal opium to the United States. That's probably down to 1 to 2 tons in the early 1980s. Before Turkey closed down in the early 1970s it produced about 70 tons of illegal opium, destined to arrive in the U.S.A. after processing. Oh yes, one more thing—the best estimate is that 150 metric tons of opium could meet the needs of all the world's narcotic addicts!

The pessimists of 1972 were right after all. A large part of the heroin now entering this country comes from the Golden Triangle. Even when countries try to do the right thing, there are problems. In Burma, in 1973, there was a sharp increase in the number of middle- and upper-class youths addicted to heroin so the government decided to increase enforcement against opium cultivation and smuggling (a la San Francisco in 1875). In 1977 the headline was: "Burma Reports Gain in its War on Opium."[63] The amount of opium produced had dropped from 450 tons in 1974-1975 to 250 tons in 1976-1977. In 1979 the headline was: "Burma Fights Growing Domestic Heroin Addiction."[64] The concern was over their 30,000 registered addicts and 100,000 users—including high school and university graduates. The 1980 headline: "A Treasure in Opium Poppies is Ripe for the Plucking in Golden Triangle."[65] The story was of a bumper crop—700 tons!

Another problem is that in the mountains of the Golden Triangle, everyone—well, almost everyone—smokes opium and grows their own. The Laotian government has been trying to eliminate that activity with American money, but with little success. An American training center in Laos flies tribesmen in "at great expense" and teaches them about the evil heroin does in the United States, gives them seeds to grow other crops, and flies them back to their home territory. Even my mother knows how successful *that* program will be. After a year and a half of operation, the center had trained 235 of some 15,000 tribesmen.[66]

Having succeeded (did I write that?) in Burma and Laos, the American juggernaut moves on. October 1981: "Yielding to U.S., Thais Target Opium Fields."[67] It's so bad. The Thai official in charge of it all says, "I'm not terribly happy about this action," to destroy opium fields in 10 of the 260 opium-growing villages but it would be, "a warning to others that this time we really mean business." Ha! And the top narcotic man in the U.S. Department of State told Thai officials that the United States could probably come up with a great deal more money for Thailand's war on narcotics if destruction took place! Yankee ingenuity triumphs again—pour money on a problem, that solves it.

It's no different in the Golden Crescent. An early 1977 report from Pakistan starts with the sentence, "American narcotics agents are worried that Pakistan may someday become a major source of heroin for the American market."[68] The Pakistan government outlawed *all* opium poppy growing in 1979. The 1980 headline: "Curbs by Pakistan Don't Halt Heroin."[69] The 1981 headline: "Heroin Output up in Pakistan Area."[70] What's a poor farmer to do? Poppy cultivation brings the farmer ten times as much as the next most profitable crop. If 150 metric tons of opium will feed the habits of all the world's addicts for a year, and if Southwest Asia produces 1600 metric tons in 1979[71] (and Southeast Asia 700 tons), and if only about 20% of American heroin comes from Southwest Asia, then the question is—what do you do with all of that opium/heroin?

You know. It's going where there are customers with money, and all the guys with the black hats are rising up again. From the story headlines of the pages of the New York Times:

> "Fast-Rising Heroin Addiction is Afflicting Western Europe" (October 30, 1977)
> "Rising Wave of Narcotic-Related Deaths Prompts West Berlin Government to Start Drug Program" (January 9, 1978)
> "West Germany Now Discovers a Deadly Monkey on its Back" (October 21, 1979)
> "Increase in Availability of Heroin Brings Drug Epidemic to Europe" (November 11, 1979)
> "Mideast Heroin Flooding Europe" (January 11, 1980)
> "New Heroin Flow Helping Revive the French Connection" (January 12, 1980)
> "Its Poppy Crop Curbed, Turkey Becomes Drug Conduit" (May 11, 1980)
> "Yugoslavs Alarmed by Sharp Rise in Drug Use" (October 4, 1981)

You're not surprised are you? Sad, sorry . . . but not surprised. Not only would you try to get new customers in areas where there's little competition—Europe—maybe you'd try to win some customers from your competitors. To do that you need to offer a better product! Up to 92% pure.[72] Usually no more than 15% to 20% pure, Persian heroin is fighting Mexican mud and Southeast Asia heroin for the market in America. And it *is* causing problems. From 1981: "Statistics Suggest U.S. Faces New Drug Abuse Problems"—the story talks of potent heroin, high-grade heroin, and the increase in emergency room heroin treatment and heroin deaths.[73]

Maybe there *is* a light at the end of the tunnel: "After more than 15 years of trying to develop ways to fight the influx and distribution of heroin in the United States, law enforcement officials say that their efforts are still not succeeding and that in some parts of the country, especially New York, the problem is worse than ever . . . only 2 to 5 percent is being kept from distribution channels" (1981).[74] The light is probably Tinkerbell. Do you believe in fairies?

A last note. The chase may be just about over. In May 1980 scientists reported that bacteria had been developed that produce large quantities of β-endorphin, a morphinelike hormone found in the brain.[75] I don't know about you, but the cops-and-robbers story of today's illegal opium trade is a lot more interesting to me than "who's got the test tube."

STREET USE

Only a glimpse of some of the mechanics of a heroin user's life can be presented here. Withdrawal signs may begin about 4 hours after the last use of the drug, but many addicts report that they begin to feel ill only 6 to 8 hours after the last dose. That puts most addicts on a schedule of 3 to 4 injections a day. Today's addict is not spending a lot of time nodding off in opium dens as in the good old days. When you have a very important appointment to keep every 6 to 8 hours, every day of the week, every day of the year, you've got to hustle not to miss one of them. Remember, there are no vacations, no weekends off for the regular user, just 1200 to 1400 appointments to keep.

And each one costs money. Heroin is frequently sold on the street in "nickel or dime" bags: $5 or $10 for a small plastic bag containing . . . Good question—what's in the bag? In 1970-1971 the material in a $5 bag might have had 3 to 5 mg of heroin. In some areas you can buy "slop dope" a little cheaper, but it contains only 1 to 2 mg of heroin. Of course, you may not get any heroin. This continually varies, but 1974 purchases in New York, Chicago, Detroit, and Los Angeles had no heroin in 3%, 0%, 7%, and 2% of the buys, and you can't complain to the Better Business Bureau. At any rate, your addiction may cost you $20 to $100 a day.

It is of some interest to note the changes in price and purity of heroin as bought on the street from 1972 to 1978. In reading Table 16-2, remember that these are national averages: purity and cost may vary greatly from region to region, city to city, and even dealer to dealer.[76] In theory high purity suggests a plentiful supply and thus low cost. As can be seen, the relationship doesn't hold up too well.

There is no FDA monitoring illegal heroin, so you never know what you are buying. A survey in New York City showed the concentration of heroin in equisized packets ranged from 1% to 77%. Variability in concentration is of recent origin and may reflect only quality control problems in an expanding market. It may also represent the impact of amateurs into an area of crime controlled through the 1960s by an efficient, international, professional organization. There have been some reports that higher amounts of heroin per bag is an effort on the part of some sellers to speed up the addiction process.

The variability in amount of heroin is also a problem because of the possibility of an overdose (OD).[77] Addicts should worry about an overdose with each new batch of drug used. A sophisticated user buying from a new or questionable source will initially try a much smaller than normal amount of the powder to evaluate its potency. There is much debate over how many overdoses result in the death of the addict.[78] Death from an overdose of an opiate will normally be from respiratory depression, suffocation.

Deaths usually attributed to a heroin overdose are much different and more rapid. Sometimes death is so rapid that the needle is still in the arm when the user is found. These deaths are almost all from asphyxiation caused by acute congestion and edema of the lungs.[79] This acute reaction may be the result of an allergic reaction to the heroin, or to quinine, but this is unlikely, since the same effect has been observed with methadone. At the least, "these deaths do not have the characteristics of a true pharmacological overdose. . . ."[79a]

Whatever the specific basis, street narcotic use is the cause of many deaths. In 1971 about 1350 deaths occurred as just described, more than in the entire decade of the 1950s. There are also deaths resulting from hepatitis, and most medical examiners group these two causes of death, along with instances in which there is no apparent cause, but all the signs of addiction and current use are present, into the category of narcotic-related deaths. About 65% to 75% of these narcotic-related deaths are an immediate reaction to the injection.

In the early 1970s narcotic-related death was the

TABLE 16-2 Price and purity of heroin, half-year averages

	1972		1973		1974		1975		1976		1977		1978	
	1st	2nd	1st	2nd	1st	2nd	1st	2nd	1st	2nd	1st	2nd	1st	2nd
Price per milligram heroin	$0.95	1.30	1.65	2.00	2.13	2.44	2.40	NA*	1.26	1.34	1.52	1.64	1.68	1.96
Purity (percent heroin in buy)	9.40	8.70	7.20	7.60	9.10	8.50	11.50	NA*	6.50	6.10	5.40	5.0	4.90	4.20

From Heroin indicators trend report, National Institute on Drug Abuse, Publication No. (ADM) 76-315, U.S. Department of Health, Education, and Welfare, Washington, D.C., 1976 and 1979, U.S. Government Printing Office.
*Not available.

largest single cause of death in New York City males between the ages of 15 and 35. Nationally there were large fluctuations in heroin-related deaths in the 1970s:

1973	1490
1974	1769
1975	2000
1976	1867
1977	767
1978	598
1979	665
1980	839

The trend will probably continue up in the early 1980s, at least.

Heroin is the drug of choice when compared to morphine and most other narcotics. It seems reasonable to believe that the faster entry into the brain by heroin, used intravenously, would increase the probability of a more intense effect.[80] One report[81] compared intramuscular injections of heroin and morphine in a nice experiment in a real clinical situation—postoperative pain of cancer patients. The equivalent of 10 mg of morphine is 4.8 mg of heroin. Both the analgesic and the mood effects were studied. Heroin produced its peak analgesic and mood effect at 1.2 hours after intramuscular administration. Morphine's peak analgesic effect came at 1.5 hours and its peak mood effect came at 1.8 hours after intramuscular injection. Fig. 16-1[82] plots the time response curves for

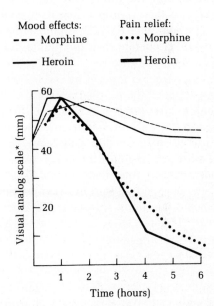

FIG. 16-1 Time action curves for pain relief and mood effects. The visual-analog scale (VAS) consisted of a 100-mm line on which the patient marked the point between extremes in effect. The extremes for relief were "no relief of pain" on the left and "complete relief of pain" on the right, and those for mood were "worst I could feel" and "best I could feel." The distance from the extreme left to the mark was the VAS score. (From Kaiko, R.F., et al.: Analgesic and mood effects of heroin and morphine in cancer patients with postoperative pain. Reprinted by permission of the New England Journal of Medicine, **304**(25):1501, 1981.

mood and analgesia for both drugs. Side effects were similar for both drugs—the only significant one being sleepiness, which occurred in 46% of the patients.

Once the user has acquired the drug, he prepares it for injection. Usually, he

mixes the powder with unsterile water, heats the mixture briefly in a spoon or bottle cap with a match or lighter, then draws the heroin into a syringe or eyedropper through cotton, thus filtering out the larger impurities. The heroin is then injected intravenously without any attempt at skin cleansing.[83]

Under these conditions it is not surprising that infections do occur. The preferred equipment today for injection is the eyedropper with a hypodermic needle attached, since the rubber bulb of the dropper is easier to operate than the plunger of a syringe.

The most common form of heroin use by male addicts is to inject the drug intravenously, that is, to "mainline" the drug. A convenient site is the left forearm (for right-handed users), and the frequent use of dirty needles will leave the arm marked with scar tissue. If the larger veins of the arm collapse, then other body areas will be used. Many beginning addicts start by "skin-popping"— subcutaneous injections. "Skin-popping" increases the danger of tetanus but decreases the risk of hepatitis compared to mainlining. Because of the lack of sterility or even cleanliness, hepatitis, tetanus, and abscesses at the site of injection are not uncommon in street users who inject drugs.

If the addict survives the perils of an overdose, escapes the dangers of contaminated equipment, and avoids being caught, there are still some dangers. Since heroin is a potent analgesic, its regular use *may* conceal the early symptoms of an illness such as pneumonia. The addict's lack of money for, or interest in, food frequently results in malnutrition. With low resistance from malnutrition and the symptoms of illness unnoticed as a result of heroin use, the addict becomes quite susceptible to serious disease.

If all these dangers are overcome, the addict may continue to use opiates to an advanced age. Sometimes, though, the addict who avoids illness, death, or arrest and who does not enter and stay in a rehabilitation program or withdraw himself from the drug may no longer feel the need for the drug and gradually stop using it. The data are still very much debated, but this "maturing out" is probably what happens to a large number of addicts. One authority reports that if an addict lives, he remains addicted for only about 8 or 9 years. This is an average, however, and according to this report the earlier a user starts, the longer he remains addicted, with maturing out generally occurring in the 35- to 45-year age period.[84] Even if he lives, the street life of an addict isn't a rose garden.

The street scene is continually shifting on all illegal drug use, and future trends are difficult to specify with certainty. As a general statement, however, and this is true of all drug use, there is a gradual homogenization of users. Every year, in drug use as in other behaviors, the differences between males and females, blacks and whites become less distinct. In the period from 1969 to 1970 four males entered drug treatment programs for every female. In 1980 the ratio was 3 to 1. Over this same period the proportion of those admitted to treatment programs who were black decreased from 55% to 30%. The proportion who were white increased from 30% to 58%. There are some changes in age at entry into the programs. Three age groupings were used: under 18, 18 to 25, and over 25. The respective percentages in 1969 were 6%, 37%, 57%. In 1980 they were 13%, 30%, 57%.

It is less true every year that the "typical" heroin user is black. It is less true that the typical user is male. The next section is on treatment, and it is clear there also that the effectiveness of rehabilitation is unrelated to these background, demographic variables.

TREATMENT AND REHABILITATION OF THE OPIATE ADDICT

I am absolutely certain that no substitute exists which, without containing opium or any of its derivatives, can cure the morphinist of his passion or even alleviate it.[85,p.69]

When Dr. Lewin wrote this in 1931, his statement was almost certainly true. Until the late 1950s few people believed that a modern opiate addict who injected heroin intravenously could ever be successfully weaned from his drug and rehabilitated into society. The data well into the 1960s seemed to be on the side of those who argued that opiate addiction is a chronic disease and that the addict patient can never be considered cured or rehabilitated. Studies of relapse rates in this period showed that many heroin addicts became readdicted following release from hospitals or institutions after treatment for the addiction.[86]

Times have changed and so have some of the facts. Several forms of treatment in use today seem to deliver some positive results, that is, social rehabilitation of the addict. Although many names are used for the various treatment modes, there are only two basic types. One approach is primarily psychosocial and emphasizes the necessity of the addict relearning certain patterns of living. There are two subgroups in this approach, with one group emphasizing the necessity for lifetime treatment and the other believing that it can accomplish true social rehabilitation and move the ex-addict completely back into the community. The second basic type of approach is pharmacological. The crucial element is the use of drugs to block the pleasurable, tension-reducing effects of heroin while also preventing the discomfort of withdrawal. There are several subgroups here, with the methadone maintenance procedure being the best-known. Another pharmacological approach involves the use of narcotic antagonists, opiate-blocking drugs such as cyclazocine. The structures of these two drugs are shown in Figs. 16-2 and 16-3. Finally, brief comment will be made on heroin maintenance and other developing programs.

General concepts

"The wide diversity of treatment methods reflects the present lack of precise knowledge as to the nature of drug addiction and abuse. Uncertainty still exists regarding the causes, whether or not it is an 'illness,' and the degree to which the condition is physical or psychological.[87,p.10] Unfortunately, this is true, and it has multiple implica-

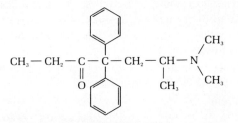

Methadone
Dolophine (Lilly)
(*dl*-6-dimethylamino-4,4-diphenyl-3-heptanone)

FIG. 16-2 Methadone.

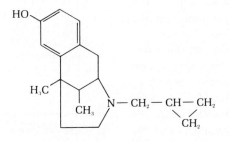

Cyclazocine
WIN 20,740 (Winthrop)
(3-[cyclopropylmethyl]-1,2,3,4,5,6-hexahydro-6,11-dimethyl-2,6-methano-3-benzazocin-8-ol)

FIG. 16-3 Cyclazocine.

tions, not the least of which has to do with money. It cost $40,000 a year to maintain a drug addict as a patient in a hospital, over $5,000 a year in a residential treatment center, $2,400 for a year of day care, and $1,750 as an outpatient. Much money is being spent, and there is no clear agreement on what a "cure" is for a drug abuser or heroin addict. Is the addict cured if drug free but dependent on the welfare system to survive? Cured if working regularly but still using drugs? Cured if there is no conflict with the law? In 1980 there were over a quarter of a million drug users being treated in more than 3000 drug abuse centers, and 38% of these clients had heroin problems.

There are many ways to define successful treatment, and the issues involved cannot be discussed here at length.[88] Some attitudes, general feelings, and beliefs of the various treatment modalities will become apparent as each is discussed. One writer has commented:

> We have been far from successful in coping with the problem of changing the addict's antisocial way of life. The resocialization of confirmed opiate abusers has proved to be a more difficult undertaking. Indeed, the term "rehabilitation" is a misnomer. Most opiate addicts have never established themselves in a legitimate adult role in society.[89]

Lending support to this are two studies that showed that addicts who have more stable backgrounds and are better socialized before they become addicted are more likely to be successfully rehabilitated.[90,91] These results are similar to those found with most behavioral change techniques: in brief, the more the individual is like what you want him to be, the more likely it is that he will achieve the goal.

Working with most addicts *is* different. The combination of a physiologically addicting drug, an addict subculture, and poor socialization make treatment (behavior change) very difficult. The necessity of constant hustling to maintain the habit, the pressures of law enforcement activities, and the physical debilitation that usually accompanies street addiction provide some motivation, albeit external, for treatment.

There is usually a delay of 4 or 5 years between the time of first use of heroin and admission to a treatment program.[92] Two out of three addicts remain in treatment less than 6 months—the data are mostly consistent: the longer an addict stays in treatment the greater the improvement (that is, likelihood of maintaining a nonheroin life-style). Some data suggest that less than 3 months in treatment is no better than no treatment.[93] One director of a methadone maintenance program has said, "The addict comes into treatment not when he wants to stop using drugs but when he can't use drugs any longer."[94] Traditional approaches do not seem generally to work,[95] and that is why specialized programs have developed.

Synanon

In 1958 an ex-alcoholic felt that an organization such as Alcoholics Anonymous should be able to help narcotic addicts who want to be rehabilitated. From quite meager beginnings Synanon has grown into a moderately successful rehabilitation program and philosophy. The Synanon concepts and practices are extensive, but a few points seem crucial. One is the belief that a narcotic addict is never cured (as AA believes an alcohol addict is never cured). Thus he should continue forever to live in the Synanon center or, after being clearly stabilized as an ex-addict, move into nearby living quarters and stay affiliated and involved with the Synanon program. As Charles Dederick, the founder of Synanon, has stated:

> I know damn well if they go out of Synanon they are dead. A few, but very few, have gone out and made it. . . . We have had 10,000 to 12,000 persons go through Synanon. Only a small handful who left became ex-drug addicts. Roughly one in ten has stayed clean outside for as much as two years.[78,p.78]

In line with this belief, Synanon counts the success of its program in terms of drug-free days. It expects relapses, since the addict is never cured, but emphasizes the time the ex-addict is free of drugs.

A second premise of this organization is that the addict must really want to be helped to discontinue drug use. To assure this motivation, there is an open door policy; a member is free to leave at any time. A third practice is the use of only ex-addicts as staff, with professionals being involved only for emergency medical service. Use of ex-addicts has two advantages, first that he's "been there" and second, that he's beaten addiction. Thus new members have someone to relate to who understands their problems. The ex-addict also has the advantage of knowing the tricks of the trade. As a result, he is able to structure the situation so that the life-style of the street is rapidly shown to be not effective at Synanon.[96,97]

Several things do make living at Synanon, and thus staying off drugs, effective. One is work; the ex-addict is kept busy. Another is faith, a religious-like belief of any kind. A third practice is to relate the type of work, the freedom, and the responsibility the individual has to the degree of his acceptance of a nondrug life-style and thus, in their terms, to his emotional maturity. Last is the assumption that an addict has difficulty in expressing his emotions and in identifying his own and others' emotions. The formal group encounters, which occur three to five times a week, are often psychologically violent but are the arena in which the ex-addict learns to stop using destructive guards to protect himself and above all learns to see himself and others as they really are.

The major objection raised to Synanon is the belief that an addict can never be cured. This means he may stay in residence for a long period and even after (if) he moves to live nearby, his world still must be centered on Synanon if he is to stay off drugs. People do leave Synanon to live *in* the community, but they are only members *of* the Synanon community. It is this lifelong commitment and absence of reentering the community that makes some wonder whether the Synanon program is moral or ethical.

There are some indications that the changing addict population is causing strains and problems for Synanon. There is less of the "we-them" kind of thinking, and this decreases cohesiveness among the members. Another factor causing stress must be the success of the various businesses that were started in order to give addicts jobs; the entire Synanon system is now a very large and profitable corporation. The glow is certainly gone from the halo that Synanon used to have. As the 1980s started a story unfolded about ripoffs of large sums of money and violence toward those who openly disagreed with, or even questioned, the rulers of Synanon. The basic ideas were good. Now—maybe there's nothing.[98]

Therapeutic communities

The many other types of psychosocial rehabilitation programs have similar kinds of residential treatment, and most are run by ex-addicts. They are also similar to Synanon in their emphasis on the necessity of the ex-addict learning a new set of social and living skills. The major difference seems to be that programs other than Synanon see themselves as waystations in the individual's life rather than a permanent home. These centers operate to make the ex-addict a member of the community where he lives when he leaves the center. These centers want to give the ex-addict an involvement in something outside the center, and their programs are geared toward social rehabilitation.[99]

Therapeutic communities do not have a good track record. One problem is that they are not research oriented and thus do not put any major effort into evaluation of results. One report stated that "it would be surprising if careful evaluation showed that more than five percent of those who come in contact with [therapeutic communities] are enabled to lead a reasonable drug-free socially productive life." Therapeutic communities are having an increasingly hard time surviving and justifying their surviving and may not make it into the 1980s. The best known is *Phoenix House*, which is the nation's largest and has several centers in New York City. Across the nation in San Francisco is the *Delancey Street Family*, which has very closely modeled its treatment techniques after Synanon. *Daytop Village* on Staten Island has achieved some attention because of its "act as if" approach to rehabilitation: Act as if . . . you're happy; . . . you don't need drugs. . . . Changing attitudes by first changing behaviors is a good rule, but Daytop Village is neither more nor less successful in rehabilitation than other therapeutic communities.[100]

Methadone maintenance

Methadone (Dolophine) is a synthetic narcotic analgesic developed in Germany during World War II and found to be a substitute for the then unavailable opium-based agents. As an analgesic it has several advantages, "which include effectiveness on oral administration, a prolonged effect, reasonable cost, and a mild withdrawal or abstinence syndrome that may pass unnoticed by the physically dependent patient."[101] Although long approved as a narcotic analgesic by the FDA, it has gained fame (notoriety?) as a drug useful in treatment programs for heroin addicts.

The initial study in this area was started in 1964 by Dole and Nyswander, a husband-wife team in New York City. In their initial work heroin addicts were given 20 to 30 mg of methadone orally every day; this was gradually increased over 4 to 6 weeks to 80 to 120 mg given orally once a day. The theory behind the use of methadone to help rehabilitate addicts is that the long-lasting effects of methadone prevent withdrawal symptoms and block the pleasurable effects of opiates. It disrupts the

pattern of swinging between the states of heroin intoxication and the withdrawal syndrome. "There are three states in the heroin addict's life," says Dr. Dole. "He's either 'straight' (feeling normal), 'high,' or 'sick.' He wakes up sick, takes a shot, and gets high. That lasts a couple of hours, maybe, until he begins coming off the high, and then he'll take another shot if he can get it. He spends very little time being straight, so he usually is not able to hold a job or live normally; he's pretty much a lost soul."[102]

The initial report of the effectiveness of this treatment program on 750 criminal addicts was spectacular.

A four year trial of methadone blockade treatment has shown 94% success in ending the criminal activity of former heroin addicts. The majority of these patients are now productively employed, living as responsible citizens, and supporting families. The results show unequivocally that criminal addicts can be rehabilitated by a well-supervised maintenance program.[103]

Methadone programs expanded steadily from the mid-sixties to the late seventies. Not without protest, however, and the ethics and morality of the methadone approach were raised early. The heart of the matter was approached in 1969:

although there is no question that methadone maintenance treatment is an effective way of reducing the criminalistic activities of drug addicts, it is a question who is being treated: society or the drug takers . . . each physician who prescribes methadone to a narcotic addict has this moral question to answer: Is he maintaining the patient on drugs for the good of society or for the good of his individual patient? Is he encouraging a kind of "cop out" by reinforcing the hopeless feeling of drug addicts when he wonders whether he can renounce drug use?[104]

Remember too that the methadone client must go to the clinic every day and take his methadone under supervision. Requiring the client to report to the clinic every day, and the expectation that the individual will stay on methadone for the rest of his life have raised questions about whether these programs are only another way for the establishment to control dissident individuals.

In spite of these concerns, things looked good for methadone maintenance as an effective program for heroin addicts. A 1970 review stated:

There are now perhaps 10,000 patients in about 50 programs. . . . About 80 percent of the patients who have started remain in the program and free of dependence on the use of opiates other than methadone. Of these 80 percent, most have resumed productive lives; the remainder, though unemployed, no longer engage in illicit enterprise. . . .[105]

A 1971 author described the overall results as "miraculous."

Appreciate that most centers use methadone maintenance only for addicts with at least a 1-year history and a substantial level of addiction. Sometimes addicts are not admitted unless they have tried other modes of rehabilitation and failed. No one has ever suggested that methadone maintenance be used with young, short-term addicts. Supporters of methadone maintenance emphasize the need for its use in a clinical setting where the addict does not control his own supply and where social support services are provided.

You should not believe that there is *a* methadone maintenance program. The general concept is widely applied but with varying emphasis: methadone to prevent withdrawal symmptoms and the cycling that occurs with heroin use, therapy to work through personal and interpersonal problems, environmental support to supply jobs, sparetime activities, etc. No one uses the high levels of methadone reported in the initial study; when comparisons were made of treatment outcomes between high, moderate, and low daily doses of methadone, no differences were found. Many methadone maintenance programs now use 40 mg a day but they don't work nearly as well as a program using 60 to 80 mg or more a day.[106]

As the programs expanded, so did costs. When costs increase and governmental money does not, something has to be stopped. What was given up in most clinics were the psychosocial aspects of the program; after all, if the delivery of the methadone stopped, there would be no methadone program. Eliminating these services diminished the effectiveness of these programs and contributed to the slow decline that methadone programs experienced in the late 1970s.[107]

Controlling the supply of methadone became an important issue in 1972 to 1974, when it developed into a major drug of abuse. Illegal sales of legally manufactured methadone boomed (over 80% was bought from an addict in a maintenance program), since $10 a day for methadone could prevent withdrawal effects from a $50-or-more-a-day heroin habit. Changes in the FDA rules controlled some of the diversion of methadone into illegal channels, but the problem continues.[108,109]

By 1972 there were 60,000 narcotic addicts in methadone maintenance programs; by 1976, about 90,000; and about the same number in the early 1980s. There were problems, however, with some of the basic data, the rationale, and the results. An excellent popular review in 1975 summarized much of the methadone work and pointed up some of the misleading (wrong) statements that had been made in the past. Both the bright and the dark spots were mentioned in a *Ten-Year Perspective* by Dole and Nyswander.[110] Interestingly there were problems from both the professionals and the addicts.

> An unfortunate consequence of the early enthusiasm for methadone treatment is today's general disenchantment with chemotherapy for addicts . . . the nearly universal reaction against the concept of substituting one drug for another, even when the second drug enabled the addict to function normally. . . . The analogous long-term use of other medications such as insulin and digitalis in medical practice has not been considered relevant.
>
> The attitude of addicts toward methadone programs is much less receptive today than it was five years ago. . . . The reason most often given by addicts for rejection of treatment was their perception of cynical and uncaring attitudes in the staff of programs, unreasonable rules, rigidity, and lack of respect. . . . It is mainly the programs rather than the addicts that have changed. . . .[110]

Perhaps what is needed is a Synanon-like concept of rehabilitation; such as emphasizing number of days worked and number of days not engaged in illegal activity. If heroin addiction is conceived of as a chronic behavioral problem, then relapses and recoveries, successes and failures should all be expected at different times within the same individuals. Cures and rehabilitation are never all-or-none processes in any chronic problem. The professional is grateful for any improvement, no matter how short lived or incomplete it may be. One report stated that of those who are now entering methadone programs, "perhaps up to 70 percent . . . return to illicit drugs at one point or another. On the other hand, the death rate for those who stay on methadone is only one-fifth to one-half that of most addicts, and the crime rate among them is twenty times lower."[111] That's better than

TABLE 16-3 Percentage of addicts remaining in methodone programs compared to therapeutic community (TC)

Aftermonth	TC	Methadone
1	64	97
2	45	85
4	30	85
6	20	80
8	5	68
12	5	64

nothing, and better than what any of the alternatives can show.[112]

One recent proposal[113] may develop into something better, since it realistically rejects the all-or-none concept of narcotic treatment success. Interweaving pharmacological and social measures, this program would start the heroin addict first on morphine maintenance, then methadone maintenance, then narcotic antagonists, and finally abstinence. In theory, if an addict fails at one level, he moves back to an earlier level, stabilizes, and then goes on again. The entire pharmacological treatment sequence would at all points be supported by social and personal rehabilitative efforts.

One excellent study[114] requires special comment because it randomly assigned male veterans (average age 31) who were heroin addicts to no treatment, therapeutic communities (TC), or methadone maintenance programs. The results are based on a follow-up of almost 100% of these men 1 year after the first assignment to a program. Several results are important. Addicts assigned to the methadone program were more likely to stay in the program than those assigned to a therapeutic community—and they stayed longer (Table 16-3).

One year after the start of treatment there were no differences in the drug use or social rehabilitation of those assigned to either program. Compared to the group that received no treatment, the veterans assigned to the therapeutic community did better than those assigned to methadone programs—but only if they stayed more than 50 days.

So methadone programs increase the likelihood of addicts staying in a program but if an addict stays in a therapeutic community it seems to do him more good than staying in the methadone program.[114]

There are two other "new ideas in treatment" coming down the pike. One is levo-alpha acetyl-methadol (LAAM), a long-acting narcotic being studied for use in methadone-like programs. The advantage to LAAM is its longer action—addicts can take it every other day, which would reduce some of the hassel we have now with the once-a-day visit to methadone clinics. There are mixed reports as to the effectiveness of LAAM in detoxification and treatment programs.

The most interesting use of pharmacology in treating narcotic addicts is the use of clonidine—a drug used widely in the treatment of hypertension.[115] It seems obvious—looking back—that, "Craving, anxiety, yawning, perspiration, lacrimation, rhinorrhea, gooseflesh, tremors, hot and cold flashes, hypertension, insomnia, restlessness, irritability, nausea, vomiting, and diarrhea are symptoms of both opiate withdrawal and increased catecholamine neurotransmitter activity."[116,p.431] You needn't worry about all the details but clonidine acts by blocking the alpha-2 adrenergic receptors, which are nonopiate receptors. Much work is going on—the best bet is that clonidine will suppress all of the signs of withdrawal from narcotic use mentioned previously—except the craving. For many addicts it seems to be adequate—the autonomic effects of withdrawal are the most aversive part of cold turkey, not the subjective discomfort.

A final idea—acupuncture has been tried and is reported effective in suppressing signs of withdrawal from narcotic use.[117] It may be effective since acupuncture stimulation in some locations seems to increase the level of enkephalins in the central nervous system.[118]

Heroin/morphine maintenance

In the late 1970s it seemed that heroin maintenance was an idea whose time had come—at least for open debate. To discuss the pros and cons requires some background, and the best place to start is in the early 1920s, when 44 clinics briefly operated in this country to provide legal morphine to addicts for the purpose of maintaining their habits. The usual comment about these clinics is that they did not work well and were closed because they increased illegal drug use. An interesting review of the activities of the clinic in Shreveport, Louisiana, used information never before available to provide a realistic assessment of the clinic operation.[119]

The characteristics of the patients served by the clinic during its 4-year life from 1919 to 1923 serve as an interesting counterpoint to today's addict. The very first addict admitted to the clinic was intravenously using 324 mg of morphine a day; the second addict used 777 mg a day.

Almost all drug use was intravenous, 90% of the clients were white, and males outnumbered females by a 3 to 1 margin. Most of the addicts were middle aged: only 39% were under 30, and only 1% under 20 years of age. Three of every four clients had become addicted as a result of medical treatment. Most people would agree that this is not a typical cross sample of today's addict population. The clinic probably did work well; one reason, according to the clinic director, was that "the clinic did not want 'bums' or 'loafers' and admission to the clinic was often refused to persons suspected of being criminal. Such persons were usually forced to leave town. . . ."[119] That's a neat way to handle the problem!

A comparison with the New York City Clinic in the same period showed two interesting differences in patient characteristics. In New York 78% were under the age of 30, and 28% were under the age of 19; three out of four had become addicted as a result of recreational drug use. These are possibly two of the important reasons that a strong advocate of morphine maintenance would say in 1919: "We are in a very bad state here in New York. Conditions are probably worse than ever . . . more opiates are peddled than ever before. The Board of Health Clinic has not been a success."[119]

With the preceding as background and the ad-

ditional facts that of the Shreveport clients, 40% had white-collar or skilled jobs, 33% were semiskilled, 6% were unskilled, 3% were professionals, and 2% owned their own business, that the Ku Klux Klan was active in this period, and that Huey Long practiced law in Shreveport, then you can evaluate the conclusions of the authors of the review[119] referred to before:

> The Shreveport experience demonstrates what could be done under a legal maintenance system very well. . . . What was done in Shreveport could very well be a model for many small cities in America.[p. 47]

> The differences between the productive, citizen-addicts of Shreveport in the 1920s and the maligned, criminal addicts of today appear to be a function of our morals, laws, and treatments rather than of the addicts themselves.[p. 48]

It is necessary always to look at what has been done, with whom, why, where, and under what conditions because all attempts to deal with drug use and abuse are relevant to today's situation. It is important to remember that relevant does not mean applicable. We can always learn something from other experiences, even if we do not learn the answers to our problems.

The British heroin maintenance system is a program we can learn from. The National Clearinghouse for Drug Abuse Information issued a report[120] in April 1973 that provides a very adequate history of the British system. Some people feel that the system is so loose that it is not a system, but that *is* the system. In Great Britain today addicts can register with a governmental agency and obtain narcotics from a clinic for the purpose of maintaining their addiction. One of the important points about the "addict register" in Great Britain is that it is so small: 1954 were receiving drugs at the beginning of 1976. This was down from 1972 a year earlier! Of most interest, however, is that in 1976, 926 were new addicts, and 532 were former addicts who had been off the rolls and registered again. Of the 1954, only 496 were on the register at both the beginning and end of 1975. Where did the other 1458 addicts go? 923 stopped seeking treatment,

69 died, and 483 were in jail! With a 50% dropout rate and a 25% penalization rate, it would not seem that the program was overly effective.

Since the British system is seen as a heroin maintenance system, you should know that at the beginning of 1976 only 4.5% were on heroin alone; 67% were on injectable methadone alone. The male/female ratio is 3 to 1, and the median age is 26. Without exhaustive documentation and many pages of text, it is impossible to develop the thesis that in spite of a common language the social situations in Great Britain and the United States are light years apart. If the two cultures are quite dissimilar, then it seems unreasonable to attempt to import their system. If, however, you believe that the two cultures are very much the same, then you might believe that a similar program should be tried in the United States.[121]

There have been some strong advocates of this in recent years. The strongest and best-formulated heroin maintenance plan was advocated in New York City in 1971 to 1972 by the Vera Institute of Justice.[122] This plan died or at least went underground in the Indian summer of heroin abuse in late 1972. It is of importance that some of the most outspoken opponents of the Vera proposal were the leaders of the black and Puerto Rican communities, where the addiction rate is highest.

In September 1976, San Diego seriously studied an experiment in supplying heroin to hard-core addicts.[123] In December 1976, the National League of Cities recommended that a study be made of a heroin maintenance system in the United States, including beginning some "research programs on heroin maintenance." One can only sympathize with the problems that those who run our cities have with drug use, abuse, and crime. It is understandable that they do not want to leave any stone unturned in their attempts to solve their problems.

The issue of heroin/morphine maintenance is going to rise up regularly as a proposal for handling what nothing else does. The practical problems alone are enormous and enough to make the other more important problems fade into the background for now.

Proposals for experimentation with heroin maintenance as a form of treatment in the United States also make little practical sense. Heroin is a short-acting drug requiring intravenous administration four or five times every day to maintain a habit. Thus, either the patient must remain virtually full-time in a clinic or he must be given take-home heroin. The current problem with methadone diversion make the latter prospect unacceptable, and the former does not seem practical from the user's or the program's point of view.[124]

Narcotic antagonists

One experimental treatment program that does not have many advocates is the use of narcotic antagonists. This type of program usually has two phases, the substitution of oral methadone for heroin and the gradual withdrawal of all methadone, which results in a narcotic-free individual. This withdrawal phase is followed by the administration of a narcotic antagonist. Although several antagonists have been used, the one that has been studied most extensively is naltrexone. The daily oral dose is gradually increased to a level where injected heroin has no effect. Mechanically the use of antagonists has the same advantages as the use of methadone in that it can be orally administered once a day after a stabilization dose level has been reached.

These antagonists have one characteristic that is both a boon and a bane. Because of low or no activity at the narcotic receptor site, the antagonists do not decrease the addict's desire for heroin. This may be a disadvantage and result in a higher failure rate than found with methadone programs. However, proponents of the narcotic antagonist treatment method emphasize the positive aspect of this characteristic. An addict on a narcotic antagonist program may continue to use heroin, since the desire to use narcotics remains high. But the heroin in this case will have no effect. Thus these proponents suggest that the addict will learn that heroin does not give pleasurable effects, and all behaviors associated with its use will become less likely to occur. (In learning terms, these other behaviors will lose their pleasurable characteristics and extinguish.) When this occurs, perhaps the regular use of the antagonist can be stopped. The concept is interesting, but clear evidence of the effectiveness of this type of program is not yet available.[125-129] Obviously such a program would not be highly desired by some addicts.

A final word on treatment

The treatment of heroin users is not a sensational success. On the other hand, it is not a flat-out bust, either. The number of good evaluations of treatment increases yearly but so does the number of attempted treatments. One report commented: *"In all three studies there were significant gross changes on all criteria in all treatments in the expected direction of reduction of socially deviant behaviors."*[130,p.105] That's a good general statement—probably true for four out of five treatment programs. Changes but not large changes. Two other points are important: one is that methadone programs retain four to six times as many of their patients for a year or more than do therapeutic communities. This increase in the length of stay in a program is a significant finding. The second point is that there are low correlations between treatment factors and treatment outcome; the available programs are equally effective (or equally ineffective) on all types of individuals. You will remember that the same result were obtained with most alcohol treatment programs. Maybe caring is enough—along with methadone.

No one of these treatment modes will be effective for all addicts. A 1972 government-supported study of all types of treatment programs concluded: "If society should decide to eliminate coercion as a means of controlling addiction, then heroin maintenance is the appropriate treatment. . . . If the goal is to achieve a given level of control with minimum . . . coercion, then it seems necessary to integrate . . . coercion and treatment into a single cooperative effort."[130] In other words, only the threat of prolonged confinement will bring many addicts into, and keep them in, treatment.

One addict who dropped out of a methadone program indicted the complexities of the problem:

"Methadone did the trick. . . . The reason I didn't stay on it was that I missed the excitement of using dope. I missed all the glamour of hustling and beating on people."[131]

CONCLUDING COMMENT

Narcotic use will wax, wane, and spread to new groups of users. Treatment programs only partially solve the problem. As with most drug use, the concern is not only with the direct effects of the drug on the individual. Rather, the present patterns of addiction to narcotic agents result in indirect harm to both the individual and society.

Harm to the individual is, in the main, indirect, arising from preoccupation with drug-taking; personal neglect, malnutrition and infection are frequent consequences. For society also, the resultant harm is chiefly related to the preoccupation of the individual with drug-taking; disruption of interpersonal relationships, economic loss, and crimes against property are frequent consequences.[132]

REFERENCES

1. Smith, R.: Status politics and the image of the addict, Issues in Criminology 2(2):157-175, 1966.
2. Lindesmith, A.R.: The addict and the law, Bloomington, Ind., 1965, Indiana University Press.
3. Historical background of the existing system of international narcotics control, International Control of Narcotic Drugs, United Nations, New York, October 1965.
4. Kramer, J.C.: Controlling narcotics in America, Drug Forum 1(1):51-69, 1971.
5. Kramer, J.C.: Controlling narcotics in America, Drug Forum 1(2):153-167, 1972.
6. Markham, J.M.: The American disease, New York Times, sec. 7, April 29, 1973.
7. Preble, E., and Casey, J.J., Jr.: Taking care of business—the heroin user's life on the street, International Journal of the Addictions 4(1):1-24, 1969.
8. Isbell, H.: Discussion, Symposium on Problems of Drug Dependence, Fourteenth Annual Conference Veterans Administration Cooperative Studies in Psychiatry, Houston, Texas, April 1, 1969, Highlights of the Conference, Veterans Administration, Washington, D.C., 1969, U.S. Government Printing Office.
9. Platt, J.J., and others: Recent trends in the demography of heroin addiction among youthful offenders, The International Journal of the Addictions 11(2):221-236, 1976.

10. The world heroin problem, Committee Print, House of Representatives, Committee on Foreign Affairs, Ninety-second Congress, First Session, May 27, 1971, Washington, D.C., 1971, U.S. Government Printing Office.

11. Inquiry into alleged drug abuse in the armed services, Report of a special subcommittee of the Committee on Armed Services, House of Representatives, Ninety-second Congress, First Session, April 23, 1971, Washington, D.C., 1971, U.S. Government Printing Office.

12. Robins, L.N.: The Vietnam drug user returns, Special Action Office for Drug Abuse Prevention Monograph, Series A, No. 2, May 1974, Contract No. HSM-42-72-75.

13. Nixon, R.M.: Message to Congress on the drug problem, July 14, 1969, U.S. News and World Report, p. 60, July 28, 1969.

14. Nixon, R.M.: Time, p. 20, June 28, 1971.

15. Heroin crisis ending? Signs point that way, Medical World News, pp. 15-17, April 13, 1973.

16. Harris, T.G.: As far as heroin is concerned, the worst is over: a conversation with Jerome H. Jaffe, Psychology Today, pp. 68-85, August 1973.

17. Gov't indicators of heroin use on upswing again; "a genuinely new situation," SAODAP chief says, Drugs and Drug Abuse Education Newsletter 5:1-2, 1974.

18. Heroin use rising U.S. official says, New York Times, March 18, 1976.

19. Federal monitoring systems show heroin at new "epidemic" levels, Washington Drug Review 6(1and 2):1, 1981.

20. DuPont, R.L.: The view around the corner. Presented at the National Issues and Strategies Symposium on the Drug Abusing Criminal Offender, Reston, Va., April 21, 1976.

21. Jurgensen, W.P.: Problems of inpatient treatment of addiction, New York State Narcotic Addiction Control Commission Reprints 1(1):2, 1968.

22. Becker, H.S.: History, culture and subjective experience: an exploration of the social bases of drug-induced experiences, Journal of Health and Social Behavior 8:175, 1967.

23. Dole, V.P.: Biochemistry of addiction, Annual Review of Biochemistry 39:821-840, 1970.

24. Kolb, L.: Pleasure and deterioration from narcotic addiction, Mental Hygiene 9:699-724, 1925.

25. Scher, J.: Patterns and profiles of addiction and drug abuse, Archives of General Psychiatry 15:539-551, 1966.

26. Lindesmith, A.R.: Addiction and opiates, Chicago, 1968, Aldine Publishing Co.

27. McAuliffe, W.E., and Gordon, R.A.: A test of Lindesmith's theory of addiction: the frequency of euphoria among long-term addicts, American Journal of Sociology 79(4):795-840, 1974.

28. Mathis, J.L.: Sexual aspects of heroin addiction, Medical Aspects of Human Sexuality 4(9):98-109, 1970.

29. Isbell, H., and White, W.M.: Clinical characteristics of addictions, The American Journal of Medicine 14:558-565, 1953.

30. Balster, R.L., and Harris, L.S.: Drugs as reinforcers in animals and humans; Symposium, Federation Proceedings 41(2):209-246, 1982.

31. Willis, J.H.: Some problems of opiate addiction, The Practitioner 200:220-225, 1968.

32. Eddy, N.B.: Analgesic and dependence-producing properties of drugs. In Wikler, A., editor: The addictive states, Baltimore, 1968, The Williams & Wilkins Co.

33. Goldstein, A.: Heroin addiction and the role of methadone in its treatment, Archives of General Psychiatry 26:291-297, 1972.

34. Powell, D.H.: A pilot study of occasional heroin users, Archives of General Psychiatry 28:586-594, 1973.

35. The epidemiology of heroin and other narcotics, National Institute on Drug Abuse Research Monograph 16, November 1977.

36. Hunt, C.G., and Zinberg, N.E.: Heroin use: a new look, Drug Abuse Council, Inc., September 1976.

37. Martin, W.R., and others: Aspects of the psychopathology and pathophysiology of addiction, Drug and Alcohol Dependence 2:185-202, 1977.

38. Penk, W.E., and Robinowitz, R.: Personality differences of volunteer and nonvolunteer heroin and nonheroin drug users, Journal of Abnormal Psychology 85(1):91-100, 1976.

39. Kurtines, W., Hogan, R., and Weiss, P.: Personality dynamics of heroin use, Journal of Abnormal Psychology 84(1):87-89, 1975.

40. Felix, R.H.: An appraisal of the personality types of the addict, American Journal of Psychiatry 100:462-467, 1944.

41. Platt, J.J.: "Addiction proneness" and personality in heroin addicts, Journal of Abnormal Psychology 84(3):303-306, 1975.

42. Wikler, A.: Opioid dependence: mechanisms and treatment, New York, 1980, Plenum Press.

43. Thompson, T., and Johanson, C.E., editors: Behavioral pharmacology of human drug dependence, NIDA Research Monograph 37, Washington, D.C., July 1981, U.S. Government Printing Office.

44. O'Brien, C.P.: "Needle freaks": psychological dependence on shooting up. In Medical World News, Psychiatry Annual, New York, 1974, McGraw-Hill Book Co.

45. Gay, G.: Heroin addiction patterns have changed, M.D. says, Drugs and Drug Abuse Education Newsletter 6:9, 1975.

46. O'Brien, C.P., and others: Conditioned narcotic withdrawal in humans, Science 195:1000-1002, 1977.

47. Siegel, S.: Morphine analgesic tolerance: its situation specificity supports a pavlovian conditioning model, Science 193:323-325, 1976.

48. Treatment of morphine-type dependence with withdrawal methods, Journal of the American Medical Association 219:1611-1615, 1972.

49. Haertzen, C.A., Meketon, M.J., and Hooks, N.T.: Subjective experiences produced by the withdrawal of opiates, British Journal of Addiction 65:245-255, 1970.

50. Bewley, T.H.: The diagnosis and management of heroin addiction, The Practitioner **200**:215-219, 1968.

51. Martin, W.R.: Personal communication, June 1977.

52. Martin, W.R., and others: Methadone—a reevaluation, Archives of General Psychiatry **28**:286-295, 1973.

53. Wilner, D.M., and Kassebaum, G.G., editors: Narcotics, New York, 1965, McGraw-Hill Book Co.

54. Simon, W., and Lumry, G.K.: Alcoholism and drug addiction among physicians—chronic self-destruction? Drug Dependence **3**:11-14, 1969.

55. Johnson, R.P., and Connelly, J.C.: Addicted physicians a closer look, Journal of the American Medical Association **245**(3):253, 1981.

56. Cline, S.: Turkish opium in perspective, Drug Abuse Council, Inc., Washington, D.C., December 1974.

57. Hess, J.L.: U.S. and France sign antidrug accord, New York Times, February 27, 1971, p. 3.

58. Thomas, H.: Turkey agrees to '72 ban on poppies, United Press International, July 1, 1971.

59. Spong, W.: Heroin: can the supply be stopped? Report to the Committee on Foreign Relations, U.S. Senate, September 18, 1972.

60. Mexico, Drug Enforcement **3**(1):6-12, Winter 1975-1976.

61. Mexican heroin flow continues unabated, Science **196**:509-510, 1977.

62. Riding, A.: Mexico making headway in war on opium poppies, New York Times, February 24, 1980, p. 1.

63. Kamm, H.: Burma reports gain in its war on opium, New York Times, October 9, 1977, p. 7.

64. Sterba, J.P.: Burma fights growing domestic heroin addiction, New York Times, June 11, 1979, p. A8.

65. Kamm, H.: A treasure in opium poppies is ripe for the plucking in Golden Triangle, New York Times, September 8, 1980.

66. Shipler, P.I.: Opium in Laos: it's hard to stop, New York Times, November 7, 1974.

67. Yielding to U.S., Thais target opium fields, New York Times, October 4, 1981, p. 21.

68. Kamm, H.: U.S. worries over Pakistani drugs, New York Times, April 17, 1977, p. 16L.

69. Kaufman, M.T.: Curbs by Pakistan don't halt heroin, New York Times, March 27, 1980, p. A11.

70. Kaufman, M.T.: Heroin output up in Pakistani area, New York Times, September 7, 1981, p. A4.

71. Wilford, J.N.: U.S. drug sleuths finally solve mystery of the deadly China white, New York Times, December 30, 1980, p. C1.

72. O'Brien, J.E.: Get ready for a surge in heroin abuse, Patient Care, **15**(3): 182, February 15, 1981.

73. Sheppard, N., Jr.: Statistics suggest U.S. faces new drug abuse problems, New York Times, September 10, 1981, p. A18.

74. Maitland, L.: Heroin trade rising despite U.S. efforts, New York Times, February 15, 1981, p. 1.

75. Check, W.A.: California team manipulates bacteria to mass-produce natural opiate, Medical News **243**(22):2273, 1980.

76. Heroin indicators trend report, National Institute on Drug Abuse, Publication No. (ADM) 76-315, U.S. Department of Health, Education, and Welfare, Washington, D.C., 1976, U.S. Government Printing Office.

77. Huber, D.H., Strivers, R.R., and Howard, L.B.: Heroin-overdose deaths in Atlanta, Journal of the American Medical Association **228**:319-322, 1974.

78. Brecher, E.M., and editors of Consumer Reports: Licit and illicit drugs, Boston, 1972, Little, Brown & Co., Chapter 12.

79. Helpern, M.: Heroin as a killer, New York Times Magazine, p. 29, December 10, 1972.

79a. Peterson, D.M, and Mahfuz, E.L.: Heroin overdose deaths: a critical examination of deaths attributed to acute reaction to dosage, Sundoz Psychiatric Spectator **10**(11):5-8, 1977.

80. Jaffe, J.H.: Treatment of drug abusers. In Clark, W.G., and del Guidice, J., editors: Principles of psychopharmacology, New York, 1970, Academic Press, Inc.

81. Kaiko, R.F., and others: Analgesic and mood effects of heroin and morphine in cancer patients with postoperative pain, New England Journal of Medicine **304**(25):1501-1505, 1981.

82. Analgesic and mood-altering effects of heroin vs. morphine, Drug Therapy Hospital, p. 9, September 1981.

83. Louria, D.B., Hensle, T., and Rose, J.: The major medical complications of heroin addiction, Annals of Internal Medicine **67**:1-22, 1967.

84. Winick, C.: Maturing out of narcotic addiction, Bulletin on Narcotics **14**(1):1-8, 1962.

85. Lewin, L.: Phantastica narcotics and stimulating drugs: their use and abuse, New York, 1931, E.P. Dutton & Co., Inc.

86. O'Donnell, J.A.: The relapse rate in narcotic addiction: a critique of follow-up studies, New York State Narcotic Addiction Control Commission Reprints **2**(1):1-21, 1968.

87. Treatment of drug abuse: an overview, National Clearinghouse for Drug Abuse Information, Report Series **34**(1), Publication No. (ADM) 75-197, U.S. Department of Health, Education, and Welfare, Washington, D.C., 1975, U.S. Government Printing Office.

88. McGlothlin, W.H., and others: Alternative approaches to opiate addiction control: costs, benefits and potential, Bureau of Narcotics and Dangerous Drugs, U.S. Department of Justice, June 1972.

89. Ball, J.C.: On the treatment of drug dependence, American Journal of Psychiatry **128**(7):873-874, 1972.

90. Bess, B., Janus, S., and Riffin, A.: Factors in successful narcotics renunciation, American Journal of Psychiatry **128**(7):861-865, 1972.

91. Bowden, C.L., and Langenauer, B.J.: Success and failure in the NARA addiction program, American Journal of Psychiatry **128**(7):853-856, 1972.

92. Egan, D.J, and Robinson, D.O.: Models of a heroin epidemic, American Journal of Psychiatry **136**(9):1162-1167, 1979.

93. Simpson, D.D.: The relation of time spent in drug abuse treatment to posttreatment outcome, American Journal of Psychiatry **136**(11):1449-1453.

94. Grafton, S., editor: Addiction and Drug Abuse Reports **5**:2-4, 1974.

95. Ketai, R.: Peer-observed psychotherapy with institutionalized narcotic addicts, Archives of General Psychiatry **29**:51-53, 1973.

96. Deissler, K.J.: Synanon—its concepts and methods, Drug Dependence **5**:28-35, 1970.

97. Yablonsky, L., and Dederich, C.E.: Synanon: an analysis of some dimensions of the social structure of an antiaddiction society. In Wilner, D.M., and Kassebaum, G.G., editors: Narcotics, New York, 1965, McGraw-Hill Book Co.

98. Lindsey, R.: Synanon's founder tells how his group changed, New York Times, December 22, 1980, p. D12.

99. Wolfe, R.C., and Boriello, R.: Drug addiction: an effective therapeutic approach, Medical Times **98**(9):185-193, 1970.

100. Perspectives in drug abuse treatment, Community Correspondents Group, NIDA, vol. 3, Washington, D.C., 1979, U.S. Government Printing Office.

101. Morgan, J.P., and Penovick, P.: Methadone: still an analgesic, Drug Therapy, pp. 18-23, January 1977.

102. Methadone maintenance: how much, for whom, for how long? Medical World News, pp. 53-63, March 17, 1972.

103. Dole, V.P., Nyswander, M.E., and Warner, A.: Successful treatment of 750 criminal addicts, Journal of the American Medical Association **206**:2708-2714, 1968.

104. Myerson, D.J.: Methadone treatment of addicts, New England Journal of Medicine **281**:390-391, 1969.

105. Kramer, J.C.: Methadone maintenance for opiate dependence, California Medicine **113**:6-11, 1970.

106. Manber, M.M.: Methadone, Medical World News, **22**(18):50, September 1, 1981.

107. Dole, V.P.: Addictive behavior, Scientific American **243**(6):138, 1980.

108. Holden, C.: Methadone: court ruling threatens FDA regulations, Science **185**:46-47, 1974.

109. Inciardi, J.A.: Methadone diversion: experiences and issues, DHEW Publication No. (ADM) 77-488, Washington, D.C., 1977, U.S. Government Printing Office.

110. Dole, V.P., and Nyswander, M.E.: Methadone maintenance treatment, a ten-year perspective, Journal of the American Medical Association **235**:2117-2119, 1976. Copyright 1976, American Medical Association.

111. Alpern, D.M., Sciolino, E., and Agrest, S.: The methadone Jones, Newsweek, p. 29, February 7, 1977.

112. Lennard, H.L., Epstein, L.J., and Rosenthal, M.S.: The methadone illusion, Science **176**:881-884, 1972.

113. Goldstein, A.: Heroin addiction, Archives of General Psychiatry **33**:353-358, 1976.

114. Bale, R.N., and others: Therapeutic communities vs. methadone maintenance, Archives of General Psychiatry **37**:179, February 1980.

115. Gold, M.S., and others: Opiate withdrawal using clonidine, Journal of the American Medical Association **243**(4):343, 1980.

116. Bourret, J.A.: Effects support noradrenergic hyperactivity hypothesis, Hospital Formulary, p. 431, April 1981.

117. Patterson, M.A.: Acupuncture and neuro-electric therapy in the treatment of drug and alcohol addiction, AJADD **2**(3):90-95, 1975.

118. Treatment of opiate-withdrawal symptoms, Lancet, **II** (8190):349, August 16, 1980.

119. Waldorf, D., Orlich, M., and Reinarman, C.: Morphine maintenance: the Shreveport Clinic 1919-1923, The Drug Abuse Council, Inc., Washington, D.C., April 1974.

120. The British narcotics system, National Clearinghouse for Drug Abuse Information, Report Series **13**(1), Publication No. (ADM) 75-153, U.S. Department of Health, Education, and Welfare, Washington, D.C., 1973, U.S. Government Printing Office.

121. Mauge, C.E., and Dragan, D.K.: Heroin maintenance: the second time around, Drug Abuse and Alcoholism Review, vol. 1, no. 3, 1978.

122. Markham, J.M.: What's all this talk? New York Times, Magazine, pp. 6-32, July 2, 1972.

123. Holles, E.R.: San Diego studies legal heroin plan, New York Times, September 12, 1976.

124. DuPont, R.L.: Response to public request for information, Boiler Plate, National Institute on Drug Abuse, Washington, D.C., 1977.

125. Freeman, A.M., and others: Clinical studies of cyclazocine in the treatment of narcotic addiction, American Journal of Psychiatry **124**:1499-1504, 1968.

126. Fink, M.: Narcotic antagonists in opiate dependence, Science **169**:1005-1006, 1970.

127. Narcotic antagonists: the search accelerates. Science **177**:56, 249-250, 1972.

128. Kurland, A.A., McCabe, L., and Hanlon, T.E.: Contingent naloxone (N-allynaroxymorphone) treatment of the paroled narcotic addict, International Pharmacopsychiatry **10**:157-168, 1975.

129. Willette, R.E., and Barnett, G., editors: Narcotic antagonists: naltrexone pharmacochemistry and sustained-release preparations, NIDA Research Monograph 28, Washington, D.C., 1981, U.S. Government Printing Office.

130. Sells, S.B.: Reflections on the epidemiology of heroin and narcotic addiction from the perspective of treatment data. In Rittenhouse, J.D., editor: the epidemiology of heroin and other narcotics, Project 4461, Stanford, Calif., 1976, Stanford Research Institute.

131. Medicine, Time, p. 60, January 4, 1971.

132. Eddy, N.B., and others: Drug dependence: its significance and characteristics, Bulletin of the World Health Organization **32**:721-733, 1965.

THE PHANTASTICANTS

CHAPTER 17

INTRODUCTION TO THE HALLUCINOGENS

She went back to the table . . . this time she found a little bottle on it . . . and tied round the neck of the bottle was a paper label with the words DRINK ME beautifully printed on it in large letters.

It was all very well to say "Drink me," but the wise little Alice was not going to do *that* in a hurry. "No, I'll look first," she said, "and see whether it's marked *poison* or not" . . . she had never forgotten that if you drink much from a bottle marked "poison," it is almost certain to disagree with you sooner or later. However, this bottle was *not* marked "poison," so Alice ventured to taste it, and finding it very nice (it had, in fact, a sort of mixed flavor of cherry-tart, custard, pineapple, roast turkey, toffy, and hot buttered toast), she very soon finished it off. "What a curious feeling!" said Alice; "I must be shutting up like a telescope." And so it was, indeed; she was now only ten inches high, and her face brightened up at the thought that she was now the right size for going through the little door into that lovely garden. [1, pp.7-8]

Alice could play many roles in the world of drugs. She certainly should be named patron saint of the OTC compounds because she compulsively read the label and followed directions. As queen of the hallucinogens she reigns supreme. For thousands of years before Alice and increasingly recently, people have believed what Alice said:

I know something interesting is sure to happen whenever I eat or drink anything.

As a result, Alice is not the only one who has eaten or drunk some substance and experienced strange and unique body sensations, changes in perceptions, and alterations of conciousness. This chapter and the next will detail some of the substances and experiences.

INTRODUCTION

Man found it necessary to try to explain these extraordinary powers of some of the plants in his environment. In all primitve cultures, this explanation invariably ascribed to the plant some particular divinity or spirit which, in many instances, was thought to be efficacious as an intermediary between man's world of humdrum reality and the supernatural or spirit realm. [2]

If God can be found through the medium of any drug, God is not worthy of being God. [3]

Over 4500 years ago a South American tribe buried one of its members and included his snuff tube and snuffing tablets. Already there must have been some expectation of an existence beyond physical death, another reality. This chapter discusses some of the ways in which people have tried to explore other realities during life by using chemicals. Many groups in the past, and some of the so-called primitive tribes today, have looked at "the beyond within" in a religious or ceremonial context. Except in more advanced cultures, people never take drugs; they use plants. This is an important distinction. Drugs and chemicals are derived from plants, but chemicals aren't used by natives; they use plants, which they believe to have a life, a resident divinity. Eating the plant means taking and acquiring the spiritual power of the plant.

The idea that plants had spirits meant that they were not used indiscriminately. Only in religious ceremonies were plants used that had power, and any plant with psychoactive properties had power. One writer comments:

> This principle was true of even so mildly psychedelic a drug as tobacco. Aboriginally, tobacco was *always* used in a sacred magicoreligious context, and never for mere secular-indulgent enjoyment. . . . And when . . . Indian chiefs . . . smoked the sacred calumet or peace pipe, the rite meant the invoking of the power of tobacco upon their sacred oath.

As we know, some of the psychoactive plants with long histories in western civilization have been adopted for "mere secular-indulgent enjoyment." Those who use drugs today in the search for religious experiences have voiced a similar concern:

> To turn on means to find a sacrament which returns you to the temple of God, your own body, to go out of your mind. To tune in means to be reborn; to drop back in, to start a new sequence of behavior that reflects your vision; in other words, to manifest in a behavioral way the religious experience you have had. . . .
>
> Today, the sacrament is LSD. However, sacraments wear out. They become part of the social game. Treasure LSD while it still works. In fifteen years it will be a tame, socialized routine.[5]

Many plants have been found that have the property of being able to transport the individual to what he feels is a new reality. In the Americas, 80 to 100 different plants have been used at different times and by different groups because of their psychoactive characteristics. The rest of the world never used more than seven species, and some feel that this is more a reflection of cultural differences than of botanical differences. Only a few of these agents can be commented on here. These plants and the psychoactive chemicals they contain are classed as hallucinogens because their distinguishing characteristic, to our society, is the ability to induce bizarre alterations in perception and states of consciousness. Most of the hallucinogens are agents that were included in Lewin's category, phantasticants. As usual the thrust will be to show the interrelationship of the drug and its effects on society as well as on the individual.[6]

CLASSIFICATION

Classification of the hallucinogens must be based on the same principles as the classification of other drugs (Chapter 6). These agents could be meaningfully grouped as naturally occurring or synthetic compounds, or on whether they have a New World or Old World origin. Some authorities use other dimensions:

> a great number of drugs can induce psychotic reactions characterized by disorders in perception (including hallucinations), thinking, feeling (affect), and behavior. These can be roughly divided into two main drug classes: (1) drugs like lysergic acid diethylamide (LSD) and mescaline that produce states something like the functional psychoses such as schizophrenia and mania, and (2) drugs like atropine and diisopropyl fluorophosphate (DFP) that produce a syndrome more like a delirium or organic psychosis. . . . The distinction between the LSD group and the deliriants is not absolute but forms two ends of a continuum. Similarly, there has been a good deal of dispute as to whether the effects of LSD do or do not resemble schizophrenia.

For most authorities there is no dispute; the drug-induced effect and schizophrenia are very different. A review summarized the work of one authority (Dr. Leo Hollister):[8,p.236]

> Withdrawal from interpersonal contacts is characteristic of schizophrenics; it is atypical of the

drug-induced psychoses. Schizophrenics and drug subjects communicate poorly, but the former seem not to care; the latter are greatly concerned about it. The nature of the hallucinations is different. In schizophrenia they tend to be auditory and threatening; in the drug-induced states they are visual and pleasant or impersonal. Subjects under drugs tend to be highly suggestible; that is why the drug tends to be cultogenic. Schizophrenics are highly resistant to suggestion. In a blind study of tape-recorded mental status interviews of six schizophrenics and six subjects under drugs, a large group of professional raters had little difficulty in distinguishing between the two groups.

For our purposes it seems most appropriate to group the hallucinogens according to the neurotransmitter through which they probably act. The three neurotransmitter substances named in Chapter 5—acetylcholine, noradrenaline, and serotonin—have very different chemical structures, each with a definite chemical nucleus. Serotonin is based on an indole nucleus:

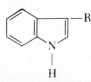

The most notorious, most maligned, and most potent hallucinogen and the agent that made this a psychedelic society is the indole-based *d*-lysergic acid diethylamide, LSD. It is a synthetic compound closely related to naturally occurring hallucinogenic agents found in some morning glory seeds. The indole nucleus is also the basic structure in psilocybin, the active ingredient of the magic mushrooms of Mexico.

Noradrenaline and the other adrenergic transmitters have a catechol nucleus:

The catechol nucleus is related to the phenethylamine structure of amphetamine, which could easily have been included in this section. The proto-

type catechol hallucinogen is mescaline, the primary active agent in the peyote cactus used in religious ceremonies by the Indians of the southwestern United States. A synthetic hallucinogen with the catechol nucleus is DOM (STP).

Acetylcholine, easily the best-established neurotransmitter, has no chemical nucleus with a specific name, but the structure does have a unique characteristic that determines its activity. This is the existence of a positively charged atom a fixed distance from a carboxyl group.

$$\begin{array}{ccccccc} & CH_3 & H & H & & O & \\ & | & | & | & & \| & \\ H_3C- & N^+ - & C - & C - & O - & C - & CH_3 \\ & | & | & | & & & \\ & CH_3 & H & H & & & \end{array}$$

Hallucinogens that act through the cholinergic system are unique because only with these agents is there poor memory for the period of altered consciousness. Three anticholinergic agents in this category occur naturally in many plants, including henbane, the deadly nightshade plant, and *Datura*. Ditran is an example of a synthetic anticholinergic hallucinogenic drug.

The hallucinogens that have attracted the most popular and scientific attention in recent years are those which most probably exert their effects by actions on the neurotransmitter serotonin. These indole-based agents span the continents and written history. They have been used in sanctuaries and on street corners, in ceremonies and in orgies. Only four of these phantasticants can be mentioned in any detail. Three are found in nature and have a rich history associated with their use. The most famous of them all was born in a test tube, but its relatives have a rich heritage.

d-LYSERGIC ACID DIETHYLAMIDE

The historical background to *d*-lysergic acid diethylamide (LSD) presented in the literature has been confusing. LSD was originally synthesized from ergot alkaloids extracted from a fungus *Claviceps purpurea*. This mold occasionally grows on grain, especially rye, and eating infected grain results in an illness called *ergotism*. LSD is a synthetic chemical and does not occur in nature under any conditions.

St. Anthony's fire

Grain that has been infected with the ergot fungus is readily identified and is usually immediately destroyed. During periods of famine, however, the grain may be used in making bread. In France between 945 AD and 1600 AD there were at least 20 outbreaks of ergotism, the illness that results from eating infected bread. A brief description of the symptoms of the illness was recorded following an outbreak in 857 AD,[9] but a better picture of the condition under which gangrenous ergot intoxication occurred in this period was that in 993 AD:

> A horrible plague raged among men, namely a hidden fire which, upon whatsoever limb it fastened, consumed it and severed it from the body. Many were consumed even in the space of a single night by these devouring flames. . . . Moreover, about the same time, a most mighty famine raged for five years throughout the Roman world, so that no region could be heard of which was not hunger-stricken for lack of bread, and many of the people were starved to death. In those days also, in many regions, the horrible famine compelled men to make their food not only of unclean beasts and creeping things, but even of men's, women's, and children's flesh, without regard even of kindred: for so fierce waxed this hunger that grown-up sons devoured their mothers, and mothers, forgetting their maternal love, ate their babes.[10,pp.2-3]

Although the cause of the illness was established before 1700, only symptomatic treatment exists even today. There are two forms of the disease. In one there are tingling sensations in the skin and muscle spasms that develop into convulsions, insomnia, and various disturbances of conciousness and thinking. In the other form, gangrenous ergotism, the limbs become swollen and inflamed, with the individual experiencing "violent burning pains" before the affected part becomes numb. Sometimes the disease moves rapidly, with less

than 24 hours between the first sign and the development of gangrene. Gangrene develops because the ergot causes a contraction of the blood vessels, cutting off blood flow to the extremities, sometimes with dramatic results.

> The separation of the gangrenous part often took place spontaneously at a joint without pain or loss of blood. It is related that a woman was riding to the hospital on an ass, and was pushed against a shrub; her leg became detached at the knee, without any bleeding, and she carried it to the hospital in her arms.[9,p.30]

It was not until 1085 that the burning sensation, the fire, was called holy *(sacro igne)*. The Order of St. Anthony was founded 8 years later, and a hospital was built in France near the church where the Saint's relics resided. During the twelfth century ergotism became associated with St. Anthony, although the reason for this is not completely clear. It may be that the hospital for the treatment of ergotism was built near the shrine of St. Anthony because he had suffered from a minor attack of ergotism. Some suggest that the demons he reported battling were the result of the disease.[11] Others believe the illness was called St. Anthony's Fire because those who made the pilgrimage to Egypt, where St. Anthony had lived, were cured. No matter, those who journeyed to Egypt as well as those who entered the hospital did lose their symptoms, probably as a result of a diet that did not include ergot-infected rye.

Two interesting articles in 1976 discussed a possible link between convulsive ergotism and the Salem village witch trials of 1692 in which 20 people were executed. The first article[12] built a very strong case that (1) the original symptoms exhibited by the "possessed" eight girls were similar to those seen in convulsive ergotism and (2) the conditions were right for the growth of the ergot fungus on the rye that was the staple cereal. The second article[13] constructed an equally convincing case that ergotism could *not* have been involved and that the "possession" was psychological in origin. In fact, we will never *know* for sure; there are, however, enough similarities and lingering doubts that ergotism seems to remain a possible basis for the Salem incident.

Special note must be made of a book[14] suggesting that there was an outbreak of ergotism in 1951 in a small French town. This suggestion has been frequently repeated in the popular literature with the symptoms of the illness attributed to ergot and/or LSD. In fact, the illness that spread rapidly through the inhabitants of the town was mercury poisoning resulting from eating bread made from mercury-treated wheat. The illness had nothing to do with the ergot alkaloids or LSD.

Discovery and early research

In the Sandoz Laboratories in Basel, Switzerland, in 1938 Dr. Albert Hofmann synthesized *lysergsaurediethylamid*, the German word from which LSD comes and the equivalent of the English *d*-lysergic acid diethylamide (Fig. 17-1). Hofmann was working on a series of compounds derived from ergot alkaloids that had as their basic structure lysergic acid. LSD was synthesized because of its chemical similarity to a known stimulant, nikethamide. It was not until 1943, however, that LSD entered the world of biochemical psychiatry when Hofmann recorded in his laboratory notebook:

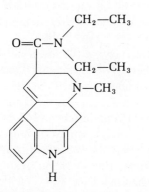

FIG. 17-1 *d*-lysergic acid diethylamide (LSD) (9,10-didehydro - *N,N* - diethyl - 6 - methyl - ergoline - 8β - carboxamide).

Last Friday, April 16, 1943, I was forced to stop my work in the laboratory in the middle of the afternoon and to go home, as I was seized by a peculiar restlessness associated with a sensation of mild dizziness. Having reached home, I lay down and sank in a kind of drunkeness which was not unpleasant and which was characterized by extreme activity of imagination. As I lay in a dazed condition with my eyes closed (I experienced daylight as disagreeably bright) there surged upon me an uninterrupted stream of fantastic images of extraordinary plasticity and vividness and accompanied by an intense, kaleidoscope-like play of colors. This condition gradually passed off after about two hours.[15,pp.184-185]

Hofmann later said, "The first experience was a very weak one, consisting of rather small changes. It had a pleasant, fairy tale–magic theater quality."[16] He was sure that the experience resulted from the accidental absorption, through the skin of his fingers, of the compound with which he was working. The next Monday morning Hofmann prepared what he thought was a very small amount of LSD, 0.25 mg, and made the following record in his notebook:

April 19, 1943: Preparation of an 0.5% aqueous solution of *d*-lysergic acid diethylamide tartrate.

4:20 P.M.: 0.5 cc (0.25 mg LSD) ingested orally. The solution is tasteless.

4:50 P.M.: no trace of any effect.

5:00 P.M.: slight dizziness, unrest, difficulty in concentration, visual disturbances, marked desire to laugh. . . .

At this point the laboratory notes are discontinued:

The last words could only be written with great difficulty. I asked my laboratory assistant to accompany me home as I believed that my condition would be a repetition of the disturbance of the previous Friday. While we were still cycling home, however, it became clear that the symptoms were much stronger than the first time. I had great difficulty in speaking coherently, my field of vision swayed before me, and objects appeared distorted like images in curved mirrors. I had the impression of being unable to move from the spot, although my assistant told me afterwards that we had cycled at a good pace. . . .

By the time the doctor arrived, the peak of the crisis had already passed. As far as I remember, the following were the most outstanding symptoms: vertigo, visual disturbances; the faces of those around me appeared as grotesque, colored masks; marked motor unrest, alternating with paresis; an intermittent heavy feeling in the head, limbs and the entire body, as if they were filled with metal; cramps in the legs, coldness and loss of feeling in the hands; a metallic taste on the tongue; dry, constricted sensation in the throat; feeling of choking; confusion alternating between clear recognition of my condition, in which state I sometimes observed, in the manner of an independent, neutral observer, that I shouted half insanely or babbled incoherent words. Occasionally I felt as if I were out of my body.
The doctor found a rather weak pulse but an otherwise normal circulation.

Six hours after ingestion of the LSD-25 my condition had already improved considerably. Only the visual disturbances were still pronounced. Everything seemed to sway and the proportions were distorted like the reflections in the surface of moving water. Moreover, all objects appeared in unpleasant, constantly changing colors, the predominant shades being sickly green and blue. When I closed my eyes, an unending series of colorful, very realistic and fantastic images surged in upon me. A remarkable feature was the manner in which all acoustic perceptions (e.g., the noise of a passing car) were transformed into optical effects, every sound causing a corresponding colored hallucination constantly changing in shape and color like pictures in a kaleidoscope. At about 1 o'clock I fell asleep and awakened next morning somewhat tired but otherwise feeling perfectly well.[15,pp.185-186]

Dr. Hofmann retired in 1971 after working 42 years for Sandoz Laboratories. In a 1976 interview he said he had taken LSD a total of 10 to 15 times but never again as high a dose as the one just described. Between 1949 and 1951 he had used LSD in his home with two very good friends, and in spite of careful preparation, at least one of the trips was a real bummer. Hofmann said that his LSD experiences had helped him realize:

> that the depth and richness of the inner and outer universe are immeasurable and inexhaustible, but that we have to return from these strange worlds to our homeland and live here in the reality that is provided by our normal, healthy senses.[16]

The amount Albert Hofmann took orally is 5 to 8 times the normal effective dose, and it was the potency of the drug that attracted attention to it. Mescaline had long been known to cause strange experiences, alter consciousness, and lead to a particularly vivid kaleidoscope of colors, but it takes 4000 times as much mescaline as LSD. LSD is usually active when only 0.05 mg is taken, and in some people a dose of 0.03 mg is effective. At this dose level it seemed possible that a physiological action was taking place, that is, an action that might occur normally in the body. Early reports suggested that LSD caused a reversible psychosis. Since LSD was active in small quantities, it seemed possible that it was mimicking the biochemical process that might normally cause schizophrenia!

The search began in earnest for the endogenous chemical that caused schizophrenia. The task still continues, and though many chemicals have been suggested, no agreement has been reached. Perhaps the major lasting impact of the psychedelics will prove to be increased study of nondrug highs and investigation of altered states of consciousness.[17-20]

Only an overview of the history of legal LSD is mentioned here. The developing illegal use of LSD and other hallucinogens will be detailed in other sections. The first report on LSD in the scientific literature came from Zurich in 1947, but it was 1949 before the first North American study on its use in humans appeared. In 1953 Sandoz applied to the Food and Drug Administration to study LSD as a new investigational drug. Between 1953 and 1966 Sandoz distributed large quantities of LSD to qualified scientists throughout the world. Most of this legal LSD was used in biochemical and animal behavior research.

In April 1966, the Sandoz Pharmaceutical Company recalled the LSD it had distributed and withdrew its sponsorship of work with LSD. Large quantities of illegally manufactured LSD of uncertain purity were being used in the street, and Sandoz decided to give the responsibility for the legal distribution of LSD to the federal government. Sandoz manufactured LSD, but research had to be approved by three agencies: the Drug Enforcement Agency, the National Institute on Drug Abuse, and the FDA.

Scientific study of the hallucinogens declined into the 1970s. The Reverend Walter Clark, a theologian and well-known advocate of controlled research on psychedelic drugs, provided data to support what he wrote in 1975[21]:

> Because of bureaucratic restrictions and public fear of the highly publicized dangers of the drugs both real and supposed, responsible investigators have too often retired from the field, despite their interest in the drugs and the conviction of many that these drugs are exceedingly promising tools in mental health and for the study of the human mind and development.

Dr. Clark was partially whistling in the dark, since research with marijuana has the same bureaucratic restrictions and is legally studied by thousands of scientists. More probably, hallucinogenic research had reached a dead end where new ideas were needed and not forthcoming. A 1974 report by an NIMH research task force on hallucinogenic research[22] stated:

> Virtually every psychological test has been used to study persons under the influence of LSD or other such hallucinogens, but the research has contributed little to our understanding of the bizarre and potent effects of this drug.

Partly as a reality-oriented response to this type of evaluation and partly because of the dead ends, the National Institute of Mental Health stopped its in-house LSD research on humans in 1968 and stopped funding university human research on LSD in 1974. The National Cancer Institute and the National Institute on Alcohol Abuse and Alcoholism stopped supporting psychedelic research in 1975 because it was nonproductive. Some animal research continues, but in 1975 there were only six investigators cleared to use LSD on humans.

Fife and drums

Out of sight, out of mind. Apart from aficionados, students, and users, LSD was almost a forgotten drug in the early 1970s. In the fall of 1975, however, a popular article could start with the sentence, "Once more LSD is in the front page news,"[23] Patty Hearst claimed she had been given LSD by her kidnapper-colleagues. Of interest here is the fact that the story of Central Intelligence Agency and army involvement with LSD research finally became public knowledge—and a public scandal.

The unraveling of the CIA/army human research programs using hallucinogens began with the June 1975 report of the Rockefeller Commission on the CIA. The incident the commission uncovered was that a 43-year-old biochemist, Frank Olson, committed suicide on November 28, 1953, less than 2 weeks after CIA agents had secretly slipped LSD into his after-dinner drink of Cointreau while he was attending a conference of government scientists. The drug caused a panic reaction in Dr. Olson, and he was taken to New York City for psychiatric treatment. There was an almost total coverup. The Olson family had been told only that he had jumped or fallen from his tenth-story hotel room in Manhattan. President Ford rapidly apologized to the Olson family at the White House and said the incident was "inexcusable and unforgiveable . . . a horrible episode in American history."[24] It was not until October 1976 that enough government red tape was cut to make it possible to award $750,000 to the Olson family. The CIA psychedelic drug project—code words *blue bird* and later *artichoke*—was modified in 1967 so that no one was given drugs without his full knowledge. In all, 139 different drugs were studied by the CIA, including coffee, marijuana, and cocaine.

Awareness of the Olson death started Congress and journalists digging for more, this time into the military as well. The army's interest in, and human experiments on, the use of psychedelics for warfare and for interrogation of prisoners and spies was not hidden. It was open knowledge in the scientific and military communities that such research was conducted at Edgewood Arsenal in Maryland, where Dr. Olson was poisoned, and at several major universities in the United States. What was not known were the low scientific standards and the complete absence of ethical considerations in the conduct of the army research. Commenting on the use of psychochemicals as offensive (!) weapons, the head of the army's chemical program wrote in 1959:

> We know the concept is feasible because we have run tests using a psychochemical on squad-sized units of soldier volunteers. They became confused, irresponsible, and were unable to carry out their missions. However, these were only temporary effects with complete recovery in all cases.[25]

It was easy to see how the military and intelligence agencies got involved in this work. "American military and intelligence officials watched men with glazed eyes pouring out rambling confessions at the Communist purge trials in Eastern Europe after World War II, and for the first time they began to worry about the threat of mind-bending drugs as weapons."[26] They worried enough to repeatedly contact Dr. Hofmann about the feasibility of large-scale production of LSD,[27] and the CIA considered buying 10 kg in 1953 for $240,000. At 10,000 doses per gram, that's a lot!

As the information kept pouring out of government files in the 1975-1976 period, it became clear that the army-sponsored research on 585 soldiers and 900 civilians between 1956 and 1967 had been very poorly done. The army and some of the university scientists had violated many of the ethical codes established as a result of the Nuremberg war crimes trials after World War II. Three failures were especially blatant: many of the volunteers were not really volunteers, many of the participants could not quit an experiment if they wanted to, and the participants were not told the nature of the experiment. This last point is a particularly valid one and points up a problem of doing any type of good human drug research. It is unethical not to tell individuals before they volunteer that they

might receive a drug, and it is unethical not to tell them the kind of effect it may have. To do this, though, would make it completely impossible to answer the army's questions: what is the effect of this drug on an individual's ability to withstand brainwashing, to follow orders, to conceal secrets, etc. In fact, these answers will never be available from research: ethical standards and controls and checks on human research are much more stringent today than ever before.

This horror story could go on almost without end; mention could be made of CIA agents picking up patrons in bars and secretly putting LSD in their drinks or of the administration of LSD to unsuspecting civilians around the world. The inspector general of the army issued a long report that criticized almost every aspect of the army's involvement with human drug research: its conception, its execution, and its productivity.[28] Perhaps a mountain has been made out of this molehill in the passing parade, but at the very least it should all too strikingly bring home the dangers of giving drugs to persons without their knowledge. These drugs can literally be mind-breaking when used incautiously.

In the spring of 1976 a senate committee that investigated the CIA's use of drugs issued a report containing a strong reprimand of the agency and reiterated stringent guidelines for all human research. Something needs to be done. The army had earlier declared its intentions to follow up and examine those 1500 individuals involved in the early drug research but by 1982 had issued only a brief comment on a study of 127 men. LSD and similar hallucinogen research on humans was discontinued in the late 1960s, but the army continued research on atropine and scopolamine until the summer of 1975. No comment was made on why they stopped the research then!

The bootleg hallucinogen story

The illegal LSD story starts with legal psilocybin, or perhaps at West Point, where Timothy Leary discovered Oriental mysticism. The eponym for the "Psychedelic Era" will certainly be Timothy Leary.

More than any other single person Leary made the mind-altering drugs newsworthy, and the media spread his gospel.

The story proper starts in the summer of 1960 in Mexico, where for the first time Leary used the magic mushrooms containing psilocybin. As he later said, he realized then that the old Timothy Leary was dead; the "Timothy Leary game" was over. A most interesting article[29] by Leary describes the entire day that Leary himself marks as the beginning of the end: Sunday, November 26, 1960, at Newton, Massachusetts. He ends the article with these words:

> From this moment on my days as a respectable establishment scientist were numbered. I just couldn't see the new society given birth by medical hands, or psychedelic sacraments as psychiatric tools.
> From this evening on my energies were offered to the ancient underground of alchemists, artists, mystics, alienated visionaries, dropouts and the disenchanted young, the sons arising.

Working at Harvard University, Leary collaborated with Dr. Richard Alpert and discussed the meaning and implication of this new world with Aldous Huxley.

During the 1960-1961 school year Leary and Alpert began a series of experiments on Harvard graduate students using pure psilocybin, which they had obtained through a physician. Leary's original work was apparently done under proper scientific controls and with a physician in attendance because drugs were used. The use of a physician was later eliminated, in opposition to state requirements, and then other controls were dropped. In fact, Leary believed strongly that not only the subject should use the drug but also the experimenter, so that he could communicate with the subject. This practice removes the experimenter from the role of an objective observer and can hardly be classified as seriously scientific.

Leary's drug taking in the role of an experimenter and the apparent abandonment of any possible former semblance of a scientific approach was definitely questioned by the Harvard authorities and other scientists and was the beginning of the end. As early as the fall of 1961 there was open question about the "research" being carried out by Leary and Alpert. There were many legitimate complaints, as noted, but attitudes were not completely unbiased. This is suggested by a memorandum by the psychologist in charge of the Center for Research in Personality, which had hired Leary. The memorandum said, in part:

> It is probably no accident that the society which consistently encourages the use of these substances, India, produced one of the sickest social orders ever created by mankind, in which thinking men spent their time lost in the Buddha position . . . while poverty, disease, social discrimination and superstition reached their highest and most organized form in all history.[30, pp. 54-55.]

Leary continued his work, and in 1963 he founded the International Federation for International Freedom (IFIF). IFIF was an organization to encourage research on psychedelic substances. Since his own research in this field was not viewed as very rigorous, the federation died for lack of outside interest or support.

All did not go well at Harvard for Leary. A combination of things not acceptable to the university gradually developed from 1961 to 1963. Some of the major issues were that no doctor was present when drugs were administered, undergraduates were used in drug experiments, and drug sessions were conducted outside the laboratory in Leary's home as well as at other places off campus.

As a result of many factors, Alpert and Leary were dismissed from their academic positions in the spring of 1963.[31] The university's reason for Leary's dismissal was his failure to meet his classes, which Leary admits he did not do since he understood he was on leave from the school.

In 1963 the White House Conference on Narcotics and Drug Abuse stated: "As yet these drugs [hallucinogens] are of minor importance in the general picture of drug abuse, in part because of their limited availability and inordinately high cost."[32, p. 288] Already, though, the illegal production of the hallucinogens had begun, and the effects of pure LSD were to be confounded with the effects of impurities and other drugs.

All was reasonably quiet in 1964 and 1965. Alpert, now known as Baba Ram Dass, separated from Leary and lectured on the West Coast,[33] while Leary settled at an estate in Millbrook, New York, which was owned by a wealthy supporter of Leary's beliefs. In 1964 Leary announced that drugs were not necessary to rise above and go beyond one's ego. He reiterated this again in 1966 after he was arrested for possession of marijuana at the Millbrook estate. He has repeatedly held since then that drugs are not necessary; they are only a help, a key to open consciousness to the inner experience he believes everyone should have.

The year 1966 was a busy one for Leary. He appeared at three Congressional hearings; one interchange with Senator Edward Kennedy about LSD is particularly interesting, first because Leary so clearly predicted what was to come, and second because Senator Kennedy and Dr. Leary didn't seem to be touching the same bases.

> *Kennedy:* Why do you not want the indiscriminate manufacture and distribution [of LSD]? Why not? Is it because it is dangerous?
>
> *Leary:* Because you do not know what you are getting.
>
> *Kennedy:* Is it because it is dangerous? Are you interested only in the consumer and whether, like truth in packaging, whether there are too many strawberries, or not enough strawberries in the pie, or is it something more dangerous than that, Dr. Leary?
>
> *Leary:* No sir; I think LSD is much less dangerous than the amphetamines and barbiturates.
>
> *Kennedy:* I am not asking that. The reason, as I would gather it, is because this is a dangerous drug; is that right?
>
> *Leary:* No, sir; LSD is not a dangerous drug.[34,p.253]

Also in 1966 Leary started his religion, the League of Spiritual Discovery, with LSD as the sacrament. The League got off to a slow start, and Leary's home base at Millbrook was under attack around the same time. Concern was that Leary would attract "drug addicts to Millbrook. When their money runs out, they will murder, rob and steal, to secure funds with which to satisfy their craving."[35]

The world moves too quickly for new prophets today. Although he was the guru of the age, Leary's sacrament was already being secularized. Increasing numbers of young people were responding to the motto of the League for Spiritual Discovery, "Turn On, Tune In, and Drop Out." Leary phrased it meaningfully:

> Turning on correctly means to understand the many levels that are brought into focus; it takes years of discipline, training, and discipleship. To turn on on a street corner is a waste. To tune in means you must harness rigorously what you are learning. . . .
>
> To drop out is the oldest message that spiritual teachers have passed on. You can get only by giving up.[36]

Noble words, perhaps, but street corner turn-ons were becoming more frequent. A combination of many things increased the use of hallucinogens, and especially LSD, during the early and mid-1960s. LSD's promise of new sensations (which were delivered), of potent aphrodisiac effects (which were not forthcoming),[37] of kinship with a friendly peer group (which occurred) spread the drug rapidly.

In the summer of 1966 delegates to the annual convention of the American Medical Association passed a resolution urging greater controls on hallucinogens. They were a little uptight, as was the nation; in part, the resolution stated that

> these drugs can produce uncontrollable violence, overwhelming panic . . . or attempted suicide or homicide, and can result, among the unstable or those with preexisting neurosis or psychosis, in severe illness demanding protracted stays in mental hospitals.[38]

The question always is, who are the unstable? Remember that the trend in all drug use is from a small selected group of individuals who probably have very clearly identifiable personal and social characteristics, to a larger group of not completely socially integrated individuals, to the population at large. The more a drug spreads to the population at large, the less likely it is that any unique characteristics can be recognized—or are relevant. What researchers find will depend on the spread of the drug among the population of their region of the country. Most of the research on the characteristics of LSD and other hallucinogen users centered on the flower children of the middle to late sixties.

Users and potential users were reported to be more suggestible on a hypnotic suggestibility test and to be less concerned about loss of self-control than those who rejected the opportunity to use hallucinogens. However, by the mid-1960s, several studies had been carried out in an attempt to characterize the personality and background of the hallucinogenic drug user. Some studies suggested there were differences between users, or those who said they were willing to use these drugs, and those who said they would not and also did not.[39,40] Another report rejected the idea that any common psychological or sociological characteristics would identify the moderate LSD user.

There is considerable support now for this attitude. Three obvious concerns in this type research will be mentioned. Most investigators search out only the chronic, heavy user of hallucinogens (much as alcoholics are studied and not just those who use alcohol). This gives a very different picture from that which would be obtained if a random selection were made from the 17% of Americans ages 18 to 25 who report having tried hallucinogens as of 1976. One 1968 study[41] compared male college students who were regular users to nonusers matched for age, education, and social class. In contrast to the nonuser, the hallucinogen user came from

a generally cold and rejecting family background which fails to develop adequate superego strength or socialization in the user who then, despite a middle class background and regular college attendance, resembles at least in some respects, the psychological test picture of the juvenile delinquent.

This picture of middle-class youths who had "slipped the traces" and become acidheads appears also in other reports.[42] Prior to heavy use of LSD, these individuals were reported to be predominantly middle class in economics and beliefs. Usually they were nonathletic, above average in intelligence, and poor in competitive situations. Frustrated with life and angry at their parents, these youths responded with passivity.

Another problem is possible regional differences in the characteristics of heavy LSD users. Is the heavy user who trips in southern California the same type as the acidhead in Minneapolis? Probably not. But there are no real data. Out of the West in the late 1960s came multiple reports of a close interaction between chronic LSD use and the supernatural. It was not enough to reject technology; a positive belief in magic, extrasensory perception, and astrology was usually acquired.

The final problem is the poor quality of most research in this area.[43] An excellent 1973 review of research on psychosocial correlates concluded: "The foregoing suggests a multitude of preproblem use correlates of adolescent psychedelic use. At the same time, there is very little consensual validation and there are many contradictory findings."[44]

While chronic users of LSD and similar drugs were being identified and studied, a decline began in the use of these drugs. LSD use reached a peak during the winter of 1967-1968 and fell thereafter. Three factors seem to be primarily responsible. One was the increasing incidence of bad trips, bummers. These bad trips probably resulted in part from the spread of LSD use into less stable and more anxious individuals. As the capacity of the individual to deal with problems decreases, or as his anxiety level increases, the probability of a bad drug experience becomes greater. Another item still contributing its share of bad trips is impure LSD. Leary's forecast was right. Not only poorly synthesized LSD but also addition of other drugs to the LSD made street acid a risky buy. It will be repeatedly emphasized that the pharmacodynamic actions of LSD and the other hallucinogens reported here are based on results obtained with legally manufactured and pure drugs. Reports from street use of these drugs—behavioral effects, adverse effects, and the like—are almost always based on an illegal product of unknown purity that may contain other chemical agents as well.

Methamphetamine was and is one of the additives. A 1967-1968 report commented that methamphetamine combined with LSD "increases the likelihood of a 'bad trip,' primarily due to the intense sympathomimetic effects of the amphetamines . . . [which are] often magnified by the LSD-sensitized mind into a panic reaction."[45]

A second factor that may have contributed to the decrease in the use of LSD was the report in 1967 that LSD damages chromosomes (p. 394). A third reason for the decline of LSD use after 1968 was the belief that other drugs were available. Mescaline and/or peyote became the hallucinogens of choice for many previous LSD users. Most users are not looking to find themselves or God through their drug experience, so mescaline is probably the drug of choice. It seems to offer less of an inner experience but an even better sensory show than LSD (see pp. 407-408, however).

The final chapter in the Timothy Leary story, but not the LSD story, is probably already written. Even as the guru announced his League for Spiritual Discovery in 1966, his position as anything more than a symbol for an era was washing away. A series of arrests on drug charges and finally sentence to a minimum security prison in 1969 helped maintain interest in the symbol of the turned-on decade. When he escaped by walking away from the prison in September 1970 he turned off the flame he ignited 10 years earlier in 1960. He had few friends and literally wandered through Europe, Asia, and Africa for 28 months before surrendering and being arrested in Aghanistan and extradited to the United States in January 1973.[46] He was given 6 months to 5 years for his escape and returned to prison.

Sequels are always curious. In the fall of 1974 his son, Jack, his early collaborator, Richard Alpert (Baba Ram Dass), and one of his former best friends, Allen Ginsberg, the poet, held a news conference in San Francisco. They did not come to praise Leary but to bury him—and they did. Calling Leary a "liar," a "paranoid schizophrenic," and a "cop informant," they "derided him harshly and bitterly for what they characterized as his betrayal in the nineteen-seventies." Although the trio were saddened by their need to discredit Leary, they apparently felt it necessary because of rumors that Leary was to tell all about his escape and his drug dealing in exchange for an early parole.

Ridiculous. Leary? The messiah of the new society? The antiestablishment man personified selling his psyche for freedom of soma? Never.

On June 7, 1976, Timothy F. Leary, Ph.D., was released from the Federal Correctional Center in San Diego. He had earlier stated he was "totally rehabilitated" and would "never, under any circumstances, advocate the use of LSD or any drug."[47]

And Galileo mumbled, "It still moves." Recanting is never for real—whether it's to the Inquisition or a federal court. Even an ex-guru has to eat. Touring college campuses in the 1980s, Leary was talking about "how to use drugs without abusing them."[48]

Pharmacodynamics

LSD is an extremely potent, odorless, colorless, and tasteless compound. One ounce contains about 300,000 human adult doses. There are no data on the lethal dose in humans, but in monkeys the LD 100 is about 5 mg/kg. In the laboratory rat the LD 50 is 16 mg/kg, while easily reproducible behavioral effects are obtained with 0.1 mg/kg.

Absorption from the gastrointestinal tract is rapid, and most human laboratory experiments administer LSD through the mouth. (Although street users primarily take the drug orally, some feel it is necessary to inject LSD intravenously.[49]) At all postingestion times, the brain contains less LSD than any of the other organs in the body, so it is not selectively taken up by the brain. Within the brain, however, the levels of the drug are highest in visual areas, parts of the limbic system, and areas of reticular system. Half of the LSD in the blood is metabolized every 3 hours, so blood levels decrease fairly rapidly. LSD is metabolized in the liver and excreted as 2-oxy-lysergic acid diethylamide, which is inactive.

Tolerance develops rapidly, repeated daily doses becoming completely ineffective in 3 to 4 days. Recovery is equally rapid, so weekly use of the same dose of LSD is possible. Cross tolerance has been shown between LSD, mescaline, and psilocybin, and the effects of each can be blocked or reversed with chlorpromazine. Physical dependence or addiction has not been shown to LSD or to any of the hallucinogens.

LSD is a sympathomimetic agent, and the autonomic signs are some of the first to appear after LSD is taken. Typical symptoms are dilated pupils, elevated temperature and blood pressure, and an increase in salivation.

The basic pharmacological mechanism through which the LSD experience is generated is not known. There is some evidence that LSD actions on both the dopaminergic and the serotonergic systems are necessary for its hallucinogenic properties.

There is now fairly general agreement that many of the primary—hallucinogenic—effects of LSD are mediated through the neurotransmitter serotonin. One problem that slowed studies on the mechanism of LSD is that there are both presynaptic and postsynaptic serotonin receptors in the brain. LSD occupies and stimulates both of these serotonin receptors but has a much greater effect on the presynaptic receptors. Stimulation of these presynaptic serotonin receptors *inhibits* the activity of this neural system (the raphe), which is important in modulating sensory inputs to the thalamus. This decrease in the modulation of sensory input combines with the actions noted next to overload the brain and impair accurate monitoring of the environment.[50]

Electrophysiological effects have been most frequently (though perhaps not correctly) associated with the hallucinogenic actions of LSD. One of its major effects is to increase the sensitivity of the sensory collaterals that feed into and activate the reticular formation. LSD is not like amphetamine. LSD lowers the threshold for reticular arousal by sensory input but does not directly increase the sensitivity of the reticular formation. By sensitizing the sensory collaterals, LSD administration makes possible activation of the central nervous system following sensory input below the normally effective level.

Although LSD apparently does not act on the sensory pathways themselves (except perhaps in the visual system), it does increase the effect of sensory input by increasing the size of the signal delivered to the cortex. This increase in the size of the signal and the increased activation of the cortex by reticular arousal could, of course, be a partial basis for the vividness of sensory experiences regularly reported following LSD ingestion. As might be anticipated from the effects on the reticular system, LSD also causes an activation of the EEG.

The reticular system is sometimes viewed as having two major functions with respect to the other areas of the brain. One is to control the activation or arousal level, and the second is to monitor and regulate the flow of sensory inputs. The reticular system can operate to increase or decrease the effect on the cortex of a given sensory signal. Thus it has a major role in determining the impact of sensory stimulation on an individual's awareness.

One of the workers in this area suggested that LSD has its effects by influencing "the processes concerned with the filtration and integration of sensory information."[7] If one recognizes that a large part of the LSD experience may be the reaction to changes in external and internal sensory inputs and to the way these inputs are integrated, then the actions of the reticular system and the previously mentioned raphe system would seem to be basic to the hallucinogenic experience.

A 1968 summary[51] of a conference that included many of those doing research on the mechanisms of action of the hallucinogens very clearly predicted what has come to pass:

> The psychotomimetic drugs, particularly LSD, may produce their complex psychic effects by the inhibition of a basic brain stem mechanism . . . the function of which is to integrate the sensory inflow and the emotional and ideational state of the organism, and in particular to suppress irrelevant information. This system may depend on

a complex interaction of serotonin and noradrenaline mechanisms. The basic requirements of a hallucinogen seem to be that it should (in specific doses) inhibit serotonin systems and potentiate noradrenaline systems. If these systems are normally mutually inhibitory, normal homeostasis might survive interruption of one of these mechanisms but would not survive simultaneous interruption of both in opposite senses. . . .

Eleven years later, in 1979, there was not much change: ". . . the most potent hallucinogenic drugs may be those that both inactivate brain serotonin and mimic brain dopamine. Serotonin inactivation may be necessary and sufficient for hallucinogenesis . . . while the dopaminergic action may modulate the intensity of the effect."[52,p.400]

Support your local travel agent

The heading for this section is from a lapel button and clearly says, "Take a Trip!" Why is an LSD experience called a trip? An excellent article starts from the premise that, among serious psychedelic drug users, the experience is viewed as "a process of self-discovery, of self-confrontation, of deep self-encounter, hopefully leading to self-acceptance, a heightened capacity to love, and spiritual harmony.[53,p.155] The essay weaves its way through Christianity's *Pilgrim's Progress* and Oriental religion to successful television shows such as *The Fugitive* to suggest that the find-yourself-by-losing-yourself theme frequently involves physical as well as psychological movement. "Every real trip is also a trip of spiritual growth, and every spiritual trip brings a heightened awareness of the real world."[53]

Some authorities reject almost categorically the idea that a religious or personally meaningful experience can be reached through hallucinogens:

As of now the self-denial, contemplation, and careful preparation that have characterized the lives of the great mystics of Eastern and Western civilizations are not likely to be replaced by the instant mysticism of a hallucinogenic trip; nor is it likely that a young college student or a beatnik in rebellion against society will discover divine truths or experience valid apocalyptical visions regarding

himself, his society, or his world merely by ingesting a drug-coated sugar cube that distorts perception and shatters reality.[54]

Others are believers whose opinion is that:

. . . the wealth of phenomena revealed in the psychedelic experience convinced us that chemicals of this type can be tools of great worth, providing the best access yet to the contents and processes of the human mind. Moreover, when a session is all that it can be, it liberates and sets in motion . . . a force and a process that not only can restore the sick to health, but can enable the normal individual to achieve a greater maturity, realize potentials, and even discover in large measure who he is and what his existence is about.[54,p.6-7]

Reactions to the LSD experience and reactions to reports of others' LSD experiences depend on the personality and history of the individual. The meaning of the experience is probably different for each individual but the fact that most hallucinogen users also use other drugs suggests that users are seeking the experience, not using the experience to seek.[55] The effects of LSD are fairly clear, and they

. . . can be divided into three general categories: somatic symptoms—dizziness, weakness, tremors, nausea, creeping or tingling sensations on the skin, and blurred vision; perceptual symptoms—altered shapes and colors, visual hallucinations, synesthesia (a mixing of senses, such as the transformation of sounds into changes in visual perception), and a distorted time sense; affective and cognitive symptoms—large and rapid mood changes, difficulty in thinking, depersonalization, and dreamlike feeling.[52,p.396]

The experience of a trip is difficult, if not impossible, to describe. Coupled with the problem of adequately verbalizing a personal inner experience is the fact that it is never-before-experienced experiences that are to be related. Gordon Wasson,[56] in speaking of the "psychic disturbance" from eating mushrooms, said:

This disturbance is wholly different from the effects of alcohol, as different as night from day. We are entering upon a discussion where the vocabulary . . . is seriously deficient. . . . We are all confined within the prison walls of our every-day vocabulary; with skill in our choice of words we may stretch accepted meanings to cover slightly new feelings and thoughts, but when a state of mind is utterly distinct, wholly novel, then all our old words fail. (How do you tell a man born blind what seeing is like?)

One summary[57] of the experience by a scientist stated:

The importance of mood, expectation, and setting on the subjective effects of LSD is well recognized. Therefore, the described effects can be quite variable from subject to subject and in the same subject at different times and under different conditions. The major effects are on sensory perception (especially visual) and emotions. Sensory changes vary with dose. At low doses mild distortions appear, with lights appearing brighter and sounds seeming clearer. Increasing the dose causes more severe distortions, often with extremely vivid coloration and the appearance of such phenomena as moving walls and moving staircases. With still larger doses pseudohallucinations appear; and, with very large doses, there is the occurrence of true hallucinations with loss of insight. Such effects as numbness, tingling, and nausea may occur. Emotionally the effects are quite variable. For some there is fear and even panic; for others there is diminution of panic; for others there is diminution of anxiety and feelings of a deep and transcendental experience. . . .

A journalist[58] phrased it a little differently:

Thirty minutes after the exploding ticket is swallowed, life is dramatically changed. Objects are luminescent, vibrating, "more real." Colors shift and split into the spectrum of charged, electric color and light. Perceptions come as killing insights—true! true! who couldn't have seen it before! There is an oceanic sense of involvement in the mortal drama in a deeply emotional new way. Colors are heard as notes of music, ideas have substance and fire. A crystal vision comes: how full is the cosmos, how sweet the flowers!

The illusions beckoned to the surface by the drug are greatly influenced by expectation, atmosphere and the traveler's mental balance. . . .

No way to say: "This is *the* description of the experience." There are as many experiences as there are drug users. Part of the wonder of these agents is that they do not give repeat performances. Although each trip differs, the general type of experience and the sequence of experiences are reasonably well delineated. When an effective dose is taken orally (0.5 to 1.5 μg/kg of body weight), the trip will last 6 to 9 hours. It can be greatly attenuated at any time through the administration of chlorpromazine intramuscularly.

The initial effects noticed are autonomic responses that develop gradually over the first 20 minutes. The individual may feel dizzy or hot and cold; his mouth may be dry. These effects diminish and, in addition, are less and less the focus of attention as alteration in sensations, perceptions, and mood begin to develop over the following 30 to 40 minutes. In one study,[59] after the initial autonomic effects, the sequence of events over the next 20 to 50 minutes was mood changes, abnormal body sensation, decrease in sensory impression, abnormal color perception, space and time disorders, and visual hallucinations. One visual effect has been described beautifully:

The guide asked me how I felt, and I responded, "Good." As I muttered the word "Good," I could see it form visually in the air. It was pink and fluffy like a cloud. The word looked "Good" in its appearance and so it had to be "Good." The word and the thing I was trying to express were one, and "Good" was floating around in the air.[59]

About 1 hour after taking LSD, the intoxication is in full bloom, but it is not until near the end of the second hour that major ego disruptions occur (if they are to occur).

Usually these changes center around a depersonalization. The individual may feel that the sensations he experiences are not from his body or that he has no body. Body distortions are common, the sort of thing suggested by the comment of one user: "I felt as if my left big toe were going to vomit!" Not unusual is a loss of self-awareness and loss of control of behavior.

In this personality disruption stage, the individual usually has the experiences that lead him, or an observer, to characterize the trip as "good" or "bad." Two frequent types of overall reactions in this stage have been characterized as "expansive" and "constricted." Some people show both. In the expansive reaction (a good trip) the individual may become hypomanic and grandiose and feel that he is uncovering secrets of the universe or profundities previously locked within himself. Feelings of creativity are not uncommon: "If I only had the time, I could write the truly great American novel." The other end of the continuum is the constricted reaction in which the user shows little movement and frequently becomes paranoid and exhibits feelings of persecution. The prototype individual in this situation is huddled in a corner fearful that some harm will come to him or that he is being threatened by some aspect of his hallucinations. Few LSD users ever reach the stage where auditory hallucinations occur. If they do, the hallucinations are usually an outgrowth of experiences in earlier phases of the trip. As the drug effect diminishes, normal psychological controls of sensations, perceptions, and mood return. As discussed in Chapter 4, there may be problems on reentry into the nonaltered reality.

A trip can be viewed in ways other than the sequential manner just discussed. One expert interpreter[60] of the hallucinogenic experience analyzes the total experience into four levels of consciousness: sensory, recollective-analytic, symbolic, integral. Each level is more difficult to attain than the one before it and is reached by fewer people. Similarly, with each succeeding level the potential of the experience increases, for good or bad.

At the sensory level, which is readily attained by all users, there are changes in the way the user perceives everything. The synesthesias, in which colors evoke musical rhythms or auditory patterns bring forth a cavalcade of forms and color, and time distortions combine with the attributing of new meanings to old sensations. These experiences have at least one major effect on many individuals that they carry back to the nondrug reality. As a result of the drug-altered perceptions, the individ-

ual frequently is forced to think and to categorize things, people, and experiences in a new way when in the nondrug condition. This new way of looking at old things is perhaps the single most important outcome of the experience at this level.

At the recollective-analytical level of consciousness, the same types of new perceptions are experienced, but now within one's own history and personality. Being forced to see oneself through LSD eyes may bring panic and anxiety or a new and fuller understanding of one's own potentials and hopes.

The symbolic and the integral levels of consciousness are further, to use a metaphor, descents and explorations into our true selves. At the symbolic level there is an appreciation of our oneness with the universal concepts expressed in myths and in the archetypes of Jungian psychology. To experience the final level, the integral level, has been likened to a religious conversion, that is, the sudden awareness that we have been accepted by God and are saved. At this level the individual feels a unity with God and/or with the essence of the universe.[61]

Some general characteristics of the entire experience that must be mentioned are the setting, use of the guide, and the dose. As mentioned in the section on pharmacodynamics, LSD and the other hallucinogens seem primarily to disrupt sensory input and processing. The more unique and stimulating the environment, the greater the effect of the drug. In a typical laboratory setting the drug experience is much different from that which occurs in a crowded room surrounded by friends, flashing lights, and acid-rock music.

How are the new experiences, sensations, and feelings to be interpreted? What do they mean? This is the primary function of the guide, although he is also available to prevent the individual from hurting himself. (You are just as dead whether you go out an upper-story window to "escape" from something or to "fly to join the beautiful stars.") The guide usually functions as an interpreter of the experience to the novice. As it is necessary to learn what you are looking at when you look through a microscope, it is necessary to learn what the drug-

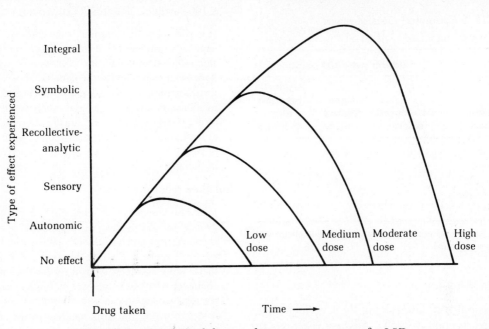

FIG. 17-2 Hypothetical dose- and time-response curve for LSD.

induced experiences mean. The guide is usually a close acquaintance or friend who has used hallucinogens and thus experienced a trip, but, while acting as a guide, he will not be using drugs. He may suggest what is happening to the user and lead him through the trip. Or, in other cases, he may only interact with the user when negative reactions seem to be appearing.

The length and depth of the experience are governed in part by the amount of the drug. As the dose increases, the experience becomes more and more like the trip to which people usually refer. With LSD and other indole hallucinogens, there does not seem to be as much euphoria associated with low doses as there is in the case of the catechol hallucinogens. Low doses of the hallucinogens do not give a miniature trip but instead produce only the autonomic and perceptual effects. An approximation of the relationship between dose and experience is indicated in Fig. 17-2.

In closing this section which attempts to describe what is impossible to describe, some points should be reemphasized. The sensations and other experiences after use of a hallucinogen are brand new to the user. As such they are very susceptible to influence by many factors; the same experience might be viewed as magnificent or horrendous, depending on these factors. The feeling of depersonalization or of certain autonomic changes may be viewed as revealing—or only cause anxiety. Since there is memory for the period of altered consciousness, the experience may have considerable impact on how the individual reacts to nondrug reality.

Adverse reactions

> In the hands of experts these agents are relatively safe but they are potent mind-shakers which should not be lightly or frivolously consumed.[62]

The adverse reactions to LSD ingestion have been repeatedly emphasized in the popular as well as scientific literature. Since there is no way of knowing how much illegal LSD is being used or how pure the LSD is that people are taking, there

TABLE 17-1 Estimated rates of major complications associated with LSD*

Groups studied	Number per 1000 persons		
	Attempted suicide	Completed suicide	Psychotic reaction over 48 hours
Subjects in experiments	0	0	0.8
Patients undergoing psychotherapy	1.2	0.4	1.8

*From Cohen, S.: Lysergic acid diethylamide: side effects and complications, Journal of Nervous and Mental Disease **130**:30-40, 1960. Copyright © 1982 The Williams & Wilkins Co.

is no possibility of determining the true incidence of adverse reactions to LSD. Adverse reactions to the street use of what is thought to be LSD may result from many factors. It is important to always remember that drugs obtained on the street frequently are not what they are claimed to be—in purity, chemical composition, or quantity.

A 1960 study surveyed most of the legal United States investigators studying LSD and mescaline effects in humans. Data were collected on 25,000 administrations of the drug to about 5000 individuals. Dosage range from 25 to 1500 µg of LSD and 200 to 1200 mg of mescaline. In some cases the drug was used in patients undergoing therapy; in other cases the drug was taken in an experimental situation to study the effects of the drug. Only LSD and mescaline used under professional supervision were surveyed. The results are noted in Table 17-1.

In reflecting on these data and others collected in the interim, a 1963 paper[63] stated:

The actual incidence of serious complications following LSD administration is not known. We believe, however, that they are infrequent. It is surprising that such a profound psychological experience leaves adverse residuals so rarely.

A 1964 article, "The LSD Controversy,"[64] stated:

It would seem that the incidence statistics better support a statement that the drug is *exceptionally safe* rather than dangerous. Although no statistics have been compiled for the dangers of psychological therapies, we would not be surprised if the incidence of adverse reactions, such as psychotic or depressive episodes and suicide attempts, were at least as high or higher in any comparable group of psychiatric patients exposed to any active form of therapy.

but then went on to say:

It is also important to distinguish between the proper use of this drug in therapeutic or experimental setting and its indiscriminate use and abuse by thrill seekers, "lunatic fringe," and drug addicts. More dangers seem likely for the unstable character who takes the drug for "kicks," curiosity, or to escape reality and responsibility than someone taking the drug for therapeutic reasons under strict medical aegis and supervision.

It is also important to emphasize that a clear distinction must be made between the pure LSD used in the "therapeutic or experimental setting" and the impure drug or combination of drugs most frequently used in the street.

Finally, a 1967 report[65] concluded:

It now appears that a variety of serious complications can result from both the therapeutic and non-therapeutic uses of LSD.

The study of adverse reactions to LSD is an emotional area, and facts are hard to obtain. One survey[66] was taken in Los Angeles of professionals treating adverse reactions in illegal users. Of those treating the users, 60% thought that half the people with adverse reactions had been emotionally disturbed prior to taking the drug. This statement goes to the heart of the real question: can LSD elicit an adverse reaction in a mentally healthy individual? The evidence is divided, and no conclusion can honestly be drawn except to ask: "Are any of us without fears and anxieties, conscious or unconscious?" Given the right dose and the right conditions, probably anyone could have one of the following adverse reactions noted in this section. However, it is probably true that the more disturbed one is in the absence of the drug, the more likely it is that one will have a bad trip or other adverse reaction.

Some believe that novices have more serious reactions than habitual users, possibly because they have not learned how to handle the altered perceptions and state of consciousness. The same reason may be the basis for reports that individuals with more rigid and constricted personalities have more problems with the drug experience.[42] An overall factor that may be of great importance in minimizing the negative effects that do develop is the realization by the individual that the distortions and effects are time limited and drug related. This realization seems to be the key to "talking someone down" from a bad trip by continually emphasizing to the person that he has not changed and that it is the drug that is causing the effects, which will soon go away.

Two types of adverse reactions that may develop during the drug-induced experience are the panic reaction and the overt psychosis. The panic reaction, which is an extreme anxiety attack, usually results from the individual's response to some particular aspects of the experience and is typified in the following case history:

> A 21-year-old woman was admitted to the hospital along with her lover. He had had a number of LSD experiences and had convinced her to take it to make her less constrained sexually. About half an hour after ingestion of approximately 200 microgm., she noticed that the bricks in the wall began to go in and out and that light affected her strangely. She became frightened when she realized that she was unable to distinguish her body from the chair she was sitting on or from her lover's body. Her fear became more marked after she thought that she would not get back into herself. At the time of admission she was hyperactive and laughed inappropriately. Stream of talk was illogical and affect labile. Two days later, this reaction had ceased. However, she was still afraid of the drug and convinced that she would not take it again because of her frightening experience.[67]

When an overt psychosis develops, remedial treatment is not usually so rapid, and the next individual to be described was hospitalized for prolonged treatment. Usually such psychosis occurs in individuals with a precarious hold on reality in the nondrug condition. The flood of new experiences and feelings is too much for this type person to integrate.

> A 23-year-old man was admitted to the hospital after he stood uncertain whether to plunge an upraised knife into his friend's back. His wife, an intelligent, nonpsychotic but masochistic woman, reported that he had been acting strangely since taking LSD approximately 3 weeks before admission. He was indecisive and often mute and shunned physical contact with her. On admission he was catatonic, mute and echopractic. He appeared to be preoccupied with auditory hallucinations of God's voice and thought he had achieved a condition of "all mind." On transfer to another hospital 1 month after admission, there was minimal improvement.
>
> During his adolescence the patient had alternated between acceptance of and rebellion against his mother's religiosity and warnings of the perils of sex and immorality. He had left college during his 1st year after excessive use of amphetamines. He attended, but did not complete, art school. His marriage of 3 years had been marked by conflict and concern about his masculinity. Increasing puzzlement about the meaning of life, his role in the universe and other cosmic problems led to his ingestion of LSD. Shortly after ingestion he was ecstatic and wrote to a friend, "We have found the peace, which is life's river which flows into the sea of Eternity." Soon afterward, in a brief essay, he showed some awareness of his developing psychosis, writing, "I am misunderstood, I cried, and was handed a complete list of my personality traits, habits, goals, and ideals, etc. I know myself now, I said in relief, and spent the rest of my life in happy cares asylum. AMEN."[67]

One of the frightening and interesting adverse reactions to LSD is the flashback. More than any other reaction, the recurrence of symptoms weeks or months after an individual has taken LSD brings up thoughts of brain damage and permanent bio-chemical changes. The next case history follows the usual pattern seen in flashback cases.

A man in his late twenties came to the admitting office in a state of panic. Although he had not taken any drug in approximately 2 months he was beginning to re-experience some of the illusory phenomena, perceptual distortions and the feeling of union with things around him that had previously occurred only under the influence of LSD. In addition, his wife had told him that he was beginning to "talk crazy," and he had become frightened. Despite a somewhat disturbed childhood and an interrupted college career he had carefully controlled his anxiety by a rigid obsessive-compulsive character structure, which had permitted him to work with reasonable success as a junior executive. Although for 6 years before admission he had felt the urge to seek help and self-understanding, he had never sought psychiatric care. He had tried marijuana, peyote and finally ground morning-glory seeds. Most of his 15 experiences with LSD had been pleasurable although he also had had 2 panic reactions, neither of which had led to hospital admission. On these occasions he thought that he was losing control and that his whole body was disappearing. At the time of admission he was concerned lest LSD have some permanent effect upon him. He wished reassurance so that he could take it again. His symptoms have subsided but tend to reappear in anxiety-provoking situations.[67]

Flashbacks consist of the recurrence of certain aspects of the drug experience after a period of normalcy and in the absence of any drug use. The frequency and duration of these flashbacks are quite variable and seem at this time to be unpredictable. One study[68] of flashbacks reported that they are most frequent just before going to sleep, while driving, and in periods of psychological stress. It was suggested that flashbacks may be attempts to resolve and master traumatic experiences. They seem to occur primarily in immature individuals and diminish in frequency and intensity with time if the individual stops using psychoactive drugs.

Where do all these reports leave us? Is LSD, or any of the better-known hallucinogens, a dangerous drug? It is clear that some people do show immediate and/or long-lasting negative reactions to a hallucinogenic experience. The evidence strongly suggests that if the individual using the drug has a marginal adjustment in the nondrug condition, there is a higher probability of a bad reaction than if he is reasonably well adjusted. However, considering the fact that even an apparently normal, mentally healthy person can have a bad trip or a prolonged adverse reaction, all these drugs must be approached with extreme caution.

Whatever happened to . . .

Everyone asks: Whatever happened to the flower children, the acidheads, the hippies, the freaks of the late sixties? Those individuals who regularly, heavily, and continually—or so it seemed—used psychedelics and other drugs. Flowers go to seed, and children grow up—but not without a trace. Tim Leary knew where they'd go; so did my daddy. There aren't many studies however. One study [69] was a 5-years-later follow-up of a large (over 100) group of hippies (hippies to the outside world; freaks if you were part of the group) who lived in the late sixties in a large eastern city.

Being a freak meant attaching oneself to a group which had to maintain itself in a hostile world of straights, schools, parents, work, police, narcs, informers, rednecks, greasers, and bikers . . . freaks could be identified more readily by their appearance and mode of behavior. Of singular importance . . . was the use of drugs.[69,p.76]

What happended to them? "These groups of adolescent hippies also dissolved as their members reached adulthood. . . . Most [over 70 percent] assumed conventional adult lives. Although all but 12 percent of the population continued to use marijuana or hashish, 97 percent . . . gave up their involvement with other drugs. . . ."[69,pp.81-82] This study concluded that two things happened to dissolve the hippies: they grew up and the world changed.

A 1974 report[70] of 16 college-age individuals who discontinued heavy use of hallucinogens sheds some light. It also provides some insight into the motivation that led to regular heavy use of hallucinogens, mostly LSD. This was a retrospective study; the previous users reported on their lives prior to the intensification of drug use:

> the period immediately preceding initial experimentation with hallucinogenic drugs was one of confusion and change. All subjects reported major life decisions being the subject of concern at that time. These concerns were often the choice of a "major" in college, choice of a graduate program, or choice of a career. All subjects seem to be searching for direction in love relationships as well as life goals. . . .[70]

The period of intense hallucinogen use lasted at least 2 years and

> was characterized by intense preoccupation with obtaining and taking drugs, and experiencing the hallucinogenic drug state. In 10 of the 16 subjects, pre-drug interpersonal relationships were exchanged for an entirely different group of peers who were largely involved in drug use. . . . Many of the subjects expressed an inability to communicate with parents, wishing to communicate more closely with them particularly about their drug experiences. When they were unable to communicate they experienced intense feelings of separation. . . . The urge to move about also increased during this period; half of the subjects traveled extensively.[70]

Bad drug experiences led only one of these individuals to discontinue psychedelic use. Usually they stopped all their drug use, except marijuana, as their interests shifted or as they were able to reach a resolution of their problems, such as marriage or a career.

> Drug use ceased as problems resolved. Relationships and goal directions were often clarified, sometimes solidified. Commitments to people, and tasks were often established, and drug experience lost prominence. Occasionally these changes were abrupt, coming with the flash of true insight; more frequently drug use gradually tapered and subjects noted that they didn't even consciously realize they had discontinued drug use. As one subject commented: "Drugs no longer seemed as important."[70]

Beliefs about LSD

LSD is truly a legend in its own time. Although there are no data, probably more people have more ideas about what LSD does and does not do than they have about any other drug. Only a few of these beliefs can be mentioned. The reader should especially note that the conclusions drawn in this section may be altered in the future, but as of now . . .

Creativity. One of the most widely occurring beliefs is that these hallucinogenic agents increase creativity or release the creativity that our inhibitions keep bottled inside us. Creativity is an ephemeral thing and not easily measured. Combining creativity with the use of a drug whose effects are very responsive to expectations and setting makes the problem very difficult to study. There have been several experiments that have attempted to study the effects of LSD on creativity, but there is no good evidence that the drug increases it. In one laboratory study using LSD at doses of 0.0025 or 0.01 mg/kg body weight, "the authors concluded that the administration of LSD-25 to a relatively unselected group of people for the purpose of enhancing their creative ability is *not* likely to be successful."[71] A 1969 report of an experiment with professional artists under the influence of LSD concluded: "for the creative artist, drugs are likely to produce more negative than positive results."[72] As always more work is needed.

Therapy. Another common belief is that LSD has therapeutic usefulness, particularly in the treatment of alcoholics, even though in the literature "reports of results with LSD in alcoholism have gradually changed from glowing and enthusiastic to cautious and disappointing."[73,p.520] One well-controlled study compared the effectiveness of one dose of either 0.6 mg of LSD or 60 mg of dextroamphetamine in reducing drinking by alcoholics. No additional therapy, physical or psychological, was used. The authors found that "LSD produced slightly better results early, but after six months the results were alike for both treatment groups."[74]

Some investigators[75] have reported considerable success with LSD in reducing the pain and depression of patients with terminal cancer. The LSD experiences were part of a several-day program involving extensive verbal interaction between the therapist and patient. Although not successful in every case, the LSD therapy was followed by a reduction in the use of narcotics, "less worry about the future," and "the appearance of a positive mood state." The authors concluded that they have a treatment "which may be highly promising for patients facing fatal illness if implemented in the context of brief, intensive, and highly specialized psychotherapy catalized by a psychedelic drug such as LSD." The potential value of the hallucinogens in the treatment of many disorders is still very much discussed and studied, and, as with most issues, a final resolution has not yet been reached.[22] The 1975 scientific peer review by NIMH[76,p.8] concluded: "Research on the therapeutic use of LSD has shown that it is not a generally useful therapeutic drug . . . as an adjunct to a routine psychotherapeutic approach . . . [or] as a treatment in and of itself. . . ."

Chromosomes. A credibility gap in the world of drugs developed in 1967 between the press and the public with the publication of a scientific report that LSD caused damage to chromosomes of white blood cells (leukocytes) in vitro. This report was quickly followed by a study showing a higher than normal incidence of chromosomal damage in the white blood cells of LSD users. These data received much attention in the mass media and are thought to be one of the reasons for the decrease in LSD use that has occurred since 1967. Not so widely publicized were the reports that did *not* show any relationship in vitro or in vivo between white blood cell chromosome damage and LSD use.

The popular reports also had a way of neglecting to emphasize (or mention) that the effects were on white blood cells and not on the germ cells, which are the only cells involved in reproduction. A poster distributed by the National Foundation—March of Dimes in this period showed a young man, in front of a possibly pregnant young woman, making the statement: "Give me one good reason why I shouldn't use LSD." The poster replies: "We can give you 46. . . . Broken chromosomes may

cause birth defects. LSD can break chromosomes. Need we say more?"

A similar misemphasis showed up in a United Press International release[77] in February of 1968, which used the headline, "Cancer linked to LSD Use." In the story, however, LSD was only one of several agents:

> Evidence was building that LSD or any other agent that causes chromosomes to break—including caffeine additives in sufficient amounts—will shorten cell life in the user and "significantly increase the chance of cancer."

Studies dealing with the effects of LSD on germ cells in animals have given both positive and negative results. Studies in mice show increased stillbirths and/or deformities when LSD is given during gestation. Data from humans are less clear, since impure, street-obtained LSD is ingested, and malnutrition and inadequate prenatal care are common. Evidence is accumulating, though, that women who use LSD during pregnancy have a higher incidence of miscarriages and babies with congenital deformities. There is no way to identify the causative factors, and some investigators do not obtain similar results.[78] It is true that:

> No one to date has conclusively proven that any birth defect is directly attributable to parental use of LSD.

And it is certainly true that:

> For the time being, it seems wiser to maintain a wait-and-see attitude.[79]

But it is most true of all that no drug used recreationally during pregnancy is good for the fetus, and some may be quite harmful (see Chapter 4 for a discussion of drugs and pregnancy).

CONCLUDING COMMENT

The hallucinogens are as fabulous in our time as coffee was a few hundred years ago in Europe. One big difference is that the hallucinogens have much more potential for personal good or harm than coffee ever had. Whether the secular and aperiodic use of hallucinogens will change the present world more than coffee and tea changed their world is a question only time can answer. The use of the hallucinogens for personal (and perhaps, therefore, social) good is an issue that is debated more and more.

An article in the *Minnesota Law Review*[80] discussed the research done with LSD. The author concluded that a solution to the problem of LSD use

is to be found, no doubt, where the answers to so many other social problems lie—in a general improvement of the quality of American society. If some such improvement came to pass, then either the need which LSD fills would disappear or its usage would become simply one very minor aspect of social life.

REFERENCES

1. Carrol, L.: Alice in Wonderland, London, 1865, The Macmillan Co.
2. Schultes, R.E.: Hallucinogenic plants of the New World, The Harvard Review 1(4):18-32, 1963.
3. Baba, M.: God speaks, New York, 1955, Dodd, Mead & Co.
4. LaBarre, W.: Old and New World narcotics: a statistical question and an ethnological reply, Botany 24(1):77,1970.
5. Smith, D.E.: Symposium: Psychedelic drugs and religion, Journal of Psychedelic Drugs 1(2):48, 1967-1968.
6. Furst, P.T.: Flesh of the gods, the ritual use of hallucinogens, New York, 1972, Praeger Publishers, Inc.
7. Smythies, J.R.: The mode of action of psychotomimetic drugs. A report on an NRP work session held on November 17-19, 1968, Neurosciences Research Program Bulletin 8(1):5, 63, 1970.
8. Lipton, M.A.: The relevance of chemically-induced psychoses to schizophrenia. In Efron, D.H., editor: Psychotomimetic drugs, New York, 1970, Raven Press.
9. Barger, G.: Ergot and ergotism, London, 1931, Gurney & Jackson.
10. Coulton, G.G.: Life in the Middle Ages, vol. 1, New York, 1928, Cambridge University Press.
11. Hordern, A.: Psychopharmacology: some historical considerations. In Joyce, C.R.B., editor: Psychopharmacology: dimensions and perspectives, Philadelphia, 1968, J.B. Lippincott Co.
12. Caporael, L.R.: Ergotism: the Satan loosed in Salem, Science 192:21-26, 1976.
13. Gottlieb, J., and Spanos, N.P.: Ergotism and the Salem village witch trials, Science 194:1390-1394, 1976.
14. Fuller, J.G.: The day of St. Anthony's fire, New York, 1968, The Macmillan Co.
15. Hofmann, A.: Psychotomimetic agents. In Burger, A., editor: Drugs affecting the central nervous system, vol. 2, New York, 1968, Marcel Dekker, Inc.
16. Horowitz, M.: Interview with Albert Hofmann, High Times, pp. 24-81, July 1976.
17. Fischer, R.: A cartography of the ecstatic and meditative states, Science 174:897-904, 1971.
18. Tart, C.T.: States of consciousness and state-specific sciences, Science 176:1203-1210, 1972.
19. Holden, C.: Altered states of consciousness: mind researchers meet to discuss exploration and mapping of "inner space," Science 179:982-983, 1973.
20. Masters, R., and Houston, J.: The varieties of post-psychedelic experience, Intellectual Digest, pp. 16-18, March 1973.
21. Clark, W.: Psychedelic research: obstacles and values, Journal of Humanistic Psychology 15(3):5-17, 1975.
22. Segal, J., editor: Research in the service of mental health, research on drug abuse, National Institute on Mental Health, Publication No. (ADM) 75-236, U.S. Department of Health, Education, and Welfare, Washington, D.C., 1975, U.S. Government Printing Office.
23. Ashley, R.: The other side of LSD, New York Times Magazine, pp.40-62, October 19, 1975.
24. Johnston, L.: Ford signs grant of $750,000 in LSD death in C.I.A. test, New York Times, October 14, 1976, p. C43.
25. Stubbs, M.: Soldier volunteers confirm psychochemical spell; CBW support is sought, Army, Navy, Air Force Journal 91:1, 27, October 31, 1959.
26. Treaster, J.B.: Mind-drug test a federal project for almost 25 years, New York Times, August 11, 1975, p. M42.
27. C.I.A. considered big LSD purchase, Washington Star, August 4, 1975. Knight, M.: LSD creator says army sought drug, New York Times, August 1, 1975.
28. Taylor, J.R., and Johnson, W.N.: Use of volunteers in chemical agent research, Inspector General Report No. DAIG-IN 21-75, Washington, D.C., March 10, 1976, U.S. Department of Army.
29. Leary, T.: In the beginning, Leary turned on Ginsberg and saw that it was good, Esquire 70:83-87, July 1968.
30. Caldwell, W.V.: LSD psychotherapy, New York, 1968, Grove Press, Inc.
31. Weil, A.T.: The strange case of the Harvard drug scandal, Look, pp.38-48, November 5, 1963.
32. White House Conference on Narcotics and Drug Abuse, Washington, D.C., 1963, U.S. Government Printing Office.
33. Dowling, C.: Confessions of an American guru, New York Times Magazine, pp. 41-43, 136-149, December 4, 1977.
34. Hearings before a special subcommittee of the Committee on the Judiciary, U.S. Senate, 89th Congress, 2nd Session, May 13, 1966.

35. Blumenthal, R.: Leary drug cult stirs Millbrook, New York Times, June 14, 1967, p. 49

36. Celebration # 1, New Yorker **42**:43, 1966.

37. Masters, R.E.L.: Sex ecstasy, and the psychedelic drugs, Playboy **14**(11):94-226, 1967.

38. Council on Mental Health and Committee on Alcoholism and Drug Dependence: Dependence on LSD and other hallucinogenic drugs, Journal of the American Medical Association **202**:141-144, 1967.

39. McGlothlin, W.H., and Cohen, S.: The use of hallucinogenic drugs among college students, American Journal of Psychiatry **122**:572-574, 1965.

40. Brehm, M.L., and Back, K.W.: Self image and attitudes toward drugs, Journal of Personality **36**:299-314, 1968.

41. Kleckner, J.H.: An investigation into the personal characteristics and family backgrounds of psychedelic drug users, Dissertation Abstracts **29B**:4380-B, 1969.

42. Ungerleider, J.T., and Fisher, D.D.: The problems of LSD^{25} and emotional disorder, California Medicine **106**:49-55, 1967.

43. Gorsuch, R.L., and Butler, M.C.: Initial drug abuse: a review of predisposing social psychological factors, Psychological Bulletin **83**(1):120-137, 1976.

44. Braucht, C.N., Brakarsh, D., Follingstad, D., and Berry, K.L.: Deviant drug use in adolescence: a review of psychosocial correlates, Psychological Bulletin **79**(2):92-106, 1973.

45. Smith, D.E.: LSD: its use, abuse, and suggested treatment, Journal of Psychedelic Drugs **1**(2):120, 1967-1968.

46. Cardoso, B.: Tim Leary and the long arm of the law, Rolling Stone, March 15, 1973.

47. Leary, once an LSD advocate, paroled, New York Times, April 21, 1976, p. 25.

48. Leary and Liddy, debating specialists, New York Times, September 3, 1981, p. B26.

49. Materson, B.J., and Barrett-Connor, E.: LSD "mainlining": a new hazard to health, Journal of the American Medical Association **200**:1126-1127, 1967.

50. Trulson, M.E., Ross, C.A., and Jacobs, B.L.: Behavioral evidence for the stimulation of CNS serotonin receptors by high doses of LSD, Psychopharmacology Communications **2**(2):149-164, 1976.

51. Action of hallucinogenic drugs, Nature **220**:961, 1968.

52. Jacobs, B.L., and Trulson, M.E.: Mechanisms of action of LSD, American Scientist **67**:396, July-August 1979.

53. Wallace, A.F.C.: The trip. In Hicks, R.E., and Fink, P.J., editors: Psychedelic drugs, Proceedings of a Hahnemann Medical College and Hospital Symposium sponsored by the Department of Psychiatry, New York, 1969, Grune & Stratton, Inc.

54. Louria, D.B.: LSD—a medical overview, Saturday Review **50**:92, 1967.

55. Metzner, R.: Reflections on LSD ten years later, Journal of Psychedelic Drugs **10**:137, April-June 1978.

56. Wasson, R.G.: The mushroom rites of Mexico, The Harvard Review **1**(4):7-17, 1963.

57. Gorodetsky, C.W.: Marihuana, LSD, and amphetamines, Drug Dependence **5**:20, 1970.

58. Farrell, B.: Scientists, theologians, mystics swept up in a psychic revolution, Life **60**:31, March 25, 1966.

59. Krippner, S.: Psychedelic experience and the language process, Journal of Psychedelic Drugs **3**(1):41-51, 1970.

60. Houston, J.: Phenomenology of the psychedelic experience. In Hicks, R.E., and Fink, P.J., editors: Psychedelic drugs, Proceedings of a Hahnemann Medical College and Hospital Symposium sponsored by the Department of Psychiatry, New York, 1969, Grune & Stratton, Inc.

61. Moody, H.: Psychedelic drugs and religious experience. In Hicks, R.E., and Fink, P.J., editors: Psychedelic drugs, Proceedings of a Hahnemann Medical College and Hospital Symposium sponsored by the Department of Psychiatry, New York, 1969, Grune & Stratton, Inc.

62. Cohen, S.: A classification of LSD complications, Psychosomatics **7**:182-186, 1966.

63. Cohen, S., and Ditman, K.S.: Prolonged adverse reactions to lysergic acid diethylamide, Archives of General Psychiatry **8**:475-480, 1963.

64. Levine, J., and Ludwig, A.M.: The LSD controversy, Comprehensive Psychiatry **5**(5):318-319, 1964.

65. Smart, R.G., and Bateman, K.: Unfavourable reactions to LSD: a review and analysis of the available case reports, Canadian Medical Association Journal **96**:1214-1221, 1967.

66. Ungerleider, J.T., and others: A statistical survey of adverse reactions to LSD in Los Angeles County, American Journal of Psychiatry **125**:108-113, 1968.

67. Frosch, W.A., Robbins, E.S., and Stern, M.: Untoward reactions to lysergic acid diethylamide (LSD) resulting in hospitalization, New England Journal of Medicine **273**:1235-1239, 1965.

68. Shick, J.F.E., and Smith, D.E.: Analysis of the LSD flashback, Journal of Psychedelic Drugs **3**(1):13-19, 1970.

69. Ramos, M., and Gould, L.C.: Where have all the flower children gone? A five-year follow up of a natural group of drug users, Journal of Drug Issues **8**:75, Winter 1978.

70. Salzman, C., and Lieff, J.: Interviews with hallucinogenic drug discontinuers, Journal of Psychedelic Drugs **6**(3):329-332, 1974.

71. Zegans, L.S., Pollard, J.C., and Brown, D.: The effects of LSD-25 on creativity and tolerance to regression, Archives of General Psychiatry **16**:740-749, 1967.

72. Painting under LSD, Time **94**(23):88, December 5, 1969.

73. Hayman, M., and del Giudice, J.: Psychotropic drugs in alcoholism. In Clark, W.G., and del Giudice, J., editors: Principles of psychopharmacology, New York, 1970, Academic Press, Inc.

74. Hollister, L.E., Shelton, J., and Krieger, G.: A controlled comparison of lysergic acid diethylamide (LSD) and dextroamphetamine in alcoholics, American Journal of Psychiatry **125**:1352-1357, 1969.

75. Pahnke, W.N., and others: Psychedelic therapy (utilizing LSD) with cancer patients, Journal of Psychedelic Drugs 3(1):63-75, 1970.
76. NIMH research on LSD, Extramural programs fiscal year 1948 to present, prepared September 1, 1975.
77. Doctor tells house of drug's dangers: cancer linked to LSD use, United Press International, February 19, 1968.
78. Maugh, T.H., II: LSD and the drug culture: new evidence of hazard, Science 179:1221-1222, 1973.
79. Egozcue, J., and Irwin, S.: LSD-25 effects on chromosomes: a review, Journal of Psychedelic Drugs 3(1):10-12, 1970.
80. Ford, S.D.: LSD and the law: a framework for policy making, Minnesota Law Review 54:775-804, 1970.

CHAPTER 18

THE MAJOR HALLUCINOGENS

PLANTS OF THE GODS.[1] Not like cocoa, just a food for the gods, but plants that are gods, or make you a god, or ". . . function as intermediaries between a person and his diety. . . ." That's what this chapter is about: "Plants regarded as sacred or magical. . . ."[2,p.647]You have to stop and think. What you study or take in an almost casual way was once a most important part of an individual's belief system. These plants and how they were used were probably a more important and immediate part of their lives than your God and your sacraments are to you!

This chapter is an adventure in time and space travel. From the soft, quiet beauty of the sacred mushroom to the cacophony of PCP tablets rattling in a bottle, from the mountains of old Mexico to the streets of Anytown, U.S.A., from the sixteenth century to the end of the twentieth, man has looked, searched, sought after the perfect aphrodisiac, religious experiences, other worlds. All this and more, and sometimes less. The hallucinogens discussed in this chapter have had important effects on man—how he sees himself, how he sees his relationship with the world. Hopscotching across centuries and over continents can only provide a hint of the importance of these drugs, but this is what must be done here.

INDOLE HALLUCINOGENS
Teonanacatl

The magic mushrooms of Mexico have a long history of religious and ceremonial use in Central America. Large stone mushrooms dating from about 1000 BC have been found in Guatemala and their importance is suggested by the figure of a god carved in the stem.

One extensive report (and the most reliable, since the author was not a professional missionary) on the pharmacopoeia and medicine of Mexico was compiled by Dr. Francisco Hernandez between 1570 and 1575. Hernandez was court physician to King Philip II of Spain, who named him Protomedico of the Indies. Philip told Hernandez to collect information about all aspects of the Mexican civilization but especially about its herbs and medicines. Mexican medicine in the sixteenth century must have been extensive because Hernandez reported 1200 remedies.

In this report Hernandez included three hallucinogenic mushrooms and a "vision-producing flower." He drew a picture of this flower, which showed it to be a morning glory, the ololiuqui described in the next section. All of these plants, as well as peyote, dropped from western sight (but not from native use) for 300 years. The mushrooms were to be particularly suppressed. The name *teo-nanacatl* can be translated as "God's flesh" or as "sacred mushroom," and either name was very offensive to the Spanish priests.

However, use was not limited to religious ceremonies. Already the secularization had begun. Summarizing some of these early reports:

> teonanacatl was not only ingested at social and festival occasions but also by witch doctors and soothsayers. The mushroom god—which the Christian missionaries called the devil—endowed them with clairvoyant properties, which enabled them, besides other things, to identify the causes of diseases and indicate the way in which they could be treated.[3,p.175]

It was not until the late 1930s that it was clearly shown that these mushrooms were still being used by natives in southern Mexico and that the first of many species was identified. The real breakthrough came in 1955. During that year a New York-banker-turned-ethnobotanist and his wife established rapport with a native group still using mushrooms in religious ceremonies. Gordon Wasson became the first outsider to participate in the ceremony and to eat of the magic mushroom. In language quite unlike a banker you can almost hear Wasson's soul cry out as he tries to describe the experience:

> It permits you to travel backwards and forward in time, to enter other planes of existence, even (as the Indians say), to know God. . . .
>
> What is happening to you seems freighted with significance, beside which the humdrum events of every day are trivial. All these things you see with an immediacy of vision that leads you to say to yourself, 'Now I am seeing for the first time, seeing direct, without the intervention of mortal eyes'. (Plato tells us that beyond this ephemeral and imperfect existence here below, there exists another ideal world of Archetypes, where the original, the true, the beautiful patterns of things, exist for evermore. Poets have pondered his words for millenia. It is clear to me where Plato found his ideas, it was clear to his contemporaries too. Plato had drunk of the potion in the Temple of Eleusis and had spent the night seeing the great vision). . .

Your body lies in the darkness, heavy as lead, but your spirit seems to soar and leave the hut, and with the speed of thought, to travel where it listeth, in time and space, accompanied by the shaman's singing . . . at last you know what the ineffable is, and what ecstasy means. Ecstasy! The mind harks back to the origin of that word. For the Greeks ekstasis meant the flight of the soul from the body. Can you find a better word to describe this state?[24]

The mushroom that seems to have the greatest psychoactive effect is *Psilocybe mexicana*. The primary active agent in this mushroom is psilocybin, which the discoverer of LSD, Albert Hofmann, isolated in 1958 and later synthesized. Before he did this, however, he ate 32 of the mushrooms (an average dose) to determine the potency of his mushroom supply. Hofmann's report of this experience is interesting because of the contrast with his experience with LSD, where he had had no prior expectations of the hallucinogenic effects. The comparison of Hofmann's experience with Wasson's account reemphasizes the importance of both the personality and the setting in trying to understand the effects of these drugs.

> Thirty minutes after taking the mushrooms the exterior world began to undergo a strange transformation. Everything assumed a Mexican character. As I was perfectly well aware that my knowledge of the Mexican origin of the mushroom would lead me to imagine only Mexican scenery, I tried deliberately to look on my environment as I knew it normally. But all voluntary efforts to look at things in their customary forms and colors proved ineffective. Whether my eyes were closed or open I saw only Mexican motifs and colors. When the doctor supervising the experiment bent over me to check my blood pressure, he was transformed into an Aztec priest and I would not have been astonished if he had drawn an obsidian knife. In spite of the seriousness of the situation it amused me to see how the Germanic face of my colleague had acquired a purely Indian expression. At the peak of the intoxication, about $1\frac{1}{2}$ hours after ingestion of the mushrooms, the rush of interior pictures, mostly abstract motifs rapidly changing in shape and color, reached such an alarming de-

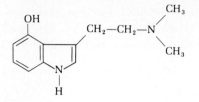

Psilocin
(3-[2-(dimethylamino)ethyl]-indol-4-ol)

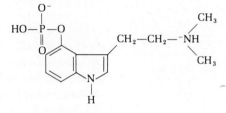

Psilocybin
(3-[2-(dimethylamino)ethyl]-indol-4-ol dihydrogen phosphate ester)

FIG. 18-1   Indole hallucinogens.

gree that I feared that I would be torn into this whirlpool of form and color and would dissolve. After about six hours the dream came to an end. Subjectively, I had no idea how long this condition had lasted. I felt my return to everyday reality to be a happy return from a strange, fantastic but quite really experienced world into an old and familiar home.[3,p.176]

The dried mushrooms contain 0.2% to 0.5% of psilocybin. Psilocybin is unique (Fig. 18-1) because it is the only known naturally occurring indole to contain phosphorus. Even so, the hallucinogenic effects of psilocybin are quite similar to those of LSD and the catechol hallucinogen mescaline, and cross-tolerance exists among these three agents.[5,6]

The psychoactive effects are clearly related to the amount used, with up to 4 mg yielding a pleasant experience, relaxation, and some body sensations. Higher doses cause considerable perceptual and body image changes with hallucinations in some individuals. Accompanying these psychic changes are dose-related sympathetic arousal symptoms. There is some evidence that psilocybin has its central nervous system effects only after it has been changed in the body to psil-

ocin. Psilocin is present in the mushroom only in trace amounts but is about one and one-half times as potent as psilocybin. Perhaps the greater CNS effect of psilocin is the result of its higher lipid solubility.

One of Leary's followers used psilocybin in the now classic Good Friday study. The Good Friday study was designed to investigate the ability of psilocybin to induce meaningful religious experiences in individuals when the drug is used in a religious setting. Twenty seminarians participated in a double-blind study, with half receiving 30 mg of psilocybin and half placebos 90 minutes before attending a religious service. Tape recordings of the subjects' experiences were made immediately after the 2½-hour service, which was held in a chapel. Within a week a questionnaire was completed, followed by a similar one 6 months later. The first was directed at determining the magnitude and type of change that occurred during the experiment, and the later one at assessing the durability of the change. Leary later summarized the outcome of the Good Friday study by saying:

the results clearly support the hypothesis that, with adequate preparation and in an environment which is supportive and religiously meaningful, subjects report mystical experiences significantly more than placebo controls.[7]

He then commented on the results of some other studies that looked at the relationship between hallucinogens and religious experiences and concluded:

data . . . indicte that (1) if the setting is supportive but not spiritual, between 40 to 75 per cent of psychedelic subjects will report intense and life-changing religious experiences; and that (2) if the set and setting are supportive and spiritual, then from 40 to 90 per cent of the experiences will be revelatory and mystico-religious.

There will always be debate over whether a religious experience associated with drug use is as real, as valid, as one that occurs in the absence of drug use. Whether you personally are pro or con on this issue, it seems essential that the following concept be integrated into your position.

On hearing reports that persons have enjoyed religious experiences following the ingestion of a mushroom, a cactus, or LSD, the typical religious person tends to dismiss such reactions as . . . dangerous forms of pseudo religion. To bring about religious experience through such artificial stimuli sounds like trying to play God. Yet those who make such suggestions see nothing amiss in trying to encourage religious experience by such artificial stimuli as organ music, Gothic architecture, Bible reading, prolonged silence, candles, ritual, or fasting; and fasting certainly has an effect on one's chemical composition.[8]

Ololiuqui

Of the psychoactive agents used freely in Mexico in the sixteenth century, ololiuqui, seeds of the morning glory plant *Rivea corymbosa*, perhaps had the greatest religious significance. In Hernandez's words, "When the priests wanted to commune with their gods and to receive a message from them, they ate this plant to induce a delirium. A thousand visions and satanic hallucinations appeared to them. . . ." When one has a good plant, it should

not be saved only for the priests; thus, ololiuqui was used medicinally "to cure flatulence, to remedy venereal troubles, to deaden pain, and to remove tumors."[3]

These seeds tie American to Europe and today because when Albert Hofmann analyzed the seeds of the morning glory, he found several active alkaloids as well as *d*-lysergic acid amide. *d*-Lysergic acid amide is about one tenth as active as LSD. The presence of *d*-lysergic acid amide is really quite amazing (to botany majors) because prior to this discovery in 1960, lysergic acid had been found only in much more primitive groups of plants such as the ergot fungus.[9]

A different species of morning glory, *Ipomoea violacea*, seems to be the primary source in the United States of most commercial morning glory seeds containing effective amounts of these alkaloids. Considering the psychoactivity of these seeds, the commercial names seem quite appropriate: Pearly Gates, Flying Saucers, Heavenly Blue!

Morning glory seeds were something quite different from mushrooms. Seeds could be bought at your nearby neighborly garden supply store, and were. When eaten, some of these commercial seeds produced psychoactive effects similar to LSD and psilocybin, according to reports in the literature, and there is at least one instance of an extract of the seeds being taken intravenously.[10-11]

DMT

Only brief mention will be made of DMT, since it is not widely used in the United States, although it has a long, if not noble, history. In fact, on a worldwide basis, DMT is probably the most important naturally occurring hallucinogenic compound, and it occurs in many plants. Dimethyltryptamine is the active agent in Cohoba snuff, which is used by some South American and Caribbean Indians. It is ineffective when taken orally, unless in the presence of a monoamine oxidase inhibitor, and must be inhaled, through snuff or smoking, or taken by injection.

The effective intramuscular dose (of the drug,

not the snuff, which is not readily available) is about 1 mg/kg of body weight. Since the effect lasts only about an hour, it can be used during lunch; the experience has been called a "businessman's trip."[12]

Amanita muscaria

It got down off the mushroom, and crawled away into the grass, merely remarking as it went, "One side will make you grow taller, and the other side will make you grow shorter."

"One side of *what?* The other side of *what?*" thought Alice to herself.

"Of the mushroom," said the Caterpillar, just as if she had asked it aloud: and in another moment it was out of sight.

Alice remained looking thoughtfully at the mushroom for a minute, trying to make out which were the two sides of it; and, as it was perfectly round, she found this a very difficult question. However, at last she stretched her arms round it as far as they would go, and broke off a bit of the edge with each hand.

"And now which is which?" she said to herself, and nibbled a little of the right hand bit to try the effect. . . .[13]

The mushrooms are personified as little men, one dwarf to a mushroom, and when under its influence one used to speak of these dwarfs as all-powerful.[14,p.415]

If Mexico has magic mushrooms, then Russia and the Scandinavian countries must lay claim to the mushroom that is reusable. The *Amanita muscaria* mushroom has been used for centuries, and Wasson[15,p.405] suggests (even though there was no tobacco in Eurasia):

It will be necessary for us all to make room in our own remote past for the part played by this mushroom, and the fly agaric will take its place by the side of alcohol, hashish, and tobacco as an outstanding inebriant utilized by *Homo sapiens* living in Eurasia.

This mushroom is also called "fly agaric," perhaps because it has insecticidal properties! It doesn't kill the flies, but when they suck its juice, it puts them into a stupor for 2 to 3 hours. Recently several authorities[16,p.441] have suggested another explanation for the name:

the association through the middle ages and earlier, of madness with the fly. People who were possessed were believed to be infested with flies. This was true throughout northern Eurasia . . . the fly spelled insanity. When you were treated, they waited for a fly to emerge from your nostril and you were cured. . . . These flies in Fly Agaric are . . . symbols for the demonic power of Fly Agaric.

The older literature suggests that eating five to ten *Amanita* mushrooms results in "severe effects of intoxication such as muscular twitching, leading to twitches of limbs; raving drunkenness with agitation and vivid hallucinations. Later, partial paralysis with sleep and dreams follow for many hours."[17,p.437] One article[18] summarizes the behavioral effects:

Effects of *Amanita muscaria* vary appreciably with individuals and at different times. An hour after the ingestion of the mushrooms, twitching and trembling of the limbs is noticeable with the onset of a period of good humor and light euphoria, characterized by macroscopia, visions of the supernatural and illusions of grandeur. Religious overtones—such as an urge to confess sins—frequently occur. Occasionally, the partaker becomes violent, dashing madly about until, exhausted, he drops into a deep sleep.

A 1963 report[19] on a case of *Amanita* intoxication comments: "In these days of drugs, pep pills, and 'goof balls' it was almost refreshing recently to encounter a revival of addiction to the old ambrosia." The authors go on to speak of the reported effects of the mushroom on the users: "They enjoyed the effects of eating the *A. muscaria*. The feeling of unreality and detachment was always pleasant. They felt an increase in power and a degree of invulnerability."

Perhaps because the written history on the mushroom is not very old, going back only to about the seventeenth century, and in part because the active chemical constituent still eludes the biochemist, there are many speculations about the role in our history of this red-topped and white-spotted poisonous fungus.

First stop is the land of the midnight sun and the Icelandic legends that describe the phenomena of *Berserksgang*—going berserk. When this happened, the warriors showed a shivering and chattering of teeth, and in battle they would fight with a tremendous rage. The rage was well known to the Christians of medieval times and is clearly reflected in one of their prayers, which has been oft-repeated in movies: "From the intolerable fury of the Norsemen, Oh Lord, deliver us!"

The intolerable fury has come down to us today in the word *berserk,* which is derived from the uniform worn in battle by one of the heroes of a Norse legend, a bear (*ber*) skin (*serk*). In the eighteenth century and again in the nineteenth, Scandinavian botanists suggested that the fury of the Norsemen resulted from eating fly agaric prior to battle.[20] There is considerable doubt today about the validity of this interpretation.

The suggestion has also been made that the ambrosia food of the gods—mentioned in the secret rites of the god Dionysius in Greece—was a solution of the *Amanita* mushroom.[21] A really far-out suggestion is that *Amanita muscaria* use formed the basis for the cult that originated about 2000 years ago and today calls itself Christianity.[22] Wasson has proposed that this fungus is the famous unidentified Soma of the Rig Veda poems written about 2000 BC,[15] and most scholars accept this interpretation.

There is no resolution of the role this magic mushroom of the North has played in our past, but its use continues today in several parts of Soviet Russian territory.

Use of the Amanita mushroom by Siberian tribes continues today largely free from social control of any sort. Use of the drug has a Shamanist aspect,

and forms the basis for orgiastic communal indulgences. Since the drug can induce murderous rages in addition to more moderate hallucinogenic experiences, serious injuries frequently result.[23]

The mushrooms are expensive; sometimes several reindeer are exchanged for an effective number of the mushrooms. They do have the unique property of being reusable, and during the long winter months they may be worth the price. The mushrooms themselves are not reusable; once eaten, they're gone. But this is a hallucinogen that is excreted unchanged in the urine. When the effect begins to wear off, "midway in the orgy the cry of 'pass the pot' goes out."[23] The active ingredient can be reused four or five times in this way!

Until a few years ago the psychoactive agent in *Amanita muscaria* was thought to be bufotenin (*N,N*-dimethylserotonin or 5-hydroxy-*N,N*-dimethyl-tryptamine). It has an indole structure and has been suspected of being a hallucinogen, but the evidence is far from clear. If bufotenin does prove to be psychoactive, it may have been the important ingredient in the witches' brew discussed in *Macbeth:*

> Round about the cauldron go;
> In the poisoned entrails throw.
> Toad that under cold stone,
> Days and nights has thirty-one.

since the skin of toads has a fair amount of bufotenin. The fly agaric mushroom, however, has very little.

The total list of active ingredients of *Amanita muscaria* is not known, but two that have much importance at this time are ibotenic acid and muscimol.

Muscimol and ibotenic acid, two psychotomimetic principles of *Amanita muscaria*, have effects similar to those of LSD on norepinephrine, dopamine and serotonin concentrations in the brains of mice and rats. The increased serotonin concentration in the hypothalamus and midbrain is probably caused by a diminished turnover or liberation of serotonin, perhaps resulting from a diminished pulse flow serotonergic neurons.[24, p. 161]

CATECHOL HALLUCINOGENS
Peyote

Peyote is truly unique among hallucinogenic agents, since it is the only American plant used in sacred and religious ceremonies from before written history that has been retained as an integral part of a recognized religious group. Peyote (peyotl) is the cactus *Lophophora williamsii*, which is a synonym for an earlier designation, *Anhalonium lewinii*. It was so named to honor Lewin, who studied the plant after his 1886 trip to the United States.[25] In 1888 Parke-Davis produced and sold a "tincture of *Anhalonium lewinii*," which they said had "marked physiological action similar to strychnine."[26]

When Cortez moved into Mexico in the early 1500s, he took with him Christian missionaries whose goal was to drive out all remnants of the Aztec civilization and religion. They were also, and rather incidentally, to save the heathens. Before the ancient religious and ceremonial customs were forced underground, many reports were made of plants being used for sacred purposes.

The peyote cactus was described by Hernandez: "The root is of nearly medium size, sending forth no branches or leaves above the ground. . . . Both men and women are said to be harmed by it . . . it causes those devouring it to be able to foresee and predict things. . . ." Earlier and later reports in the sixteenth century emphasized even more the psychoactive aspects of its use: "those who eat or chew it see visions either frightful or laughable . . ." and "see visions of terrifying sights like the devil. . . ." Briefly:

> Peyote (from the Aztec *peyotl*) is a small, spineless, carrot-shaped cactus, *Lophophora williamsii* Lemaire, which grows wild in the Rio Grande Valley and southward. It is mostly subterranean, and only the grayish-green pincushion-like top appears above ground. . . .[27]

> In pre-Columbian times the Aztec, Huichol, and other Mexican Indians ate the plant ceremonially either in the dried or green state. This produces profound sensory and psychic derangements last-

ing twenty-four hours, a property which led the natives to value and use it religiously.[28,p.7]

Only the part of the cactus that is above ground is easily edible, but the entire plant is psychoactive. This upper portion, or crown, is sliced into disks that dry and are known as "mescal buttons." These slices of the peyote cactus remain psychoactive indefinitely and are the source of the cactus between the yearly harvests. The journey by Indians in November and December to harvest the peyote is an elaborate ceremony, sometimes taking almost a month and a half. When the mescal buttons are to be used, they are soaked in the mouth until soft, then formed by hand into a bolus and swallowed.

Mescal buttons should not be confused with the mescal beans or with mescal liquor, which is distilled from the fermentation of the agave cactus. Mescal buttons are slices of the peyote cactus and contain mescaline as the primary active agent. Mescal beans, however, are dark red seeds from the shrub *Sophora secundiflora*. "These seeds, formerly the basis of a vision-seeking cult, contain a highly toxic alkaloid, cystisine, the effects of which somewhat resemble nicotine, causing nausea, convulsions, hallucinations and occasional death from respiratory failure."[3] The mescal bean has a long history, and there is some evidence that use of the bean diminished and ceased when the safer peyote became available in the southwestern United States. In the transition from a mescal bean to a mescal button cult there appeared, in some tribes, a period in which a mixture of peyote and mescal seeds was concocted and drunk. These factors contributed to considerable confusion in the early (and some recent) literature.[9]

It would be a serious error if an anthropologist or ethnobotanist confused the two. In a legislative situation such a confusion could have a devastating impact. In a weighty report to the House of Representatives in 1918 on "Prohibition of Use of Peyote," one of the supporting documents was a 1909 letter by an Indian agent who confused the two. (Compare his description with those of the mescal bean and mescal button effects noted previously.) In part, his report[29] said:

with reference to the effects of the peyote, commonly known as mescal . . .

Several deaths have been reported to me which were clearly caused by the use of peyote; two, in particular, which resulted from an apparently healthy Indian dying while in the stupor from the use of peyote.

The customary dose for beginners is eight peyote beans, taken in the form prescribed below, together with from two to five drinks of the water in which the beans have been steeped. . . .

Death is caused from malnutrition and by a violent disturbance of the digestive organs, and also by action on the respiratory centers.

The users of the peyote have described to me a feeling which they say they experience after using it a short time resembling that of suffocation. . . .

It is most commonly used among the Indians of this agency by first steeping the bean in hot water; then the bean is mashed and rolled in the fingers, and from 8 to 50 are taken at one time or during one meeting of the peyote users. In addition to eating the bean, they also drink the water in which the bean has been steeped. . . .

Use in religion. Peyote played an important role in some of the religious groups in Mexico. The early missionaries attempted to stop its use. A Spanish missionary, Padre de Leon, had priests include the following questions in the confessional to be used with penitent Indians:

Art thou a sooth-sayer? Dost thou foretell events by reading omens, interpreting dreams, or by tracing circles and figures on water? . . . Dost thou suck the blood of others? Dost thou wander about at night, calling upon demons to help thee? Hast thou drunk peyotl, or given it to others to drink. . . .[28,p.23]

Nothing succeeded in eliminating its use, but peyote did go underground, along with the other magic plants of Mexico, only recently to reemerge. Although there was evidence that the use of peyote had moved north into the United States as early as 1760, it was not until the late nineteenth century

that a peyote cult was widely established among the Indians of the plains.

From that time to the present, Indian missionaries have spread the peyote religion to almost a quarter of a million Indians, some as far north as Canada. The development of the present form of this sect has been summarized:

the independent groups of the Peyote Religion have federated into the Native American Church during the 20th century, like the independent congregations of the Jesus Cult federated into the Catholic Church during the 4th century. However, just as not all congregations accepting the basic doctrines of Christianity belonged to the Catholic Church, so not all groups accepting the basic doctrines of Peyotism belong to the Native American Church.[30]

In 1960 peyotism was "the major religious cult of most Indians of the United States between the Rocky Mountains and the Mississippi. . . ."[27]

One version of how this variant of Christianity developed was told by a member of one tribe:

A long time ago Indians were fighting: they killed each other and one woman was left from the tribes. She walked over the Desert—there was no food nor water: she was almost starved. Then a voice was heard from the sky. It was Jesus, and said, "Look down at this thing (pointing to Father Peyote, a large peyote disc) and you will get food and drink." She walked over a hill and on the other side she found water—it was her food from the skies, and the voice said this, peyote, was her food.[31]

The Native American Church of the United States was first chartered in Oklahoma in 1918 and is an amalgamation of Christianity and traditional beliefs and practices of the Indians. Its basic beliefs are simply stated in the articles of incorporation:

The purpose for which this corporation is formed is to foster and promote religious believers in Almighty God and the customs of the several Tribes of Indians throughout the United States in the worship of a Heavenly Father and to promote morality, sobriety, industry, charity, and right living and cultivate a spirit of self-respect and brotherly love and union among the members of the several Tribes of Indians throughout the United States . . . with and through the sacramental use of peyote.[32]

As in all religions there has developed a whole series of rituals surrounding the use of peyote in religious ceremonies. Peyote is also used in other ways because the Indians attribute spiritual power to the peyote plant. As such, peyote is believed to be helpful, along with prayers and modern medicines, in curing illnesses. It is also worn as an amulet, much as some Christians wear a St. Christopher's medal, to protect the wearer from harm.

In the charter year, 1918, bills were introduced into the United States Congress, as they had been before, to restrict the use of peyote by the Indians. The entire report to the House of Representatives on "Prohibition of Use of Peyote" is interesting, but only a few of the more relevant issues can be mentioned here.

Reviewing some of the clear thinking presented by those advocating restricting the use of peyote, it is surprising that the bill was not enacted. For example, considering the question of whether alcohol or peyote is more harmful, the report of a physician says:

So far as its results upon the human economy are concerned from a pathological standpoint, alcohol is altogether the safest and least harmful. The alcoholic subject may, by careful system of dietetics, escape physical and mental weakness, but the mescal fiend travels to absolute incompetency. It is a vicious thing.[29]

Some testimony was solicited from scientific authorities, and Dr. H.W. Wiley, who spearheaded the enactment of the 1906 Pure Food and Drugs Act, sent a letter that said, in part:

It is driving many of them to ruin. Its effects may be compared in some particulars to those of cocaine. It causes the victim, who becomes semi-conscious, to have the most wonderful sensations of delight and pleasure, especially through the visions of flowers, sunshine, and verdure, which rise before him. The intoxication lasts from 24 to 48

hours and then gradually passes away. During its continuation the person is totally unfit for any useful purpose. It is a typically habit-forming drug, and to those who indulge in it the desire for its use becomes uncontrollable. The active principle is probably a resin or a glucoside. It probably is of the same nature of the poison in Indian hemp. Its use can no more be regarded in the light of a religious rite than that of alcohol, morphine, or cocaine. Its entire prohibition would conserve the financial, physical, mental, and spiritual welfare of the Indians.[33]

A petition to the Commissioner of Indian Affairs to prohibit peyote on Indian reservations was rejected by the Secretary of Interior, who prohibited "absolutely any interference by the Indian Bureau with the religious practices of the Native American Church."[34] This proved to be a good decision.[35]

Over 30 years later as "the baby-with-the-bathwater" type of thinking reemerged in the drug world, five famous anthropologists[32] believed it necessary to issue a statement on peyote, which begins:

there has been some propaganda to declare illegal the peyote used by many Indian tribes. . . . our duty to protest against a campaign which only reveals the ignorance of the propagandists concerned.

After a thousand well-chosen words this distinguished group concluded that

the Native American Church of the United States is a legitimate religious organization deserving of the same right to religious freedom as other churches; also, that peyote is used sacramentally in a manner corresponding to the bread and wine of white Christians.[32]

Hallucinogenic use. Near the end of the nineteenth century, Heffter isolated several alkaloids from peyote and showed that mescaline was the primary agent only for the visual effect induced by peyote. Spath in 1919 finally synthesized mescaline and most experiments on the psychoactive and/or behavioral effects since then have used synthesized mescaline. There have now been over 30 psychoactive alkaloids identified in peyote, but mescaline does seem to be the agent responsible for the vivid colors and other visual effects. The fact that mescaline is not equivalent to peyote is not always made clear in the literature.[36]

One of the early investigators of the effects of peyote was Dr. Weir Mitchell, who used an extract of peyote and who reported, in part:

> The display which for an enchanted two hours followed was such as I find it hopeless to describe in language which shall convey to others the beauty and splendor of what I saw. Stars, delicate floating films of color, then an abrupt rush of countless points of white light swept across the field of view, as if the unseen millions of the Milky Way were to flow in a sparkling river before my eyes . . . zigzag lines of very bright colors . . . the wonderful loveliness of swelling clouds of more vivid colors gone before I could name them.[37,p.34]

Another early experimenter was Havelock Ellis. Interestingly, he took his peyote on Good Friday in 1897, 65 years before the much noted Good Friday experiment with psilocybin. His experience is described in detail in a 1902 article titled "Mescal: A Study of a Divine Plant"[38] in *Popular Science Monthly*, but a brief quotation gives the essence of the experience:

> . . . On the whole, if I had to describe the visions in one word, I should say that they were living arabesques. There was generally a certain incomplete tendency to symmetry, the effect being somewhat as if the underlying mechanism consisted of a large number of polished facets acting as mirrors. It constantly happened that the same image was repeated over a large part of the field, though this holds good mainly of the forms, for in the colors there would still remain all sorts of delicious varieties. Thus at a moment when uniformly jewelled flowers seemed to be springing up and extending all over the field of vision, the flowers still showed every variety of delicate tone and tint.

In reflecting on his experience Ellis[38] comments:

> It should be added that a sense of well-being is not an essential part of these sensory manifestations. In this respect mescal is entirely unlike those drugs of which alcohol is the supreme type. Under the influence of a moderate dose of alcohol the specific senses are not obviously affected at all, but there is a vague and massive consciousness of emotional well-being, a sense of satisfaction tending to a conviction that 'all's well with the world.' Alcohol has a dulling influence on sensory activity and on the intellectual centers. . . . Mescal, on the other hand, is not mainly emotional in its effects but mainly sensory and it leaves the intellect almost unimpaired even in large doses. It is true that at one stage of mescal intoxication, and more especially in quite healthy persons, there is a feeling of well-being, and even of beatitude, accompanied by an illusory sense of quite unusual intellectual activity; but there is no stage of maudlin emotionality; on the whole there is a condition of fairly unimpaired and alert intellect, untiringly absorbed in the contemplation of the strange world of new sensory phenomena into which the subject has been introduced.

In an earlier article (1897) titled "Mescal: A New Artificial Paradise,"[39] Ellis concluded by stating that

> unlike the other chief substances to which it may be compared, mescal does not wholly carry us away from the actual world, or plunge us into oblivion; a large part of its charm lies in the halo of beauty which it casts around the simplest and commonest things. . . .

> The few observations recorded in America and my own experiments in England do not enable us to say anything regarding the habitual consumption of mescal in large amounts. That such consumption would be gravely injurious I can not doubt. Its safeguard seems to lie in the fact that a certain degree of robust health is required to obtain any real enjoyment from its visionary gifts. It may at least be claimed that for a healthy person to be once or twice admitted to the rites of mescal is not only an unforgettable delight, but an educational influence of no mean value.

It may well be that not every healthy individual wants every educational opportunity that is offered him. William James, surprisingly, was one who did not. He wrote to his brother Henry: "I ate one but three days ago, was violently sick for twenty-four hours, and had no other symptoms whatever except that and the Katzenjammer the following day. I

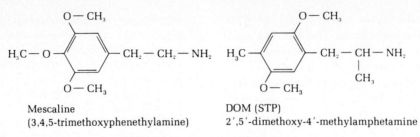

FIG. 18-2 Catechol hallucinogens.

will take the visions on trust." Even Dr. Weir Mitchell, who had the effect previously recorded, said: "These shows are expensive. . . . The experience, however, was worth one such headache and indigestion but was not worth a second."

Even if you get by without too much nausea and physical discomfort, which the Indians also report, all may not go well. Huxley, whose 1954 *The Doors of Perception*[40] made him a guru in this area, admitted: "Along with the happily transfigured majority of mescaline takers there is a minority that finds in the drug only hell and purgatory." It is reported that natives sometimes wished for "bad trips" when taking this or other plants. By meeting their personal demons, much like Saint Anthony, they hoped to conquer them and remove problems from their lives.

Pharmacodynamics of mescaline. Mescaline is readily absorbed if taken orally, but only very poorly passes the blood-brain barrier (which explains the high doses required). There is a maximal concentration of the drug in the brain after 30 to 120 minutes. About half of it is removed from the body in 6 hours, and there is evidence that some mescaline persists in the brain for up to 9 to 10 hours. Similar to the indole hallucinogens, the effects obtained with low doses, about 3mg/kg, are primarily euphoric, while doses in the range of 5mg/kg give rise to a full set of hallucinations. Most of the mescaline is excreted unchanged in the urine, and the metabolites identified thus far are not psychoactive. A study [41] of peyote-using Indians showed no effect of long-term regular use of peyote on white cell chromosomes.

A dose that is psychoeffective in humans causes pupil dilation, pulse rate and blood pressure increases, and an elevation in body temperature. All of these effects are similar to those induced by LSD, psilocybin, and most other alkaloidal hallucinogens. There are other signs of central stimulation, such as EEG arousal, following mescaline intake. In rats the LD 50 is about 370 mg/kg, 10 to 30 times the dose that causes behavioral effects. Death results from convulsions and respiratory arrest. Tolerance develops more slowly to mescaline than to LSD, and even though these drugs appear to act through different mechanisms, there is cross-tolerance between them. As with LSD, mescaline intoxication can be blocked with chlorpromazine.

Fig. 18-2 contains the chemical structures of mescaline and DOM and clearly shows their relationship to the phenethylamine structure and the catechol nucleus.

DOM (STP)

DOM is 2,5-dimethoxy-4-methylamphetamine. According to most users, DOM is called STP, and street talk is that the initials stand for serenity, tranquility, and peace. Little human work has been done with this drug in controlled laboratory situations.[42,43] Its actions and effects, however, are highly similar to mescaline and LSD, with a total dose of 1 to 3 mg yielding euphoria most often, and 3 to 5 mg a 6- to 8-hour hallucinogenic period. This makes DOM about a hundred times as potent as mescaline but only one thirtieth as potent as LSD.

DOM has a reputation of inducing an extraordinarily long experience, but this seems to be caused by the very large amounts being used. Pills of DOM bought on the street contain about 10 mg—a very big dose. Reports by users had suggested that DOM was unlike other hallucinogens and that its effects were enhanced rather than blocked by chlorpromazine. Controlled laboratory work with normal volunteers, however, has clearly shown that the effects of DOM are similar to those of other hallucinogens and that chlorpromazine does attenuate the DOM experience.[44]

An early report[45] and an excellent review from the Haight-Ashbury Clinic[46] contains most of the essential information about the rise and fall of DOM use. The latter paper concluded:

> It appears then that DOM produces a higher incidence of acute and chronic toxic reactions than any of the other commonly used hallucinogens. . . . It appears that the effects of DOM are like a combination of amphetamine and LSD with the hallucinogenic effects of the drug very often putting the peripheral amphetamine like physiological effects out of perspective. . . .[46,p.4]
> DOM may be taken more frequently than is known. It is often substituted for mescaline. In one study none of 23 "mescaline" purchases contained mescaline, but several were DOM.[47]

ANTICHOLINERGIC HALLUCINOGENS

It may be a bit discouraging to those whose ancestors came from Europe that so far only one of the hallucinogens has had its noble, or ignoble, history in traditional western culture. Unfortunately, now it is necessary to deal with the drugs that poisoned Hamlet's father as well as the Roman Emperor Claudius. Strange that they should be the same agents that probably made Cleopatra bright-eyed if not bushy-tailed and the same magic potions that gave witches liftoff power and put the kick in Vietnam marijuana.

The potato family contains all the naturally occurring agents to be discussed here. Three of the genera—*Atropa, Hyoscyamus,* and *Mandragora*—have a single species of importance and were primarily restricted to Europe. The fourth genus, *Datura,* is world-wide and has many species containing the active agents.

The family of plants in which all these genera are found is *Solanaceae,* herbs of consolation, and three pharmacologically active alkaloids are responsible for the effects of these plants. Atroprine, which is *dl*-hyoscyamine, scopolamine or *l*-hyoscine, and *l*-hyoscyamine are all potent central and peripheral cholinergic blocking agents. These drugs occupy the acetylcholine receptor site but do not activate it; thus, their effect is primarily to block cholinergic neurons, including the parasympathetic system. The relative potencies of atropine and scopolamine vary at different structures. In their central actions scopolamine may be as much as a hundred times as potent as atropine. The *l* form of hyoscyamine is up to 50 times as potent centrally as atropine, which is a combination of the *d* and *l* forms of hyoscyamine. The structures of the two most widely studied anticholinergic agents, atropine and scopolamine, are shown in Fig. 18-3.

These agents have potent peripheral as well as central effects, and some of the psychological responses to these drugs are probably a reaction to peripheral changes. These alkaloids are frequently ingredients in cold symptom remedies because they block the production of mucus in the nose and throat. They also prevent salivation, so the mouth becomes uncommonly dry, and perspiration stops. Temperature may increase to fever levels (109° F has been reported in infants with atropine poisoning), and heart rate may show a 50-beat-per-minute increase with atropine. Even at moderate doses these chemicals cause considerable dilation of the pupils of the eyes with a resulting inability to focus on nearby objects.

Centrally these drugs depress the reticular formation and cause a slowing of the EEG. With large enough doses, a behavioral pattern develops which resembles that of a toxic psychosis; there is delirium, mental confusion, loss of attention, drowsiness, and loss of memory for recent events. It was the loss of memory and confusion that was the basis for Lewin's classification of these agents as hypnotics rather than as phantasticants. These two characteristics—a clouding of consciousness and no memory for the period of intoxication—plus the absence of vivid sensory effects separate these

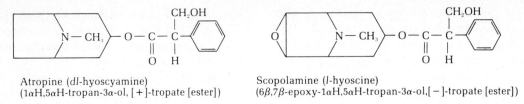

Atropine (*dl*-hyoscyamine)
(1αH,5αH-tropan-3α-ol, [+]-tropate [ester])

Scopolamine (*l*-hyoscine)
(6β,7β-epoxy-1αH,5αH-tropan-3α-ol,[−]-tropate [ester])

FIG. 18-3 Naturally occurring anticholinergic hallucinogens.

drugs from the indole and catechol hallucinogens.

These agents are rapidly absorbed from the gastrointestinal tract and from the mucous membranes of the body. There are no definitive studies, but up to 50% of atropine may be excreted unchanged in the urine. At high doses death results from paralysis of the respiratory muscles.

All of these anticholinergic effects, from both central and peripheral nervous system actions, can be reversed by administration of physostigmine (eserine). Physostigmine has anticholinesterase activity, which results in an accumulation of acetylcholine to levels where the receptor blockade (by atropine or scopolamine) is overridden. When given in the absence of anticholinergic agents, physostigmine can be quite toxic and causes an increase in the activity of the cholinergic-parasympathetic system. The toxicity is clearly suggested by the fact that physotigmine was originally derived from the "ordeal bean" of Calabar, West Africa. An individual accused of a crime was made to drink a potion made from the beans; if he survived, he was innocent. If not, the verdict and sentence were delivered together.

Atropa belladonna

The deadly nightshade, *Atropa belladonna*, has as its active ingredient atropine, which was isolated in 1831. The name of the plant reflects two of its major uses in the Middle Ages and before. The genus name reflects its use as a poison. Atropos was the oldest of the three Fates in Greek mythology, and it was her duty to cut the thread of life when the time came. The deadly nightshade was one of the plants used extensively by both professional and amateur poisoners, since 14 of its berries contain enough of the alkaloid to cause death.

Belladonna, the species name, refers to the "beautiful woman," a term that is a result of the use of the extract of this plant to dilate the pupils of the eyes. Interestingly, Roman and Egyptian women knew something that science did not learn until quite recently. In the 1950s it was demonstrated, by using pairs of photographs identical except for the amount of pupil dilation, that most people judge the girl with the most dilated eyes as the prettiest.

Of more interest here than pretty girls or poisoned men is the sensation of flying reported by witches. The first step toward completing this experiment is to make an ointment. Although there are many recipes, a good one seems to be baby's fat, juice of water parsnip, aconite, cinquefoile, deadly nightshade, and soot. The soot makes the mixture black and, when rubbed on, serves to camouflage the body at night. The baby fat is added in amounts to suit the individual and makes the concoction adhere to the skin. The water parsnip is most likely not the kind used in salads but rather hemlock (yes, the same hemlock Socrates was forced to use), which is quite similar in appearance. Aconite is a pretty plant from the buttercup family and the deadly poison that killed Romeo. In very small doses the *Aconitum napellus* plant will cause a slowing and irregular heartbeat. The deadly nightshade containing atropine is the only other active ingredient in our flying recipe. With moderate doses there is some excitement and delirium along with impaired vision because of the pupillary dilation.

When the ointment is made, it is rubbed on the body and especially liberally between the legs and on a stick that is to be straddled. This stick served as a phallic symbol during the ceremony of the Sabbat. The Sabbat, or Black Mass, worshipped Satan, and both males and females engaged in a nightlong orgy. Straddling the stick and hopping and shrieking around a circle they felt able "to be carried in the aire, to feasting, singing, dansing, kissing, culling and other acts of venerie, with such youthes as they loue and desire most!"[48,p.81] The feeling of levitation perhaps comes from the irregular hearbeat in conjunction with drowsiness. Some have reported that changes in heart rate coupled with falling asleep sometimes results in a sensation of falling (or flying?)[49] but a more likely explanation is simply the power of suggestion.

Other actions were important in causing the effects of the Sabbat. The pounding of the heart would certainly convey excitement, and the excitement might cause sexual arousal. One of the reputations of belladonna was as an aphrodisiac, so it may all fit together. Perhaps the physiological effects of the agents coupled with a good placebo effect was enough for the witches who attended the Sabbat. It is to be noted that, unfortunately, the recipe will not work on the well-scrubbed American of today. Few agents are absorbed through unbroken skin, but in the typical individual of the Middle Ages—unwashed and with vermin bites, open sores, and the like—there is a good chance that the alkaloids would get into the bloodstream from the ointment.

Mandragora officinarum

The famous mandrake plant (*Mandragora officinarum*) contains all three alkaloids. One writer suggests that the root may contain up to 0.4% of the agents, a healthy dose. Although many drugs could be traced to the Bible, it is particularly important to do so with the mandrake because of its close association with love and lovemaking has persisted from Genesis to recent times.

In the time of wheat-harvest Reuben went out and found some mandrakes in the open country and brought them to his mother Leah. Then Rachel asked Leah for some of her son's mandrakes, but Leah said, "Is it so small a thing to have taken away my husband, that you should take my son's mandrakes as well?" But Rachel said, "Very well, let him sleep with you tonight in exchange for your son's mandrakes." So when Jacob came in from the country in the evening, Leah went out to meet him and said, "You are to sleep with me tonight; I have hired you with my son's mandrakes." That night he slept with her. . . .[50,p.33]

The root of the mandrake is forked and, if you have a vivid imagination, resembles a human body. The root contains the psychoactive agents and was endowed with all sorts of magical and medical properties as a result of the "Doctrine of Signatures," which was phrased nicely by Mr. Stone in Chapter 11. It was the association with the human form that led Juliet in her farewell to use the phrase: "And shrieks like mandrakes torn out of the earth, That living mortals hearing them run mad."

One of the foremost experts[51] in the field of psychoactive plants, in referring to the mandrake, states:

Its intricate history as a magic plant has hardly been equalled by any other species. . . . Folk medicine regarded *Mandragora* as a panacea and recommended its use, notwithstanding its great toxicity, as a sedative and hypnotic agent in treating nervous conditions and pain. . . . It was employed further for many other illnesses and abnormal conditions, and, in many regions was considered to be an effective aphrodisiac.

Hyoscyamus niger

Compared to the deadly nightshade and the mandrake, the *Hyoscyamus niger* has had a most uninteresting life. This is strange, since it is pharmacologically quite active and contains both scopolamine and *l*-hyoscyamine. There are other plants of this genus that contain effective levels of the alkaloids, but it is *Hyoscyamus niger* that appears throughout history as henbane, a highly poisonous substance and truly the bane of hens as well as other animals.

Pliny in 60 AD said: "For this is certainly known,

that, if one takes it in drink more than four leaves, it will put him beside himself." Hamlet's father must have had more than four leaves because it was henbane that was used to poison him.

Henbane may also have been used for socially popular purposes. This is brought home in the following quotation, in which a close relationship is suggested between the orgies of the ancients and the Sabbats of the Middle Ages:

> These plants were undoubtedly used in the ancient world in connection with orgiastic rites characterized by sexual excess. Thus at the Bacchanalia, when the wild-eyed Bacchantes with their flowing locks flung themselves naked into the arms of the eager men, one can be reasonably certain that the wine which produced such sexual frenzy was not a plain fermented grape juice. Intoxication of this kind was almost certainly a result of doctoring the wine with leaves or berries of belladonna or henbane. The orgiastic rites were never totally suppressed by the Church and persisted in secret forms through the Middle Ages. Being under the shadow of the Church's displeasure, they were inevitably associated with the Devil, and those who took part in them were considered to be either witches or wizards.[37]

Datura

The distribution of the many *Datura* species is worldwide, but they all contain the three alkaloids under discussion—atropine, scopolamine, and hyoscyamine—in varying amounts. Almost as extensive as the distribution are its uses and its history. Some hint of the length of this history is seen in a quote from a 1970 article:[51] "The Chinese valued this drug far back into ancient times. A comparatively recent Chinese medical text, published in 1590, reported that 'when Buddha preaches a sermon, the heavens bedew the petals of this plant with rain drops.' " The text does suggest the importance of the plant, *Datura metel*, by associating it with Buddha, much as tea and Daruma were related in legend.

Halfway around the world 2500 years before the Chinese text, virgins sat in the temple to Apollo in Delphi and, probably under the influence of *Datura*,[51] mumbled sounds that holy men phrased as predictions that always came true. The procedure was straightforward, and:

> preliminary to the divine possession, she appears to have chewed leaves of the sacred laurel . . . [prior to speaking] . . . she was supposed to be inspired by a mystic vapour that arose from a fissure in the ground.[52,p.831]

Probably either the plant material eaten was one of the *Datura* species or the burning seeds and leaves of the *Datura* plant formed the mystic vapor she inhaled. It should not go unnoticed, as we search for the beyond within, that engraved on the temple at Delphi were the words, "Know thyself."

Datura was and is part of love potions in India, and the practice of mixing the crushed seeds of *Datura metel* in tobacco and food in Asia persists even today. But, as one writer[51] stated:

> The real centre of the hallucinogenic use of *Datura* lies in the New World, where many more species play major roles in magic, medicine and religion in sundry cultures.

The ever-busy chronicler Hernandez mentioned the use of *Datura inoxia* by the Aztecs, and the use of various *Datura* species by Indians of the United States Southwest for magical and religious purposes is well substantiated.[48] One of the interesting uses of *Datura stramonium*, which is native and grows wild in eastern United States, was devised by the Algonquin Indians. They used the plant to solve the problem of the adolescent search for identity.

> The youths are confined for long periods, given " . . . no other substance but the infusion or decoction of some poisonous, intoxicating roots . . . " and "they became stark, staring mad, in which raving condition they were kept eighteen or twenty days. . . .". These poor creatures drink so much of that water of Lethe that they perfectly lose the remembrance of all former things, even of their parents, their treasure and their language. When the doctors find that they have drunk sufficiently of the wysoccan . . . they gradually restore them to their senses again. . . . Thus they unlive their

former lives and commence men by forgetting that they ever have been boys.[51]

This same plant is now called Jamestown weed, or shortened to jimsonweed, as a result of an incident that happened in the seventeenth century. This was fortunately recorded for history in the famous book *The History and Present State of Virginia*,[53,p.139] published first in 1705 by Robert Beverly.

The *James-Town* Weed (which resembles the Thorny Apple of *Peru*, and I take to be the Plant so call'd) is supposed to be one of the greatest Coolers in the World. This being an early Plant, was gather'd very young for a boil'd Salad, by some of the Soldiers sent thither, to pacifie the Troubles of *Bacon*; and some of them eat plentifully of it, the Effect of which was a very pleasant Comedy; for they turn'd natural Fools upon it for several Days: One would blow up a Feather in the Air; another wou'd dart Straws at it with much Fury; and another stark naked was sitting up in a Corner, like a Monkey, grinning and making Mows at them; a Fourth would fondly kiss, and paw his Companions, and snear in their Faces, with a Countenance more antick, than any in a *Dutch* Droll. In this frantick Condition they were confined, lest they should in their Folly destroy themselves; though it was observed, that all their Actions were full of Innocence and good Nature. Indeed, they were not very cleanly; for they would have wallow'd in their own Excrements, if they had not been prevented. A thousand such simple Tricks they play'd, and after Eleven Days, return'd to themselves again, not remembring any thing that had pass'd.

Some authorities[54] believe that some of the marijuana used in Southeast Asia is spiked with *Datura*. Reports of these marijuana users and observation of their behavior fit nicely into the type of syndrome discussed here. There may also be marijuana liberally laced with opium or hashish, but *Datura* probably is part of the mixture in some of the cigarettes.

Products containing stramonium are used in the treatment of asthma; prior to 1968 many could be purchased as OTC drugs. Use of these products to produce hallucinations led the FDA to make them all prescription-only compounds. Publication of several widely read books by Carlos Castaneda on Mexican Indian mysticism[55] resulted in increased use of jimsonweed. As should by now be evident, it is easy to misuse, and hospitalizations occurred; it is not a good trip.[56]

Synthetics

Both atropine and scopolamine are found in many prescription drugs and preparations, but they are most easily available in some OTC cold remedies and sleeping preparations.[57] There are some reports that atropine is effective in the treatment of some neuroses and psychoses, but its use has not been widespread.[58]

Ditran is a synthetic anticholinergic agent that causes a toxic psychosis much like that induced by atropine or scopolamine. Doses, orally, are in the range of

2-20 mg in adult males. The autonomic effects of Ditran exceed those of LSD. Mydriasis, flushing, nausea, vomiting, dryness of the mouth, tachycardia, hyperreflexia, and ataxia are encountered. More mental confusion, speech disturbances, and disorientation are seen than with other hallucinogens. Blocking, amnesias, thought disorganization, and feelings of strangeness are often mentioned. All contact with reality and insight into the cause of the mental disruptions may be lost.[59,p.503]

To this time this agent has not been reported in use illegally. Not so with PCP.

PHENCYCLIDINE

Phencyclidine hydrochloride, PCP (see Fig. 18-4), was never sacred, is never found in a plant, is still in its twenties, and yet is *the* hallucinogen of our time. It is difficult to figure out just why this is, but that's what we'll try to do here. In the middle to late 1960s PCP was everywhere but the trip was so bad that people stopped using it—or so they thought. PCP went underground—it was sold as mescaline, LSD, THC, you name it. It is now believed that the bad experiences reported in the

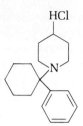

FIG. 18-4 Phencyclidine [1-(1-phenylcyclohexyl) piperidine hydrochloride].

sixties were the result of using overly large doses. PCP is the only hallucinogen in wide use that continues to increase in use. This is probably because it is available, can be taken in many ways, is fairly cheap, and has a dose range for effects that promises something for every taste—including those who are looking for danger. Another thing that PCP has going for it is a "good press"—lots of play by the media. The basic rule in publicity is: Say anything you want, but spell the name right. The media did and use went up, as was done with marijuana, with LSD, with heroin, with. . . . The media told stories about PCP that either weren't true or were distorted.[60]

Phencyclidine was synthesized in 1957 by Parke-Davis as part of a program that was looking for new nonvolatile anesthetics and analgesics. Phencyclidine was a pretty good analgesic (brand name Sernyl), and the first report[61] of its use stated that

> it can produce a profound state of analgesia. . . . The only drawback was relatively poor muscular relaxation. During the operation the animal had its eyes open and looked about unconcernedly.

> It . . . does not depress circulation or respiration. . . . It produces profound analgesia to a degree that even some major surgical procedures may be done without supplemental drugs. It has the decided disadvantage of producing in some patients severe excitement on emergence and severe hallucinatory disturbances.

The advantages of an effective, potent, intravenous, short-acting anesthetic are obvious, but there was never a way to reduce the incidence of the

hallucinatory experience as the anesthetic wore off. One later writer[62] commented that the major disadvantage "was the high incidence of dissociative phenomena. . . . These reactions, severe enough to be characterized as 'hallucinatory' in some instances, were seen in about 40 per cent of the patients anesthetized by phencyclidine and were frequently of long duration." Because of the aftereffects of this group of drugs when used for anesthesia, Parke-Davis withdrew Sernyl as an investigational drug in 1965, and in 1967 licensed another company to manufacture and sell Sernylan as a primate anesthetic. It is not and never has been an animal tranquilizer; it was an analgesic-anesthetic, and a good one for animals. This was taken off the market in the late 1970s. The PCP that is now on the street is illegally manufactured. Unfortunately, it is very easy and very inexpensive to make, and you don't even need a chemistry background. Because of this, the increased use, and the effects PCP has on the user, PCP was moved from Schedule III to Schedule II to Schedule I as of 1980.

In the late 1950s some investigators in Detroit[63] studied the effect of Sernyl on a group of normal individuals and on schizophrenic patients. They concluded that:

> There is an impressive similarity between the psychopathology resulting from . . . Sernyl and certain primary symptoms of the schizophrenic process. The disturbance in associations, inability to maintain a set, and concreteness produced by the drug were accompanied by none of the kaleidoscopic, visual, hallucinatory phenomena so characteristic of LSD-25 and mescaline. This would seem to distinguish Sernyl from the psychotomimetic agents, which might be said to mimic the secondary or restitutional symptoms of schizophrenia, while only minimally impairing the ability to associate, abstract, and maintain attention.

About 20 years later a study[64] compared hospitalized patients: PCP psychotics and acute schizophrenics. Those clinicians reported that what seems most striking . . . is a lack of interesting significant differences between the PCP psychotics and acute schizophrenics. . . . PCP psychotics do not appear to be more violent, panicky, resistant to treatment or 'organic' (for example, disoriented, confused, or ataxic) than acute schizophrenics."[64,p.242] A 1981 study[65] from the Los Angeles County Psychiatric Hospital Emergency Room identified (via blood tests) 63 PCP users in a 48-hour weekend and concluded that these patients" . . . revealed a wide variety of psychotic clinical pictures resembling mania, depression or schizophrenia with relatively few of the supposedly characteristics of PCP intoxication. . . . Each of the patients had at least one manifestation of toxic psychosis and/or acute delirium. . . . [65,p.193]

One experimenter[66] used Sernyl with schizophrenics and found that (1) they didn't like the effects and refused to take the drug again, although they would take LSD and mescaline more than once (2) many felt that they were dead or dying and became quite fearful, and (3) there were many body image disturbances. The same effects are reported by street users.

Some reports in the scientific literature associate violence with PCP use.[67] Users, however, do not. A large series of interviews with PCP users summarized the user's feelings: "In almost all cases, however, PCP users were baffled by the connection of PCP and violence. Most of them believed that PCP was so powerful that the kind of coordination and ability required in a fight situation would be lost."[68,p.11] When violence occurred it was either against property or a panic reaction to restraint attempts. Remember, it is true that PCP is an effective analgesic-anesthetic so pain is not a big deterrent under high doses of PCP.

No one has yet determined the mechanism or site of action of PCP. There are some signs of both peripheral and CNS sympathetic effects, but this is not the primary mechanism. There is evidence, both research and clinical, that "the drug is presumed to have a relatively selective action on thalamus and mid-brain, resulting in demonstrable impairment of pain, touch, proprioception and discriminative aspects of sensation."[63] Some believe that PCP prevents the individual from filtering sensory input, and the individual is overwhelmed by the stimulation. Whether the filtering system or the association system is disrupted, it is true that one of the factors that reduces the intensity of the PCP reaction is a decrease in environmental stimulation. This fact suggests that it may not be the best to try to "talk down" a PCP tripper; perhaps the less stimulation, the better. Maybe just sitting with the user in a quiet environment is best.

Onset of the action is 30 to 60 minutes after oral ingestion of 2 to 10 mg, with the maximum effect 2 to 5 hours after intake; recovery to predrug condition may take 12 or more hours. Tolerance does develop in animals. There may be a sharp transient increase in blood pressure and a mild short-duration depression of respiration, but these are not usually significant, although deaths have been reported.[69,70] Street users report the same collection of symptoms mentioned first in 1959,[71,72] although, of course, individual effects may vary greatly from these general statements. Take note: "Phencyclidine appears to be unique in action compared to other psychedelic drugs and its effects are less dependent upon the individual's personality than are the effects of LSD or mescaline."[73,p.1234] The most characteristic effect of the drug is an alteration in body image ("my arms feel like a 20-mile pole with a pen at the end"), and this is frequently accompanied by uncomfortable feelings of unreality. This effect, as well as others, is very compatible with the idea that PCP acts especially on proprioceptive feedback from the extremities and the skeleto-muscular system. The discomfort frequently reported is increased by a second effect in some individuals, a feeling of loneliness and isolation. The disorganization of thought that makes the person appear to have brain damage is another general effect, and this may be further emphasized by the appearance of repetitive motor behavior. Some users report a euphoria, a cheap drunk; at higher doses the euphoria-related loss of inhibition may result in uncontrollable rage and/or convulsions. Others may report numbness and analgesia in some parts of the body, which probably gives rise to the "I'm dying" and "I'm dead" type of thoughts.

A few final comments. PCP can be used in pill or liquid form and taken orally but more often it is smoked (by dusting it on marijuana) or snorted. Smoking and snorting provide more rapid effects and better control of the dose. Since the dose and the effects can be readily adjusted, PCP can appeal to those looking for: euphoria (a low dose); a wasted, body-wide anesthetic effect with supersensitivity to sensations—the out-of-the-body stage (a moderate dose); or an incoherent, immobile, conscious state (a high dose). If you're having trouble getting a feel for PCP, you're in good company. Even users can't agree on what the experience is like. One third of PCP users say it's unique, another third say it's like the hallucinogens or marijuana, and the last third isn't sure. When neither the users, the researchers, nor the clinicians can agree on the the experience, the mechanisms, or the symptoms, you know that more research is needed.

CONCLUDING COMMENT

One final item. In these days of expanding drug use, the search for new highs, and the desire for less hassle with the police, it should not be surprising that American capitalism rears its head. A nonprofit organization that has closely monitored and analyzed street-drug purchases noted that

a new industry has evolved over the past 10 years—the selling of so-called "legal highs" in retail stores or by mail. Nationally distributed magazines now exist to champion and promote the merchandising of these agents. The Food and Drug Administration appears reluctant to monitor the apparently profitable "legal high" industry. Do "legal highs" deliver full value? Or do they represent just another commercially profitable rip-off?[75]

This group surveyed the literature and purchased and carried out chemical and pharmacological evaluations of many "legal high" products. The results were overwhelming, and you know what they found:

In the case of "legal highs," as with many recreational pursuits, value received appears to be in proportion to what the purchaser expects, rather than what he *actually* purchases.[75]

Caveat emptor.

REFERENCES

1. Shultes, R.E., and Hofman, A.: Plants of the gods, New York, 1979, McGraw-Hill Book Co.
2. Diaz, J.L.: Ethnopharmacology of sacred psychoactive plants used by the Indians of Mexico, Annual Review Pharmacological Toxicology **17**:647, 1977.
3. Hofmann, A.: Psychotomimetic agents. In Burger, A., editor: Drugs affecting the central nervous system, vol. 2, New York, 1968, Marcel Dekker, Inc.
4. Crahan, M.E.: God's flesh and other preColumbian phantastica, Bulletin of the Los Angeles County Medical Association **99**:17, 1969.
5. Wolbach, A.B. Jr., Isbell, H., and Miner, E.J.: Cross tolerance between mescaline and LSD-25, with a comparison of the mescaline and LSD reactions, Psychopharmacologia **3**:1-14, 1962.
6. Isbell, H., and others: Cross tolerance between LSD and psilocybin, Psychopharmacologia **2**:147-159, 1961.
7. Leary, T.: The religious experience: its production and interpretation, Journal of Psychedelic Drugs **1**(2):3-23, 1967-1968.
8. Clark, W.H.: The religious significance of psychedelic substances, Religion in Life **36**:393-403, 1967.
9. Schultes, R.E.: The plant kingdom and halluncinogens (Part II), Bulletin on Narcotics **21**(4):26-27, 1969.
10. Fink, P.J., Goldman, M.J., and Lyons, I.: Morning glory seed psychosis, Archives of General Psychiatry **15**:209-213, 1966.
11. Cohen, S.: Suicide following morning glory seed ingestion, American Journal of Psychiatry **120**:1024-1025, 1964.
12. Szara, S.: DMT (N,N-dimethyltryptamine) and homologues: clinical and pharmacological considerations. In Efron, D.H., editor: Psychotomimetic drugs, New York, 1970, Raven Press.
13. Carroll, L.: Alice in Wonderland, London, 1865, The Macmillan Co.
14. Brekhman, I.I., and Sam, Y.A.: Ethnopharmacological investigation of some psychoactive drugs used by Siberian and Far-Eastern minor nationalities of USSR. In Efron, D.H., editor: Ethnopharmacologic search for psychoactive drugs, Washington, D.C., 1967, National Institute of Mental Health.
15. Wasson, R.G.: Fly agaric and man. In Efron, D.H., editor: Ethnopharmacologic search for psychoactive drugs, Washington, D.C., 1967, National Institute of Mental Health. (See also Wasson, R.G.: Soma, divine mushroom of immortality, New York, 1971, Harcourt, Brace, Jovanovich.)
16. Wasson, R.G., and Eugster, C.H.: Discussion. In Efron, D.H.: Ethnopharmacologic search for psychoactive drugs, Washington, D.C., 1967, National Institute of Mental Health.
17. Waser, P.G.: The pharmacology of *Amanita muscaria*. In Efron, D.H., editor: Ethnopharmacologic search for psychoactive drugs, Washington, D.C., 1967, National Institute of Mental Health.

18. Schultes, R.E.: Hallucinogens of plant origin, Science **163**:245-254, 1969.

19. Horne, C.H.W., and McCluskie, J.A.W.: The food of the gods, Scottish Medical Journal **8**:489-491, 1963.

20. Fabing, H.D.: On going berserk, The Prescriber **3**:30-31, 1956.

21. Graves, R.: Steps, London, 1958, Cassell & Co.

22. Allegro, J.M.: the sacred mushroom and the cross, New York, 1970, Doubleday & Co., Inc.

23. Hallucinogens, Columbia Law Review **68**(3):521-560, 1968.

24. Waser, P.G., and Bersin, P.: Turnover of monoamines in brain under the influence of muscimol and ibotenic acid, two psychoactive principles of *Amanita muscaria*. In Efron, D.H., editor: Psychotomimetic drugs, New York, 1970, Raven Press.

25. Bender, G.A.: Rough and ready research—1887 style, Journal of the History of Medicine **23**:159-166, April 1968.

26. Bruhn, J.G.: Three men and a drug: peyote research in the 1980s, Pacific Information Service on Street Drugs—**6**(3-4):20, 1978.

27. LaBarre, W.: Twenty years of peyote studies, Current Anthropology **1**(1):45, 1960.

28. LaBarre, W.: The peyote cult, Hamden, Conn., 1964, The Shoe String Press.

29. Thackery, F.A.: Prohibition of use of peyote, House Reports (Public) No. 560 **2**:17-19, 1917-1918.

30. Slotkin, J.S.: Religious defenses (the Native American Church), Journal of Psychedelic Drugs **1**(2):77-95, 1967-1968.

31. Bromberg, W., and Tranter, C.L.: Peyote intoxication: some psychological aspects of the peyote rite, Journal of Nervous and Mental Disease **97**:518-527, 1943.

32. LaBarre, W., and others: Statement on peyote, Science **114**:524, 582-583, 1951.

33. Wiley, H.W. Quoted in Congressional Record—Senate **56**:4130, 1918.

34. Collier, J.: The peyote cult, Science **115**:503, 1952.

35. Bergman, R.L.: Navajo peyote use: its apparent safety, American Journal of Psychiatry **128**:695-699, 1971.

36. Kapadia, G.J., and Goyez, M.B.E.: Peyote constituents: chemistry, biogenese, and biological effects, Journal of Pharmaceutical Sciences **59**:1699-1727, 1970.

37. De Ropp, R.S.: Drugs and the mind, New York, 1957, Grove Press, Inc.

38. Ellis, H.: Mescal: a study of a divine plant, Popular Science Monthly **61**:59,65, 1902.

39. Ellis, H.: Mescal: a new artificial paradise, Annual Report of the Smithsonian Institution **52**:547-548, 1897.

40. Huxley, A.: The doors of perception, New York, 1954, Harper & Row, Publishers.

41. Dorrance, D.L., Janiger, O., and Teplitz, R.L.: Effect of peyote on human chromosomes, Journal of the American Medical Association **234**:299-306, 1973.

42. Synder, S.H., Faillace, L.A., and Weingartner, H.: DOM (STP), a new hallucinogenic drug, and DOET: effects in normal subjects, American Journal of Psychiatry **125**:357-363, 1968.

43. Hollister, L.E., Macnicol, M.F., and Gillispie, H.K.: An hallucinogenic amphetamine analog (DOM) in man, Psychopharmacologica **14**:62-73, 1967.

44. Snyder, S.H., Faillace, L., and Hollister, L.: 2,5-Dimethoxy-4-methyl-amphetamine (STP): a new hallucinogenic drug, Science **158**:669-670, 1967.

45. Meyers, F.H., Rose, A.J., and Smith, D.E.: Incidents involving the Haight-Ashbury population and some uncommonly used drugs, Journal of Psychedelic Drugs **1**(2):140-146, 1967-1968.

46. Smith, D., and Meyers, F.: The psychotomimetic amphetamine with special reference to STP (DOM) toxicity. In Smith, D., editor: Drug abuse papers, 1969, Section 4, Berkeley, 1969, University of California.

47. 70% burns: street drugs analyzed, Rolling Stone, February 17, 1972.

48. Briggs, K.M.: Pale Hecate's team, New York, 1962, The Humanities Press.

49. Langdon-Brown, W.: From witchcraft to chemotherapy, Cambridge, 1941, Cambridge University Press.

50. Gen. 30:14-16, The New English Bible, Oxford University Press and Cambridge University Press, 1970.

51. Schultes, R.E.: The plant kingdom and hallucinogens (Part III), Bulletin on Narcotics **22**(1):43-46, 1970.

52. Encyclopedia Brittanica, vol. 16, 1929.

53. Beverly, R.: The history and present state of Virginia, 1705, Chapel Hill, N.C., 1947, University of North Carolina Press.

54. Evans, W.O., and Kline, N.S., chairmen: Symposium and Panel Discussion on Social Patterns of Drug Use, Historically and in Nonwestern Cultures, San Juan, Puerto Rico, December 10, 1970, American College of Neuropsychopharmacology.

55. Castaneda, C.: The teachings of Don Juan: a Yaqui way of knowledge, Los Angeles, 1968, University of California Press. A separate reality, 1971; Journey to Ixtlan, 1973; Tales of power, 1974; Second ring of power, 1977, New York, Simon & Schuster.

56. Shervette, R.E., and others: Jimson "Loco" weed abuse in adolescents, Pediatrics **63**(4):520, 1979.

57. Long, R.E., and Penna, R.: Drugs of abuse. In Drug abuse education, ed. 2, Washington, D.C., 1969, American Pharmaceutical Association.

58. Lynch, H.D., and Anderson, M.H.: Atropine coma therapy in psychiatry: clinical observations over a 20-year period and a review of the literature, Diseases of the Nervous System **36**:648-652, 1975.

59. Cohen, S.: The hallucinogens. In Clark, W.G., and del Giudice, J., editors: Principles of psychopharmacology, New York, 1970, Academic Press, Inc.

60. Morgan, J.P., and Kagan, D.: The dusting of America: the image of phencyclidine (PCP) in the popular media, Journal of Psychedelic Drugs **12**(3-4):195, 1980.

61. Greifenstein, F.E., and others: A study of a l-dryl cycle hexyl amine for anesthesia, Anesthesia and Analgesia **37**(5):283-294, 1958.

62. Corssen, G., and Domino, E.F.: Dissociative anesthesia: further pharmacological studies and first clinical experience with the phencyclidine derivative Cl-581, Anesthesia and Analgesia **45**(1):29-40, 1966.

63. Luby, E., and others: Study of a new schizophrenomimetic drug—Sernyl, A.M.A. Archives of Neurology and Psychiatry **81**:113-119, March 1959.

64. Erard, R., and others: The PCP psychosis: prolonged intoxication or drug-precipitated functional illness? Journal of Psychedelic Drugs **12**(3-4):235, 1980.

65. Yago, K.B., and others: The urban epidemic of phencyclidine (PCP) use: clinical and laboratory evidence from a public psychiatric hospital emergency service, Journal of Clinical Psychiatry **42**(5):193, May 1981.

66. Ban, T.A., Lohrenz, J.J., and Lehmann, H.E.: Observations on the action of Sernyl—a new psychotropic drug, Canadian Psychiatric Association Journal **6**:150-157, June 1961.

67. Siegel, R.K.: PCP and violent crime: the people vs. peace, Journal of Psychedelic Drugs **12**(3-4):317, 1980.

68. Angel dust in four American cities, Services Research Report, HHS Publication (ADM) 81-1039, Washington, D.C., 1980, U.S. Government Printing Office.

69. Bibb, J.: Drug overdose kills student, The All State (published by Austin Peay State University) **46**(15):1, February 4, 1976.

70. PCP: a terror of a drug, Time, p. 53, December 19, 1977.

71. Liden, C.B., Lovejoy, F.H., and Costello, C.E.: Phencyclidine. Nine cases of poisoning, Journal of the American Medical Association **234**:513-516, 1975.

72. Tong, T.G., and others: Phencyclidine poisoning, Journal of the American Medical Association **234**:512-513, 1975.

73. Showalter, C.V., and Thornton, W.E.: Clinical pharmacology of phencyclidine toxicity, American Journal of Psychiatry **134**(11):1234, November 1977.

74. Peterson, R., and Stillman, R.: Phencyclidine (PCP) abuse: an appraisal, NIDA Research Monograph 21, August 1978.

75. Brown, J.K., and Malone, M.H.: "Legal highs"—constituents, activity, toxicology, and herbal folklore, Pacific Information on Street Drugs **5**(3-6):11-53, May 1977.

CHAPTER 19

MARIJUANA AND HASHISH

Marijuana has now won middle-class respectability, as have blue jeans, long hair, feminism, health foods, group therapy, The Rolling Stones, and sexual practices of various kinds. The American counter-culture, once viewed as extremely threatening, has become the over-the-counter culture. . . .[1]

You can close your eyes, you can bark at the moon, you can wail and moan and gnash your teeth, or you can rub your hands with glee, roll back on your heels, snap your suspenders and smile. . . . It doesn't much matter what you, me, the feds, or anyone else does: America has a new recreational drug—a nondrug drug to the 50 million plus that have tried it. It's not a safe drug—but then neither are alcohol and nicotine. It's not a drug that everyone will use—ditto for booze and cigarettes. The fight has been long and hard, like the Crusades, and many good people have fallen on both sides. And like the Crusades—I'm still not sure if anyone won or lost . . . but I do know there was a battle!

Does this mean that it's all over but the shouting? No, the outcome seems clear but you will still hear. . . .

Marijuana perhaps more than any other drug is the NOW generation.[2] Not just the hippies or the dropouts or the alienated but the doctors, lawyers, and all kinds of chiefs of tomorrow say marijuana is it. It is better than booze: no hangover. It is a mind drug, not a body drug, as is alcohol. It is a harmless drug, whereas alcohol and nicotine are known to be responsible directly or indirectly for much illness and many deaths. It is a euphoriant in a world that needs joy, not the obliteration of sensation that accompanies alcohol. It is not addicting, whereas hard liquor is. No one dies when they stop using it; some have died when they stopped drinking. It represents and is part of a new attitude toward life while alcohol is regressive.

On the otherhand . . .

Nonsense. Marijuana smoking is frequently the first step toward dropping out of life. It sometimes leads to the use of even more dangerous drugs. It has not been studied enough to say it is harmless. It is a symbol of an attitude that will destroy our country and lower everyone's standard of living. Alcohol does present problems, but it is the drug of choice in all of the more technologically advanced countries, so it cannot be too bad. Marijuana, on the other hand, is used only in the backwater countries of the world.

This chapter will detail some of the stories, the facts, and the history of the coming of age of marijuana. Whether you support or condemn its use, believe it should be decriminalized, legalized or fought tooth and nail—you need to understand why

419

some have called marijuana a "harmless giggle"[3] while others call it the "killer weed." And most of all . . . you need to understand that, in part, both are right.

CANNABIS

As we all know, marijuana is a preparation of leafy material from the *Cannabis* plant that is used by smoking. The question is which *Cannabis* plant, since there is still botanical debate over whether there is one, three, or more species of *Cannabis*. There are many legal implications over the number of species that are recognzied, and the evidence is strong that there are three species of *Cannabis*. *Cannabis sativa* originated in the Orient but now grows worldwide and primarily has been used for its fibers, from which hemp rope is made. This is the species that grows as a weed in the United States and Canada. *C. indica* is grown for its psychoactive resins and is cultivated in many areas of the world, including selected planters and backyards of the United States. The third species, *C. ruderalis*, grows primarily in Russia and not at all in America. The plant Linnaeus named *C. sativa* in 1753 is what is still known as *C. sativa*.[4]

It was *C. sativa* that George Washington grew at Mount Vernon, most likely not to get high but to make rope. From his fields and many others like it, *C. sativa* spread across the nation, growing spontaneously. Assays of marijuana from weedy *C. sativa* in mid-America generally show less than 1% of the psychoactive material. This makes it easy to understand why some neophytes, who have been harvesting their marijuana wherever they find it, could be ripped off by a street purchase of a mixture of ground oak tree leaves and oregano. Marijuana from the leaves of *C. indica* will usually contain from 2% to 5% of the psychoactive material. There is some evidence that the amount of psychoactivity is related more to genetic factors than to environment.

The primary psychoactive agent, Δ-9 tetrahydrocannabinol (THC), is concentrated in the resin of the plant, with most of the resin in the flowering tops, less in the leaves, and very little in the fibrous parts. The psychoactive potency of a *Cannabis* preparation depends on the amount as well as the strength of the resin present and therefore varies depending on the part of the plant used. *Hash*, or *hashish*, in this country is a concentrate of resin from the flowering tops of the plant and thus is highly potent. Hash is eaten or smoked. Marijuana is much less potent, perhaps one third to one tenth as potent as hash. In 1975 street marijuana averaged about 1% THC, by 1979 5% THC was not uncommon. In 1972 hash oil, an old form of *Cannabis* made by boiling hash in a solvent and filtering out the solids, appeared on American streets—some of it with a THC content of 63%.[5] The hash oil on the street in 1979 was usually between 15% and 20% THC—very potent. THC in adequate amounts will produce the same kind of experience as LSD.

Even within *C. indica* there are large differences in the amount and potency of the resin. It now seems clear that these differences are primarily the result of genetic differences, not the environmental conditions where the plant is grown. These ideas, and many other agricultural and biochemical facts, have come from research carried out at the federally supported marijuana farm near Biloxi, Mississippi. Started in 1968, *Cannabis* is being grown and studied behind a high fence topped with barbed wire.[6] A variety of seeds gives a variety of plants, and even the nonbotanist can see differences in leaves, branches, and other characteristics. At maturity some plants are 2 feet tall, some 20. Some grow slowly, others 3 feet a week. Even when the seeds are all from *C. indica*, there are great morphological variations in the plant. It will interest the serious student of botany that the seeds of *C. sativa* are longer, flatter, and lighter in color than those of *C. indica*.

EARLY HISTORY

The history of the use of the plant *Cannabis* is difficult to give because so little of it is known.[7] *Cannabis* was never a staple in the doctor's black bag, so there are not extensive references to it in medical history. The earliest reference to *Cannabis* is in a pharmacy book written in 2737 BC by the Chinese emperor Shen Nung. Referring to the euphoriant effects of *Cannabis*, he called it the "Liberator of Sin." There were some medical uses, however, and he recommended it for "female weakness, gout, rheumatism, malaria, beriberi, constipation and absent-mindedness"![8]

Since the earliest record is Chinese, a slight credibility gap exists in noting that the most popular story of marijuana's discovery is a legend from the Arabic world. The hero is Haider, a very stoic, seclusive monk, who built a monastery in the desert and made a point of never enjoying any pleasures. Things changed for Haider when

> One burning summer's day when the fiery sun glared angrily upon Mother Earth as if he wished to wither up her breasts, Haider stepped out from his cloister and walked alone to the fields. All around him lay the vegetation weary and without life, but one plant danced in the heat with joy. Haider plucked it, partook of it, and returned to the convent a happier man. The monks who saw him immediately noticed the change in their chief. He encouraged conversation, and acted boisterously. He then led his companions to the fields, and the holy men partook of the hasheesh, and were transformed from austere ascetics into jolly good fellows.[9,p.23]

The same characteristics of the plant to which Haider responded spread its use around the world. There are scatterd references to *Cannabis* in India, China, and the Middle East between 2737 BC and recent years. One writer commented:

> Opium is mentioned in many medical texts because of its ability to relieve pain, references to hashish are confined to a more fanciful, vague world of religious and mystical experience. The drug's wondrous ability to set man's imagination free, to change the shape and color of his world, has caused it to be used quite differently from opium and for purposes more related to man's spiritual existence.[10,pp.44-45]

Some of the early references were to the use of *Cannabis* as an inebriant. In 430 BC Herodotus reported that the Scythians burned hemp seeds and inhaled the smoke to induce intoxication. Since the seeds contain little if any of the psychoactive agent, probably the entire top of the plant was used. The scattered reports of *Cannabis* as an intoxicant are of little importance here, but social use of the plant spread to the Moslem world and North Africa by 1000 AD. Its social use increased to the point where it was considered epidemic in the twelfth century.[11]

In this period in the eastern Mediterranean area a legend developed around a religious cult that committed murder for political reasons. The cult was called "hashishiyya," from which our word "assassin" developed. In 1299 Marco Polo told the story he had heard of this group and their leader. It was a marvelous tale and had all the ingredients for surviving through the ages: intrigue, murder, sex, the use of drugs, mysterious lands. The story of this group and their activities was told in many ways over the years, and Boccaccio's *Decameron* contained one story based on it. Stories of this cult, combined with the frequent reference to the power and wonderment of hashish in *The Arabian Nights*, were widely circulated in Europe over the years.

MIDDLE HISTORY

At the turn of the nineteenth century, world commerce was expanding. New and exciting reports from the world travelers of the seventeenth and eighteenth centuries introduced new cultures and new ideas to Europe. The Orient and the Middle East had yielded exotic spices as well as the stimulants coffee and tea. Europe was ready for another new sensation, and she got it. The returning veteran, as usual, gets part of the blame for introducing what Europe was ready to receive.

> Napoleon's campaign to Egypt at the beginning of the nineteenth century increased the Romantic's acquaintance with hashish and caused them to associate it with the Near East. . . . Napoleon was forced to give an order forbidding all French soldiers to indulge in hashish. Some of the soldiers brought the habit to France, however, as did many other Frenchmen who worked for the government or traveled in the Near East.[10,p.63]

By the 1830s and 1840s, everyone who was any-one was using, thinking about using, or decrying the use of mind-tickling agents such as opium and hashish. One of the earliest (1844) popular accounts of the use of hashish is in *The Count of Monte Cristo* by Alexander Dumas. The story includes a refer-ence to the Assassin story and contains statements about the characteristics of the drug that still sound contemporary.

Throughout the middle of the nineteenth cen-tury the great French writers of the period were in constant communication with each other. During the 1840s a group of artists and writers gathered monthly at the Hotel Pimodan in Paris' Latin Quarter to use drugs. This group became famous because one of the participants, Gautier, wrote a book, *Le Club de Hachischins*, that described their activities. From this group have come some of the best literary descriptions of hashish intoxication. These French Romantics, like the impressionistic painters of a later period, were searching for new experiences, new sources of creativity from within, new ways of seeing the world outside. A few of the regulars are well-known writers such as Baudelaire, Gautier, and Dumas. Balzac was pretty much of an antidrug man and even warned against the use of coffee, tea, alcohol, and sugar!

Baudelaire was addicted to opium, but at the time of his death at an early age as a result of syphilis, he was opposed to the use of drugs. His writings, however, contain much of value for those who want to understand the use and attraction of *Cannabis*. The drug being used was hashish, one of the most potent forms of the psychoactive ma-terial of *Cannabis* available at that time. (A more potent oil "extracted from hashish by distil-lation"[12,p.41] was known but not used by Baude-laire.) The two *Cannabis* species were clearly known to him, and "every attempt to date has failed"[p.16] to produce hashish with French hemp; only Indian or Egyptian hemp could be used. Two types of hashish were described; one included "a small quantity of opium,"[p.16] a fact which should be remembered when reading any of the reports of this period, including those of Baudelaire and Du-mas. The other

Hashish *concentrate*, such as the Arabs prepare it, is obtained by boiling the tops of the flowering plant in butter with a little water. Following com-plete evaporation of all moisture, it is strained, and yields a preparation that looks like a greenish-yellow pomade, and retains the disagreeable odor of hashish and rancid butter. . . . Because of the repugnant odor, which increases with time, the Arabs set the concentrate in the form of jellies.

. . . a mixture of concentrate, sugar, and various aromatics, such as vanilla, cinnamon, pistachio, almond, or musk.[p.39]

Baudelaire repeatedly used this drug and was an astute observer of the effects in himself and in others. In his book *Artificial Paradises*[12,pp.41-43] he echoes what Dumas had written about the kind of effect to expect from hashish:

the uninitiated . . . imagine hashish intoxication as a wondrous land, a vast theater of magic and juggling where everything is miraculous and un-expected. That is a preconceived notion, a total misconception. . . . The intoxication will be noth-ing but one immense dream, thanks to intensity of color and the rapidity of conceptions; but it will always preserve the particular tonality of the in-dividual. . . . The dream will certainly reflect its dreamer. . . . He is only the same man grown larger . . . sophisticate and ingénu . . . will find nothing miraculous, absolutely nothing but the natural to an extreme. The mind and body upon which hashish operates will yield only their ordi-nary, personal phenomena, increased, it is true, in amount and vitality, but still faithful to their original. Man will not escape the fate of his physical and mental nature: to his impressions and intimate thoughts, hashish will be a magnifying mirror, but a *true* mirror, nonetheless.

The extent of Baudelaire's actual experience with hashish is debatable, but he did identify (and ex-aggerate) three stages of intoxication following oral intake.[12] These are still being rediscovered.

At first, a certain absurd, irresistible hilarity over-comes you. The most ordinary words, the simplest ideas assume a new and bizarre aspect. This mirth is intolerable to you; but it is useless to resist. The demon has invaded you. . . . You laugh at your own foolishness and nonsense; your companions laugh in your face, but you do not mind, because the characteristic good will is beginning to manifest itself.

It sometimes happens that people completely unsuited for word-play will improvise an endless string of puns and wholly improbable idea relationships fit to outdo the ablest masters of this preposterous craft. But after a few minutes, the relation between ideas becomes so vague, and the thread of your thoughts grows so tenuous, that only your cohorts . . . can understand you.[pp. 18-19]

The second stage is ushered in by a sensation of coldness in the extremities, and a great over-all weakness. You are all thumbs, as they say; your head is heavy, and there is a general numbness throughout your being.

. . . Your senses become extraordinarily keen and acute. Your sight is infinite. Your ear can discern the slightest perceptible sound, even through the shrillest of noises.

The strangest ambiguities, the most inexplicable transpositions of ideas take place. In sounds there is color; in colors there is a music. . . . You are sitting and smoking; you believe that you are sitting in your pipe, and that *your pipe* is smoking *you;* you are exhaling *yourself* in bluish clouds.

This fantasy goes on for an eternity. A lucid interval, and a great expenditure of effort, permit you to look at the clock. The eternity turns out to have been only a minute. Another stream of ideas sweeps you away; it will carry you along for a moment in its rushing whirlpool; and this moment, too, will seem an eternity. . . . One lives several lifetimes in the space of an hour.

From time to time, your personality will vanish . . . your identity will blend with things outside yourself. Here you are, as a tree, moaning in the wind, whining plant melodies to nature. . . . Now you are soaring through the immense blue expanses of the sky. . . . By and by, your sense of time will vanish completely.[pp. 21,22]

The third phase . . . is something beyond description. It is what the Orientals call *kef;* it is complete happiness. There is nothing whirling and tumultuous about it. It is a calm and placid beatitude. Every philosophical problem is resolved. Every difficult question that presents a point of contention for theologians, and brings despair to thoughtful men, becomes clear and transparent. Every contradiction is reconciled. Man has surpassed the gods.[p. 23]

As the end of the nineteenth century approached, the use of anxiety-relieving drugs increased, but the hashish experience held little interest for the dweller in middle America. Just beginning, however, was the new science of psychology, whose interest was in the workings of the mind. The writings of William James and others introduced the possibility of using psychoactive agents in studying psychological processes. In 1899 one of the psychologists who had been using *Cannabis* in experiments said, "To the psychologist it [*Cannabis*] was as useful as the microscope to the naturalist; it magnifies psychological states and in this way is an aid to its study."[13]

This psychologist, E.B. Delabarre, delivered a public lecture titled "Hashish and Its Effects" in January 1899. He read from *The Count of Monte Cristo* and commented that at least 5 grains of hashish was necessary to produce psychological effects. The newspaper report[13] of his talk said in part:

The outward symptoms noted after taking hashish were seen in the pulse, breathing and temperature. The pulse rose on one occasion from 70 to 156. Breathing is quickened and is superficial, while the muscular strength is diminished, although the one under the influence of the drug thinks his strength is vast, and feels as if he was making extraordinary muscular efforts. The steadiness of the hand is decreased, and there is also a tendency to move about and to make rhythmical movements. . . .

An interesting thing which is found detailed in many of the accounts of hashish is the tendency to overestimate and to underestimate. This is true of heat, space, muscular efforts and of number of objects.

Mentally the power of association is much increased. During the period of increase it is from 30 to 40 per cent larger. Along with the ease and rapidity of this action comes the richness of images—they are fuller of detail and thoughts. . . .

Emotions, too, are very much intensified, both as to pleasure and pain. Apparently the drug had no effect on the memory; if anything it was decreased. Usually the accuracy of mental processes was the same as under normal condition. To sum up his observations, Prof. Delabarre stated that the effects noted were due to hyper-excitability of the nervous system. In the process from the normal to the maximum excitement there is a wave or rhythmical increase; it generally takes about seven hours for the full influence to be felt after the drug has been taken, and when its effect passes off there is no period of depression.

He spoke of the symptoms, the thrills, glows, the increase in mental power and visions, which would vary with individuals. . . . The only danger attending its use is that of becoming an habitual user, aside from the danger to the health from this strain. One may think while under the influence of the drug that he is surely going to die, but on its effects passing off no harm has been incurred, so far as is known.

In conclusion, a warning was given against danger attending the habitual use, although it was stated that none was apparent if a sufficient period elapsed in making tests with it.

This is still a reasonable summary of the effects of a moderate amount of hashish or of a large amount of marijuana. In spite of the promised potential of the use of drugs to study the mind, their use decreased in early years of this century. In part this resulted from the passage of the 1906 Pure Food and Drugs Act.

THE COMING OF "MARIJUANA, ASSASSIN OF YOUTH"

During the beginning of the twentieth century, public interest in marijuana and its use was not very widespread. In the early 1920s there were a few references in the mass media to the use of marijuana by Mexican-Americans, but public concern was not aroused. In 1926, however, a series of articles associating marijuana and crime appeared in a New Orleans newspaper. As a result, the public began to take an interest in the drug.

Enough concern developed that one news agency sought out a government authority on plants and interviewed him about the reported episodes involving the use of marijuana. This plant scientist[14] commented:

It made me smile a little when I saw the first reports that a young Mexican was "concealing" his patch of hemp plants in a New York park. The plant grows from six to ten feet tall and requires plenty of open sunlight; concealment would not have been easy.

Recent reports of the smuggling and use in this country of the Mexican hemp derivative "marijuana" or "marihuana" were no news to us. . . . We have had correspondence with El Paso and other border cities in Texas for a good many years about this situation. The reported effects of the drug on Mexicans, making them want to "clean up the town," do not jibe very well with the effects of cannabis, which so far as we have reports, simply causes temporary elation, followed by depression and heavy sleep.

The no-cause-for-alarm attitude expressed by this scientist seemed to be prevalent in government circles, although 16 states included *Cannabis sativa* in their antinarcotic laws by 1929. The Commissioner of Narcotics, Harry Anslinger, said that in 1931, when 23 states had antimarijuana laws, the Bureau of Narcotics' file on marijuana was less than 2 inches thick. The same year, the Treasury Department stated:

A great deal of public interest has been aroused by the newspaper articles appearing from time to time on the evils of the abuse of marijuana, or Indian hemp. . . . This publicity tends to magnify the extent of the evil and lends color to an inference that there is an alarming spread of the improper use of the drug, whereas the actual increase in such use may not have been inordinately large.[8, p. 130]

Even so, by 1935 there were 36 states with laws regulating the use, sale, and/or possession of marijuana. By the end of 1936 all 48 states had similar laws. The federal worm had also turned. In 1937, at congressional hearings, Anslinger stated that "traffic in marihuana is increasing to such an extent that it has come to be the cause for the greatest national concern."[15] In the 1931-1937 period it is true that the use of marijuana had spread throughout the country, but there is no evidence that there was wide use. The primary motivation for the congressional hearings on marijuana came not because of the use of marijuana as an inebriant or a euphoriant but because of reports by police and in the popular literature stating: "Most crimes of violence . . . are laid to users of marihuana."[16]

When *Scientific American*[17] reported in March 1936 that:

Marijuana produces a wide variety of symptoms in the user, including hilarity, swooning, and sexual excitement. Combined with intoxicants, it often makes the smoker vicious, with a desire to fight and kill.

and *Popular Science Monthly*[18] in May 1936 contained a lengthy article including such statements as:

the chief of Philadelphia County detectives declared that whenever any particularly horrible crime was committed—and especially one pointing to perversion—his officers searched first in marijuana dens and questioned marijuana smokers for suspects.

it hardly seemed necessary for the reader to be told that marijuana had arrived as "the foremost menace to life, health, and morals in the list of drugs used in America."[18]

The association was repeatedly made in this period between crime, particularly violent and/or perverted crime, and marijuana use. A typical report,[19] cautiously phrased as were all of them, follows:

In Los Angeles, Calif., a youth was walking along a downtown street after inhaling a marijuana cigarette. For many addicts, merely a portion of a "reefer" is enough to induce intoxication. Suddenly, for no reason, he decided that someone had threatened to kill him and that his life at that very moment was in danger. Wildly he looked about him. The only person in sight was an aged bootblack. Drug-crazed nerve centers conjured the in-

nocent old shoe-shiner into a destroying monster. Mad with fright, the addict hurried to his room and got a gun. He killed the old man, and then, later, babbled his grief over what had been wanton, uncontrolled murder.

"I thought someone was after me," he said. "That's the only reason I did it. I had never seen the old fellow before. Something just told me to kill him!"

That's marijuana!

However, not all articles condemned marijuana as the precipitator of violent crimes. An article in *The Literary Digest* reported that the chief psychiatrist at Bellevue Hospital in New York City had reviewed the cases of over 2200 criminals convicted of felonies. Referring to marijuana he said, "None of the assault cases could be said to have been committed under the drug's influence. Of the sexual crimes, there was none due to marihuana intoxication. . . . It is quite probable that alcohol is more responsible as an agent for crime than is marihuana."[20]

There was very poor documentation of the marijuana-crime relationship, which was stated as proved in the 1930s. A thorough review[21] of Anslinger's writings, including the marijuana and vicious crime cases related throughout this period, concluded that:

In the works of Mr. Anslinger, there are either no references or references to volumes which my assistants and I have checked and which, in our checking, we find to be based upon much hearsay and little or no experimentation. We found a mythology in which later writers cite the authority of earlier writers, who also had little evidence. We have found, by and large, what can most charitably be described as a pyramid of prejudice, with each level of the structure built upon the shaky foundations of earlier distortions.

With such poor evidence supporting the relationship between marijuana use and crime, it seems strange that the true story was never told. There are probably several reasons. One was the Great Depression, which made everyone acutely sensitive to, and wary of, any new and particularly foreign influences. The fact that it was the lower-class Mexican-Americans and Negroes who had initiated use of the drug made the drug doubly dangerous to the white middle class. These factors, combined with the broad cultural attitudes about marijuana use, further increased anxiety levels.

> Cannabis has been accepted for centuries in India and other eastern countries where cultural and religious teachings support introspection, meditation, and bodily passivity. On the other hand, the West, with its cultural emphasis on achievement, activity, and aggressiveness, has elected alcohol as its acceptable, almost semi-official euphoriant. These cultural differences are consonant with some of the important, pharmacological differences between the two drugs. Clearly the more introspective, meditative, non-aggressive stereotype associated with marihuana goes against our cultural mainstream. And while this contributes to its attractiveness to some, it makes it repellent, even threatening, to many others who identify with the active, aggressive, manly stereotype.[22]

There were other issues operating to build marijuana into a national menace. Perhaps some of the negative beliefs about marijuana stemmed from the opinion that it offered pleasure without penalty.

> In the years which preceded the passage of the Marijuana Tax Act, the specter of "demon rum" was still quite clear in the minds of the moral entrepreneurs of this nation, when a new menace, the "killer weed" raised its ugly head. Like alcohol, it was an intoxicant which was sought after primarily because of the pleasure it gave the user, but unlike alcohol, it did not provide for the spiritually-redeeming morning-after hangover. Its use, like alcohol, is a pleasurable, hedonistic, nonproductive, and above all, a sinful practice.[23]

Another contributing factor probably was the regular reference in associating marijuana and crime to the murdering cult of Assassins as suggestive of the characteristics of the drug.[24] The 1936 *Popular Science Monthly*[18] reference to the Assassins is the most concise.

> The origin of the word "assassin" has two explanations, but either demonstrates the menace of Indian hemp. According to one version, members

of a band of Persian terrorists committed their worst atrocities while under the influence of hashish. In the other version, Saracens who opposed the Crusaders were said to employ the services of hashish addicts to secure secret murderers of the leaders of the Crusades. In both versions, the murderers were known as "haschischin," "hashshash" or "hashishi" and from those terms comes the modern and ominous "assassin."

In none of the original stories and legends were the murders committed by individuals under the influence of hashish; rather, it was part of the reward for carrying out the murders.

No matter. As the thirties rolled on, fear of the marijuana user increased, as did state marijuana-control laws. In the mid-1930s the Narcotics Bureau acted to support federal legislation, and in the spring of 1937 congressional hearings were held.

Passage of the Marijuana Tax Act was a foregone conclusion. There were few witnesses to testify other than law enforcement officers. The birdseed people had the act modified so they could import sterilized *Cannabis* seed for use in their product. An official of the American Medical Association (AMA) testified on his own behalf, not representing the AMA, against the bill. His reasons for opposing the bill were multiple. Primarily, though, he thought the state antimarijuana laws were adequate enough and, also, that the social menace case against marijuana had not been proved at all. The bill was passed in August and became effective on October 1, 1937.

The general characteristics of the law followed the regulation-by-taxation theme of the Harrison Act of 1914. The federal law did not outlaw *Cannabis* or its preparations, it just taxed the grower, distributor, seller, and buyer and made it, administratively, almost impossible to have anything to do with *Cannabis!* In addition, the Bureau of Narcotics prepared a uniform law that many states adopted. The uniform law on marijuana specifically named *C. sativa* as the species of plant whose leafy material is illegal. In recent years there have been some court cases in which the defense has argued that the material confiscated by the police came from *C. indica* and thus was not illegal. In the usual specimens obtained by police and/or presented in court, all distinguishing characters between species are either not present or are obliterated by drying and crushing. Since the cannabinols are generic, present in all species, there is no way of telling what species one has at hand with most confiscated *Cannabis* material. Sometimes the spirit and sometimes the letter of the law wins. Britain was smarter: they refer only to *Cannabis*.

The state laws made possession and use of marijuana illegal per se. In May 1969, 32 years later, the United States Supreme Court declared the Marijuana Tax Act unconstitutional and overturned the conviction of Timothy Leary because there was:

in the Federal anti-marijuana law—a section that requires the suspect to pay a tax on the drug, thus incriminating himself, in violation of the Fifth Amendment: and a section that assumes (rather than requiring proof) that a person with foreign-grown marijuana in his possession knows it is smuggled.[25]

AFTER THE ACT

Passage of the Marijuana Tax Act had an amazing effect. Almost immediately there was a sharp reduction in the reports of heinous crimes committed under the influence of marijuana! The price of the merchandise increased rapidly (the war came along, too), so that 5 years after the act the cost of a marijuana cigarette, a reefer, had increased 6 to 12 times and cost about a dollar.

The year after the law was enacted, 1938, Mayor Fiorello LaGuardia of New York City remembered what no one else wanted to recall. What he recalled were two army studies on marijuana use by soldiers in the Panama Canal Zone around 1930. Both reports found marijuana to be innocuous and that its reputation as a troublemaker "was due to its association with alcohol which . . . was always found the prime agent."[26]

Mayor LaGuardia asked the New York Academy of Medicine to study marijuana, its use, its effects, and the necessity for control. The report, issued in 1944, was intensive and extensive and a very good study for its time. The complete report is available[27]

and widely discussed, so only a part of the summary is quoted. (See also references 28 and 29.)

It was found that marihuana in an effective dose impairs intellectual functioning in general. . . .

Marihuana does not change the basic personality structure of the individual. It lessens inhibition and this brings out what is latent in his thoughts and emotions but it does not evoke responses which would otherwise be totally alien to him. It induces a feeling of self-confidence, but this expressed in thought rather than in performance. There is, in fact, evidence of a diminution in physical activity. . . .

Those who have been smoking marihuana for a period of years showed no mental or physical deterioration which may be attributed to the drug.[27,p.408]

This 1944 report, which was completed by a very reputable committee of the New York Academy of Medicine, brought a violent reaction. The AMA stated in a 1945 editorial[30]:

For many years medical scientists have considered cannabis a dangerous drug. Nevertheless, a book called "Marihuana Problems" by New York City Mayor's Committee on Marihuana submits an analysis by seventeen doctors of tests on 77 prisoners and, on this narrow and thoroughly unscientific foundation, draws sweeping and inadequate conclusions which minimize the harmfulness of marijuana. Already the book has done harm. One investigator has described some tearful parents who brought their 16 year old son to a physician after he had been detected in the act of smoking marihuana. A noticeable mental deterioration had been evident for some time even to their lay minds. The boy said he had read an account of the La Guardia Committee report and that this was his justification for using marihuana. He read in *Down Beat*, a musical journal, an analysis of this report under the caption "Light Up Gates, Report Finds 'Tea' a Good Kick." . . . Public officials will do well to disregard this unscientific, uncritical study, and continue to regard marihuana as a menace wherever it is purveyed.

As in all such reports and reactions to reports, there is little dispute over the facts, only over the interpretation. Since the LaGuardia Report is in substantial agreement with the Indian Hemp Commission Report of the 1890s,[31] the Panama Canal Zone reports of the 1930s,[32] and the comprehensive reports in the 1970s by the governments of New Zealand,[33] Canada,[34] Great Britain,[35] and the United States,[36,37] in addition to the 1981 report to the World Health Organization[38] and the 1982 report by the National Academy of Science to the Congress of the United States,[39] it is likely that the conclusions of the LaGuardia Report were and are for the most part valid.

The conflict between the LaGuardia Report and its opponents was debated in the mass media, and usually the LaGuardia Report lost. A 1945 article[40] in a popular monthly, *Magazine Digest*, asks, "How 'Mild' is Marihuana?" and, to its credit, adds some new horror stories to the list of those possibly completed by individuals perhaps under the influence of marijuana. Place particular attention on the wording of the story; nowhere does it even say the man used marijuana!

> That there is a certain anesthetic effect from marihuana cannot be denied. In medical records there is the case of a man from Texas who, out on bail pending appeal from a conviction for raping a 12-year-old girl, slashed to death two respectable women, and then turned the knife on himself, slashing his own body so severely and repeatedly that a doctor who examined him before he died declared that marijuana was the only thing which could have desensitized his nerves sufficiently to allow him to carry out such self-mutilation without fainting from pain after the first cut. Opiates in a sufficient dose for this anesthetic effect would have rendered the man unconscious.

This post–Marijuana Tax Act period is best closed with the realization that in 1945 "the narcotic law enforcement officials are also faced with the problem of returned servicemen bringing home with them the 'hemp habit' from other countries."[40] C'est la vie, Napoleon!

The 1950s and 1960s form a unique period in the history of marijuana. There was a hiatus in scientific research on marijuana and *Cannabis*, but experimentation in the streets increased continually.

There were some rational reports in the mass media,[41] but they were easy to ignore. With the arrival of the "psychedelic sixties," the popular press could and did emphasize the more sensational hallucinogens. Marijuana, however, was everywhere the action was in the youth culture, but for the most part the major concern was on the more potent agents.

Toward the end of the 1960s, LSD use declined, heroin use increased rapidly in and out of the ghetto, and marijuana use was becoming the initiation rite of the turned-on generation.[42,43] Discussion of the drug, however, no longer had the one-sidedness of the 1930s. Advocates of the decriminalization of marijuana, if not of marijuana itself, spoke out clearly, even at Senate hearings.[44]

MEDICAL USES OF *CANNABIS*

Since *Cannabis* never attained the medical status of opium, its medical report is spotted, but the first report of medical use was by Shen Nung in 2737 BC. Some 2900 years after the Shen Nung report, another Chinese physician, Hoa-tho (200 AD) recommended *Cannabis* resin mixed with wine as a surgical anesthetic. Although *Cannabis* preparations were used extensively in medicine in India and after about 900 AD in the Near East, there was almost nothing about it in European medicine until the 1800s.

Early reports in European medical journals, such as de Sacy's 1809 article titled "Intoxicating Preparations made with Cannabis," awakened more interest in the writers and artists of the period than in medical men. In 1839, however, a lengthy article, "On the Preparations of the Indian Hemp, or Gunjah," was published by a British physician working in India.[45] He reviewed the use of *Cannabis* in Indian medicine and reported on his own work with animals, which suggested that *Cannabis* preparations were quite safe. Having shown *Cannabis* to be nontoxic, he used it clinically and found it to be an effective anticonvulsant and muscle relaxant, as well as a valuable drug for the relief of the pain of rheumatism.

This article by W.B. O'Shaughnessy started the

up-and-down history of the medical use of *Cannabis* in Europe and the United States. In 1860 the Ohio State Medical Society's Committee on *C. indica* reported its successful use in the treatment of stomach pain, chronic cough, and gonorrhea. One physician felt he had to "assign to the Indian hemp a place among the so-called hypnotic medicines next to opium. . . ."[46] By the 1890s a medical text included the statement: "Cannabis is very valuable for the relief of pain, particularly that depending on nerve disturbances. . . ."[8] It certainly was never true that "there was a time in the United States when extracts of cannabis were almost as commonly used for medical purposes as is aspirin today."[47,p.3]

In 1938 a book-size review of the literature titled *Marijuana, America's New Drug Problem*[48] attributed the rapid increase in the medical use of *Cannabis* drugs in the last half of the nineteenth century to several causes.

> This popularity of the hemp drugs can be attributed partly to the fact that they were introduced before the synthetic hypnotics and analgesics. Chloral hydrate was not introduced until 1869 and was followed in the next 30 years by paraldehyde, sulfonal and the barbitals. Antipyrine and acetanilide, the first of their particular group of analgesics, were introduced about 1884. For general sedative and analgesic purposes, the only drugs commonly used at this time were the morphine derivatives and their disadvantages were very well known. In fact, the most attractive feature of the hemp narcotics was probably the fact that they did not exhibit certain of the notorious disadvantages of the opiates.[p.152]

Interestingly, although used widely, therapeutic doses of *Cannabis* were seldom reported to have intoxicating properties. One recent writer comments that the patients receiving *Cannabis* never "were 'stoned,' changed their attitudes about work, love, their fellow men or patriotism."[8]

One of the difficulties that has always plagued the scientific, medical, and social use of *Cannabis* is the variability of the product. An 1898 brochure[49] reviewed the assay and standardization techniques used with many of the common plant drugs and stated: "In Cannabis Indica we have a drug of great importance and one which all of materia medica is undoubtedly the most variable."[50] Four years later Parke, Davis & Company,[50] using new standardization procedures, claimed that "each lot sent out upon the market by us is of full potency and to be relied upon." They listed a variety of *Cannabis* products available for medical use, including "a Chocolate Coated Tablet Extract Indian Cannabis ¼ grain"!

In spite of improved standardization of potency and an increased number of preparations, the use of *Cannabis* declined.

> In 1885 there were 5 prescriptions out of every 10,000 as fluid extract; in 1895, 11.6; in 1907, 8 out of every 10,000; in 1926, 2.3, and in 1933, the last figures we have 0.4 out of every 10,000.[51,p.114]

Passage of the 1937 law resulted in all 28 of the legal *Cannabis* preparations being withdrawn from the market, and in 1941 *Cannabis* was dropped from *The National Formulary* and *The U.S. Pharmacopeia*. Note well that the decline in the medical use of *Cannabis* occurred long before 1937 and that the law did not eliminate an actively used therapeutic agent. Four factors, however, certainly contributed to the declining prescription rate of this plant. One was the development of new and better drugs for most illnesses. Second was the variability of the available medicinal preparations of *Cannabis*, which was repeatedly mentioned in the 1937 hearings.[51] Third, *Cannabis* is very insoluble in water and thus not amenable to injectable preparations. Last, taken orally it has an unusually long (1- to 2-hour) latency to onset of action.

With the recent renewed interest in marijuana as a social drug has come some reevaluation and rethinking of the implications of some of the older therapeutic reports.[52] Scientists are looking again at some of the more interesting reported therapeutic effects of *Cannabis*. One is its anticonvulsant activity. A 1949 report[53] found it effective in some cases where phenytoin (Dilantin), the anticonvulsant of choice both then and now, was ineffective. Another area being explored is the bactericidal characteristics of *Cannabis;* maybe it is effective against gonorrhea! The fact that both Queen Victoria's physician and Sir William Osler, as well as others, found *Cannabis* to be very effective against tension headaches and/or migraine will probably be investigated in the future.[8,54] Similarly, old and new reports that *Cannabis* can be used in the treatment of narcotic withdrawal are also sure to be further investigated.[55,56] It is really true that there is nothing new under the sun.[57]

Three medical uses are of particular interest. A 1972 report showed that marijuana smoking was effective in reducing the fluid pressure of the eye in a glaucoma patient.[58] That report became a cause célèbre in 1975 when a glaucoma patient was arrested for growing marijuana plants on his back porch for medical purposes. This man 15 months later (1) had the charges against him dropped, (2) had his physician certify that the only way for him to prevent blindness was to smoke five joints a day, and (3) had these marijuana joints legally supplied to him by the United States government.[59] The second possible important medical use was reported in 1975. Medication containing THC, the active ingredient in marijuana, was the only kind that was effective in reducing the severe nausea caused by certain drugs used to treat cancer. The third medical finding points out the differences between the acute and chronic use of marijuana. Chronic use of marijuana decreases the diameter of the air passageways in the lungs, but taken on an acute basis it increases their diameter and makes it easier for individuals with asthma to breathe.

You need to know that as of 1982, 32 states have said THC/marijuana can be used—with proper controls—in investigational (experimental) medical treatment. State laws don't mean much since THC is still a Schedule I drug. THC is handled as an investigational drug (see Chapter 3) and an IND must be obtained by the clinician-researcher. To do that the clinician-researcher must be approved by the NIDA and the FDA. The hospital pharmacy that is to hold and dispense the THC has to be approved by the DEA. For work with cancer patients the NIDA and the FDA have given authority for issuing quantities of THC to the National Can-

cer Institute. As of mid-1981 over 1000 physicians and 400 pharmacies were approved for THC work with cancer patients.[60,61] THC is available in several forms: 2.5-, 5-, and 10-mg capsules, 5 mg/ml injectable, and almost any THC-content marijuana cigarettes. (The NIDA turns out about 1 million cigarettes a year and has capsules made as needed.) The 1980 production quota (set by the Attorney General) for tetrahydrocannabinols was 5000 g.

Obviously we're a lot fancier today than 10 or 100 years ago—do we know any more? As of 1982:

> Cannabis and its derivatives have shown promise in the treatment of a variety of disorders. The evidence is most impressive in glaucoma. . . ; in asthma. . . ; and in the nausea and vomiting of cancer chemotherapy . . . [and] might also be useful in seizures, spasticity, and other nervous system disorders. . . .[39,p.150]

Not much new but perhaps even more important is the fact that *Cannabis* seems to act by different mechanisms than the standard therapies—this finding may open new worlds for the development of more effective treatments.

EFFECTS OF *CANNABIS* ON HUMANS

The *Cannabis* plant has separate male and female plants, and both manufacture the psychoactive material in usable amounts. The psychoactive material is most concentrated in the resin of the plant, and this resin is secreted in highest quantity by the unfertilized flowers of the female. It is this highly resinous mixture of female flowering tops that is called hashish or hash in the United States and *charas* in India.

The term *marijuana* comes from a Spanish or Portuguese word meaning "intoxicant" and refers to a smoking preparation containing chopped leaves and perhaps flowers and stems of either the male or the female plant or both. The leaves contain between 10% and 20% as much of the psychoactive material as is found in the resin.

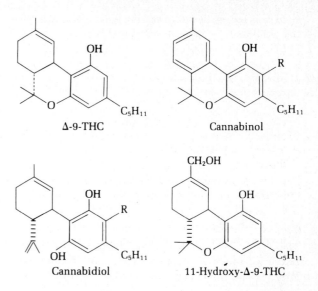

FIG. 19-1 Cannabinoid structures.

Pharmacodynamics

The chemistry of *Cannabis* is quite complex, and isolation and extraction of the active ingredient are difficult even today. *Cannabis* is unique among psychoactive plant materials in that it contains no nitrogen and thus is not an alkaloid. This fact was established over 100 years ago by two chemists, the Smith brothers (yes, it's those Smith brothers). Because of its nonnitrogen content, the nineteenth-century chemists who had been so successful in isolating the active agents from other plants were unable to identify the active component of *Cannabis*.

There are over 400 different chemicals in marijuana but only 61 of them are unique to the *Cannabis* plant—these are called cannabinoids. One of them, Δ-9-tetrahydrocannibinol (THC), was isolated and synthesized in 1964 and is clearly the most pharmacologically active. Structures of some of these chemicals are shown in Fig. 19-1. 11-Hydroxy-Δ-9-THC is the major active metabolite in the body of THC.

Take special note that the relationship of THC to *Cannabis* is probably more similar to the relationship of mescaline to peyote than of alcohol to beer, wine, or distilled spirits. Alcohol is the *only*

behaviorally active agent in alcoholic beverages, but mescaline is the most important of many in peyote. There may be more than one active agent in *Cannabis*: street lore suggests that cannabinol is responsible for the "munchies," the appetite increase reported by some marijuana users.

Thus far the study of the effects of THC on the physiology of the body has done little more than quantify earlier reports in which resin extracts were used. The established physiological effects of *Cannabis* are dose related, for the most part minor, of indeterminate importance for the psychological effects, and of unknown toxicological significance. The 1982 National Academy of Sciences Summary[39] is not much different from the 1971 federal government summary[62] of physiological effects, which is not much different from a 1942 summary.[28] For many years there has been substantial agreement on the short-term physiological effects of *Cannabis*. From the 1982 summary:

> Physiological changes accompanying marijuana use at typical levels of American social usage are relatively few. One of the most consistent is an increase in pulse rate. Another is reddening of the eyes at the time of use. Dryness of the mouth and throat are uniformly reported. Although enlarge-

ment of the pupils was an earlier impression, more careful study has indicated that this does not occur. Blood pressure effects have been inconsistent.[62]

Except for bronchodilation, acute exposure to marijuana has little effect on breathing as measured by conventional pulmonary tests.[39,p.58] Heavy marijuana smoking over a much longer period could lead to clinically significant and less readily reversible impairment of pulmonary function.[p.59] The smoking of marijuana causes changes in the heart and circulation that are characteristic of stress. But there is no evidence to indicate that it exerts a permanently deleterious effect on the normal cardiovascular system. . . . Marijuana increases the work of the heart, usually by increasing heart rate, and in some persons by increasing blood pressure. This increase in workload poses a threat to patients with hypertension, cerebrovascular disease, and coronary atherosclerosis.[p.72]

Additional information has been accumulating, but the basic, hard-core data are unchanged. The lethal dose of THC has not been extensively studied, and no human deaths have been reported from the use of *Cannabis*. There is general consensus, though, that the LD/ED (lethal dose/effective dose) ratio is much higher for *Cannabis* than it is for alcohol, for which the ratio is about 10. Perhaps the same type of relationship holds true for physical addiction. Addiction does occur to THC, but, unlike alcohol, only at dose and use levels far above what is now used recreationally. The withdrawal signs are irritability, restlessness, vomiting, nausea, diarrhea, and sleep disturbances, as well as other symptoms. The 1976 report on *Marihuana and Health*[36] notes that this withdrawal syndrome has been observed only once outside of a research setting.

For years there was debate over whether tolerance developed to the effects of THC and/or marijuana. The debate is over, and it is now clear that tolerance does develop with prolonged use at recreational levels.[36,p.25] As some have said, tolerance had to develop. "How else could people take the huge doses of hashish that are taken in other countries without some of the 'zonked' effects that we see when somebody takes a lot of hash here?"[63]

There are reports of reverse tolerance or sensitization occurring, that is, less drug being necessary with each succeeding use of the drug. With an accumulation of the active agent in the body, less and less new drug would be needed to reach a threshold level.[64]

The evidence supports this as a possibility. When smoked, THC is rapidly absorbed into the blood and distributed to tissues so that within 30 minutes much is gone from the blood. The psychological and cardiovascular effects occur together, usually within 5 to 10 minutes. The THC remaining in blood has a half-life of about 19 hours but metabolites (of which there are at least 45), primarily 11-hydroxy-THC, are formed in the liver and have a half-life of 50 hours. Complete elimination of one dose of THC and its metabolites may take 30 days. After 1 week 25% to 30% of the THC and its metabolites may remain in the body. THC taken orally is slowly absorbed and the liver transforms it to 11-hydroxy-THC, so little THC reaches the brain after oral ingestion.

The high lipid solubility of THC means that it (and its metabolites) is selectively taken up and stored in fatty tissue to be released slowly. Excretion is primarily through the feces. All of this has two important implications: (1) there is no easy way to monitor (in urine or blood) THC/metabolite levels and relate them to behavioral and/or physiological effects, as can be done with alcohol and (2) the long-lasting, steady, low concentration of THC/metabolites on the brain and other organs may have effects not yet thought of—note that this is a very different action from that of alcohol, nicotine, and caffeine, which ". . .are rapidly metabolized and leave no trace a few hours after moderate intake."[39,p.23]

With the advent of isolated THC, dose-response relationships could be determined, and the differential response to oral and inhalation modes of intake evaluated.

Threshold doses of 2 mg. smoked and 5 mg. orally produced mild euphoria; 7 mg. smoked and 17 mg. orally, some perceptual and time sense changes occurred; and at 15 mg. smoked and 25 mg. orally, subjects reported marked changes in body image, perceptual distortions, delusions and hallucinations.[62]

Oral intake is more frequently followed by nausea, physical discomfort, and hangover, and the dose level cannot be titrated as accurately as is possible when smoking. There may be other differences in effects between comparable oral and smoking intake, although this has not been studied extensively.

One of the major problems in communicating about *Cannabis* is that it is not readily placed in any of the usual pharmacological categories. It is not possible to summarize the effects of the drug with a single word, such as depressant or hallucinogen.

> The pharmacological action of marihuana has some similarities to properties of the stimulant, sedative, analgesic and psychotomimetic classes of drugs.
>
> In large doses, cannabis drugs bear many similarities to the psychotomimetics. Isbell described marked distortion of auditory and visual perception, hallucinations and depersonalization. He found LSD was 160 times more potent as a psychotomimetic than Delta-9-THC. . . .
>
> In low doses, the effects of marihuana and alcohol are similar. Both produce an early excitant and later sedated phase, and are commonly used as euphoriants, relaxants and intoxicants. At low doses, subjects experience difficulty differentiating the effects of alcohol from marihuana and placebo.[62,pp.105-106]

Some users disagree very much with the implication that the marijuana and alcohol experiences are difficult to distinguish. One user[65] has said:

> A pot high is quite different from a liquor high. Alcohol dulls the senses whereas pot sets them on edge. If a child were screaming in the next room, I'd take a drink, not a joint. If I were sitting with an arm around Jane Fonda and she had just told me I had beautiful eyes, I'd light up. Drink is for tuning out. Pot is for tuning in.

A reminder: *Cannabis* is a drug that has primarily been used in two dosage forms of very different potency. Hashish and *Cannabis* extracts that give rise to the experiences reported by Baudelaire and others are potent hallucinogenic agents. The drug delivery system that spread through the country in the 1920s and 1930s was a much less potent form, marijuana. The active ingredient is the same; the amount differs. Both marijuana and hashish are available and used in the United States today, although the great majority of users restrict themselves to marijuana.

Behavioral effects

Almost all writers emphasize that a new user has to learn how to smoke marijuana. They elaborate on three stages in the learning process.[66] The first step involves deeply inhaling the smoke and holding it in the lungs for 20 to 40 seconds. Then the user has to learn to identify and control the effects, and, finally, he has to learn to label the effects as pleasant. Because of this learning process, most first-time users do not achieve the euphoric "stoned" or "high" condition of the repeater.

The effects accompanying marijuana smoking by the experienced user are relatively well established.

> A cannabis "high" typically involves several phases. The initial effects are often somewhat stimulating and, in some individuals, may elicit mild tension or anxiety which usually is replaced by a pleasant feeling of well-being. The later effects usually tend to make the user introspective and tranquil. Rapid mood changes often occur. A period of enormous hilarity may be followed by a contemplative silence.[34,p.174]

One investigator had experienced marijuana smokers indicate how frequently their marijuana intoxication included each of 206 effects listed on a sheet. Although there are great difficulties in looking for generalizations among idiosyncratic responses, the investigator was able to summarize 124 common subjective effects.

Sense perception is often improved, both in intensity and in scope. Imagery is usually stronger but well controlled, although people often care less about controlling their actions. Great changes in perception of space and time are common, as are changes in psychological processes such as understanding, memory, emotion, and sense of identity. . . .

To the extent that the described effects are delusory or inaccurate, the delusions and inaccuracy· are widely shared. It is interesting, too, that nearly all the common effects seem either emotionally pleasing or cognitively interesting, and it is easy to see why marijuana users find the effects desirable regardless of what happens to their external behavior.[67]

The subjective effects of smoking marijuana, the high, are quite difficult to study. First, since tolerance does develop, experienced smokers should show *less* effect than beginning smokers. But almost everyone suggests that you have to learn to use marijuana, and you have to learn to appreciate the psychological effects that occur. This would mean that experienced smokers should show *more* effect than beginning smokers. In addition to these factors, or maybe as part of them, there is much learning and association of the high with the smell, feel, taste, and rituals of using marijuana. This would suggest that an experienced user would report *more* effect from a placebo cigarette than would a beginning user. The placebo cigarette would elicit the feelings associated with (conditioned to) the use of marijuana, and there should be more of these associations in the experienced user. It might also be expected that frequent marijuana users would be *less* sensitive than infrequent users to THC itself, since more of their expectations are involved in the factors related to smoking marijuana. Tables 19-1 and 19-2 speak to these issues.

Placebo cigarettes were made for these studies by extracting the THC and other cannabinols from marijuana with alcohol. The marijuana contained 0.9% THC, and the cigarettes were made so that they contained 9 mg of THC, of which about 5 mg would be delivered to the user. This was midrange potency compared to what was being sold on the

TABLE 19-1 Reports of intoxication and measured physiological changes from experienced users smoking marijuana and placebo cigarettes (n = 100)*

Intoxication level (0 sober, 100 maximum)	Number of subjects reporting	
	Marijuana	Placebo
0-19	15	35
20-39	11	28
40-59	20	21
60-79	32	12
80-100	22	4
Average	61	34

Average physiological change (pre- to post-smoking)	Marijuana†	Placebo‡
Pulse rate (beats/minute)	+24.00	−4.00
Salivary flow (cc/5 minutes)	−1.60	+0.80
Redness of eye (0-4 scale)	+1.92	+0.04

*Modified from Jones, R.T.: Tetrahydrocannabinol and the marijuana-induced social "high," or the effects of the mind on marijuana. In Singer, A.J., editor: Marijuana: chemistry, pharmacology, and patterns of social use, Annals of the New York Academy of Sciences **191**:155-165, 1971.
†All significant, $p < 0.05$.
‡None significant.

streets of San Francisco where these double-blind studies were done.[68]

Table 19-1 shows very nicely that, although experienced users report more intoxication from using a THC-containing marijuana cigarette, there is a moderate level of intoxication reported after the use of a similar smelling, tasting, and feeling cigarette without THC. This should not be too surprising, since some experienced users report that they can turn themselves on just by thinking about it. It may be possible to fool the psyche, but not the soma. The physiological changes from use of the active cigarette are what you would expect: increase in heart rate, drying of mouth, reddening of eyes. These changes do not occur with the placebo.

TABLE 19-2 Reports of intoxication and measured physiological changes in frequent and infrequent marijuana users*

	Infrequent users (less than 2 cigarettes a month)	Frequent users (more than 2 cigarettes a month)
Reported level of intoxication after using (averages, range 0-100)		
A. Marijuana cigarette	67	52
Placebo cigarette	22	48
B. Marijuana cigarette	62	56
Oral extract (25 mg THC)	72	32
Placebo cigarette	26	51
Placebo oral extract	2	5
Physiological changes		
Pulse-rate (beats/minute)	+31.0†	+17.0
Salivary flow (cc/5 minutes)	−1.8†	−0.9
Redness of eye (0-4 scale)	+2.1	+1.5

*Modified from Jones, R.T.: Tetrahydrocannabinol and the marijuana-induced social "high," or the effects of the mind on marijuana. In Singer, A.J., editor: Marijuana: chemistry, pharmacology, and patterns of social use, Annals of the New York Academy of Sciences **191**:155-165, 1971.
†Significant differences, $p < 0.05$, between infrequent and frequent users.

The interaction of learning (reverse tolerance?) and of tolerance are clear in Table 19-2. Frequent users report less effect when using an active cigarette but more effect to the placebo. Infrequent users do not get as high a high from using the placebo but do report more effect from using the THC-containing cigarette. The same type of response shows up in part B of Table 19-2, but of most interest is the finding that frequent users respond much less to the oral THC than do the infrequent users. This is probably a combination of pharmacodynamic tolerance and absence of the usual associations with getting high. (If I don't see, smell, and feel these things, then I can't be intoxicated.) Even though the subjective effects vary with expectancy and other factors, the physiological effects follow the physiology, and the frequent users show smaller physiological changes to the oral THC than infrequent users.

At the level of social intoxication there is a dose-related impairment in scores of psychomotor and cognitive tests with "moderate impairment . . . during the period of peak intoxication."[62] In laboratory studies naive users report fewer subjective effects but show greater decrement in test performance.[69]

One of the consistent alterations in function is on short-term memory that is, tasks such as learning and remembering new information or remembering and following a sequence of directions. In everyday use while intoxicated, the marijuana user is unable to easily recall information he just learned seconds or minutes before. This memory lapse affects the general thread of conversation among a group of users, as Baudelaire noted. On this issue one of the truly grand old men of the study of drug effects, A. Wikler, commented that to understand the effects and actions of a drug, you must measure the pertinent variables, the important effects. He summarizes the areas in which much more research needs to be done on alcohol and marijuana with the couplet:

> The drunkard staggers—
>   only when he walks,
> The pothead forgets—
>   only when he talks.

Perhaps police will still continue to have the drunk-ard try to walk a straight line, but they will have to ask the pothead to engage in a goal-directed, sequential, verbal task.

This impairment of short-term memory is prob-ably the basis for the changes in time sense fre-quently reported. The user feels that more time has passed than actually has. Such overestimation of the passage of time is the most commonly re-ported psychological effect of marijuana smoking and has been validated in many experiments.

One particularly important finding is that while reaction time is not greatly affected, if affected at all, there is a great impairment in the ability to engage in *tracking behavior*. Tracking behavior re-quires sustained attention and this ability is de-creased considerably by marijuana. Loss of con-centration is perhaps also demonstrated by the finding that the quality of interpersonal commu-nication (the richness of the language and attention to feedback from the other person) goes down un-der the influence of marijuana.

Many users report increased sensory awareness and sensitivity. For the most part changes in the sensory system have not been shown in laboratory experiments; probably it is the response to sensory input, not the input per se, that is altered.

In summary, there are a few statements con-cerning the behavioral effects of marijuana use for which relatively widespread consensus of opinion exists. First, a marijuana high requires learning on the part of the user. Second, the drug does impair short-term memory. Third, the user experiences an overestimation of the passage of time. Fourth, there is a loss in the ability to maintain a focused attention on a task, that is, to maintain vigilance. It should be clear, as mentioned in Chapter 4, that driving an automobile is impaired by marijuana, that the impairment is dose-related, and that the impairment is significant at dose levels reached by social users of marijuana. However, each of these effects must be viewed in light of the conclusions of one reviewer[70] who stated:

> The most consistently striking finding in all of these studies is that marijuana produced no strik-ing findings. Indeed, one is impressed with how easily subjects could suppress the marijuana "high."

Adverse reactions

A whole host of adverse reactions to normal mar-ijuana use can be mentioned rapidly to show that there are no completely safe drugs. Flashbacks have been reported by several investigators and apparently occur under the same conditions as LSD flashbacks.[71] Marijuana-precipitated psychosis has been long known. Psychotic reactions occurred in some of the prisoners studied for the LaGuardia Report, but the comment in that report is still true: "A characteristic marihuana psychosis does not ex-ist. Marihuana will not produce a psychosis *de novo* in a well-integrated, stable person."[29] The psychosis that does appear is "clinically indistinguishable from an acute schizophrenic reaction."[72]

The most common adverse reaction to marijuana use is panic; usually this occurs after high-level use. Much like many of the bad head trips to the more potent phantasticants, the reaction is usually fear of loss of control, fear that things will not return to normal. Even our, by now, old friend Baudelaire understood about bad trips and advised his readers to surround themselves with friends and a pleasant environment before using hashish. The most ef-fective method of dealing with a panic response is talking down (see Chapter 4). There are other mi-nor adverse responses, such as nausea, vomiting, and dizziness, but these are easily handled by most users and have no lasting effects.

Two reports require brief comment. One is that there have been serious physical effects from in-travenous injections of a water extract of mari-juana.[73] The second report warns against the use of marijuana that has been treated with liquid fer-tilizer, since it "may result in the formation of N-nitrosamines which are among the most potent of the known carcinogens."[74] Enough said.

There are four major medical concerns that con-tinually arise about the recreational use of mari-juana. Although some were briefly mentioned be-fore, they need emphasis. Usually the concern is with use that is more frequent than two or three joints a week. Some people, however, will be rel-atively sensitive and others relatively insensitive to these and other effects of marijuana use, so every-one should be aware of them. It should be clear at the outset that there are no obvious, high-frequency, serious physiological effects of moderate use of marijuana over a 5- to-10-year period. If there were, we would see the results all around us. But then, there are no obvious, high-frequency, serious effects of moderate use of cigarettes or alcohol over a 5- to-10-year period. Chapters 8 and 9 speak to the aftermath of this kind of thinking. It seems fairly clear that as more people use more potent marijuana more often for longer periods of time, there will be more and more serious medical problems identified. The incidence of these problems will not be high, but they will occur in a certain percentage of users.

Because of the ideas expressed in the preceding paragraph, no objective scientist or worker in the area of drug use worried very much about the 1971 report of brain atrophy in a group of young marijuana smokers.[75] If brain damage occurred after moderate use for a moderate period (3 to 11 years), many individuals would have reported it years ago, and marijuana would not be the choice of millions. Finally, in 1977, two reports confirmed what everyone knew: moderate marijuana smoking does not cause changes in the physical structure of the brain.[76,77] The 1982 report concluded, "There is no persuasive evidence that marijuana causes morphological changes in the brain."[39,p.89]

The concern over the effects of marijuana use on chromosome abnormalities is a standoff. There are research and clinical reports on both sides; some find abnormalities, some do not. Most probably THC will have a dose-related effect on chromosomes, as do many other drugs (p. 394). As with these other drugs, the significance of the effect on chromosomes is unclear. Again, however, there must be the warning that it is unwise for a pregnant woman to use any nonessential drug at any level because of the possibility of effects on the fetus.[39,p.105]

Another potentially serious medical problem that is actively debated is the clinical significance (and even the validity) of the finding that marijuana use reduces testosterone levels in males.[78] Many researchers agree that after 4 to 6 weeks of daily marijuana use testosterone levels decrease, but still stay within what are acceptable normal ranges. Some argue that if a 220-pound, 6-foot-tall football player loses 50 to 60 pounds, his weight may still be in the normal range, but it is a significant decrease for that individual. Work continues, since the final answer will be of great importance for the preadolescent and adolescent male from 11 to 16 years of age. Still undetermined is whether regular use of marijuana by a pregnant woman would have serious specific effects on a male fetus.[79] We do know that "In men, sperm number and motility are decreased during chronic marijuana use"[39,p.104] as defined before. As of now there is no clear effect on fertility, and the effect seems to be reversed when marijuana use stops.

The last medical problem to be mentioned is still a fuzzy issue: it is the action of marijuana use on the immune systems of the body, those which help us fight off illnesses. Although there is controversy, "The data from animal studies suggest that Δ-9-THC and some of its analogues have a mild transient, immunosuppressent effect."[39,p.105] There is no evidence that the suppression has any clinical significance. That is, marijuana users do not show a higher incidence of viral infections or cancer. Whether there will be significant long-term effects will have to wait 20 to 40 years for an answer, as was done with cigarette smoking.

This is a difficult section to write objectively. There are many contradictions in the scientific and clinical literature. If you want to present a strongly antimarijuana position, you might start with a quote from one of the very active and productive scientists working with marijuana and THC who has very strong opinions on the issue:

> The brain is the organ of the mind. Can one repetitively disturb the mental function without impairing the brain?
> The brain, like all other organs of the human body, has very large functional reserves which allow it to resist and adapt to stressful abnormal demands. It seems that chronic use of psychotropic drugs, including *Cannabis* derivatives, slowly erodes these reserves.[80,p.249]

The position taken here on the adverse medical effects of marijuana use should be clear. The sixth annual report on *Marihuana and Health*[36,p.26] phrased it:

> While, it now appears that infrequent, experimental use at typical U.S. levels is usually without significant hazard, more frequent, and especially chronic use, may have quite different implications.

MARIJUANA USE TODAY AND TOMORROW

Remember that our patterns of drug use are but one facet of our evolving society. Our drug use affects, and is affected by, other social trends in our life. You should at least make note of three of these themes and keep them in mind as you try to read the tea leaves for a glimpse of the future. One trend is the increased emphasis on physical health—the change, particularly since the early 1970s, is well documented in the 1980 report: *Health, United States*.[81] Jogging, exercising, dieting, eating health foods, lowering cholesterol, etc. are all reflections of our national concern over shaping up. I don't know anyone who believes drug use is healthy so the "health trend" operates against increasing drug use. Second, when you're bent in one direction almost to the breaking point you react by moving rapidly in the other direction. Politically, Lyndon Johnson's Great Society was reacted to with the landslide victory for Nixon but the jump to the conservative side was clearest in the early 1980s. A conservative ideology, and all that is encompassed in it, operates to decrease the expansion of drug use. Last, there is always the question of economics. Drug use expands in expanding, affluent economies. When times are tough most people—since they are drug users, not drug abusers—decrease their drug use and focus on survival and stabilizing their life and their world.

The future may be fuzzy but in 1982 it's easy to see where we are with respect to marijuana use. Fig. 19-2 contains data from in-school high school seniors from 1975 through 1981 and plots four measures of drug use. The decline in use from the peak in 1978-1979 is obvious, significant, and meaningful. Of particular importance is the decline in the percentage of daily users since these are the ones

most likely to have both physical and psychosocial problems from their drug-taking behavior. These frequent marijuana users are also those who are most likely to try, and misuse, other illegal drugs. In line with that, you should know that in one study[39,p.41] of those who drop out or are "absentees" from school, 56% reported marijuana use—compared to 38% of in-class students. You need to remember that 93% of these 1981 high school seniors had tried alcohol, and 71% had tried cigarettes. Daily marijuana use is about the same as alcohol use (6%), and marijuana use in school occurs more often than alcohol use in school.

The high school seniors who are daily users of marijuana (that is, who are using marijuana 20 or more times a month) have some characteristics that seem important. They are more often residents of larger cities; males outnumber females almost 2 to 1; 11% of whites and 5% of blacks are daily users; daily use is associated with poor performance in school; 13% of non-college-bound students are daily users—in contrast to 7% of the college-bound; as belief in religion and law abiding behavior goes up, daily use is less frequent; and those who date more have higher daily use. These characteristics fit in well with those elaborated for young drug users in Chapter 1.

It is true that high school seniors leave school and get older—and they carry some of their drug-taking behavior with them. A national survey in 1979 showed that over 50 million Americans had at least tried marijuana: 31% of those 12 to 17 (7 million); 68% of those 18 to 25 (21 million); and 20% of those 26 and older (25 million). There was about a 10% increase in current marijuana users (within the last month) from 1977 to 1979 in the young adult group (18 to 25) and most of the increase was in white, southern, non-high-school graduate, non-metropolitan area males. In the older adult group the increase was primarily a result of increase in use by white, southern, college educated males. Drug use moved from the ghetto, the city, the North and oozed into the Sunbelt—along with a thousand other social changes.

A 1981 report[82] made two interesting sets of comparisons: one was of the characteristics of college

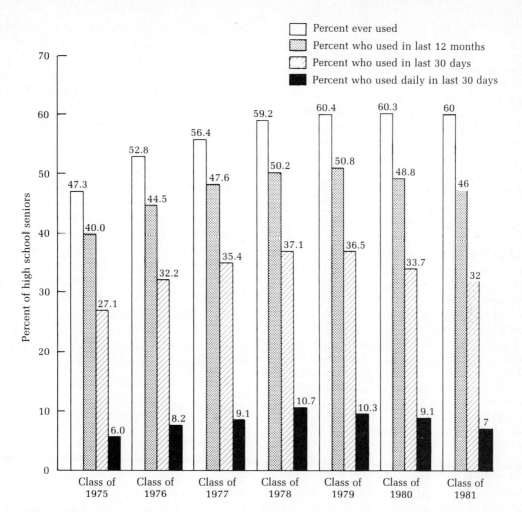

FIG. 19-2 Trends in prevalence of marijuana use by high school seniors, 1975-1981 (in school). (Adapted from Johnson, L.D., Bachman, J.G., and O'Malley, P.M.: Highlights from student drug use in America, 1975-1981.)

students using drugs in 1978 compared to those using drugs in 1969; the other comparison was between drug-using and non-drug-using college students. "Differences between users and nonusers, already modest in 1969, had narrowed further by 1978, users and nonusers were indistinguishable on grades, athletics, other college activities, career plans, and subjective alienation. Only heterosexual activity and visits to a psychiatrist still distinguish users from nonusers."[82,p.588] Drug users do more of the latter two, and the authors comment, ". . . it

is differences in self-concept, attitudes, and values in the user, and not the drug use itself, that creates these differences."[82,p.591] At the college level it *is* impossible to separate users from nonusers—unless you ask.

The world does move swiftly. In 1955 a major textbook in pharmacology could reasonably state that the marijuana user was

usually a person 20 to 30 years of age, idle and lacking in initiative, with a history of repeated frustrations and deprivations, sexually maladjusted (often homosexual) who seeks distraction, escape and sometimes conviviality by smoking the drug. He almost uniformly has major personality defects and is often psychopathic.[83,p.174]

In the 1960s, however, things changed, and use increased rapidly, even though the drug was illegal and severe penalties were mandated. In part the increased use in recent years may result from

a contagion effect. The more users the less viable the official line on marihuana and to a lesser extent other drugs. The less respected the rationale for such sanctions, the greater the experimentation. Greater experimentation increases the number of those who use and makes it easier for novices to obtain drugs. The more varied the user groups the less any potential user has to change his identity to begin using. The more users the more jobs open for drug traffickers and the more sellers will operate among their own kind; the more they blend with their clientele the more difficult it becomes to catch them. This leads to the perception of less risk and greater desirability of dealing. Over time the contagion reaches a point where serious doubt about official positions is replaced by contemptuous disregard.[84]

The spread of marijuana use probably reached its near maximum in the middle and late seventies. Some evidence of the plateauing is evident even in the 1975 and 1976 data. It is unlikely that large percentages of adults over the age of 30 will start using marijuana, even if it is completely legalized. Remember, too, that 20% of the adults in the United States believe that alcohol prohibition should be brought back. That suggests that there may be a large group of individuals who do not support the recreational use of any psychoactive drug. With marijuana use now in the 50% to 60% incidence range in the age group of highest susceptibility, there is not much more opportunity for marijuana use to spread. It is certainly true that each succeeding year will see a higher percentage of those over 30 using marijuana.

There are other forces at work in opposition to the previously mentioned trends. You should go back and read the section on the physiological and intellectual effects of marijuana use. Then you will appreciate that it *is* true that marijuana is not a safe drug, that at social use levels the overt behavioral effects of marijuana and alcohol are comparable, and that a high from either drug impairs performance.[69] It also seems true that there has not been much change in what we know about the adverse consequences of moderate marijuana use, and that there is a relative lack of acute physiological and/or psychological effects.

With all that as background, in the Spring of 1981, the Director of the NIDA reported that ". . . five different national sources of data on attitudes have reported an increase in the proportion of teenagers perceiving the negative consequences of cigarette and drug use, and a significant increase in the number of high school students 'who would disapprove of friends who use drugs.'"[85] Why the change? Conservatism? Health concerns? A slowing economy? A leveling in the proportion of adolescents in the population? The impact of prevention programs? Parents beginning to be more concerned and involved with their children? I don't know, nor does anyone, and I don't know if the trend will persist. It pleases me, as it must any responsible citizen—who can be in favor of adolescents using drugs, except those adolescents who are using drugs? But mark well, the change occurred in the absence of new information on adverse effects of drug use. That's important.

CHRONIC *CANNABIS* USE

People are really neat. Dozens of studies—lasting over 20 years and conducted on tens of thousands of people who live the same kind of life, eat the same kinds of food, work at the same kinds of jobs, breathe the same kinds of air, and have the same kinds of health problems—are ignored or denied by people very much like those studied, and cigarette smoking continues.

Three studies—which were retrospective and conducted on a total of 117 people who live very different kinds of lives, eat different kinds of food, work at different kinds of jobs, breathe different kinds of air, and have different kinds of health problems—are acclaimed and make newspaper headlines by people very much unlike those studied, and marijuana use increases.

I just think it's amusing.

The three studies referred to are, of course, the studies of the effect of chronic marijuana use on health problems and behavior. The studies were done in Greece, Costa Rica, and Jamaica.[86] The reader will already know that "there aren't major health consequences that occur in a high percentage of chronic users of marihuana."[87] In fact, compared to what we already knew medically:

> they are terribly limited studies. They were studies in less complex, more traditional societies. They were studies where people who had many of the health problems which might have been related to marihuana use were excluded through the sample selection process. . . . We wanted to study fairly healthy people. . . . I'm not at all sure that if you took alcohol and tobacco and put them to the same test they would show up bad either.[87]

The behavioral effects were somewhat more interesting in the Jamaica study, although few people commented on them. There is always the question of the relevance of these results to the American marijuana-using society. The Jamaicans studied were field workers and farmers who did manual labor hoeing and harvesting crops. Their work performance was studied by "microanalysis of movements." The farmers believed that they were doing a better weeding job after smoking. In fact, they worked harder but accomplished less:

> Total hoeing or soil-turning space covered, or work accomplished in number of plants reaped, was usually reduced per unit of time after smoking. The number of body movements per minute was often greater after smoking, but more movements were required to complete a given task.[88]

These results are not unlike those reported in Chapter 4: under the influence of a drug many of us feel that we are performing well, even better than without the drug. Frequently that is not so; we do worse. The fact that few of the Jamaican users reported subjective effects similar to those American users experience—enhancement of perception of color, taste, sound—should not surprise anyone. Expectancies play an important role in these drug effects In middle-class consuming-oriented America we look for ways to increase our joy of consumption. Probably not so in field workers in Jamaica.

The inadequacies of these three "chronic" studies are well appreciated by the federal government, so they have started several large-scale, American-based studies that should provide some of the answers we need over the next generation. Moderate-length studies (for example, 94 days) so far confirm the facts as reported elsewhere in this chapter.[89]

THE WRITING ON THE WALL

In retrospect some decisions seem easy. It is fairly easy to believe that the drug scene today might be less disruptive and less anxiety arousing if the Marijuana Tax Act of 1937 had never happened. Marijuana use was slowly moving across the United States, and the relatively mild psychoactive drug was becoming acculturated. Society would have adapted to marijuana and would have adapted marijuana to society. Soon it would have been part and parcel of society: most people would know how to use it; some, of course, would have abused it. It happened before with coffee, tea, and tobacco. It is the only way to introduce a new psychoactive drug—slowly and easily.

The 1937 law changed all that. The dam that was built to stop a trickle was required to hold back the pressure of a tidal wave in the 1960s and early 1970s. Marijuana was not the catch phrase at the start of the psychedelic era; LSD was. Acid came first; the gentler high of marijuana followed later. And so did the arrests. There were state and federal laws against the possession, use, sale, or purchase of marijuana. As is always the case with social problems, you could find experts at both extremes. Some argued for legalization,[90] some for even more stringent penalties.[91] Everyone had his favorite story about the innocent youth of 18 or 19, usually a former altar boy supporting his widowed mother by working at two jobs, who was busted by the police and given 20 years in prison for the possession of 1 ounce of marijuana. Even in Texas that seemed a little steep to some people.

A dialogue did start, however, on the pros and cons of marijuana, or at least two simultaneous monologues.

No one obeys the law against marijuana, and everyone is learning disrespect for all laws.

Did you ever know anyone who was into hard drugs who didn't start with marijuana?

We all started with our mother's milk—should we outlaw that too?

Once you try one drug, then you'll try another; it all starts with marijuana.

Police money can be better spent on real crimes, not on chasing marijuana experimenters.

All the while things were changing. The counterculture thoughts, dress, and attitudes, as well as their drugs, were slowly moving into the establishment mainstream. Everything in America was loosening up, but only a little! Thousands of Everytown, U.S.A., citizens worried about the morality of Vietnam. And people were still being busted for possession of marijuana. Everyone knew why the arrests were made: possession of marijuana was illegal. The question was, why was marijuana illegal?

That was a tougher question to answer; there is no rational medical or legal answer, only a psychosocial answer, and that involves value judgments (Chapter 2). Few laws are passed, repealed, or changed unless there is strong pressure. Democracy works on the "status quo is best" theory: Leave it alone unless some group forces us to change it. Voice was given to the millions of marijuana users in 1970 when a young Washington lawyer established NORML, the National Organization for the Reform of Marijuana Law, with a grant from the Playboy Foundation. As the founder of NORML[92] put it: "The only people working for reform then were freaks who wanted to turn on the world, an approach that was obviously doomed to failure. I wanted an effective, middle-class approach, not pro-grass but antijail. . . ."

Things moved in fits and starts in the early years, and NORML had an important impact on the move to decriminalize marijuana possession—done in 10 states—and to reduce marijuana possession from a felony to a misdemeanor—done in all but two of the remaining states. In 1979 NORML changed its tune and is now calling for the legalization of the use and sale of marijuana. The action of NORML that had brought the most joy to college students is their distribution of the 1936 movie *Reefer Madness*. The film "depicts a group of high-school students trying marijuana, with murder, rape, prostitution and madness as the swift result of their folly."[92] It is so bad, it is really good and should help young people understand some of the factors that shaped attitudes about marijuana in the 1930s. NORML has grown in membership and influence since the early seventies and has been *the* national organization urging the decriminalization of marijuana use and possesion for personal use.[93]

The year 1972 was a turning point in the fight to decriminalize marijuana. There are many variations on the theme, but the basic concept of decriminalization is that there should be no prison sentences for the possession of a small amount of marijuana for personal use. Usually any amount less than an ounce is considered to be for personal use and not for sale or resale. Possession for personal use may still be illegal, as is exceeding the speed limit on the highway, but the penalty is a fine, not prison, and the individual who is fined does not have a police record.

If you remember, the Comprehensive Drug Abuse Prevention and Control Act of 1970 established a Commission on Marijuana and Drug Abuse (Chapter 2). It was to study the issues comprehensively and make "recommendations for legislative and administrative actions" within 2 years. The commission members were known to be very conservative on questions of drug use, so not much was expected. And even if the report was balanced or liberal on various drug issues, what would happen? The 1962 President's Ad Hoc Panel on Drug Abuse had concluded "that the hazards of marijuana per se have been exaggerated and that long criminal sentences imposed on an occasional user or possessor of the drug are in poor social perspective." Nothing happened.

The wheel turns. Time marches on. Things look different when you change your position. Both the interim and the first reports[62] of the Marijuana Commission not only agreed with the 1962 panel, but recommended legislative changes.

> The Commission recommended that federal and state laws be changed so that private possession of small amounts of marihuana for personal use, and casual distribution of small amounts without monetary profit, would no longer be offenses, though marihuana possessed in public would remain contraband. Cultivation, distribution for profit, and possession with intent to sell would remain felonies. Criminal penalties would be retained for disorderly conduct associated with marihuana intoxication and driving under the influence of marihuana, and a plea of marihuana intoxication would not be a defense to any criminal act committed under its influence.[94]

The 184-page report was excellent. It provided a social and historical perspective and an honest evaluation of the status of marijuana research at that time. The sluice gates were lifted a little, and some of the pressure behind the dam was released. In May 1972, the Canadian government commission issued its report, the LeDain report,[34] and recommended that possession of marijuana be *legalized*. It seems that every month in that year some action was taken that either actually or symbolically expressed a different attitude toward marijuana and its users. Throughout the year, states began releasing some of the 2000 individuals previously jailed for marijuana possession.[95] Not only was amnesty for those in prison catching on, but so was leniency for those arrested (but sometimes not even charged) with small amounts of marijuana. In September, Ann Arbor, Michigan, changed its city laws so that possession of marijuana was only a $5 fine, and smoking in public increased.

Because most people had concerns about the effects of marijuana on health, it was of special significance that in June 1972 the AMA came out in favor of dropping criminal penalties for possession of "insignificant amounts" of marijuana and noted that "there is no evidence supporting the idea that marijuana leads to violence, aggressive behavior or crime."[96] This was a very significant change from the 1968 AMA position that declared, "Cannabis is a dangerous drug and as such is a public health concern."[97,98]

In August 1972 the American Bar Association (ABA) called for the reduction of criminal penalties for possession but did not recommend decriminalization, although it did a year later.

In November 1977, the AMA and the ABA issued a joint (!) statement endorsing the decriminalization of marijuana for personal use.

A week before Christmas in 1972 it came to pass that the best-known and most literate of American conservatives[99] proclaimed in favor of the decriminalization of marijuana, saying:

> It isn't silly to say that the user should not be molested, even though the pusher should be put in jail. It was so, mostly, under prohibition, when the speakeasy operators were prosecuted, not so the patrons. Thus it is, by and large, in the case of prostitution; and even with gambling; and most explicitly with pornography, the Supreme Court having ruled that you can't molest the owner, even though you can go after the peddler.

In 1973 the United States passed into the eye of the hurricane. First the storm before the calm. In that year there were 420,700 people arrested on marijuana charges in the United States. That was a slight increase from 8 years earlier, 1965, when 18,815 were arrested! Of the 420,000 arrests, 93% were for possession. How many were jailed, fined, etc., is unknown. These marijuana arrests accounted for 67% of all drug arrests in 1973. (Although marijuana arrests reached 445,600 in 1974, the worst was over, and in 1973 America began to march to a different drummer.) Then the calm. "In October, 1973, Oregon abolished criminal penalties for marijuana use, substituting civil fines of up to $100. Marijuana offenders are given citations that are processed like traffic tickets."[100]

Oregon was a good place to start the drive to decriminalize the possession of marijuana, although it wasn't conscious, well-thought-out, or part of a national plan. Oregon is both a progressive and a conservative state. Marijuana use by adults in Oregon in 1973 was lower than that of either

California or Washington. As one Oregon lawyer[101] put it in 1977:

> Where, but in Oregon, is it possible to threaten a supermarket store manager with a $1,000 fine and a year in jail if he dares sell even one bottle of beer without that bottle having a refund value of at least two cents but, at the same time, to threaten a hippie hitchhiker with only a $100 fine if he carries his "pot" in small amounts.

Did marijuana use increase in Oregon as a result of the decriminalization? Yes. By leaps and bounds? No. From the fall of 1974, a year after decriminalization, to the fall of 1977, the percentage of adults over 18 who had "ever used" marijuana went from 19% to 25%. "Current users" went from 9% to 10% over the same period. Of most interest, though, was the increase of "ever used" in the 18-to-29-year age group: from 46% in 1974 to 62% in 1977; 30% of those sampled in this age range in 1977 said they were current users.[102] The most important data relevant to the decriminalization question was never obtained: what is the change in the incidence of use in those under 18 years of age?

Was the Oregon law important? The first of anything is always important, and the director of NORML[103] said it clearly:

> When Oregon said private use wasn't a crime, it in effect said marijuana wasn't immoral. Ever since then we've considered the war to be over.

Nine other states have made possession of a small amount of marijuana only a civil offense: Alaska, Maine, Colorado, California, Ohio, Minnesota, Mississippi, New York, and North Carolina. South Dakota has passed a decriminalization law, but even before the law went into effect, it was repealed when conservatives gained control of the legislature. "In four of these states—California, Colorado, Minnesota, and Ohio—not-for-profit transfers of small amounts of marijuana also are regarded as civil offenses, punishable by fine."[102,p.1]

At the federal level, action picked up in 1977. In January, "Rosalynn Carter joined her husband, the President, in calling for the decriminalization of marijuana . . ." and revealed that their oldest son had been discharged from the navy for smoking marijuana. Bills to decriminalize marijuana possession were introduced into both houses of Congress, and in August President Carter sent a message to Congress in which he asked them to abolish all federal criminal penalties for the possession of small amounts of marijuana. The only organizations that continued to speak against the decriminalization movement were police and narcotic control organizations. Some of these organizations point out that the United States will be violating its international treaty obligations if it reduces criminal penalties on marijuana.[104] Whether this is true will depend on the specific law passed. Be that as it may, President Carter's adviser on drug issues told a congressional committee that the administration "will continue to discourage marijuana use, but we feel criminal penalties that brand otherwise law-abiding people for life are neither effective nor an appropriate deterrent."[105]

At the practical, law enforcement level, the simple decriminalization of marijuana possession by the federal government would have little impact other than psychological. (The psychological effect would be very great.) Rarely is an arrest for possession only or a small-amount sale made by federal law enforcement officers. These arrests (which are made less and less often) are carried out by local and state officials under local and state laws. Action by Congress could, however, be such that the federal decriminalization law would eliminate all state laws that mandate criminal penalties for possession for personal use. If that type of law were passed, there might be multiple court cases arguing that control of marijuana within a state's borders is the responsibility of the state.

If the truth were known, in the late 1970s de facto decriminalization had already occurred in many areas of the country. Law enforcement agencies in many of the larger cities of the United States have stopped arresting marijuana users and do not search out those with small amounts for personal use. The states have long known what a 1977 report of the National Governor's Conference said: states that have decriminalized marijuana possession have shown a substantial saving of tax dollars.[106]

Those who view the decriminalization of marijuana possession as an isolated event in the social movement of our culture need a better perspective. Just as drug use cannot be separated from other social trends, marijuana laws and attitudes cannot be isolated from laws and attitudes toward other drugs. In 1975 a Drug Enforcement Administration official predicted what may come:

> If you talk about decreasing penalties and decriminalization, people think you're saying drugs are not so bad . . . when you decriminalize marijuana . . . people are now waiting for the next step. . . . It's one package. The basic concept . . . is: Let's stop trying so hard to prevent people from using drugs.[107]

The director of the National Institute on Drug Abuse agreed with part of that. "It's now clear to me that the leading edge of change in drug-using behavior for the American population—and I think this is true worldwide—is marijuana."[87] As marijuana goes, so goes the drug scene? In spite of this, the director still believed that decriminalization was the way to go. The relevant question is the wisdom of using the criminal sanction as a means of discouraging consumption, when considerably less costly avenues of discouragement are available."[108]

It is interesting to see everyone tiptoe around and try to be right, on both sides of the issue. In 1978 the director of NIDA realized that if possession is basically not illegal, then there will have to be a large, illegal procurement, transport, and sales force, unless everyone grows their own. Speaking to Congress, "he urged a reduced penalty for cultivation of small amounts in the home [while] stressing that he is not advocating a 'grow-your-own' philosophy. . . ."[108] *I* understand that, don't you? The issue was phrased best during the New York State decriminalization debate. The director of the Bureau of Narcotics Enforcement said, "We are creating a demand by easing the penalties for users while at the same time making it illegal to

satisfy that demand."[109] Maybe that's one of the reasons alcohol prohibition didn't work. NORML agreed and urged "the right of private cultivation of marijuana."

Creating a demand . . . creating a demand . . . hmmm—there's always money to be made when you satisfy a demand. It may not be easy but there's a lot of money. Carrying eggs across the Yukon in the Alaskan Gold Rush in 1897—they were worth $5 each delivered. It's always been true—satisfy a demand and add on a profit to cover the risk (the greater the risk, the greater the profit). If you luck out you're rich. In the game we're about to describe, if you lose you may be dead, in jail, or broke.

Yes, marijuana is big business. Of the $90 billion illicit drug retail market in 1979 the DEA estimates that about 35% of sales is for marijuana, 1% for hashish, 27% for cocaine, 23% for dangerous drugs, and 14% for heroin. Appreciate all the production and use figures in this section are best estimates based on street buys, raids, larger purchases abroad, informers, etc.

The 1980 estimate of marijuana use in the United States was 15,000 tons for the year—that's 480 million ounces. If you're a user, you're probably saying, "That's too low, why last month . . ."; if you're not a user, "Why so high? *I* didn't use any and neither did mom or dad. . . ." In addition to the marijuana probably 200 tons of hashish was smuggled into the United States in 1978. No one knows how much marijuana is smuggled in each year but during a 45-day period in the fall of 1979 the federal government made an all-out push to stop the inflow of marijuana. During that 45-day period they confiscated 900,000 pounds of marijuana—maybe one third of the flow.[110]

Probably about 10,000 tons plus of the marijuana that reaches the United States each year comes from Colombia. In 1980 Colombian marijuana sold for $40 to $50 an ounce ($600 a pound) on the street, in dormitories, discos, and dives. The Colombian farmer gets about $1 a pound for the marijuana in its rough state at the field; that gives him five to six times what he could make raising coffee, corn, or cotton! One guess is that in 1979 Colombia harvested 6 billion pounds of marijuana, which was raised on 300,000 acres. It grows well in Colombia; in 6 months it can reach a height of 15 feet. In case you don't already know it: if you can grow tomatoes, you can grow marijuana. Marijuana will grow any place a dandelion will grow. (I keep checking my front yard.)

Until 1977 most of our imported (!) marijuana came from Mexico—now it's only 1000 to 2000 tons a year. The Middle East—Lebanon—contributes a similar amount. Since the late 1970s marijuana has become a major cash crop in several states and maybe 10% to 20% of what we smoke is home-grown. The most famous state of course is California, particularly Northern California, and most especially Mendocino County. The emphasis there is on quality, not quantity. *Sinsemilla* is Spanish for "without seeds" and is the current designation for quality, high-potency marijuana. It sells for $100 to $200 an ounce.

> The high-potency marijuana is produced by weeding out the male cannabis plants before they can pollinate the female plants. This causes the female plant to produce more and more resin in its flowering buds. Leaves are also carefully plucked to produce a bushier plant loaded with buds and reaching a height of 20 feet.[110,p.36]

Properly watered, fertilized, tended, and loved you can cultivate a sinsemilla plant in a 3 × 3 foot area, which will produce 1 to 3 pounds of 6% to 8% THC marijuana for the luxury market. The farmers here are not an itinerate downtrodden group of serfs. "Some of the growers have organized themselves into cooperatives." One ironic twist, some farmers do their cultivating on isolated land owned by the federal government.

One final bit of information. A difficulty with the simple "let's decriminalize marijuana" is—which marijuana?

Type/origin	Percent THC
Nepal	2.8
Mexico	1.7
Colombia	3.0
Jamaica	2.8
United States	0.4
Sinsemilla	6.3

The variation[39,p.16] in THC content is over 15-fold. If you're used to less than 0.5% and you get 6%, that's enough to cause an anxiety attack or a panic state in most novitiates. You can have fun and play with numbers all you want—how much tax money could 12 billion reefers bring into Uncle Sam? Sales tax dollars? How many THC levels would be needed? Etc., etc.

ONE LAST TOKE

Can you read the writing on the wall yet? If you can't, here is what it says:

> The Age of Pot is upon us. The Day of the Reefer has dawned. After 40 years of trying to stamp out the dread weed with a steadily escalating law-enforcement campaign that has become virtually a war, the various states of these United States are beginning to sue for peace. After spending millions of dollars, ruining thousands of young lives, and clogging our already overworked judicial and police apparatus with hundreds of thousands of petty crimes and misdemeanors, the men who make our laws are saying: "Let them smoke pot."[111]

Slowly, slowly. "What whiskey did to the Indians, marijuana may do to white, middle-class America."[111]

I hope not.

CONCLUDING COMMENT

Has the world gone to pot? It sure has! It looks very much as if the United States will soon embark on a large-scale social experiment, but I don't know how soon. There's no rush; it has been developing for many years, but its impact is still difficult to predict. The other side of the coin, the prohibition of alcohol, also developed slowly over several decades. That was a disaster after a few years.

As my daddy used to say: Keep your eyes and ears open—big things are about to happen!

I believe it, since:

> Marijuana is symbolic of a more passive, contemplative, and less competitive attitude toward life than has been traditional in the United States. It

is usually denounced by people who like things the way they are. Whether society accepts or rejects the drug will undoubtedly have some influence on the evolution of our national character.[47,p.x]

REFERENCES

1. Dionne, E.J.: Dedicated to dope, In Anderson, P.: Review of high in America, NY Times Book Review, p. 11, April 12, 1981.
2. Grass grows more acceptable, Time, September 10, 1973.
3. Marijuana: bad, but . . . , Drug Topics, p. 20, February 1, 1980.
4. Emboden, W.A.: The genus *Cannabis* and the correct use of toxonomic categories, Journal of Psychoactive Drugs **13**(1):15-21, 1981.
5. Hashish oil, Drug Enforcement, pp. 24-25, Fall 1973.
6. Stone, B.: Grass farm, Drug Enforcement **7**(1):11-15, 1980.
7. Toaw, M.: The religious and medicinal uses of *Cannabis* in China, India, and Tibet, Journal of Psychoative Drugs **13**(1):23-34 1981.
8. Snyder, S.H.: What we have forgotten about pot, New York Times Magazine, pp. 27, 121, 124, 130, December 13, 1970.
9. Robinson, V.: An essay on hasheesh, ed. 2, New York, 1925, E.H. Ringer, Publisher.
10. Mickel, E.J.: The artificial paradises in French literature, Chapel Hill, N.C., 1969, University of North Carolina Press.
11. Cannabis study group (chairman: Alfred Freedman): The Ninth Annual Meeting of the American College of Neuropsychopharmacology, San Juan, Puerto Rico, December 8-11, 1970.
12. Baudelaire, C.P.: Artificial paradises; on hashish and wine as means of expanding individuality, translated by Ellen Fox, New York, 1971, Herder & Herder.
13. Unpublished material in the Archives of the American Psychological Association, Department of Psychology, University of Akron, Akron, Ohio.
14. Our home hasheesh crop, The Literary Digest, p. 64, April 3, 1929.
15. Taxation of marihuana, hearings before the Committee on Ways and Means, House of Representatives, Seventy-fifth Congress, First Session, on H.R. 6385, April 27-30 and May 4, 1937, Washington, D.C., U.S. Government Printing Office.
16. Parry, A.: The menace of marihuana, American Mercury **36**:487-488, 1935.
17. Marihuana menaces youth, Scientific American **154**:151, 1936.
18. Wolf, W.: Uncle Sam fights a new drug menace . . . marijuana, Popular Science Monthly **128**:14-119, 1936.
19. Anslinger, H.J., and Cooper, C.R.: Marijuana: assassin of youth, American Magazine **124**:19, 153, 1937.
20. Facts and fancies about marihuana, Literary Digest **122**:7-8, 1936.
21. Whitlock, L.: Review: marijuana, Crime and Delinquency Literature **2**(3):367, 1970.
22. Grinspoon, L.: Marihuana, International Journal of Psychiatry **9**:488-516, 1970-1971.
23. Smith, R.: U.S. marijuana legislation and the creation of a social problem, Journal of Psychedelic Drugs **2**(1):93-103, 1968.
24. Mandel, J.: Hashish, assassins, and the love of God, Issues in Criminology **2**(2):149-156, 1966.
25. Fort, J.: Pot: a rational approach, Playboy, pp. 131, 154, October 1969.
26. The marihuana bugaboo, Military Surgeon **93**:95, 1943.
27. Mayor LaGuardia's Committee on Marijuana. In Solomon, D., editor: The marihuana papers, New York, 1966, The New American Library.
28. Adams, R.: Marihuana, Bulletin of the New York Academy of Medicine **18**:705-730, 1942.
29. Allentuck, S., and Bowman, K.M.: The psychiatric aspects of marihuana intoxication, American Journal of Psychiatry **99**:248-251, 1942.
30. Marijuana problems, Journal of the American Medical Association **127**:1129, 1945.
31. Marijuana. Report of the Indian Hemp Drugs Commission 1893-1894, Baltimore, 1969, Waverly Press. (Originally published in 1894.)
32. Editorial: The marihuana bugaboo, Military Surgeon **93**:94, 1943.
33. Drug dependency and drug abuse in New Zealand, first report, Board of Health, Report Series No. 14, Wellington, New Zealand, 1970, A.R. Shearer, Government Printer.
34. Interim report of the Commission of Inquiry into the Non-medical Use of Drugs, Ottawa, 1970, Queen's Printer for Canada. (Also called the LeDain Report.)
35. Cannabis, Report by the Advisory Committee on Drug Dependence, London, 1968, Her Majesty's Stationery Office. (Also known as the Wooton Committee Report.)
36. Marihuana and health, sixth annual report to the U.S. Congress from the Secretary of Health, Education, and Welfare, Publication No. (ADM) 77-443, Washington, D.C., 1976, U.S. Government Printing Office.
37. Task force report: narcotics and drug abuse, President's Commission on Law Enforcement and Administration of Justice, Washington, D.C., 1967, U.S. Government Printing Office.
38. Report of an ARF/WHO scientific meeting on adverse health and behavioral consequences of *Cannabis* use, Toronto, 1981, Addiction Research Foundation.
39. Marijuana and health, Institute of Medicine, National Academy of Sciences, Washington, D.C., 1982, National Academy Press.

40. Esrati, A.E.: How "mild" is marijuana? Magazine Digest, pp. 81, 85-86, June 1945.

41. Kolb, L.: Let's stop this narcotics hysteria! Saturday Evening Post 229:19-55, 1956.

42. McGlothlin, W.H., and West, L.J.: The marihuana problem: an overview, American Journal of Psychiatry 125:370-378, 1968.

43. Kaufman, J., Allen, J.R., and West, L.J.: Runaways, hippies, and marihuana, American Journal of Psychiatry 126:717-720, 1969.

44. Competitive problems in the drug industry, hearings before the Subcommittee on Monopoly of the Select Committee on Small Business, United States Senate, Ninety-first Congress, First Session (July 16, 29, 30 and October 27, 1969), Part 13, Psychotropic Drugs, Washington, D.C., 1969, U.S. Government Printing Office.

45. O'Shaughnessy, W.B.: On the preparations of the Indian hemp, or gunja, Trans. Med. m. Phys. Soc., Bengal, pp. 71-102, 1838-1840; pp. 421-461, 1842.

46. Mikuriya, T.H.: Marijuana in medicine: past, present and future, California Medicine 110:34-40, 1969.

47. Synder, S.H.: Uses of marijuana, New York, 1972, Oxford University Press.

48. Walton, R.P.: Marihuana, America's new drug problem, Philadelphia, 1938, J.B. Lippincott Co.

49. Standardization of drug extracts, promotional brochure, Detroit, 1898, Parke, Davis & Co.

50. Letter to E.P. Delabarre, 9 Arlington Ave., Providence, R.I., from Parke, Davis & Co., Manufacturing Department, Main Laboratories, Detroit, Superintendent's Office, Control Department, March 10, 1902.

51. Taxation of marijuana, House of Representatives, Committee on Ways and Means, Washington, D.C., 1937.

52. Mikuriya, T.H., editor: Marihuana: medical papers 1839-1972, Oakland, Calif., 1973, Medi-Comp.

53. Davis, J.P., and Ramsey, H.H.: Antiepileptic action of marihuana-active substances, Federation Proceedings 8:284-285, 1949.

54. Lieberman, C.M., and Lieberman, B.W.: Marihuana—a medical review, New England Journal of Medicine 284:88-91, 1971.

55. Hine, B., Friedman, E., Torrelio, M., and Gershon, S.: Morphine-dependent rats: blockade of precipated abstinence by tetrahydrocannibinol, Science 187:443-445, 1975.

56. Maugh, T.H., II: Marihuana: the grass may no longer be greener, Science 185:683-685, 1974.

57. Carlson, E.T.: Cannabis indica in 19th-century psychiatry, American Journal of Psychiatry 131:1004, September 1974.

58. Marijuana smoking said to have power to deter glaucoma, New York Times, July 28, 1972.

59. Medical therapy, legalization issues debated at Marijuana Reform Conference, National Drug Reporter 7(1):3-5, 1977.

60. Procedure for obtaining THC for cancer patients, Medical News 246(1):15, 1981.

61. Gunby, P.: Many cancer patients receiving THC as antiemetic, Medical News 245(15):1515, 1981.

62. Marihuana and health, Department of Health, Education, and Welfare, Washington, D.C., 1971, U.S. Government Printing Office.

63. Faltermayer, E.K.: What we know about marijuana—so far, Fortune 83(3):96-132, 1971.

64. Lemberger, L., and others: Marihuana; studies on the disposition and metabolism of delta-9-tetrahydrocannabinol in man. Science 170:1320-1322, 1970.

65. Pop drugs: the high as a way of life, Time, p. 73, September 26, 1969.

66. Becker, H.S.: Outsiders, studies in the sociology of deviance, New York, 1963, The Free Press.

67. Tart, C.T.: Marijuana intoxication: common experiences, Nature 226:701-704, 1970.

68. Jones, R.T.: Tetrahydrocannabinol and the marijuana-induced social "high," or the effects of the mind on marijuana. In Singer, A.J., editor: Marijuana: chemistry, pharmacology, and patterns of social use, Annals of the New York Academy of Sciences 191:155-165, 1971.

69. Rafaelsen, O.J., Cannabis and alcohol: effects on simulated car driving, Science 179:920-923, 1973.

70. Brill, N.Q., and others: The marijuana problem (UCLA Interdepartmental Conference), Annals of Internal Medicine 73:449-465, 1970.

71. Keeler, M.H., Reifler, C.B., and Liptzin, M.B.: Spontaneous recurrence of marihuana effect, American Journal of Psychiatry 125:384-386, 1968.

72. Kaplan, H.S.: Psychosis associated with marijuana, Psychiatry Digest, pp. 26-27, January 1972.

73. Payne, R.J., and Brand, S.N.: The toxicity of intravenously used marihuana, Journal of the American Medical Association 233:351-354, 1975.

74. Farnsworth, N.R., and Cordell, G.A.: New potential hazard regarding use of marijuana—treatment of plants with liquid fertilizers, Journal of Psychedelic Drugs 8(2):151-155, 1976.

75. Campbell, A.M.G., Thomson, J.L.G., Evans, M., and Williams, M.J.: Cerebral atrophy in young cannabis smokers, Lancet 1:202-203, 1972.

76. Co, B.T., and others: Absence of cerebral atrophy in chronic cannbis users, Journal of the American Medical Association 237:1229-1230, 1977.

77. Kuehnle, J., Mendelson, J.H., Davis, K.R., and New, P.F.J.: Computed tomographic examination of heavy marijuana smokers, Journal of the American Medical Association 237:1231-1232, 1977.

78. Tinklenberg, J.R., editor: Marijuana and health hazards: Methodological issues in current research, New York, 1975, Academic Press, Inc., chapters 8-11.

79. Tinklenberg, J.R., editor: Marijuana and health hazards:

methodological issues in current research, New York, 1975, Academic Press, Inc., chapters 1-4.

80. Nahas, G.G.: Marihuana—deceptive weed, New York, 1973, Raven Press.

81. Health United States, 1980 U.S. Department of Health and Human Services, DHHS Publ. No. 81-1232, Washington, D.C. December 1980, U.S. Government Printing Office.

82. Pope, H.G., and others: Drug use and life-style among college undergraduates, Archives of General Psychiatry **38**:588, May 1981.

83. Goodman, L.S., and Gilman, A.: The pharmacological basis of therapeutics, ed. 2, New York, 1955, The Macmillan Co.

84. Carey, J.T.: Marihuana use among the new bohemians, Journal of Psychedelic Drugs **2**(1):80- 81, 1968.

85. Drug scene changing: NIDA boss, The U.S. Journal, p. 13, May 1981.

86. Dornbush, R.L., Freedman, A.M., and Fink, M., editors: Chronic cannabis use, Annals of the New York Academy of Sciences **282**:vii-viii, 1976.

87. Maugh, T.H., II: Marihuana: a conversation with NIDA's Robert L. DuPont, Science **192**:647-649, 1976.

88. Study of chronic use of marijuana demonstrates no chromosome breaks, brain damage, or untoward effects. Medical Tribune **14**(39):1, 34, 36, 1973.

89. Authority on drug abuse, MD, pp. 65-67, April 1976.

90. Kaplan, J.: Marihuana—the new prohibition. New York, 1970, World Publishing Co.

91. Blackly, P.H.: Effects of decriminalization of marijuana in Oregon. In Dornbush, R.L., Freedman, A.M., and Fink, M., editors: Chronic cannabis use, Annals of The New York Academy of Sciences **282**:405-415, 1976.

92. Anderson, P.: The pot lobby, New York Times Magazine, pp. 8-9, January 21, 1973.

93. Anderson, P.: High in America, New York, 1981, Viking Press.

94. Farnsworth, D.L.: Summary of the Report of the National Commission on Marihuana and Drug Abuse, Tracks, No. 9, pp. 1-2, 1972.

95. Knight, M.: Easing of marijuana laws stirs wide concern over those in prison, New York Times, May 28, 1972, p. 27.

96. Lyons, R.P.: A.M.A. would drop serious penalties, New York Times, June 21, 1972.

97. Marijuana and society (editorial), Journal of the American Medical Association **204**:91-92, 1968.

98. The AMA and pot, Stash Capsules **4**(4), August 1972.

99. Buckley, W.F., Jr.: Pot, legalization of, conservative division, New York Times, December 18, 1972.

100. Parachini, A.: Legal hostility to "Pot" fades, New York Times, December 8, 1974.

101. Titus, H.W.: Oregon marijuana decriminalization, the moral question, Journal of Drug Issues **7**:23-34, 1977.

102. Marijuana survey—state of Oregon Drug Abuse Council, Inc., News Release, January 4, 1978.

103. The private use of "pot"—a growing public issue, U.S. News and World Report, pp. 37-38, April 28, 1975.

104. Decriminalization would violate international law: police chiefs, U.S. Journal, p. 13, April 1977.

105. Carter seeks end of marijuana curb; cocaine examined, New York Times, March 15, 1977, p. 30.

106. States are found to save money by marijuana decriminalization, New York Times, April 1, 1977, p. A10.

107. Grafton, S., editor: The continuing marijuana story, Addiction and Drug Abuse Report **6**(8):1, August 1975.

108. Decriminalize marijuana says DuPont, National Drug Reporter **7**(3):1-2, March 1977.

109. Bird, D.: Shortcomings cited in marijuana curbs, New York Times, May 6, 1977, p. B5M.

110. Drug Enforcement, vol. 7, March 1980.

111. Goldman, A.: Entering the new age of pot: what will happen when middle-class America gets the straight dope? New York, pp. 28-41, August 25, 1975.

UNIT **7**

CONCLUSION

CHAPTER 20

A RATIONAL LOOK AT DRUG USE

HAPPINESS IS a last chapter that can be a beginning. One of the bright things about a book is that the concluding chapter does not have to be the end. Some readers will remember some of the facts, the stories, and the ideas and use them in looking at the drug scene now and tomorrow. A concluding chapter should offer a beginning, a new view as well as an overview of the problem.

This chapter will serve several purposes. First, it will summarize the themes and principles that have been everywhere evident. And we've been almost everywhere—from the Andes to Vienna, from Turkey to the suburbs, from the laboratory to the streets of every city. To what end? Why? Why not just the here and now? For one reason, to know that the drug situation is not new; we have been where we are now many times before. At the same time, we have never been where we are now, never in 4000 years. That is what this chapter is about. How are we the same and how are we different from earlier periods of high drug use? What general principles can be derived about the use of psychoactive drugs? Not concepts about specific drugs in specific societies, but broad principles about the interactions that occur repeatedly among drugs, individuals, and society. Three of these principles are so pervasive and fundamental that they have

appeared repeatedly in the preceding chapters. Remember them well.

Basic to any understanding of the problems in the area of drug use, misuse, and abuse is the realization that drug taking is behavior. As such it follows the same rules and can be understood and modified to the same extent as any other kind of behavior. The most basic rule is that drug taking follows the Minimax Principle: behavior persists if it *minimizes* discomfort or *maximizes* pleasure and satisfaction. People don't take drugs for the hell of it; they use drugs because they provide an increase in satisfaction or a reduction in discomfort. Nothing will reduce the spread of drug use unless there is an adequate substitute for the feelings that drugs provide.

Drug use does not occur in isolation; it occurs in and is understandable only within a context. Drug use is not foreign to the American heritage or the present social milieu. The drug problem is not a tumor that can be plucked from the bosom of society. Drug use and abuse are an integral part of the fabric of our evolving social philosophy. To change patterns of drug use requires changing the social context.

It is not true that the drug problem is a war to be won or lost. Much past and present thinking has been based on the idea that *we* are fighting *them*—the enemy, drug abuse. Unfortunately, Pogo was right: We have met the enemy . . .and they is us. There is no war to be won; like death, taxes, and poverty, there will always be drug problems. Only in the bicentennial year did the federal bureaucracy finally face this fact and liken the drug problem to a garden: it will always need tending.

A major goal of this chapter is to consider all of the general principles and to draw some conclusions. Of particular importance are the implications of these principles for the present culture. Finally, after reviewing the major themes and considering their implications, a rational view of drug use today in our society seems possible.

THEMES AND PRINCIPLES
Dimensions and determinants of drug effects

What are the determinants of the behavioral effects of a psychoactive drug? They are multiple and range from pharmacological and biochemical factors to the cultural history and social setting of the user. There is no simple answer to the general question, what is *the* behavioral effect of *this* drug? Nevertheless, at the most fundamental level, all drugs used recreationally on a regular basis directly or indirectly either increase pleasure or decrease discomfort. However, individuals and cultures may differ greatly in whether a particular effect is experienced as pleasant or unpleasant.

To find the common physiological threads weaving through the psychoactive drug experiences, only two broad dimensions of brain activity need be considered for our purposes: level of arousal and information processing. The activity level of the brain is increased by stimulants, such as caffeine, amphetamine, and cocaine, and decreased by depressants, including alcohol and barbiturates. The action of these drugs seems primarily to be through their effect on the reticular formation. Some agents, such as LSD, have an alteration of activation level as a secondary rather than a primary effect.

Most of the drugs that have been adopted by western culture are those primarily affecting arousal level. Perhaps stimulation or depression, and thus a loss of inhibitions, has been compatible with our aggressively achieving but tightly moral society. Whether speeded up or slowed down, the user is still focused on the outside "real world."

The distortion-of-information-processing dimension results from one of two types of actions on the nervous system. The distortion can result from alterations of the primary or secondary sensory input pathways, or it can result from impaired retrieval and processing of memories. The hallucinogens, LSD, mescaline, and hashish have their primary effect on the information-processing systems. Images, colors—all experiences—are partly unreal when hallucinogenic drugs are employed. Only at the extremes of the arousal dimension—high activation or extreme depression—does distortion of information processing become an important feature of drugs that primarily influence level of arousal.

Drugs that alter information processing have been foreign to western civilization. There are probably many reasons for this fact, but one of them certainly has to be that by providing "multiple realities," hallucinogens would impair the single focus that is essential for rapid scientific and technological progress. It may be that the present movement away from such a single cultural focus will be coupled with an increase in the use of this class of agents.

Throughout the book it has been demonstrated that to discuss drug use meaningfully it is essential to specify dosage range, mode of administration, frequency of drug use, and setting in which the use occurs. The low oral dose of amphetamine that helps bored blimps make it through the day is a far cry from shooting speed, even though some people simply categorize both as drug misuse. The mild temporal and spatial distortions and the euphoria accompanying marijuana smoking have only a tenuous behavioral connection with the very personal hallucinations of hashish. Use of LSD and other hallucinogens in a laboratory setting certainly alters their effects from those obtained when they are used in a social situation surrounded by friends and containing pulsating lights and music.

Expectations are of great importance in determining the effects of an agent, as seen most vividly in work done with placebos. The belief that an authority, the physician, is giving a medicine that will have a specific effect is frequently enough to *in fact* produce the effect, even though an inert agent has been used. The expectations an individual has about various drugs obviously develop from his personal history of experiences and needs that occur in a social context. For this reason it is important that the social context present accurate and credible information about what a drug can and cannot do.

It cannot be emphasized too much that the greater the role played by mechanisms of consciousness and the integration of information in producing a drug's effects, the more variable these effects can be. A drug may have very specific biochemical actions and still have quite variable behavioral effects. Such variability results because drugs do not create new patterns of nervous system activity. Rather, they only serve to modify already existing patterns, most of which are the result of an individual's unique personal experiences. That is, these psychoactive drugs act by altering *ongoing information processing* and retrieval of *already stored memories*.

Psychoactive drugs, then, do not add new components to experience, or awareness, or consciousness. They may shape the existing components differently, distort them, mute or intensify them, but the drugs do not take the user beyond himself and his environment. If, in fact, each of us carries some of his own personal heaven or hell, then these agents may make it easier to experience each of these.

In spite of the uniqueness of the drug experience resulting from an interplay of all these factors, generalizations about the effects of these chemicals can be made because of three facts. First, the drugs do have specific biochemical actions (even if they are in part unknown) on areas, functions, or processes of the brain. This means that the range of effects an agent can produce is somewhat restricted. Second, the general culture, as well as the small subgroups in which each of us lives, presents a narrow range of experiences, hopes, and fears. It is from this set of possible experiences that drug effects must be selected. Last, one is taught which drug effects should be sought and emphasized and which are to be minimized. We learned, to some extent, whether the drug-induced effects are to be labeled as desirable or undesirable.

How safe are drugs?

There are at least three ways in which the harmfulness of a drug can be considered. One is the common medical usage referring to the toxic effects and lethality resulting from the use of the drug. Both short-term and long-term toxic effects need to be identified (these may be different). Furthermore, all statements refer only to what is now known. Toxic effects that may appear tomorrow cannot be predicted today. Therefore, medically speaking, the basic rule is to approach all drugs with respect and with caution.

From a medical point of view no drug is safe. With some doses, modes of administration, and frequency of use, all drugs cause toxic effects and even death. It is equally true that at some doses, modes of administration, and frequency of use all drugs are safe. The concern here is whether a drug, *used the way most people use it today*, is physically harmful. From this position, alcohol and marijuana are relatively safe drugs the way most people use them. Nicotine, in contrast, is a very harmful drug, since the usual amount of cigarette smoking does increase mortality rate. (Appreciate, however, that when cigarette smoking began, the lethal effects were much less; people smoked fewer cigarettes and also did not live long enough for much of the cigarette-induced mortality to appear! If cigarettes appeared today for the first time, it would probably be no more than 5 to 10 years before their contribution to mortality would be identified.)

The regular, nonseptic use of intravenous injections makes any drug dangerous. The possibility of hepatitis, general infection, or an overdose clearly labels the usual form of heroin or injectable stimulant as medically dangerous. The fact that the users of these drugs frequently are also malnourished, with all that implies, only contributes to making the usual use of these agents clearly medically harmful.

Not so easy to categorize as medically safe or dangerous are hallucinogens. In the normal, illegal, street use of these agents there is no way of knowing what drug is actually being used, or the purity of the agent, or the dosage, or whether one or more drugs are contained in the dose as taken. Under these conditions it is not surprising that bad trips, deaths, and long-term psychiatric hospitalizations do occur. Perhaps this situation parallels that seen in the realm of the over-the-counter drugs—safe if used as directed. When purity, dose, and other factors are controlled, hallucinogens have not resulted in a high incidence of adverse effects. Aspirin is a reasonably safe drug even though about 100 youngsters a year die because of misuse. Oral use of pure hallucinogens is medically more dangerous than oral use of aspirin but not as physically dangerous as regular, moderate cigarette smoking.

An increasing number of individuals are beginning to emphasize other implications of the word "harmful." This position considers the personal-social aspect of a drug's use to be of paramount importance. The question here is, to what extent does use of the drug lead to, or contribute to, a major disruption of the individual's relationship to society? That is, does the use of the drug impair the interaction of the user and the existing culture?

When concern is directed to the degree of drug-induced impairment of the relationship between a user and society, different pictures appear. Nicotine is used regularly without greatly impairing the user's interaction with the world (up to the point where cigarette smoking causes hospitalization or death). Alcohol, however, is not harmless, since at least 10% of those who use it at all use it to an extent that they are unable to function in society. The data are not as well established with respect to marijuana, but many feel that the incidence and

extent of social impairment are about the same for users of alcohol and marijuana.

The injected agents also score high as dangerous drugs when impairment of social functioning is considered. Few heroin or intravenous stimulant users manage to maintain a useful relationship with society. It is not easy to categorize the use of hallucinogens, since the data are fragmentary. Users who center their life, for one reason or another, around the use of these drugs become dropouts and certainly fail to make any contribution to the present society. However, there must also be many occasional and irregular users who do maintain their positions in society, but a percentage division is not possible.

A third possibility is that the use of a drug may also have important interrelations with social trends in the culture. Concern is not with the medical effects of the drug or with the possible personal consequences of drug use but with the implications that extensive use of the drug may have for the society. Drug consumption by a large number of individuals may be important to the extent that a drug's effects support or oppose certain themes in the culture. That is, does the use of certain drugs fit more compatibly with certain philosophies of life?

It is suggested that two of the main threads of the American culture have been aggressive achievement and tight inhibition of impulses. As a result of these closely knit threads, American society is at a standard of technology unmatched anywhere. All our social institutions have reflected and supported these threads. For example, the schools supported these themes with the emphasis on grades (learn facts, you are not here to think) and winning sports teams (it is not how you play, it is whether you win or lose that counts) and a fairly rigid lock-step method of advancement through the system. The churches have reflected the national ethos by actively proselytizing and sending missionaries to foreign lands. Occasionally a sermon on Christian capitalism would be punctuated by a few verses of "Onward Christian Soldiers," which reaffirms the central themes of society. The emphasis on impulse control, from "nice boys don't fight" and "don't show your emotions" to the series of "thou shalt not's" that formed the basis of yesterday's religion, made it necessary to attack the environment and the problems of science and technology.

Even the drugs have contributed. All drugs that have become widespread through western societies have been those which alter arousal level. Not one drug whose primary action is to distort information processing has been part of the developing American scene. Within the class of drugs affecting arousal level, there have been some restrictions on their use, depending on their potency, but those of mild to moderate potency are generally attainable. Caffeine, amphetamines, alcohol and barbiturates are clearly the drugs of choice for an outwardly oriented, achieving, inhibited society. Even oral opiates did not detract from the on-moving thrust of this society.

The hallucinogens, drugs that alter information processing, seem to be more supportive and more compatible with a different set of values. Drugs offering multiple realities and suggesting internal rewards far beyond those in the outside world seem hard to fit into a focused, accomplish-it-because-it's-there orientation. Instead of outward achievements and activation, these drugs would seem to offer inner exploration and passivity. Rather than a communion of individuals joining together to fight the infidels out there, these agents promise a personal, solitary adventure inside the soul. Hallucinogens are potent drugs. Their danger, though, seems primarily to be to the achievement themes of our society. However, the point must be re-emphasized that when any aspect of drug use is considered, all pharmacological and social variables must be specified if the total range of implications is to be detailed.

Perspective of history

Drug use has affected society, but social changes also affect the use of drugs. One overriding theme has certainly been that the perspective of history and of other cultures is needed to properly view drug use in America today. Drug use, as with other behaviors, takes place and has meaning only in a context, and the context for all social phenomena must be historical. For example, an important part of the context in which drug use occurs consists of the attitudes held about the drug and the user of the drug. Only by knowing how drugs have been used and viewed in the past can present attitudes toward the use of any drug be fully appreciated.

Lewin's sentiment, which is quoted in the frontispiece, seems almost axiomatic. Throughout history, when a psychoactive drug has been introduced to a culture, its use has spread without stopping. However, until recently, most drugs started in the medicine man's bag of tricks and took years or centuries to disperse. From the chemist's test tube to the hamlets in the hills is now only a matter of weeks or months. Everything moves faster.

The transition from a select group of users of a drug to its acceptance as a critical component of the culture has been seen already with caffeine, nicotine, and distilled spirits. The recent flow of antipsychotic, antianxiety, and antidepressant drugs from the hospital pharmacy to the home medicine cabinet is but a modern version of the spread of a drug. The question still to be answered, of course, is which, if any, of the present illicit drugs will move into the homes of America.

In our society, the spread of a greater and greater number of drugs has been seen. From coffee in the morning through an aspirin during the day to the final nightcap—liquid or pill—we use drugs. Drugs are seen as problem solvers, and for some people they are. They make us feel good, forget the bad; they lift us from the rat race of life to the ecstasy of eternity and remove the boredom of the banal and replace it with the excitement of the evernew. Drugs are also viewed as causing problems, and for some they do this. They make us ill, kill us, take a bad world and make it worse, and take a bright future and turn it into a dull haze. For most drug users, no matter what drug they use, none of this will happen. Whether legal or illegal, most of us use drugs in such amounts and frequencies that our lives are not seriously altered by our use of drugs. We are, however, engaging in pharmacological promiscuity and becoming much more casual about our use of drugs.

Another principle abstracted from history is that if a psychoactive drug is to be widely used in a society, it must be integrated into and fill some need in that society. Once the agent occupies a niche, it cannot be dislodged except by changing the culture or offering a substitute to meet the same need. For example, in primitive groups the use of psychoactive plants was almost exclusively in a religious or spiritual setting. The active ingredient provided many of the experiences necessary for the participant to maintain the faith that sustained the group structure.

When a particular drug is widely used and used in a particular way, it seems to be a part of the glue that holds a culture together. Whether it is *Datura* in initiation rites or martinis at a business lunch, the drug is a part of and a supporter of that society's prevailing world view. When the drug no longer contributes to and supports the culture, the drug is dropped. More likely, however, the form of the drug use will shift to adjust to the changing culture. In some cases the culture shifts so as to incorporate the use of the drug.

The failure of the Eighteenth Amendment to dislodge alcohol from our society shows clearly that alcohol is firmly entrenched in our culture. It will not be eliminated without an acceptable substitute being offered or a major change occurring in our attitudes about life. The shifting pattern of caffeine use, from the formal and generally less convenient use of coffee to the casual and everywhere available colas, both reflects and supports our changing concepts of work and play. Therefore, the psychoactive drugs a culture selects for regular use and the form of this use can tell much about the culture. Each drug widely used in a particular way is as much of a supporting institution of the society as is its form of government, its churches, and its schools.

There are a number of reasons for the increase in the number of drugs used in our society. Only a few of the more obvious and important will be sketched here. In our generally affluent society each individual learns early that science and technology will supply answers to problems once the

problems are identified. Because of the present rate of social and technological change and the great publicity given to even minor discoveries, the expectation of quick solutions to problems is now well ingrained in our culture. Drugs provide these quick solutions. The priming in the medical area was carried out over the first half of this century, so that by the post–World War II period it was easy to believe that drugs would take care of everything, from a cold to cancer.

Throughout the 1950s and 1960s the United States was flooded with drugs that promised to solve most personal problems. Sniffles? Take a pill. Bad day at school or office? Take two pills. Trouble relating to those around you? Take a tablet. The pressures for increased use of legal drugs to solve problems have been well identified throughout the book, and their effectiveness is clear. The marketplace is replete with exhortations to use this or that drug to remedy a variety of uncomfortable situations. Such advertisements are not false, just misleading. The pill does not cure the cold; it just removes some symptoms! The tablet does not solve the problems you are having with other people, but it does make you less concerned about them.

However, the drugs that were being rapidly developed and marketed did temporarily solve some major problems for one group of individuals, the physicians. Physicians were confronted with increasing demands on their time, and over half of their patients presented symptoms resulting in large part from nonphysical problems. The drugs of the 1950s and 1960s made it possible for the physician to process a lot of patients and make most of them feel at least temporarily better. Cure, no. Resolution of problems, no. Relief for both the patient and the physician, yes. Little wonder that physicians dispense medication in large amounts.

Another factor that contributes to the increased drug use is simply the availability of more drugs. Not only are there more things to try, but each of the agents offers, and partially delivers, a different effect, and thus different needs of more individuals may be met. Also, an affluent society such as this one may be conducive to increasing drug use. In an economically wealthy society it is possible to drop out and be a reaonably heavy drug user and still survive. This fact may be an important determinant of some individuals' behavior.

Another general cultural trend that seems to interact importantly with the increase in the use of illegal psychoactive drugs is the diminishing importance of the traditional arbiters of public and private behavior. Accepted patterns of behavior are shifting rapidly in many areas of society. The old black-and-white guidelines have been breeched and the social institutions—church, school, family—have not yet found their way out of the gray area where many behaviors "sound wrong, but I guess they are all right."

Closely intertwined with the fact that these groups no longer speak with authority on matters of individual behavior is the increase in personal freedom and rights that has accompanied the civil rights and woman's liberation movements. Such an emphasis on personal freedom has already had a major impact on what is moral, legal, and acceptable in the areas of sex and censorship. It seems probable that the expansion of individual rights, that is, the absence of restrictions on behavior that does not immediately and directly harm another peron, might soon come to include drug-taking behavior. This thesis has already been repeatedly presented by those advocating reform of the current drug laws. It does appear difficult to justify expanding each individual's personal freedom in every area except that of drug use.

In addition to the dissolving traditional moral standards, which in the past have partially countered increased drug use by labeling it as *bad*, *immoral*, or *sinful*, the shifting patterns of drug use today make it difficult to combine opposition to drug use with already existing prejudices. Identifying the use of alcohol and saloons with the lower class, immigrant Catholic made it easy for the middle-class, second-generation Protestant to vote for prohibition in the early part of the century. Marijuana prohibition was easy in the 1930s; the drug had an obviously foreign name, it was primarily introduced into this country by Mexicans, and its usage was spread by lower-class blacks. There was little conflict when the heroin problem of the 1950s

was considered. The high incidence of use was in the black ghettos, and the drugs were smuggled and sold by a foreign-dominated group, the Mafia. One could nicely compartmentalize the drug, the user, and the seller and be against all three with no problem.

One of the conflicts about drug use today, in contrast to previous times, is that patterns of use are changing, and things are not so easily compartmentalized. Marijuana—a bad drug—is being used by white middle-class students and workers—good groups. The heroin—bad drug—problem has partly moved to the country club in the suburbs—nice people. All sorts of psychoactive drugs are being used by more and more people. No longer is it possible to categorically label those who experiment with drug use as bad, or degenerate, or sick.

Increased pressure for drug use may reflect the fact that the era of instant communication is upon us. The mass media have done an excellent job of spreading the word about the use of drugs, perhaps too good. Perhaps most stories about the use of drugs serve only to increase curiosity about the drugs and thus increase experimentation. Rarely reaching the level of news is the occasional user of any drug or the socially impaired user whose life *is* drugs. What makes the news is the exciting, the adventurous, the dramatic drug episode. Perhaps, as some have said, this is the time to cool it.

Similar comment could be made about the exploding number of ill-conceived, rapidly established, and poorly aimed drug education programs in this country. By emphasizing drug use only in a moral and legal context (which is not accepted by many people today), it seems probable that drug education programs will increase the amount of drug experimentation. If these programs only emphasize the dramatic and then say *"don't!"*, it is difficult to see how they can do more than support the confusion and interest already started by the news media.

A final aspect of our present society that must be briefly mentioned is the federal government. The national government is playing a pivotal and conflicting role in the expansion of illegal drug use in several ways. It is clear that there is now no consensus at the national level on the medical, personal, or societal meaning of drug use and abuse. Several issues are of concern. Many pronouncements still insist on considering the drug problem as primarily one of law enforcement, when it clearly goes beyond that to become a matter of social philosophy. Similarly, the decrease in penalties for marijuana possession and the developing emphasis on education and rehabilitation has not been paralleled by a shift in the thinking of those responsible for implementing the laws. The most basic flaw in the foundation of our federal policy is the emphasis on reactions to problems rather than proposals for the society in which we all live. This is the heart of the issue. It is the sociocultural problems that must be addressed; the questions we ask shape the answers and the actions we take. Rather than devote all our energies and resources to battling the fire that rages around us, we must devote some time and effort to developing a strategy for the future.

A RATIONAL VIEW OF DRUG USE

One of the first steps that must be taken to look rationally at drug use is to clarify terms. The legal aspects of drug usage must be kept separate from the concept of abuse. Only by identifying the different patterns of drug usage do the problems stand out and make it possible to develop solutions.

There are two major ways of looking at patterns of drug use: the legality of the drug use and the

psychosocial effects that accompany drug use. These two dimensions are shown in Fig. 20-1. The use-misuse-abuse dimension is clearly a continuum. Most of us use drugs in ways that complement rather than detract from our lives. Some individuals, however, become so involved in drug use that personal or social problems develop for them. This is drug misuse: using drugs causes significant transient or chronic minor problems for users. Drug abuse, the end of the continuum, occurs when individuals use drugs in such a way that the drugs cause a major and lasting disruption of relationships with society, peers, or themselves. The term *drug abuse* should be restricted to patterns of drug use that impair the individual's ability to function optimally in his personal, social, and vocational life. It complicates rather than clarifies the issues to label a 17-year-old moderate alcohol drinker as a drug abuser, when in fact he is only an illegal drug user. Use of an illegal drug should not automatically be considered drug abuse. Similarly, misuse of a drug, as by overweight, bored, frustrated, depressed suburban housewives who continue to function as adequate wives and mothers, should not be labeled as drug abuse.

The legal-illegal dimension is usually seen as a dichotomy. There are, though, varying degrees of legality or illegality. It is illegal for a 16-year-old to buy cigarettes from a vending machine, but no one is ever arrested for it. The trend toward the decriminalization of marijuana has added another gray zone: legal to have and use, illegal to sell. The major immediate problem for society is the drug abuser,

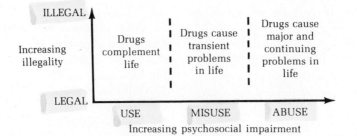

FIG. 20-1 Dimensions of drug use.

whether he abuses a legal drug, such as alcohol, or an illegal drug, such as heroin. These abusers are individuals whose life-style is most disruptive and expensive to society.

With terminology clarified, some basic premises should be enunciated. Some are facts, and some are, I believe, reasonable conclusions drawn from the available facts. Being conclusions, they are debatable. Some people may feel that the conclusions do not follow from the facts, or that relevant facts were not considered, or that the assumptions made in moving from the facts to the conclusions were wrong. However, I believe these conclusions to be valid and justifiable. The basis for these premises will not be elaborated in detail. Either they appear reasonable enough from the material already presented so that a conceptualization can be suggested, or all the collecting of facts that is possible would have little hope of convincing the reader.

There is an overemphasis on the medical and pharmacological effects of drug use as a basis for making psychosocial and political decisions about drugs. This is everywhere evident; the relative medical safety of marijuana is given as the justification for decriminalization. There is a continuing emphasis on methadone maintenance programs, even though many of the essential psychosocial support systems have been eliminated because of budget cuts. The talk of seriously considering the decriminalization of cocaine is another example of fools and federal officials rushing in where angels fear to tread: the land of inadequate data and misplaced emphasis.

The physical and medical reasons against using some of the presently illegal drugs are valid only for the impure street variety drug. The current, regular intravenous use of heroin, stimulants, or any drug is clearly dangerous and frequently leads to hospitalization and/or death. Used orally and on an occasional basis the potent hallucinogens sometimes result in hospitalization, but with moderate doses of pure drugs there are only infrequent adverse effects. Marijuana, up to now, appears to be as safe (and as dangerous) in moderate social use as alcohol.

Drug-taking behavior seems to belong in the same category of personal freedom as does sexual behavior. It is probably easier, though, for non-users to understand and accept the motivations behind increased individual rather than societal responsibility for one's sexual behavior than to understand or accept personal freedom in drug use. Nevertheless, it seems unlikely that the area of personal rights and freedoms can be increased much further without the right to use certain now-illegal drugs becoming an open question for society and the law.

Among individuals who are satisfactorily integrated into the present culture, there is a low incidence of use of most illegal drugs. *There is extensive use of a drug only when the drug meets unfilled needs of the individuals in a society.* It seems clear that to diminish drug use or to prevent its further increase, the needs of individuals must be satisfied in a nondrug setting. Society must offer attractive alternatives to a drug-using lifestyle if there is to be a decrease in drug use.

Evidence has been frequently presented that, historically, *drug use has initially altered society and then functioned as one of the stabilizing and supporting forces of the altered culture.* Changing patterns of drug use do change society. Once the change has occurred, the behaviors that develop around the use of the drug oppose additional change. The more unique the drug and the behaviors associated with its use, the more difficult the drug is to assimilate into society, and the greater the change required by society. It is debatable whether the decriminalization of marijuana would greatly alter today's culture. On the other hand, general use of the more potent hallucinogens most likely would result in considerable changes in today's society.

One of the major differences between today and the previous periods is that the stabilizing social institutions have lost some of their stability as well as their influence. *In every previous period of high drug use there have been potent forces countering the extensive use of drugs.* This assured a relatively slow spread of usage and some rational social debate on the meaning of the use of the drug. Today, even the federal government has not thought through the question of widespread drug use and, as such, is not an effective counteragent to recreational drug use.

There seems little debate over the fact that *for every psychoactive drug in use, legal or illegal, there will be a certain percentage of the users who are abusers*. It does not seem possible for a drug to be used without it also being abused by some. This seems a fact of life. As new psychoactive drugs are developed, their abusers will spring up. What is not known is whether each new drug will add to the total number of abusers or whether the number of abusers will remain constant, with only the specific drug being used changing.

One of the amazing things is the almost magical belief many people have that the law and law enforcement are something separate from and independent of society. Failure to appreciate that the law is but one of the reflections of the culture is one of the points of contention in the drug scene today. *Law enforcement works as a social control only when the society wants it to work and that occurs only when the law is in agreement with the major themes and beliefs of the society*. This is the difficulty with considering the drug problem to be a law-enforcement problem. Until a resolution is reached about the role of drug-taking behavior in our culture, the role of law enforcement will be ambiguous.

Another component of this sociocultural, historical approach is that *education can change patterns of behavior*, but *only* if the education is early and is compatible with the life-style and realities of the learner. We must appreciate that the best drug prevention programs may never even mention drugs but instead emphasize life-styles and coping behaviors incompatible with more than occasional drug use. We must appreciate that different ages require different messages, different regions of the country require different approaches, different sociocultural groups require different solutions because they have different problems. Some people do drugs because they have too many

problems, some because they don't have enough.

The educational problem is not how to prevent illegal drug use and stop drug abuse. No reasonable and informed peron believes that either can be done in today's world. What is critical is that we develop strategies, rationales, and actions for minimizing the destructive social and personal impact of recreational drug use.

The most serious problem for all of us is the possible increase in drug use by the very young, those 10 to 14 years old. These are the beginning critical years in which individuals learn the social skills and personal self-concept that enable them to grow into a socially meaningful and personally rewarding life. It's a hard job to do well. Drugs are so much easier and more fun, for a while at least. Of primary importance is that no actions be taken which increase the availability of drugs for these individuals or increase social sanctions for adolescent recreational drug use.

Beginning use of illegal drugs in the early years of secondary school is a sign of an unhappy, unsuccessful youth and is midway in the development of a deviant life-style, not the beginning. The evidence is clear from many studies: early drug use results from personality and background factors that result in the rejection of social values and goals. The use of illegal drugs also increases the rate of development of other asocial and antisocial behavior. The prevention of drug use by the young lies in the socialization process and in family relationships.

The basic question in the area of drug use is one of social philosophy: what kind of society do we aspire to, how can we increase the opportunities and specify realistic, socially integrative goals for our citizens to reach out for? The real issues and the hard ones are psychosocial and behavioral and will be solved only with that perspective. The medical problems associated with the illegal use of street drugs can easily be solved if we decide that is what we want to do. Before any actions are taken in prevention, law enforcement, or treatment, we must answer the philosophical questions about our social goals that the drug scene has posed for us.

CONCLUDING COMMENT

The difficulty today in obtaining a clear picture of the changing patterns of drug-taking behavior seems primarily to be a result of viewing drug use as an isolated phenomenon. The facts about the actions and behavioral effects of psychoactive drugs are meaningful only when considered in the context of social history. It is necessary to identify and debate cultural trends that foster and oppose the current increase and diversification of drug-taking behavior if society is to understand and resolve the present crisis in drug use.

Finally, it is important that we address ourselves to the ways in which recreational drug use can remain as punctuation marks on a socially integrated and personally meaningful life, rather than becoming the theme around which our lives are woven. To deal with today's problems of drug use and drug users requires new concepts, new actions, new perspectives. To understand drug use in today's society, it is necessary to look beyond drugs— to look beyond drugs to the broad panorama of our developing social beliefs.

INDEX

Italics indicate figures; ˮtˮ indicates table.

464

NOTES

NOTES

NOTES

NOTES

NOTES

NOTES

NOTES

NOTES

CHECKLIST FOR KNOWLEDGE OF AND INTEREST IN DRUGS AND DRUG USE

TO THE INSTRUCTOR

This checklist is to secure student appraisal of knowledge and interest in various topics and issues in the area of drugs and drug use. When used at the beginning of a semester, this checklist can help appraise student interest and understanding to facilitate your planning the organization and emphases of the course. The checklist will also provide the student with an orientation to the breadth of the area of drugs and drug use.

TO THE STUDENT

The results of this questionnaire will not be used for grading purposes. The purpose of this checklist is to allow you to indicate your present knowledge and interest in the various areas and issues involved in drugs and drug use. Your replies will be useful in planning the course so that the emphasis and time allotments will best meet most of your needs and interests.

Directions: Read each item carefully. There are no right or wrong answers. Answer each item as honestly as you can. After each item put an X in the space that represents your knowledge on the topic and an X in the space that represents the degree of interest you have in the topic.

Terminology

KNOWLEDGE

None	You have little or no knowledge of this topic.
Some	You know something about the topic but would like to have more information.
Adequate	You are satisfied that you know enough about this topic.

INTEREST

None	You have no interest in this topic.
Some	You have a moderate interest in this topic and, if time were available, would like to learn more about the subject.
Great	You have considerable interest in this topic and would like to explore the subject in some detail.

Example

6. **Impact of society's drug use**

    b. Effect on laws . . . .

              (Answer would indicate that the individual had some knowledge and considerable interest in this topic.)

	KNOWLEDGE			INTEREST		
	none	some	adequate	none	some	great

1. Philosophical issues surrounding drug use
   a. The debate over an individual's personal right to use drugs. . . . .
   b. The debate over the responsibility of society to place restrictions on an individual's private drug use . . . .
   c. The debate over the shift in responsibility for control of drug use from society to the individual. . . .
   d. The debate over the relationship between personal freedom in sexual behavior and in drug-taking behavior. . . . .

2. Causes of illegal drug use
   a. Personal reasons. . . . .
   b. Social pressures . . . .
   c. Cultural changes . . . .
   d. Availability. . . . .

3. Social issues
   a. Ways in which drug use can be an integral and integrating part of a society. . . . .
   b. Ways in which drug use can disrupt a society . . . .
   c. Factors in the American culture that encourage and promote drug use. . . . .
   d. Factors in the American culture that discourage drug use . . . .

4. Cross-cultural factors in drug use
   a. Drug use in ancient western cultures. . . . .
   b. Drug use in primitive cultures . . . .
   c. Drug use today in other countries . . . .
   d. Drug use in the United States before 1950. . . . .

5. The spread of illegal drug use
   a. From country to country. . . . .
   b. From state to state in the United States. . . . .
   c. From one area of a city to another. . . . .
   d. From one type of user to another . . . .
   e. From one individual to another. . . . .

6. Impact of a society's drug use
   a. Effect on mores and morals. . . . .
   b. Effect on laws . . . .
   c. Effect on educational systems . . . .
   d. Effect on art and literature . . . .

	KNOWLEDGE			INTEREST		
	none	some	adequate	none	some	great

7. Importance of drug use
  a. Influence on directions in which
     society moves. . . . .
  b. Influence on the generation gap . . . .
  c. Influence on women's liberation
  d. Influence on the sexual freedom
     revolution . . . .

8. Impact of wars on drug use
  a. Disruption and modification of drug supply lines
     and supply sources . . . .
  b. Introduction of soldiers to new cultures . . . .
  c. Use of drugs in treatment of war-related
     illness and disease . . . .
  d. Search for mind-altering drugs for use
     in chemical warfare. . . . .

**9. Importance to society of the search for
    new drugs**
  a. In the laboratory . . . .
  b. As motivation for the fifteenth- to
     twentieth-century explorers. . . . .

10. Patent medicines
  a. Drug content. . . . .
  b. Value in treatment of illness . . . .
  c. Importance of nineteenth-century America. . . . .
  d. Government regulation. . . . .

11. Prohibition of alcohol, 1919 to 1933
  a. Factors leading to prohibition . . . .
  b. Factors leading to end of prohibition . . . .
  c. Effectiveness of prohibition in
     regulating alcohol consumption . . . .
  d. Social changes between 1919 and 1933
     resulting from prohibition . . . .
  e. Lasting social changes resulting from
     the prohibition period. . . . .

12. Literature
  a. Influence of drug use on writers and
     their writing. . . . .
  b. Incidental reporting of drug use in
     nondrug literature . . . .
  c. Literature oriented around drug use . . . .
  d. Influence of literature on drug use in a society . . . .

	KNOWLEDGE			INTEREST		
	none	some	adequate	none	some	great

13. Religion
    a. Use of drugs in traditional religions . . . .
    b. Use of drugs in primitive religions. . . . .
    c. Religions centered around drug use. . . . .
    d. Political freedom for religious use of drugs . . . .

14. Possible ways of influencing patterns of drug use
    a. Legislation. . . . .
    b. Education . . . .
    c. Control of source . . . .
    d. Religion. . . . .
    e. Social sanctions . . . .

15. Social background and precipitating causes for legislation
    a. Passage of 1906 Pure Food and Drugs Act . . . .
    b. Passage of 1914 Harrison Narcotic Act . . . .
    c. Passage of 1937 Marijuana Tax Act. . . . .
    d. Passage of 1938 Food, Drug, and Cosmetic Act. . . . .
    e. Passage of 1962 Food and Drug Act Amendments . . . .
    f. Passage of 1970 Comprehensive Drug Abuse Law. . . . .

16. Social behavior
    a. Factors determining an individual's behavior . . . .
    b. Similarity of drug-taking behavior to other behaviors . . . .
    c. Differences between drug-taking behavior and other behaviors . . . .
    d. Drug use as a means to an end and as an end itself. . . . .

17. Relationship between driving skill, automobile accidents, and
    a. Use of alcohol . . . .
    b. Use of marijuana . . . .
    c. Use of narcotics . . . .
    d. Use of antianxiety drugs (minor tranquilizers) . . . .
    e. Use of stimulants . . . .
    f. Use of barbiturates and nonbarbiturate sedatives . . . .
    g. Use of OTC drugs . . . .

	KNOWLEDGE			INTEREST		
	none	some	adequate	none	some	great

18. Relationship between criminal activity and
a. Use of alcohol . . . .
b. Use of marijuana . . . .
c. Use of narcotics . . . .
d. Use of antianxiety drugs (minor
   tranquilizers) . . . .
e. Use of stimulants . . . .
f. Use of barbiturates and nonbarbiturate
   sedatives . . . .

19. Relationship between violence and
a. Use of alcohol . . . .
b. Use of marijuana . . . .
c. Use of narcotics . . . .
d. Use of antianxiety drugs (minor
   tranquilizers) . . . .
e. Use of stimulants . . . .
f. Use of barbiturates and nonbarbiturate
   sedatives . . . .

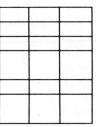

20. Relationship between athletic performance and
a. Use of alcohol . . . .
b. Use of marijuana . . . .
c. Use of narcotics . . . .
d. Use of antianxiety drugs (minor
   tranquilizers) . . . .
e. Use of stimulants . . . .
f. Use of barbiturates and nonbarbiturate
   sedatives . . . .

21. Relationship between sexual behavior and
a. Use of alcohol . . . .
b. Use of marijuana . . . .
c. Use of narcotics . . . .
d. Use of antianxiety drugs (minor
   tranquilizers) . . . .
e. Use of stimulants . . . .
f. Use of barbiturates and nonbarbiturate
   sedatives . . . .

22. Relationship between pregnancy and
a. Use of alcohol . . . .
b. Use of marijuana . . . .
c. Use of narcotics . . . .
d. Use of antianxiety drugs (minor
   tranquilizers) . . . .
e. Use of stimulants . . . .
f. Use of barbiturates and nonbarbiturate
   sedatives . . . .

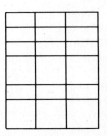

	KNOWLEDGE			INTEREST		
	none	some	adequate	none	some	great

23. The nervous system
   a. How the nervous system works . . . .
   b. How drugs affect the nervous system . . . .
   c. How drug actions on the nervous system
      alter sensation, feeling, and thinking . . . .
   d. How drugs can permanently damage the
      nervous system . . . .

24. How drugs get into the body
   a. Effectiveness of oral, injection, and
      inhalation methods of intake . . . .
   b. Advantages and disadvantages of
      different methods of drug intake . . . .

**25. Relationship between drug overdose
and/or bad drug experiences and**
   a. Possibility of permanent physiological
      damage . . . .
   b. Possibility of death . . . .
   c. When to call in a physician . . . .
   d. What you can and should do . . . .

26. Developing and testing new drugs
   a. How new drugs are created or discovered . . . .
   b. How new drugs are tested . . . .
   c. How new drugs are marketed . . . .
   d. How new drugs are controlled by the government . . . . .

27. Drug classification
   a. As safe to sell without a prescription . . . .
   b. As safe to sell only with a prescription . . . .
   c. As not being drugs at all . . . .
   d. As narcotic drugs . . . .
   e. As dangerous drugs . . . .

28. Commercial drugs and street drugs
   a. Differences in purity . . . .
   b. Differences in potency . . . .
   c. Differences in profit to the seller . . . .
   d. Differences in adverse reactions . . . .

29. Treatment of mentally ill
   a. Changing concepts of mental illness . . . .
   b. Effectiveness of drugs in treating
      mental illness . . . .
   c. Changes in other treatments as a result
      of use of drugs . . . .
   d. Kinds of drugs used for different forms of
      mental illness and personality disruption . . . .

	KNOWLEDGE			INTEREST		
	none	some	adequate	none	some	great

30. Consequences of addiction
 a. To alcohol . . . .
 b. To barbiturates. . . . .
 c. To minor tranquilizers . . . .
 d. To opiates (morphine, heroin) . . . .

**31. Rationale, procedures, and effectiveness
 of therapeutic programs**
 a. Alcoholics Anonymous for alcohol addicts . . . .
 b. Antabuse for alcohol addicts . . . .
 c. Psychotherapy for alcohol addicts. . . . .
 d. Synanon and other social therapies for
   opiate addicts. . . . .
 e. Methadone maintenance for opiate addicts . . . .
 f. Narcotic antagonists for opiate addicts . . . .
 g. Psychotherapy for opiate addicts . . . .

32. Legal drug use
 a. Relationship with personality factors . . . .
 b. Relationship with mental illness. . . . .
 c. Relationship with level of income . . . .
 d. Relationship with stressful environment . . . .
 e. Relationship with race . . . .
 f. Relationship with religious beliefs . . . .
 g. Relationship with education . . . .
 h. Relationship with crime . . . .

33. Illegal drug use
 a. Relationship with personality factors . . . .
 b. Relationship with mental illness. . . . .
 c. Relationship with level of income . . . .
 d. Relationship with stressful environment . . . .
 e. Relationship with race . . . .
 f. Relationship with religious beliefs . . . .
 g. Relationship with education . . . .
 h. Relationship with crime . . . .

34. Use of drugs
 a. To reduce appetite . . . .
 b. To reduce anxiety. . . . .
 c. To increase wakefulness . . . .
 d. To aid in falling asleep . . . .
 e. To reduce symptoms of mental illness . . . .
 f. To reduce cold and allergy symptoms. . . . .
 g. To reduce aches and pains. . . . .
 h. To reduce mania. . . . .
 i. To modify learning ability . . . .
 j. To increase pleasure. . . . .

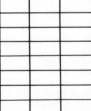
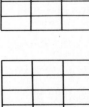

<table>
<tr><th colspan="3">KNOWLEDGE</th><th colspan="3">INTEREST</th></tr>
<tr><th>none</th><th>some</th><th>adequate</th><th>none</th><th>some</th><th>great</th></tr>
</table>

35. Alcohol
a. Physiological effects . . . .
b. Use for medical purposes . . . .
c. Use for nonmedical (recreational-social)
   purposes . . . .
d. Possible adverse effects with moderate use. . . . .
e. Possible adverse effects with excessive or
   long-term use. . . . .

36. Caffeine
a. Physiological effects . . . .
b. Use for medical purposes . . . .
c. Use for nonmedical (recreational-social)
   purposes . . . .
d. Possible adverse effects with moderate use. . . . .
e. Possible adverse effects with excessive or
   long-term use. . . . .

37. Nicotine
a. Physiological effects . . . .
b. Use for medical purposes . . . .
c. Use for nonmedical (recreational-social)
   purposes . . . .
d. Possible adverse effects with moderate use. . . . .
e. Possible adverse effects with excessive or
   long-term use. . . . .

38. Aspirin
a. Physiological effects
b. Use for medical purposes . . . .
c. Use for nonmedical (recreational-social)
   purposes . . . .
d. Possible adverse effects with moderate use. . . . .
e. Possible adverse effects with excessive or
   long-term use. . . . .

39. Relationship between the use of oral contraceptives and
a. Body chemistry . . . .
b. Increased medical problems . . . .
c. Probability of cancer. . . . .
d. Sex drive and sexual activity . . . .
e. Probability of pregnancy when use
   is stopped . . . .
f. Possibility of damage to fetus if
   pregnancy occurs . . . .
g. Population growth . . . .
h. Religion. . . . .

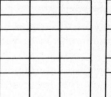
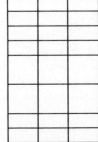

	KNOWLEDGE			INTEREST		
	none	some	adequate	none	some	great

40. Amphetamines
  a. Physiological effects . . . .
  b. Use for medical purposes . . . .
  c. Use for nonmedical (recreational-social)
     purposes . . . .
  d. Possible adverse effects with moderate use. . . . .
  e. Possible adverse effects with excessive or
     long-term use. . . . .

41. Cocaine
  a. Physiological effects . . . .
  b. Use for medical purposes . . . .
  c. Use for nonmedical (recreational-social)
     purposes . . . .
  d. Possible adverse effects with moderate use. . . . .
  e. Possible adverse effects with excessive or
     long-term use. . . . .

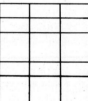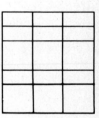

42. Barbiturates
  a. Physiological effects . . . .
  b. Use for medical purposes . . . .
  c. Use for nonmedical (recreational-social)
     purposes . . . .
  d. Possible adverse effects with moderate use. . . . .
  e. Possible adverse effects with excessive or
     long-term use. . . . .

43. Heroin, morphine, and other narcotic drugs
  a. Physiological effects . . . .
  b. Use for medical purposes . . . .
  c. Use for nonmedical (recreational-social)
     purposes . . . .
  d. Possible adverse effects with moderate use. . . . .
  e. Possible adverse effects with excessive or
     long-term use. . . . .

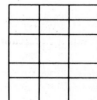

	KNOWLEDGE			INTEREST		
	none	some	adequate	none	some	great

44. LSD, mescaline, and other hallucinogens
   a. Physiological effects . . . .
   b. Use for medical purposes . . . .
   c. Use for nonmedical (recreational-social)
      purposes . . . .
   d. Possible adverse effects with moderate use . . . .
   e. Possible adverse effects with excessive or
      long-term use . . . .

45. Phencyclidine (PCP)
   a. Physiological effects . . . .
   b. Use for medical purposes . . . .
   c. Use for nonmedical (recreational-social)
      purposes . . . .
   d. Possible adverse effects with moderate use . . . .
   e. Possible adverse effects with excessive or
      long-term use . . . .

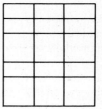

46. Marijuana
   a. Physiological effects . . . .
   b. Use for medical purposes . . . .
   c. Use for nonmedical (recreational-social)
      purposes . . . .
   d. Possible adverse effects with moderate use . . . .
   e. Possible adverse effects with excessive or
      long-term use . . . .

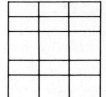

47. Hashish
   a. Physiological effects . . . .
   b. Use for medical purposes . . . .
   c. Use for nonmedical (recreational-social)
      purposes . . . .
   d. Possible adverse effects with moderate use . . . .
   e. Possible adverse effects with excessive or
      long-term use . . . .

MAJOR INTERESTS

The following drugs are mentioned in the text. In planning major blocks of time it will be helpful to the instructor to know their order of interest to the students. In the spaces at the left, please number the topic most interesting as 1 and number the remaining topics from 2 to 17 in the order of their declining interest.

_____ Alcohol
_____ Amphetamines
_____ Antianxiety drugs
_____ Antidepressant drugs

_____ Antipsychosis drugs
_____ Aspirin
_____ Barbiturates
_____ Caffeine
_____ Cocaine
_____ Hashish
_____ Heroin, morphine, and other narcotics
_____ LSD, mescaline, and other hallucinogens
_____ Marijuana
_____ Nicotine
_____ Oral contraceptives
_____ Over-the-counter drugs
_____ Phencyclidine (PCP)